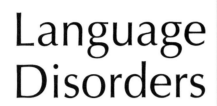

Language
Disorders

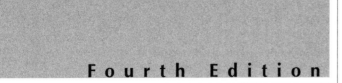

Fourth Edition

Language Disorders

A Functional Approach to Assessment and Intervention

Robert E. Owens, Jr.
State University of New York at Geneseo

PEARSON

Boston • New York • San Francisco
Mexico City • Montreal • Toronto • London • Madrid • Munich • Paris
Hong Kong • Singapore • Tokyo • Cape Town • Sydney

Executive Editor and Publisher: Stephen D. Dragin
Senior Editorial Assistant: Barbara Strickland
Production Supervisor: Joe Sweeney
Editorial–Production Service: Walsh & Associates, Inc.
Composition and Prepress Buyer: Linda Cox
Manufacturing Buyer: Andrew Turso
Cover Administrator: Kristina Mose-Libon
Photo Researcher: PoYee Oster
Electronic Composition: Omegatype Typography, Inc.

For related titles and support materials, visit our online catalog at www.ablongman.com.

Library of Congress Cataloging-in-Publication Data

Owens, Robert E.
    Language disorders : a functional approach to assessment and intervention / Robert E.
Owens, Jr. — 4th ed.
      p. cm.
    Includes bibliographical references and index.
    ISBN 0-205-38153-7
    1. Language disorders in children.   I. Title.

RJ496.L35O94 2003
618.92'855—dc21

2003050280

Photo credits: p. 3, Syracuse Newspapers/AVID LASSMAN/The Image Works; pp. 18, 277, Will Hart; pp. 57, 345, Bob Daemmrich/The Image Works; p. 97, Ellen Senisi/The Image Works; p. 117, Jeff Greenberg/The Image Works; p. 141, T. Lindfors Photography; p. 172, Najlah Feanny/Stock Boston; p. 212, Jeff Greenberg/PhotoEdit; p. 237, David Young Wolff/Photo Edit; p. 262, Robin Sachs/Photo Edit; p. 381, Bob Daemmrich/Stock Boston.

Printed in the United States of America

10 9 8 7 6 5 4 3   09 08 07 06 05

Contents

Preface

The fourth edition of *Language Disorders: A Functional Approach to Assessment and Intervention* is the result of an exhaustive compilation of studies conducted by my professional colleagues and of several years of clinical work in speech-language pathology with both presymbolic and symbolic children and adults. In this book, I concentrate on children because of the special problems they exhibit in learning language. Adults who are acquiring language, or who have lost language and are attempting to regain it, represent a much more diverse group and would be difficult to address in this text. This statement does not imply that children with language impairment are a homogeneous group or that intervention with this group is easy. Any school speech-language pathologist will attest otherwise. This heterogeneity is reflected in Chapter 2, which describes various identifiable language impairments.

I call the model of assessment and intervention presented in this text *functional language.* This approach goes by other names, such as environmental or conversational, and includes elements of several other models. Where I have borrowed someone's model, ideas, or techniques, full credit is given to that person. I find assessment and intervention to be an adaptation of a little of this and a little of that within an overall theoretical framework. Readers should approach this text with this in mind. Some ideas presented are very practical and easy to implement, whereas others may not apply to particular intervention settings. Readers should use what they can, keeping in mind the overall model of using the natural environment and natural conversations as the context for training language. I am the first to acknowledge that I do not have a monopoly on assessment and intervention methods, nor do I pretend to have all of the answers.

Within *Language Disorders,* I have made some content decisions that should be explained. I group all children with language problems, both delays and disorders, under the general rubric of *language-impaired.* This expedient decision was made recognizing that this text would not be addressing specific disorder populations except in a tangential manner.

The fourth edition of this text is updated and more inclusive. Readers will find expanded coverage of assessment and intervention with culturally, linguistically diverse children. The chapter on classroom intervention (Chapter 12) has been modified to reflect current realities in intervention services and to enhance the overall model of using the child's communicative contexts in intervention. A new chapter has been added addressing reading and writing and the role of speech-language pathologists with disorders of each. Finally, I have deleted coverage of phonology in recognition that the topic deserves more in-depth discussion than is possible here.

Acknowledgments

No text is written without the aid of other people. First, I thank the reviewers of this edition: Debra W. Bankston, Stephen F. Austin State University; Donna J. Crowley, Florida State University; Karen L. McComas, Marshall University; and Laura E. Sargent, University of Washington. I have tried to heed their sound advice.

I also acknowledge the advice and counsel of Dr. Shirley Szekeres, chair, Department of Speech Pathology and Audiology, Nazareth College, a knowledgeable professional and a genuinely warm person; and Dr. Addie Haas, Department of Communication Disorders, State University of New York at New Paltz, a constant inspiration and breath of freshness and someone who helps me stretch my imagination and explore new possibilities. My many conference presentations and long hikes in the woods with Dr. Haas are always a learning experience and a joy. Linda Deats, a colleague at State University of New York and a dear friend, has offered constant encouragement and lots of laughs. In addition, special thanks and much love to my partner at O and M Education, Moon Byung Choon, for his patience, support, and perseverence. Other supporters include Dr. Linda House, chair, and Dr. Dale Metz and Irene Belyakov of the Department of Speech Pathology and Audiology, State University of New York at Geneseo; and Donna Cooperman, Department of Speech Pathology and Audiology, College of St. Rose. Finally, my deepest gratitude to Dr. James MacDonald, Department of Speech Pathology and Audiology, The Ohio State University, for introducing me to the potential of the environment in communication intervention. Thanks, Jim!

Language Disorders

Introduction

1

A Functional
Language Approach

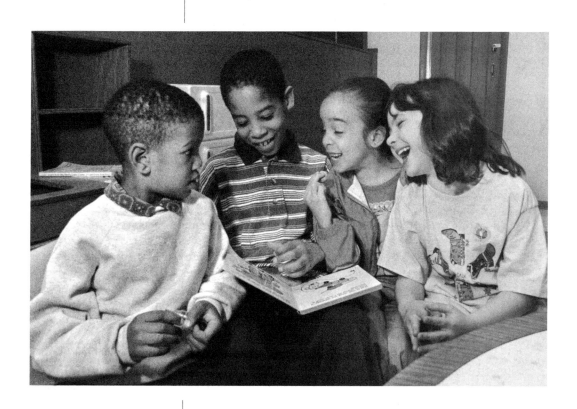

Language is a vehicle for communication primarily used in conversations. As such, language is the social tool that we use to accomplish our goals when we communicate. In other words, language can be viewed as a dynamic process. If we take this view, it changes our approach to language intervention. We become interested in the *how* more than in the *what*. It is that aspect of language intervention that I wish to explore with you through this book. At times the going will get tough. I've packed a lot into this text. I don't believe in wasting your time. But you can do it. You're intelligent and, hopefully, motivated. Before we begin, let's define some terms, **language impairment** and **functional language intervention.** I have chosen to use the term *language impairment* to refer to both language disorders and language delays. The term seems inclusive and will help us avoid arguments such as whether children with mental retardation exhibit disorders or delays.

The American Speech-Language-Hearing Association, the professional organization for speech-language pathologists, defines *language disorder* as follows:

> A LANGUAGE DISORDER is impaired comprehension and/or use of spoken, written and/or other symbol systems. This disorder may involve (1) the form of language (phonology, morphology, syntax), (2) the content of language (semantics), and/or (3) the function of language in communication (pragmatics) in any combination. (Ad Hoc Committee on Service Delivery in the Schools, 1993, p. 40)

To this very language-specific definition, we will add more description and causal information and assert the primacy of pragmatics, discussed later in this chapter. In addition, I feel more comfortable saying what language impairment is not. Specifically, it is not just a difference. For our purposes, we shall consider the term language impairment to apply to a *heterogeneous group of developmental disorders, acquired disorders, delays, or any combination of these principally characterized by deficits and/or immaturities in the use of spoken or written language for comprehension and/or production purposes that may involve the form, content, or function of language in any combination.* Language impairment may persist across the lifetime of the individual and may vary in symptoms, manifestations, effects, and severity over time and as a consequence of context, content, and learning task. Language differences, such as those found in some individuals with limited English proficiency and with different dialects, do not in themselves constitute language impairments.

In attempting to clarify the definition of language impairment, we have, no doubt, raised more questions than we have answered. For example, causal factors, such as prematurity, although important, are omitted from the definition because of their diverse nature and the lack of clear causal links in many children with language impairment (LI). In general, causal categories are not directly related to later language attributes (Lahey, 1988). Likewise, diagnostic categories, such as mental retardation, are not included for many of the same reasons. The definition also states that language differences are not disorders or delays, although the general public and some professionals often confuse them. We explore all of these issues in Chapter 2 and the chapters that follow.

The professional with primary responsibility for habilitation or rehabilitation of language impairment is the speech-language pathologist (SLP). The wearer of many hats, the SLP serves as team member, team teacher, teacher and parent trainer, and language facilitator. Language intervention is as likely to occur within the class as in a separate therapy room.

There is also a growing recognition that viewing the child and his or her communication as the problem is an outmoded concept, and increasingly, language intervention is becoming family centered or environmentally based. Professional concern is shifting from individual morphological endings or vocabulary words to a more functional, holistic approach and broadening to a concern for the child's overall communication effectiveness.

A functional language approach to assessment and intervention, as described in this text, targets language used as a vehicle for communication. A functional approach is a communication-first approach. The focus is the overall communication of the child with language impairment and of those who communicate with the child. As stated, the goal is better communication that works in the client's natural communicative contexts. The speech-language pathologist needs to ensure that the language skills that are targeted and trained generalize to the everyday environment of the child. This concern for language use necessitates a new primacy for pragmatics and the interrelatedness of all aspects of language in intervention protocols.

In short, in a functional language approach, conversation between children and their communication partners becomes the vehicle for change. By manipulating the linguistic and nonlinguistic contexts within which a child's utterances occur, the partner facilitates the use of certain structures and provides evaluative feedback while maintaining the conversational flow. From the early data collection stages through target selection to the intervention process, the speech-language pathologist and other communication partners are concerned with the enhancement of overall communication.

Functional language approaches have been used to increase mean length of utterance and multiword utterance production; the overall quantity of spontaneous communication; pragmatic skills; vocabulary growth; language complexity; receptive labeling; and intelligibility and the use of trained forms in novel utterances in children with mental retardation, autism, specific language impairment, language learning disability, developmental delay, emotional and behavioral disorders, and multiple handicaps (Camarata, Nelson, & Camarata, 1994; Dyer, Williams, & Luce, 1991; Girolometto, 1988; Nye, Foster, & Seaman, 1987; Scherer & Olswang, 1989; Schwartz et al., 1985; Theodore, Maher, & Prizant, 1990; Whitehurst et al., 1991). Even minimally symbolic children who require a more structured approach benefit from a conversational milieu (Owens et al., 1987; Yoder et al., 1994). In addition, functional interactive approaches improve generalization even when the immediate results differ little from those of more direct instructional methods (Cole & Dale, 1986; Rogers-Warren & Warren, 1985; Warren & Kaiser, 1986a). Finally, a conversational approach yields more positive behaviors from the child, such as smiling, laughing, and engagement in activities, with significantly more verbal initiation than does an imitation approach. In contrast, the child learning through an imitation approach is more likely to be quiet and passive (Haley, Camarata, & Nelson, 1994).

In the past, language-training programs have focused on language form and content, with little consideration given to pragmatics or language use. Form consists of syntax, morphology, and phonology; content is semantics or meaning; and pragmatics is use. The typical approach to teaching language forms has been a highly structured, behavioral one emphasizing the teaching of specific behaviors within a stimulus-response-reinforcement model (Fey, 1986). Thus, language is not a process but a product or response elicited by a stimulus or produced in anticipation of reinforcement.

Stimulus-response-reinforcement models of intervention often take the form of questions by the SLP and answers by the child or directives by the SLP for the child to respond. Typical stimulus utterances by the SLP might include the following:

Which one sounds better...or...?
Did I say that correctly?
Tell me the whole thing.
Say that three times correctly.

Consequences are based on the correctness of production and might include *Good, Good talking, Repeat it again three times, Listen to me again,* and so on. Table 1.1 contrasts the more structured, stimulus-response-reinforcement paradigm with a more functional approach.

Many SLPs prefer structured approaches because they can predict accurately the response of the child with LI to the training stimuli. In addition, structured behavioral approaches increase the probability that the client will make the appropriate, desired response. Language lessons usually are scripted as drills and, therefore, are repetitive and predictable for the SLP.

The child becomes a passive learner as the SLP manipulates structured stimuli in order to elicit responses and dispenses reinforcement. The SLP's overall style is highly directive (Ripich & Panagos, 1985; Ripich & Spinelli, 1985). In other words, the clinical procedure is unidirectional. These "trainer-oriented" approaches (Fey, 1986) are inadequate for developing meaningful uses for the newly acquired language feature.

Structured behavioral approaches that exhibit intensity, consistency, and organization have been successful in teaching some language skills to children with mental retardation and with language learning disability (LLD). A major problem is generalization from clinical to more natural contexts (Hunt & Goetz, 1988). Such generalization usually is not automatic.

Lack of generalization can be a function of the material selected for training, the learning characteristics of the child, or the design of the training. Stimuli present in the clinical setting that directly or indirectly affect the behavior being trained may not be found in other settings. Some of these stimuli, such as training cues, have intended effects, whereas others, such as the SLP, may have quite unintended ones. In addition, clinical cues or consequences used for teaching may be very different from those encountered in everyday situations. This lack of natural consequences also may remove the motivation to use the behavior elsewhere.

In contrast, functional approaches give more control to the child and decrease the amount of structure in intervention activities. Indices of improvement are an increase in successful communication,

TABLE 1.1   Comparison of traditional and functional intervention models

Traditional Model	Functional Model
Individual or small group setting using artificial situations.	Individual or small or large group setting within contextually appropriate setting.
Isolated linguistic constructs with little attention to the interrelationship of linguistic skills.	Relationship of aspects of communication stressed through spontaneous conversational paradigm.
Intervention stresses modeling imitation, practice, and drill.	Conversational techniques stress message transmission and communication.
Little attention to the use of language as a social tool during intervention sessions.	The use of language to communicate is optimized during intervention sessions.
Little chance or opportunity to develop linguistic constructs not targeted for intervention.	Increased opportunity to develop a wide range of language structures and communication skills through spontaneous conversation and social interaction.
Little opportunity to interact verbally with others during intervention.	Increased opportunity to develop communication skills by interacting with a wide variety of partners.

Source: Adapted from Gullo & Gullo (1984).

rather than the number of correct responses. Procedures used by the SLP and the child's communication partners more closely resemble those in the language-learning environment of children developing typically. In addition, the everyday environment of the child with LI is also included in training.

Naturally, the effectiveness of any language-teaching strategy will vary with the characteristics of the child with LI and the content of training. For example, children with LLD seem to benefit more from specific language training than do other children with language impairment (Nye et al., 1987). Likewise, children with more severe LI initially benefit more from a structured imitative approach.

In this chapter, we explore a rationale for a functional language approach. This rationale is based on the primacy of pragmatics in language and language intervention and on the generalization of language intervention to everyday contexts. Generalization is discussed in terms of the variables that influence it. After the rationale is established, we discuss in following chapters various LIs and assessment and intervention methods within the functional model.

Role of Pragmatics in Intervention

Pragmatics consists of the intentions or communication goals of each speaker and of the linguistic adjustments made by each speaker for the listener in order to accomplish these goals. Most features of language are affected by pragmatic aspects of the conversational context. For example, the selection of pronouns, verb tenses, articles, and adverbs or adverbial phrases of time involves more than syntactic and semantic considerations. The conversational partners must be aware of the preceding linguistic information and of each other's point of reference.

An earlier interest by SLPs in psycholinguistics has led to the present therapeutic emphasis on increasing syntactic complexity. The SLP's role has been to discover each child's individual learning strategies and to use these within the unidirectional, SLP-directed approach mentioned previously.

With the therapeutic shift in interest to semantics or meaning in the early 1970s came a new recognition of the importance of cognitive or intellectual readiness but little understanding of the importance of the social environment. Most intervention approaches maintained structural behavioral teaching techniques. Cognitive process-based approaches were ignored or nonexistent.

The influence of sociolinguistics and pragmatics in the late 1970s and 1980s has led to interest in conversational rules and contextual factors. Everyday contexts have provided a backdrop for explanations of linguistic performance.

In working with special populations, the focus shifted to the communication process, rather than to treating specific symptoms of disorder. Previously, for example, children's behaviors were considered either appropriate or inappropriate to the stimulus-reinforcement situation, rather than as a part of the interaction. Echolalia and unusual language patterns considered inappropriate were extinguished or punished. When emphasis shifts to pragmatics and to the processes that underlie behavior, however, the child's language can be considered on its own terms.

Older approaches tend to emphasize childrens' deficits with the goal of fixing what's wrong (Duchan, 1997). In contrast, a functional approach stresses a child's needs in order to accomplish his or her communication goals. It follows that intervention should provide contexts for actively engaging children in communication. In shifting the focus from the disorder to supporting the child's communication, the goal becomes increasing opportunities and support for the child to participate in everyday communication situations. The natural outgrowth is to involve families and teachers in training programs.

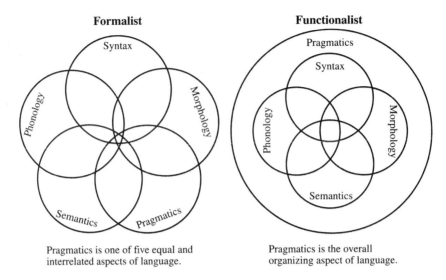

Formalist

Pragmatics is one of five equal and
interrelated aspects of language.

Functionalist

Pragmatics is the overall
organizing aspect of language.

FIGURE 1.1   Relationship of the aspects of language.

The traditional, or *formalist,* view of language as a composite of various rule systems, consisting of syntax, morphology, phonology, semantics, and pragmatics (Figure 1.1), may be inadequate. This approach has given way to a *functional* model and to a more holistic approach to intervention. Language is a social tool, and, as such, considerations of its use are paramount. The formalist model has been replaced by one in which pragmatics is the overall organizing framework. Increasingly, SLPs are recognizing that structure and content are influenced heavily by the conversational constraints of the communication context.

This view of language necessitates a very different approach to language intervention. In effect, intervention has moved from an *entity approach,* which targets discrete isolated bits of language, to a *systems* or *holistic approach,* which targets language within the overall communication process (Norris & Hoffman, 1990a). The major implication is a change in both the targets and the methods of training. If, as formalists contend, pragmatics is just one of five equal aspects of language, then it offers yet another set of rules for training. Thus, there will be additional training goals, but the methodology need not change. The training still can emphasize the *what* with little change in the *how,* which can continue in a structured behavioral paradigm.

In contrast, an approach in which pragmatics is the organizing aspect of language necessitates a more interactive conversational training approach, one that mirrors the environment in which the language will be used. Therapy becomes bidirectional and child oriented, and conversation is viewed as both the teaching *and* transfer environment.

Dimensions of Communication Context

Language is purposeful and takes place within a dynamic context. Context affects form and content and may, in turn, be affected by them. *Context* consists of a complex interaction of the following eight factors (Dudley-Marling & Rhodes, 1987):

Purpose. Language users begin with a purpose that affects what to say and how to say it.

Content. We use language to communicate about something. The topic of discourse will affect the form and the style.

Type of discourse. Certain types of discourse, such as a debate or a speech, use a characteristic type of structure related to the purpose.

Participant characteristics. Participant characteristics that affect context are background knowledge, roles, life experiences, moods, willingness to take risks, relative age, status, familiarity, and relationship in time and space.

Setting. Setting includes the circumstances under which the language occurs.

Activity. The activity in which the language users are engaged will affect language, especially the choice of vocabulary.

Speech community. The speech community is that group with whom we share certain rules of language. It may be as large as the speakers of a language, such as English, or as small as two people who share a secret language of their own.

Mode of discourse. The purpose and the relations of language users in time and space usually are determined by the mode of discourse. Speech and writing are modes that require very different types of interaction from the participants.

Within a conversation, participants continually must assess these factors and their changing relationships.

The SLP must be a master of the conversational context. Unfortunately, it is too easy to rely on overworked verbal cues, such as "Tell me about this picture" or "What do you want?" to elicit certain language structures. As simple a behavior as waiting can be an effective intervention tool when appropriate. Similarly, a seemingly nonclinical utterance, such as "Boy, that's a beautiful red sweater," can easily elicit negative constructions when directed at a child's green socks. SLPs who know the dimensions of communication context understand these dimensions more effectively and manipulate them more efficiently.

At least five dimensions of the communication context must be considered by the SLP (Prutting, 1982). They are the cognitive context, the social context, the physical context, the linguistic context, and the nonlinguistic context.

The *cognitive context* includes the communication partners' shared knowledge about the physical world. Obviously, two individuals cannot share exactly the same knowledge base. A toddler and her mother, for example, have very different knowledge bases, and yet they can communicate.

Parents adapt their behavior to the assumed knowledge level of their child. The child provides feedback that is used, in turn, by the parents in structuring the conversation. In the clinical setting, SLPs must modify their behavior as well.

The *social context* includes each communication partner's knowledge of the social world. Such knowledge encompasses the communication setting, the partner, and the interactional rules used by each partner. In the clinic, the SLP should consider each child's social skills. Preschoolers who seem unaware of the need to self-monitor and to repair their production may not have social knowledge of listener needs.

In the *physical context* are each partner's perceptions of the people, places, and objects that form that context. For example, pictures are very concrete for adults but may be very abstract for young preschoolers. The SLP can manipulate the variables within this context to resemble more closely the transfer environment. Better still, intervention can occur in everyday settings in which the training targets are likely to occur.

The *linguistic context* consists of the verbal features that precede, accompany, and follow a verbalization and that are used by each partner for processing. For example, a question usually is followed by an answer; there is an obligation to reply. These verbal features can be manipulated by the SLP.

Finally, the *nonlinguistic context* contains the nonlinguistic and paralinguistic events that surround a verbal production—that is, the activity in which the conversational partners are engaged. Some activities, such as group projects, encourage conversation; others, such as silent reading, do not. The importance of this context as a facilitator of verbal production cannot be overlooked in the clinical setting.

Summary

In the clinical setting, SLPs need to be aware of the effects of context on communication. How well children with LI regulate their relationships with other people depends on their ability to monitor context (Prutting, 1982). Given the dynamic nature of conversational contexts, it is essential that intervention also address generalization to the child's everyday communication contexts.

Role of Generalization in Intervention

One of the most difficult aspects of therapeutic intervention in speech-language pathology is generalization, or carryover, to nontraining situations (Fey, 1988; Halle, 1987; Hunt & Goetz, 1988; Warren, 1988). For our purposes, let us consider *generalization* to be the ongoing interactive process of clients and of their newly acquired language feature with the communication environment (Figure 1.2). For example, if we are trying to teach a child the new word *doggie,* we might repeat the word several times in the presence of the family dog and then cue the child with "Say doggie." If the child repeats the word only in this situation, he has not learned to use the word. If he says the word spontaneously and in the presence of other dogs, however, then we can reasonably assume that the child can produce the word without a model and thus has learned the word. The trained content has generalized.

The factors that affect generalization lie within the training content, the learner, and the teaching program and environment but will vary as particular aspects of the teaching situation change. If a response is to occur in a nontraining situation, then some aspects of that situation should be present in the training situation to signal that the response should occur. In other words, the SLP must consider the effects of the various teaching contexts on generalization to everyday contexts.

Time and again, we SLPs bemoan the fact that although Johnny performed correctly 100 percent of the time in therapy, he could not transfer this performance to the playground, classroom, or home. When language features taught in one setting are not generalized to other content and contexts, the goal of communicative competence is not realized.

Some SLPs hope that the training will generalize but exercise little influence over that possibility. This condition reflects a failure to manipulate the variables that affect generalization. Language training may not generalize because it is taught out of context, does not represent either the child's communicative functions or linguistic knowledge or experiences, or presents few communicative

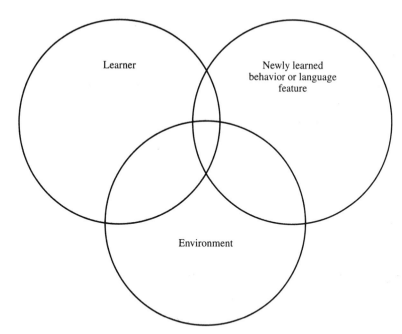

Generalization is the interaction of the individual, the newly trained behavior or
language feature, and the environment. All three must be present for
generalization to occur.

FIGURE 1.2   Generalization schematic.

opportunities. To some extent, generalization is also a result of the procedures used and of the variables manipulated in language training. Finally, the very targets chosen for remediation may contribute to a lack of carryover.

    With each client, the SLP needs to ask: Will this procedure (or target) work in the child's everyday
environment? Is there a need within the everyday communication of the client for the feature that is
being trained, and do the methods used in its teaching reflect that everyday context? In a recent meeting
with a student SLP, the answer to these questions was no. As a result, we decided to forego auxiliary
verb training with a middle-aged adult with mental retardation in favor of communication features
more likely to be used within the client's everyday communication environment, such as ordering at a
fast-food restaurant, asking directions, and using the telephone. In other words, we opted for a more
functional approach that targeted useful skills in the everyday environment of the client.

Variables That Affect Generalization

Generalization is an essential part of learning. Even the young child using his or her first word must
learn to generalize its use to novel content. The word *doggie* may be used with other four-legged animals. Eventually, the child abstracts those cases in which the word *doggie* is correct and those in
which it is not. The child is learning those contexts that obligate the use of *doggie* and those that preclude its use. Contexts regulate application of language rules.

Likewise, the young child who can say, "May I have a cookie, please?" has not learned this new utterance until it is used in the appropriate contexts. The child learns the appropriate contextual cues, such as the presence of cookies, that govern use of the utterance.

The contexts in which training takes place influence what the child actually learns. In fact, correctness is not inherent in the child's response itself but is found in the response in context, as illustrated in the "May I have a cookie, please?" example. The relationship of context to learning is not a simple one, and the stimuli controlling a response may be multiple.

Generalization is also an integral part of the language intervention process. Thoughts on generalization should not be left until after the intervention program is designed. Generalization is not a single-line entry at the end of the lesson plan, nor is it homework.

To facilitate the acquisition of truly functional language—language that works for the child—it is essential that SLPs manipulate the variables related to generalization throughout the therapeutic process. In the functional model, generalization is an essential element at every step. Table 1.2 includes a list of the major generalization variables.

Generalizations are of two broad types: *content generalization* and *context generalization*. Content is the *what* of training. Content generalization occurs when the child with LI induces a language rule from examples and from actual use. Thus, the new feature (e.g., plural *-s*) may be used with content not previously trained, such as words not used in the therapy situation. Content generalization is affected by the *targets* chosen for training, such as the use of negatives, and by the specific choice of *training items*, such as the words and sentences used to train negation.

Overall, the content selected for training reflects an SLP's theoretical concept of language and of strategies for learning and the communication needs of the child. When grammatical units are targeted, different uses or functions for those units are essential to meet the child's needs.

Context is the *how* of training. Context generalization occurs when the client uses the new feature, such as the use of auxiliary verbs in questions, within everyday communication, such as in the classroom, at home, or in play. In each of these contexts are differences in persons present and in the location, as well as in the linguistic events that precede and follow the newly learned behavior. Generalization can be facilitated when the communication contexts of the training environment and of the natural environment are similar.

Context includes an intrapersonal component unique to each individual and an interpersonal component shared by all persons in the communication setting (Spinelli & Terrell, 1984). *Intrapersonal variables* include each partner's cognitive and social knowledge or context, variables that may differ greatly. These variables influence intervention decisions on the selection of content and the individualization of program design.

TABLE 1.2 Variables that affect generalization of language training

Content generalization	Training targets
	Training items
Context generalization	Method of training
	Language facilitators
	Training cues
	Consequences
	Location of training

Interpersonal variables include situational factors (e.g., method of training, personnel involved, training cues, reinforcement method, location and time of training, and objects present) and participant factors (e.g., conversational roles of the participants). The effects of some of these variables on generalization are discussed in detail in the following sections.

Training Targets

The very complexity of language makes it impossible for the SLP to teach everything that a child with LI needs to become a competent communicator. Obviously, some language features must be ignored. Target selection, therefore, is a conscious process with far-reaching implications.

Training target selection should be based on the actual needs and interests of each child within his or her communication environments. The focus of instruction should be on increasing the effectiveness of child-initiated communication. Because language is a dynamic process that is influenced heavily by context, language features selected for training should be functional or useful for the child in the communication environment.

Generalization is also a function of the scope of the training target and of the child's characteristics and linguistic experience with the target. In general, language rules with broad scope generalize more easily than those with more restricted scope (Kamhi, 1988).

The scope of rule application can be a function of the way it is taught. Narrow, restricted teaching reduces training targets to easily identifiable and observable units. Rules interpreted by the child as applying to a limited set of lexical items combined in a very specific manner will involve little generalization (Johnston, 1988a).

The child's prior knowledge of language also influences generalization. The failure of training to generalize may reflect training targets that are inappropriate for the knowledge level of the child. For example, it would be inappropriate to train indirect commands prior to the child's understanding and using yes/no questions and direct commands.

In conclusion, training targets should be selected on the basis of each child's actual communication needs and abilities, rather than on some preconceived agenda. The targets selected for training should be functional or useful in the client's everyday communication environment.

Training Items

The actual items selected for intervention, such as the specific verbs to be used in training past tense or the sentences to be used in training negation, and the linguistic complexity of these intervention items also can influence generalization. In general, it is best if these items come from the natural communication environment of the child with LI. Structured observation of this environment can aid intervention programming. For example, the active child may use the verbs *walk, jump,* and *hop* frequently. It is more likely that use of the past-tense *-ed* will generalize if these frequently occurring words are used in the training.

Individualization is important because of the many potentially different use environments. The child who is institutionalized may have very different content to discuss than does the child who resides at home. The interests of younger children are also very different from those of adolescents.

Targeted linguistic forms, whether word classes or larger linguistic structures, can be trained across several functions. For example, negatives used with auxiliary verbs can occur in declaratives ("That doesn't fit"), imperatives ("Don't touch that"), and interrogatives ("Don't you want to go?") and in functions, such as denying ("I didn't do it") or requesting information ("Why didn't you go?").

For optimum generalization, then, it is necessary to select training items from the child's everyday environment. In addition, these items should be trained across linguistic forms and/or functions and across linguistic and nonlinguistic contexts.

Method of Training

The training of discrete bits of language devoid of the communication context actually may retard learning and growth (Damico, 1988; N. Nelson, 1993). Such fragmentation allows minute analysis units to eclipse the essential language qualities of intentionality and synergy (Damico, 1988). In other words, language use in communication is lost. Intervention that focuses on these specific, discrete, structural entities fosters drills and didactic training. These adversely affect the flow, intentionality, and meaningfulness of language (Oller, 1983).

If language is viewed holistically, then the training of language involves much more than just training words and structures. Clients learn strategies for comprehending language directed at them and for generating novel utterances within several conversational contexts.

Training should occur in actual use within a conversational context. Prutting (1983) states that language intervention should meet the "Bubba" criterion. *Bubba* is Yiddish for "grandmother." If we were to explain our intervention approach to our Jewish grandmother, she would reply: "Oh, I could have told you that. It just makes sense to use conversations to train. Why didn't you ask me?" In other words, the training regimen should make sense. Training in context makes sense.

Our intervention methodology should flow logically from our concept of language. If language is a social tool and if the goal is to train for generalized use, then it follows that language should be trained in conditions similar to the ultimate use environment. Thus, the SLP modifies the interactional context within which language is trained so that it closely resembles or actually takes place within the child's ongoing everyday communication. It is important, therefore, to view context not as a backdrop but as an ongoing *process.*

Discussion of the method of training leads naturally to consideration of the other contextual variables. For optimum generalization, training should occur within a conversational context with varying numbers of facilitators, cues, consequences, and locations.

Language Facilitators

Language facilitators are "adults who increase the child's potential for communication success" (Craig, 1983, p. 110). Parents, teachers, aides, and unit personnel, in addition to the SLP, should act as language facilitators because of their relationship with and the amount of time each spends with the child. Interactional partners form communication environments for each other, and it is essential that the client experience newly learned language in a number of these. Because language is contextually variable, it will differ within the context created by the child with each communication partner. Thus, generalization depends on the number of communication partners we can involve in the intervention process (Craig, 1983). For children developing typically, the number of individuals they see during the day or week is positively correlated with the rate of language development (K. Nelson, 1973).

Programs that involve the child's communication partners, especially parents, produce greater gains for children than do programs that do not. Parents offer a channel for generalizing to the natural environment of the home. With parent or caregiver training, both parents and teachers can function on a continuum from paraprofessionals to general language facilitators (Adler, 1988; McDade & Varnedoe, 1987; Owens, 1982d).

With these additional language facilitators, the traditional role of the SLP changes. In essence, the SLP becomes a programmer of the child's environment, manipulating the variables to ensure successful communication and generalization. To be effective, the SLP needs to recognize that the child's communication partners are also clients, as well as agents of change (MacDonald, 1985). The SLP acts as a consultant, helping each child-parent dyad fine-tune its conversational behaviors.

Training Cues

Goals for the child should include both initiating and responding behaviors in the situations in which each is appropriate. Therefore, the SLP considers training language through a great variety of both linguistic and nonlinguistic cues.

The adult encourages child utterances by subtle manipulation of the context and responds to the child in a conversational manner. A functional language approach adapts these techniques as naturally as possible to intervention.

Contingencies

The nature of the reinforcement used in training is also a strong determiner of generalization. Everyday, natural consequences are best. If the child requests a paintbrush, she should be given one, unless, of course, there is a good reason not to give it. If that is the case, then the child should not have been required to learn that request.

Weaning the child away from edible or tangible reinforcers in favor of social ones is commendable as long as the social reinforcer is found in the natural communication environment. Verbal or social training consequences such as "Good talking," encountered only rarely in the course of everyday conversations, should be discontinued as soon as possible in favor of more natural responses.

Verbal responses that combine feedback about correctness/incorrectness with additional information can be both a language-learning opportunity and a communicative turn while maintaining the conversational flow. "Good talking" ends social interaction by commenting on the correctness of the child's utterance only and leaving little that the child can say in return.

Not every utterance is reinforced in the natural environment. In the course of everyday conversations, many utterances are not reinforced. In typical language intervention, however, every utterance by the child may be reinforced. Behaviors continuously reinforced are easy to extinguish. Intermittently reinforced responses are much more resistant and more closely resemble patterns found in the real world.

Location

The location of training involves not only places but also events. For maximum generalization, language should be trained in the locations, such as the home, clinic, school, or unit, and in the activities in which it is used, such as play or household chores. Children removed from familiar contexts may not exhibit their most creative language uses (Lieven, 1984).

Language should be trained within the daily activities of the client. Daily routines can provide a familiar framework within which conversation can occur. The familiar situation provides a frame that allows for a degree of automatization important in the acquisition of such skills as language. Often called *incidental teaching,* this approach attempts to ensure that children learn and have ample opportunity to use language within naturally occurring activities (McCormick, 1986; Owens, 1982d; Warren & Rogers-Warren, 1985). Generalization increases with the similarity of the original learning situation to the transfer situation. If the conditions for training and use are the same, the need for contrived generalization strategies is alleviated.

The ideal training situation is one in which the child with LI is engaged in some meaningful activity with a conversational partner who models appropriate language forms and functions (Staab, 1983). In this way, the child learns language in the conversational context in which it is likely to occur. It is within these everyday events that language is acquired naturally and to these events that the newly trained language is to generalize.

Within these daily events are naturally occurring communication sequences (Craig, 1983). Daily events, such as phone calls, friendly meetings, dinner preparation, and even dressing, can provide a framework for language and for language training. The frame provides a guide to help the participants organize their language and their language learning. Routines and familiar situations provide support (Lieven, 1984). The SLP can plan conversational roles and language training through the use of such daily events.

Summary

Language training can be a dynamic process of exchange that occurs during natural events in different environments and with different conversational partners. Reinforcement can be the intrinsic conversational success of the child. The variables relative to content and context can, if manipulated carefully, facilitate generalization of newly learned language features and make intervention seem more natural.

Unfortunately, in practice, generalization is too often the final step in planning client training. Instead, "communication goals and effects should be preserved and considered the first, pervasive, and most basic step in intervention planning" (Craig, 1983, p. 110).

Conclusion

A functional approach emphasizes nurturant and naturalistic approaches (Duchan & Weitzner-Lin, 1987). The nurturant aspect requires the SLP/facilitator to relinquish control to the child and to respond to the child's communication initiations. The naturalistic aspect emphasizes everyday events and context because language makes sense only when used within a communication context. The SLP becomes a master in the manipulation of that context in order to facilitate communication and generalization. Language is trained while it is actually used in everyday contexts. As a result, the training generalizes.

Learning and generalization are the result of good planning based on a knowledge of the variables that affect generalization and the individual needs of each child. The content selected for training and the context within which this training takes place are both important aspects of the generalization process. The SLP helps the child determine the best response to fulfill his or her initiations within contexts that facilitate his or her intervention targets.

Although the role of the SLP within the functional language paradigm changes from primary direct service provider to language facilitator and consultant, the SLP still has primary responsibility for planning and implementing intervention. Recognizing the need to meet these responsibilities more effectively, many professionals have proposed more functional intervention goals and procedures, such as those outlined in this text.

It is easy to deride functional approaches as offering no framework for learning, allowing the child total freedom. Yet, the approach outlined in this chapter is not one in which the SLP and child converse with little intervention occurring. Under such conditions, there is little development on the part of the child and little generalization.

Some professionals cast a wary eye on implementation of such conversational and communication-based approaches to language intervention. The fear is that intervention will deteriorate into a "Hey, man, what's happenin'?" approach, too open-ended to be effective in changing client behavior. Although this danger does exist, it is not inherent in functional approaches. As this text progresses, we discuss assessment and training procedures that enable SLPs to maintain a teaching momentum within the more natural context of conversation. It's productive and fun.

In the following chapters, we explore LIs, assessment, and intervention. After a discussion of children with LIs, we discuss the assessment process and the collection and analysis of conversational and narrative data. In the following chapters, an intervention paradigm and various techniques are presented, along with discussion of special applications to the classroom environment.

CHAPTER 2

Language Impairments

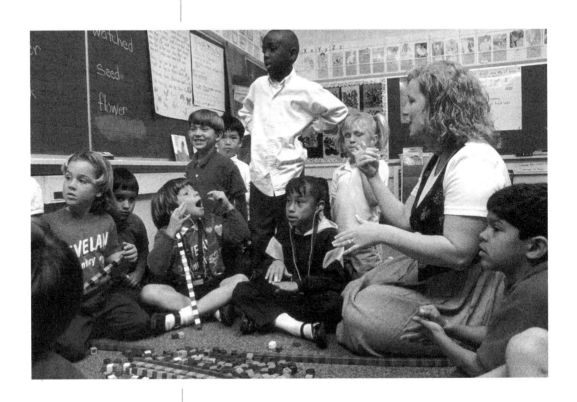

> *What's wrong, Juan? You seem upset.*
>> *Took them things.*
> *Who did, honey? What?*
>> *That boy.*
> *Which one? Show me.*
>> *Him.* (points) *Him took thems.*
> *Timmy? Timmy took something?*
>> (nods affirmatively) *Thems!*
> *What? I don't see anything.*
>> *Thems, thems things that I build.*
> *Oh, Timmy took your legos? Timmy took your legos.*

Obviously, we have a communication breakdown. Juan, at age 8, is unable to communicate the simple concept *Timmy took my legos.* Juan has a language impairment.

Juan, like many of the children described in this chapter, may have impairments in other areas of development as well. For example, children with mental retardation are going to experience slower maturity in all developmental areas, not just language. It is also reported that some children with LI have nonverbal deficits in identifying an object after it has been rotated, in analogies (A is to B as C is to _____), and in rapidly repetitive manual motor tasks (Swisher, Plante, & Lowell, 1994). This and other reported differences may reflect actual deficits or may be confounded by the linguistic aspects of these tasks (Casby, 1997). We still have much to learn from these children.

In this chapter, I describe the most common diagnostic categories of children with LI. I attempt to personalize this discussion whenever possible, but readers should remember that we are examining groups of children, not individuals. For example, no one child with a language learning disability may exhibit all of the characteristics ascribed to these children. I'll try to explain commonalities and differences across various disorders and to explore the most common language problems seen by SLPs.

Diagnostic Categories

Many categories of disability have language components. In this section, we discuss some of these categories in detail, attempting to describe both similarities and differences.

Typical language learning requires the following (Johnston, 1991):

1. The ability to perceive sequenced acoustic events of short duration
2. The ability to attend actively, to be responsive, and to anticipate stimuli
3. The ability to use symbols
4. The ability to invent syntax from the language of the environment
5. Enough mental energy to do all of the above simultaneously

Because language is learned naturally from another person in the course of conversation, let's add an additional requirement:

6. The ability to interact and communicate with others

Many of the children described in the following section have problems in one or more of these areas. As we discuss each language impairment, try to keep these abilities in mind.

There is a danger in describing categories of children and then assigning children to these categories. In general, such categories are helpful for discussion, but there is a danger that the category can become self-fulfilling. Children assigned to the category then are treated as the category, not as individuals. It is important to remember that the child is not *mentally retarded,* but rather is a child *with mental retardation.*

Discussing of LI categories can also cause us to overlook the similarities that exist between children classified by different categories. Many assessment and intervention strategies and techniques can be used across children.

Many children with LI cannot be described easily by any of the categories discussed in this chapter. Such children may have either more than one primary diagnostic category or characteristics that do not fit into any category. Each child represents a unique set of circumstances, so language assessment and intervention should be individualized.

Within each disorder category below, we limit the discussion to general characteristics, language characteristics, and possible causal factors. Unfortunately, we will be unable to discuss all possible language impairments. Some identifiable disorders have been omitted because of the small numbers of children or the paucity of research data. Others—for example, Tourette syndrome, a neurological movement disorder that affects up to 3 percent of children and consists of uncontrolled motor and phonic tics (Jankovic, 2001)—have been omitted because concomitant behaviors place the disorder in a somewhat specialized category and because language impairment is tangential to the primary disorder. In addition, language impairments resulting from low birth weight, prolonged hospitalization, or multiple births are not discussed separately and can be found within other categories described in this chapter (Bishop & Bishop, 1998; Hemphill et al., 2002; Tomblin & Buckwalter, 1998). Finally, deafness has also been omitted because of the very broad range of issues relative to hearing, speech, and language. Issues of deafness deserve their own text.

Information Processing

Prior to discussing specific disorders, it may be helpful to quickly review the information processing system that serves both thought and language. New research is indicating the importance for both language development and language impairment of this system and of the process of handling information.

Each individual processes information in a somewhat different manner. These differences can be explained by structural differences in individual brains and by learned differences, such as the way in which each of us approaches new information or problem solving. These learned differences influence, among other things, decisions about attending, schemes for organization, and rules and strategies for handling information.

Information processing can be divided into four steps: attention, discrimination, organization, and memory or retrieval. These are presented in Figure 2.1. Attention includes automatic activation of the brain, orientation that focuses awareness, and focus (Cowan, 1995). When the brain focuses on a stimulus, a neural or mental "model" is formed in working memory that allows further processing to occur.

We do not attend to all possible stimuli, as can be noted in Stimulus D in Figure 2.1. The child with poor attending skills may not attend to important stimuli, with the result that he or she will have poor discrimination.

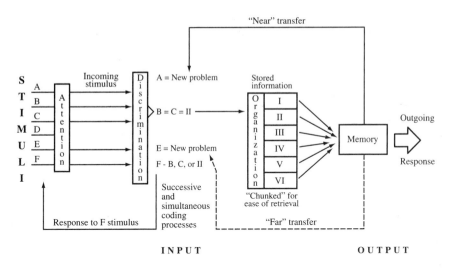

FIGURE 2.1   Schematic representation of information processing.

Discrimination is the ability to identify stimuli from a field of competing stimuli. Decisions are made on the similarity or dissimilarity of stimuli based on the "model" in working memory. In Figure 2.1, Stimuli B and C are perceived to be similar to each other and to information previously stored in Area II, a fictitious location in the brain.

Incoming linguistic information undergoes two types of synthesis: simultaneous and successive. Simultaneous coding is related to higher thought, and separate elements of the message are synthesized into groups so that all members are retrieved simultaneously. Overall meaning of the message is coded. In contrast, successive coding occurs in linear fashion, one at a time. Language is processed at the unit level rather than holistically. Both processes are used for decoding and encoding of linguistic and nonlinguistic information.

Organization is the categorization of information for storage and later retrieval. Information that is organized is more easily retrievable. Material that is unorganized or poorly organized will hinder later recall and quickly overload memory capacity. More efficient processing requires increasingly better organization, which, in turn, leaves room for more information. In this fashion, capacity for long-term storage becomes virtually unlimited.

It would be erroneous to think of storage as simply filing of information. Information is stored in networks that relate to all aspects of stored information. The more associations formed, the better memory and retrieval function.

Memory is the storing and retrieval of information. The capacity for storage and the speed and accuracy of retrieval increases with maturity. Retrieval is limited and dependent on environmental cues, the frequency of previous retrieval, competition from other memory items, and the age of learned information. All else being equal, it is easiest to retrieve information that has been frequently retrieved, has few competing memory items, has distinct environmental cues, and was learned recently and well.

Although not one of the four steps, transfer or generalization—the application of learned material to previously unlearned information or to new contexts—is important for learning. Transfer exists along a continuum of near to far. Near transfer involves only minimal difference between known information and the new problem. In contrast, far transfer involves substantial difference. Both types are represented in Figure 2.1. As you might assume, near transfer is easier for people functioning typically.

The simplicity of this discussion so far doesn't do justice to the process. Actually, processing occurs on many levels simultaneously (Snyder, Dabasinskas, & O'Connor, 2002). At bottom levels, processing is shallow and involves primarily perceptual analysis. In contrast, top levels of processing are more elaborate and associate the new information with knowledge already stored in the brain. As you might surmise, top processing results in better memory because of the associations formed (Hamman & Squire, 1996, 1997).

Less complex stimuli are initially processed via perceptual analysis at bottom levels then forwarded to working memory for more elaborate encoding—a process called bottom-up processing—and storage in long-term memory. For more elaborate stimuli, such as language, the brain activates higher or top-level processes, such as linguistic and word knowledge. Through these processes, the brain formulates "guesses" of what's coming next, and the low-level processes analyze incoming information perceptually to see how it fits. This process is called top-down. In other words, language is "heard" in accordance with the guesses that are based on stored linguistic information and the message so far (Samuel, 2001). It's unknown whether the two processes are dependent, interdependent, independent, or if they function simultaneously (Von Berger et al., 1996).

It's believed that working memory is the "place" where information is kept active through a system of coding, storage, access, and retrieval (Gillam & Bedore, 2000). The brain's central executive function (CEF) determines the cognitive resources needed and monitors and evaluates their application while controlling the flow of information. Thus, the CEF is responsible for selective attention and for the coordination and inhibition of stimuli and concepts (Baddeley, 1996). Children with LI may have difficulty because of the ways in which they attend to and perceive information and the ways in which concepts are represented (Gillam et al., 2002).

In addition, the processes may operate either automatically or in a controlled fashion based on the amount and type of information incoming, the demands of the task, and the capacity of the individual. In contrast to automatic processes, controlled ones are performed consciously and intentionally and make considerable demands on the resources of the brain.

Now let's pull this all together. And this is important. If a child must use controlled processes in bottom-level analyses, he or she may be limiting the amount of language processed. In other words, the child may not have the resources available for automatic top-level analysis (Ellis Weismer, 1994; Ellis Weismer & Hesketh, 1996; Johnston, 1995). Too much energy expended in bottom-level controlled analysis—because of poor attending, poor working memory, poor discrimination, or poor organization and/or retrieval—may limit the child's ability to process language automatically at higher levels of functioning. As we discuss information processing in each disorder, remember the overall process and the effects that each step in the process has on the others.

Mental Retardation

The American Association on Mental Retardation (AAMR) defines *mental retardation* as the following:

> …substantial limitations in present functioning
>
> …significantly subaverage intellectual functioning, existing concurrently with related limitations in two or more of the following applicable adaptive areas: communication, self-care, home

living, social skills, community use, self-direction, health and safety, functional academics, leisure, and work

…manifests before age 18 (AAMR, 1992)

This definition needs some explanation.

Significantly subaverage means two standard deviations below the mean of 100, a position at the extreme of the human intelligence curve. Approximately 3 percent of the population is below this point, which is at an IQ of 68. The definition is concerned with more than IQ, which is a measure of past learning, and considers *intellectual functioning* plus *adaptive areas*. Finally, individuals with mental retardation are considered to be developmental beings, so the definition covers the period during which humans develop into adults. Only individuals who meet all of the criteria are considered to have mental retardation.

The exact number of individuals who have mental retardation is unknown. Estimates vary from 1 to 3 percent of the population, or approximately 2.7 to 8 million people in the United States.

Severity varies among individuals, and usually changes little over time. Severity typically is associated with IQ, as noted in Table 2.1. Nearly 90 percent of the population with mental retardation is classified as mildly retarded.

Not every child with mental retardation (MR) is similar. Differences in severity occur, and other factors, such as amount of home support, living environment, education, type of retardation, mode of communication, and age, must be considered. I have worked with very social, very verbal preschoolers and with adolescents with severe multiple disabilities and very little usable communication behaviors.

Language Characteristics

Language is often one of the most impaired areas for the child with MR and may be the single most important characteristic of the disorder. Even when compared with typically developing children of the same mental age, children with MR often exhibit poorer language skills.

TABLE 2.1   Severity of mental retardation

Severity	IQ Range	% of MR	Characteristics
Mild	52–68	89	Usually live and work independently within the regular community. Often have families.
Moderate	36–51	6	Capable of some semi-independence at work and in residence. As adults, many work in supportive environments and live with relatives or in community residences.
Severe	20–35	3.5	Capable of learning some self-care skills and are not totally dependent. Some adults are able to work in a supportive environment and live with relatives or in community residences.
Profound	19 and below	1.5	Capable of learning some basic living skills but will require continual care and supervision. Often exhibit multiple handicaps.

Source: Adapted from American Association on Mental Retardation (1992).

Although some of this language difference may be attributed to low intellectual functioning, this factor alone does not fully explain the phenomenon. In addition, the cognition-language relationship is an inconsistent one among individuals with MR. For approximately half of the retarded population, both language comprehension and production levels are similar to cognitive levels. In other words, a 6-year-old child with MR might have both a mental age and a language age of 42 months. In 25 percent of the population, both language comprehension and production are below the level of cognition. Finally, in another 25 percent, language comprehension and cognition are at similar levels but language production is below both.

Both qualitative and quantitative differences occur between the language of children with MR and of children developing typically (Table 2.2) (Weiss, Weisz, & Bromfield, 1986). In general, below a mental age of 10 years, children with MR and those without follow similar developmental paths, although children with MR seem to produce shorter, less elaborated utterances—a quantitative difference. After a mental age of 10 years, the developmental paths begin to differ more, and the differences between the two groups become more qualitative.

TABLE 2.2   Language characteristics of children with mental retardation

Pragmatics	Gestural and intentional developmental patterns similar to those of children developing normally. Delayed gestural requesting. May take less dominant conversational role. No difference in clarification skills from mental-age-matched peers developing typically.
Semantics	More concrete word meanings. Slow vocabulary growth. More limited use of a variety of semantic units. Children with Down syndrome able to learn word meanings from exposure in context as well as mental-age-matched peers developing typically.
Syntax/Morphology	Length–complexity relationship similar to that of preschoolers developing typically. Same sequence of general sentence development as children developing typically. Shorter, less complex sentences with fewer subject elaborations or relative clauses than mental-age-matched peers developing typically. Sentence word order takes precedence over word relationships. Reliance on less mature forms, though capable of more advanced. Same order of morpheme development as preschoolers developing typically.
Phonology	Phonological rules similar to those of preschoolers developing typically but reliance on less mature forms, though capable of more advanced ones.
Comprehension	Poorer receptive language skills, especially children with Down syndrome, than mental-age-matched peers developing typically. Poorer sentence recall than mental-age-matched peers. More reliance on context to extract meaning.

Source: Based on Abbeduto, Davies, Solesby, & Furman (1991); Abbeduto, Short-Meyerson, Benson, & Dolish (1997); Chapman, Kay-Raining Bird, & Schwartz (1990); Chapman, Schwartz, & Kay-Raining Bird (1988); Kernan (1990); Klink, Gerstman, Raphael, Schlanger, & Newsome (1986); Merrill & Bilsky (1990); Mervis (1988); Moran, Money, & Leonard (1984); Mundy, Kasari, Sigman, & Ruskin (1995); Owens & MacDonald (1982); Rondal, Ghiotto, Bredart, & Bachelet (1988); Rosin, Swift, Bless, & Vetter (1988); Shriberg & Widder (1990).

As stated, prior to a mental age of 10, the overall sequence of development of children with MR is similar to that of children developing typically, although the rate is slower (Pruess, Vadasy, & Fewell, 1987). This pattern can be seen in development of intentions, role taking, presupposition, sentence forms, morphological markers, and phonological processes (Mundy et al., 1995; Owens & MacDonald, 1982; Shriberg & Widder, 1990). **Presupposition** is the speaker's assumption of the listener's perspective, what she or he knows and needs to know. In addition to the above, children with Down syndrome, a chromosomal disorder, are also as skilled as their mental-age-matched peers developing typically in inferring novel word meanings and in producing these words correctly thereafter (Chapman, Kay-Raining Bird, & Schwartz, 1990).

Even when children are matched for mental age, however, children with MR seem to use more immature forms than do their peers developing typically. The utterances of children with MR tend to be shorter and less complex. Although the narratives of children and adults with Down syndrome are of the same length and complexity as those of mental-age-matched peers developing typically, the linguistic devices and cohesion are poorer (Boudreau & Chapman, 2000). Children with Down syndrome produce fewer words, fewer different words, and shorter utterances while engaging in more verbal perseveration than mental-age-matched peers developing typically (Rein & Kernan, 1989). **Perseveration** is excessive talking on a topic when it is inappropriate or previously addressed. Males with fragile X, or Martin-Bell, syndrome, a disorder associated with the X, or female, chromosome resulting in severe to moderate-to-severe retardation, perseverate more than children with Down syndrome and exhibit more **jargon,** or meaningless unintelligible speech, and more echolalia, or repetition of a partner's speech. Although children with MR are capable of learning syntactic rules, they tend to rely on less mature word-order rules and a less mature and simpler method of interpretation. Likewise, although capable of requesting clarification, children with MR are less likely to do so within conversations (Abbeduto et al., 1991).

It is possible that the difficulties noted in the language of children with MR reflect problems integrating learning into ongoing events. Possibly these children are using their available cognitive energy to monitor and understand the conversation, leaving little for integration of language skills. All of us experience this phenomenon with newly acquired skills until they become more automatic.

Finally, some children with MR, especially those with Down syndrome, exhibit poorer receptive language skills than do their mental-age-matched peers developing typically (Abbeduto, Furman, & Davies, 1989; Chapman, Schwartz, & Kay-Raining Bird, 1988; Mervis, 1988; Rosin et al., 1988). The context seems particularly important for these children in aiding comprehension (Ezell & Goldstein, 1991).

Possible Causal Factors

Possible causal factors for MR are many and varied, including, but not limited to, biological and social-environmental causes of retardation and language impairments and information-processing differences related to language comprehension and production (Table 2.3). Any discussion of causality must be tempered with the recognition that for many children the cause of mental retardation is unknown. In addition, more than one causal factor may be at work. In any case, causal factors rarely are related directly to the performance level of the child in question.

Biological Factors.   Biological causes are most likely a factor for a majority of children with MR. These include genetic and chromosomal causes, such as Down syndrome; maternal infections, such as rubella or measles; toxins and chemical agents, causing, for example, fetal alcohol syndrome;

TABLE 2.3   Causal factors related to mental retardation (Adapted from AAMR)

Type	Examples	Characteristics
Biologic		
Genetic and chromosomal	Down syndrome (Trisomy 21)	Broad head and characteristic facial features, small stature, mental retardation
	Fragile X syndrome	Mental retardation in males, possible learning disabilities in females; 4:1 males to females
	Cri-du-chat syndrome	Catlike cry, microcephaly, mental retardation
Infectious processes	Maternal rubella	Cardiac defects, cataracts, hearing loss, microcephaly, possible mental retardation
	Congenital syphilis	Deafness, vision problems, possible epilepsy or cerebral palsy, mental retardation
Toxins and chemical agents	Fetal alcohol syndrome	Persistently deficient growth, low brain weight, facial abnormalities, cardiac defects, mental retardation
	Lead poisoning	Central nervous system and kidney damage, hyperactivity
Nutrition and metabolism	Phenylketonuria (PKU)	Reduced pigmentation, motor coordination problems, convulsions, microcephaly, mental retardation
	Tay-Sachs disease	Progressive deterioration of nervous system and vision, mental retardation, death in preschool years
	Inadequate diet	Small stature, possible mental retardation
Gestational disorders	Hydrocephalus	Enlarged head caused by increased volume of cerebral-spinal fluid, visual defects, epilepsy, mental retardation
	Cerebral malformation	Absence or underdevelopment of cerebral cortex and resultant mental retardation
	Craniofacial anomalies	Malformed skull and associated mental retardation
Complications of pregnancy and delivery	Extreme immaturity or preterm infant	Low birth weight, higher prevalence of central nervous system disorders
	Exceptionally large baby	Possible birth injury to central nervous system
	Maternal nutritional disorders	Low birth weight, higher prevalence of central nervous system disorders
Gross brain diseases	Tumors and tuberous sclerosis	Tumors in heart, seizures, tuberous "bumps" on nose and cheeks, mental retardation
	Huntington disease	Degenerative neurological functioning evidenced in progressive dementia and cerebral palsy
Social-Environmental		
Psychosocial disadvantage	Subnormal intellectual functioning in immediate family and/or impoverished environment	Functional retardation
Sensory deprivation	Maternal deprivation Prolonged isolation	Functional retardation and failure to thrive

Source: Owens, R. (1997). Mental retardation. In D. Bernstein & E. Tiegerman-Farber, *Language and communication disorders in children* (4th ed.). Boston: Allyn & Bacon. Reprinted by permission.

nutritional and metabolic causes, such as phenylketonuria, or PKU; gestational disorders, primarily in the formation of the brain or skull; complications from pregnancy and delivery; and gross brain diseases, including tumors. In general, a strong correlation exists between biological factors and severity of retardation. Remember that although biological causal factors may explain resultant retardation in part, they tell us very little about development, specifically language acquisition.

Social-Environmental Factors.   Social-environmental causal factors of retardation are more difficult to identify and may involve many interactive variables. Deprivation, poor housing and diet, poor hygiene, and lack of medical care can affect the development of the child adversely, although the exact effect of each is unknown and varies with each child.

Despite the fact that children with MR display only limited behaviors, there is no evidence that their mothers interact with them less. In general, maternal behavior varies with the child's language level, whether the child has MR or is developing typically. Mothers of children with MR do talk more to their children. By attributing more meaning to their children's less frequent behaviors, these mothers are able to interact more frequently (Yoder & Feagans, 1988). In short, mothers of children with MR interpret more of their children's behaviors as communicative than do mothers of children developing typically.

Mothers of children with MR match their verbal behavior to the child's language ability while adopting a teaching role (Davis, Stroud, & Green, 1988). Although they exert more control in play than do mothers of children developing typically, mothers of children with Down syndrome are equally or more responsive (Tannock, 1988a, 1988b). Their control behavior includes trying to elicit more responses from their children.

Processing Factors.   There may be differences in the cognitive, or information-processing, abilities of the MR population that cannot be attributed to low IQ alone. Children with MR do not seem to process information in the same manner as mental-age-matched peers developing typically. This difference is especially critical for learning. Cognitive abilities important for learning are attention, discrimination, organization, memory, and transfer.

Attention.   In general, individuals with MR can sustain attention as well as mental age-matched peers who are nonretarded. Difficulty comes for the individual with MR in the scanning and selection of stimuli to which to attend.

Discrimination.   Individuals with MR have difficulty identifying relevant stimulus cues. This difficulty reflects, in part, the tendency of individuals with MR to attend to fewer dimensions of a task than do individuals who are nonretarded. If the stimulus dimensions chosen are not the salient ones, the individual's ability to discriminate and to compare new information to stored information is limited. Discrimination can be taught, however, and individuals with MR can apply this information to discrimination tasks as well as can individuals who are nonretarded.

In general, discrimination ability and speed are related to severity of MR. The more severe the retardation, the slower and less accurate the discrimination. Persons with severe or profound MR have more limited attentional capacity and are less efficient at attention allocation (Nugent & Mosley, 1987).

Organization.   Individuals with mild-moderate MR have difficulty developing organizational strategies to aid storage and retrieval. They do not seem to rely on either mediational or associative strategies or to use them as efficiently as individuals developing typically. In **mediational strategies,** a word or a symbol, such as a category name, forms a link between two entities. In **associative strategies,** one word or symbol aids in recall of another, as in "bacon and _____" or "salt and _____."

Individuals with mild MR exhibit both simultaneous and successive coding; however, these individuals may use these processes differently from individuals who are nonretarded, especially in complex tasks. Individuals with Down syndrome seem to have greater difficulty with successive processing than do other mental-age-matched retarded individuals. This deficit may be explained in part by the poor verbal auditory memory abilities of individuals with Down syndrome. It is interesting to note, however, that the reported sequential processing difficulties of children with Down syndrome do not affect number sequential recall (Kay-Raining Bird & Chapman, 1994). The element of meaning present in language may complicate verbal sequential processing.

Memory.   Memory involves the retrieval of previously stored information. In general, individuals with MR demonstrate poorer recall than individuals developing typically. The more severe the retardation, the poorer the memory skills. Individuals with mild-moderate MR are able to retain information within long-term memory as well as individuals who are nonretarded, although the retrieval process is slower (Merrill, 1985). No doubt, organizational deficits contribute to difficulty retrieving information.

More obvious differences can be seen in short-term memory (Gutowski & Chechile, 1987). Poor performance by individuals with mild MR may reflect a limited use of associational strategies and organizational/storage deficits. It may be affected also by the rapid rate of forgetting found in the retarded population, especially within the first 10 seconds (N. Ellis, Deacon, & Wooldridge, 1985). Information is retained by rehearsal. It appears that individuals with MR do not spontaneously rehearse and that they need more time than individuals who are nonretarded to do so (Turner & Bray, 1985).

Memory can be affected also by the type of information. Individuals with MR do more poorly with auditory information than with visual (N. Ellis, Woodley-Zanthos, & Dulaney, 1989). Within auditory information, nonlinguistic signals, such as a car horn or a doorbell, are much easier for individuals with MR to remember than linguistic information. In general, nonlinguistic signals can be recognized and recalled similarly by individuals with mild retardation and without. It is in the recall of linguistic information that differences become evident.

Sentence recall involves reproduction from memory and editing of the recalled text. For individuals with mild MR, difficulty probably is encountered in the second stage.

Auditory memory deficits are exhibited more by individuals with Down syndrome than by those with other types of retardation (Marcell & Weeks, 1988). Phonological short-term recall seems to be especially affected (Seung & Chapman, 2000). This difficulty may be related to poor verbal working memory, a process that enables the hearer to continue to hear a sound after it has ceased. The "echo" may decay more rapidly among individuals with Down syndrome than among individuals developing typically. The memory deficit among individuals with Down syndrome is specific to verbal information and seems unrelated to receptive vocabulary or auditory or speech difficulties (Jarrold, Baddeley, & Phillips, 2002).

Transfer.   Transfer, or generalization, is an area of processing especially difficult for individuals with MR. Although learning may enhance performance, it does not enhance generalization. In general, the more severe a person's MR, the weaker that person's transfer abilities. In addition, persons with MR have difficulty with both near and far transfer, in part because of an inability to detect similarities. Thus, generalization deficits may reflect discrimination and organization problems mentioned previously.

Problems in information processing help us understand MR and other disorders but do not explain these disorders. Differences may represent the cause, the result, or a concurrent problem (Leonard, 1987). In any case, the differences found in the population with mental retardation suggest certain intervention techniques to be used when working with children with MR. These are represented in Table 2.4.

Conclusion

Generalizations about the language skills of the retarded population are complicated by the many causes of MR and by different severities. Overall, language development follows a path similar to typical development but at a slower pace. Still, differences occur, such as the reliance on less mature forms and the overuse of others. These differences may reflect the information-processing difference found in individuals with MR, especially in the areas of organization and memory.

Language Learning Disability

The National Joint Committee on Learning Disabilities (1991) has adopted the following definition of learning disabilities:

> Learning disability is a general term that refers to a heterogeneous group of disorders manifested by significant difficulties in the acquisition and use of listening, speaking, reading, writing, reasoning, or mathematical abilities. These disorders are intrinsic to the individual, presumed to be due to central nervous system dysfunction, and may occur across the lifespan. Problems in self-regulatory behaviors, social perception, and social interaction may exist with learning disabilities but do not by themselves constitute a learning disability. Although learning disabilities may occur concomitantly with other handicapping conditions...or with extrinsic influences..., they are not the result of those conditions or influences. (p. 19)

Let's explore this wordy definition a bit. First, as with other disorders, learning disability (LD) is characterized by heterogeneity. It is also important to note that the cause is presumed to be *central nervous system dysfunction*, although other conditions also may be present. Thus, the cause of learning difficulties is not environmental, nor is it these other accompanying conditions. Although not stated, it is assumed that children with learning disabilities have normal or near-normal intelligence.

Most children with learning disabilities will not have all of the characteristics. For example, approximately 15 percent have difficulty with motor learning and coordination. More than 75 percent have difficulty learning and using symbols (Miniutti, 1991). These children are considered to have a *language learning disability* (LLD).

The characteristics of children with learning disabilities are many and varied. In general, they divide into six categories: motor, attention, perception, symbol, memory, and emotion. Symbol difficulties are discussed under language characteristics.

Motor difficulties usually involve **hyperactivity,** a condition of overactivity in which children seem to be constantly in motion. Approximately 5 percent of all children have hyperactivity, but the condition is nine times as prevalent in boys as in girls (Sattler, 1988). Not all children with hyperactivity have learning disabilities, nor do all children with learning disabilities have hyperactivity. The condition is difficult to assess, especially among preschoolers, in part because of the wide range of variability (S. Campbell, 1985).

TABLE 2.4   Techniques to use with individuals with mental retardation

Attention

1. Aid attending by visually or auditorily highlighting stimulus cues. Likewise, gestures used to highlight important information can enhance the auditory message. Cues should be gradually decreased.
2. Teach child to scan stimuli for relevant cues.

Discrimination

1. Highlight and explain similarities and differences that will aid discrimination. Preschoolers do not understand terms such as same and different. Teachers must demonstrate likenesses and differences, such as hair/no-hair. *Meaningful* sorting tasks with real objects can be helpful. Overall size and shape (**not** *circle, square,* or *triangle*) and function are relevant characteristics for preschoolers.

Organization

1. "Pre-organize" information for easier processing and storage. No "winging it" here. Visual and spatial cues may be helpful.
2. Train associate strategies. What things go together? Why?
3. Use short-term memory tasks, such as repetition of important information, to aid simultaneous and successive processing. Repetition *and* interpretation are helpful.

Memory

1. Train rehearsal strategies, such as physical imitation. Gradually shift to more symbolic rehearsal tasks.
2. Use overlearning and lots of examples.
3. Train both signal (sounds, smells, tastes, sights) and symbol recall of events. Signals, which are easier to recall, can be gradually reduced.
4. Word associations for new words will improve recall of the words. Likewise sentential and narrative associations will improve recall.
5. Highlight important information to be remembered, thus enhancing selective attending.
6. Use visual memory to enhance auditory memory.

Transfer

1. Training situations should be very similar or identical to the generalization context. Use real items in training, at least initially.
2. Highlight similarities between situations, especially if training and generalization contexts differ. Help child recall similarities.
3. Help child recall previous tasks when approaching new problems.
4. Use people in child's everyday contexts for training.

Source: Adapted from Owens (1989).

Children with hyperactivity have difficulty attending and concentrating for more than very short periods of time. Unlike children with autism spectrum disorder, who may be hyperactive at one time and hypoactive (underactive) at another, children with hyperactivity are always active. Other motor difficulties of LD may include poor sense of body movement, poorly defined handedness, poor eye-hand coordination, and poorly defined concepts of space and time.

Attentional difficulties include a short attention span and inattentiveness. Children with LD seem easily distracted by irrelevant stimuli and easily overstimulated. At present, we are in the middle of a labeling frenzy regarding children and their ability to learn. More and more children are being labeled with **attention deficit hyperactivity disorder** or ADHD, characterized by overactivity and an inability to attend for more than a very short period but without many of the associated difficulties of learning disability. ADHD is most likely an impairment in the executive function of the brain that regulates behavior, especially impulsivity. Although these children have difficulty using language for social and educational purposes, their language deficits are difficult to measure with standardized testing (Oram, Fine, Okamoto, & Tannock, 1999). Such testing may be inappropriate. Although this explosion of identification of kids with ADHD reflects some real differences, it also reflects our rigid one-size-fits-all educational system (Wallach & Butler, 1995), sedentary lifestyle, junk food, and hectic, overworked parents and teachers.

Some children with learning disabilities may become fixed on a single task or behavior and repeat it. This fixation is called **perseveration.** Several children with whom I have worked would repeat an utterance over and over, seemingly unaware that they were doing it.

Perception and reception are not the same. Learning disability is not a sensory or reception disorder. Perceptual difficulties are interpretational difficulties. These occur after the stimuli are received. As might be assumed, children with learning disabilities may confuse similar sounds and words and similar printed letters and words. In addition, these children may have difficulty in *figure-ground perception* and in *sensory integration*. **Figure-ground perception** involves being able to isolate a stimulus against a background of competing stimuli. For example, figure-ground discrimination would include being able to listen to the teacher while other things are occurring in the classroom. **Sensory integration,** on the other hand, involves being able to make sense of visual and auditory stimuli occurring at the same time. Each may carry part of the message. For example, gestures, facial expression, body language, intonation, and verbal language may be used to convey information. Each alone may be insufficient.

Memory difficulties include short-term storage and retrieval problems. Children with LD often have difficulty remembering directions, names, and sequences. Word-finding problems are also common.

Finally, emotional problems also may accompany learning disabilities but are not a causal factor. Rather, emotional problems are a reaction to or an accompaniment to the frustrating situation in which these children find themselves. Children with LD have been described as aggressive, impulsive, unpredictable, withdrawn, and impatient. Some children may exercise poor judgment, have unusual fears, and/or adjust poorly to change. I worked with a child with learning disabilities who was afraid of shoes, a rather unusual fear. In others, poor adjustment to change may reflect dependence on routines when one has difficulty interpreting language in those contexts.

Language Characteristics

Usually all aspects of language, spoken and written, are affected in children with language learning disabilities (LLD) (Wallach & Butler, 1995). It should be stressed again that although these children may play the TV or radio at a loud volume, or seem to talk too loudly, or squint and rub their eyes when reading, *the problem is not sensory*. Although hearing or vision difficulties may or may not be present, they are not central to the disorder. Difficulties are perceptual.

Children with LLD may have difficulty with the give-and-take of conversation and with the form and content of language (Table 2.5). Synthesizing of language rules seems to be particularly difficult, resulting in delays in morphological rule acquisition and in the development of syntactic complexity. Problems with morphological markers are found both in speaking and writing, with the

TABLE 2.5 Language characteristics of children with language learning disability

Pragmatics	Little problem with turn taking. Difficulty answering questions or requesting clarification. Difficulty initiating or maintaining a conversation.
Semantics	Relational term difficulty (comparative, spatial, temporal). Figurative language and dual definition problems. Word-finding and definitional problems. Conjunction (*and, but, so, because,* etc.) confusion.
Syntax/Morphology	Difficulty with negative and passive constructions, relative clauses, contractions, and adjectival forms. Difficulty with verb tense markers, possession, and pronouns. Able to repeat sentences but often in reduced form, indicating difficulty learning different sentence forms. Article (*a, an, the*) confusion.
Phonology	Inconsistent sound production, especially as complexity increases.
Comprehension	*Wh-* question confusion. Receptive vocabulary similar to that of chronological-age-matched peers developing normally. Poor strategies for interacting with printed information. Confusion of letters that look similar and words that sound similar.

Source: Based on Baker, Ceci, & Hermann (1987); Catts (1986); Kail & Leonard (1986); Lieberman, Meskill, Chatillon, & Schupack (1985); Seidenberg & Bernstein (1986); Wiig & Wilson (1994).

most common error being omission (Windsor, Scott, & Street, 2000). In short, all areas of language are affected.

Overall oral language development for children with LLD may be slow (Reed, 1986). Their language is often like that of younger children, although children with LLD may use mature structures less frequently. As preschoolers, these children may exhibit little interest in language and may be unable to follow a story or be disinterested in books.

Word-finding is a particular problem found in both conversations and narratives (German, 1987), resulting in greater time needed to respond verbally. Retrieval difficulties may result in more communication breakdown (MacLachlan & Chapman, 1988), characterized by repetitions, especially of pronouns before words seemingly difficult to retrieve ("*He, he, he…*John was…"), reformulations, substitutions of indefinite pronouns (*it*), empty words (*one, thing*), delays, and insertions ("He was…*oh, I can't remember…*") (German & Simon, 1991).

Word-retrieval difficulties may be complicated by the deficient vocabularies of children with LLD (Leonard, 1990; Wiig, 1990). Young children with LLD have poor understanding of literal meanings. As these children age, they experience difficulties with multiple and figurative meanings (R. Lee & Kamhi, 1990; Lutzer, 1988; Seidenberg & Bernstein, 1986; Wiig, 1990).

The linguistic demands of the classroom are often well above the oral language abilities of these children. The well-documented academic underachievement of children with LLD demonstrates the link between language deficits and learning disabilities (Catts & Kamhi, 1986). Oral language skills are the single best indicator of reading and writing success in school. Difficulty with oral language skills among children with LLD is evidenced later in written-language problems, called **dyslexia** and **dysgraphia.**

Affecting males at twice the rate as females, dyslexia is a reading disorder characterized by word recognition and/or reading comprehension abilities two years below the expected level due to no known emotional, environmental, intellectual, perceptual, or obvious neurological problem. The lack of obvious signs does not change the fact that dyslexia—like learning disability in general—is the result of central nervous system dysfunction, most likely in the left temporal area of the brain, right frontal area, or in subcortical areas connecting the two hemispheres (Riccio & Hynd, 1996). The lack of a single affected area leads to the heterogeneity seen among children with dyslexia.

In addition to reading difficulties, children with dyslexia exhibit delayed language development and problems with listening comprehension, phonological awareness, and rapid oral naming (Catts, 1996). Word-recognition problems may reflect deficits that underlie both reading and word finding (Casby, 1992; Wolf & Segal, 1992). In fact, naming and reading problems co-occur in dyslexia, indicating a relationship between the two (Ackerman, Dykman, & Gardner, 1990; Bowers, Steffy, & Swanson, 1986). Naming speed and reading seem independent of phonological awareness but related to each other, possibly sharing processes related to speed (Bowers & Swanson, 1991; Felton & Brown, 1990). Slower letter- and word-naming speeds may impede decoding and word-recognition processes (Wolf & Segal, 1992).

Dysgraphia is difficulty writing, especially with the motor skills involved. Obviously, writing involves much more than speaking, including the integration of linguistic, cognitive, and motor skills. Writing problems among these children often persist into adolescence and adulthood (Isaacson, 1987). Difficulties include spelling errors, word omission and substitution, punctuation, agrammatical sentences, and lack of organization (Englert & Thomas, 1987; Gerber, 1986). These errors often reflect an underlying deficiency in syntactic and morphological knowledge (Rubin, Patterson, & Kantor, 1991). Writing difficulties become even more evident as the child progresses through school.

Although reading and writing are different, certain underlying processes influence both. For example, often there is no overall organization to the writing of children with LLD. In reading, they also fail to understand the underlying organization, thus treating each sentence as separate and unrelated to the whole (Raphael & Englert, 1990; Seidenberg, 1989).

The behavior of children with LLD also demonstrates the interrelatedness of cognition and language. This relationship can be seen in analogical reasoning skills in which known concepts are used to solve novel problems. In verbal proposition (A is to B as C is to ___), one type of analogical reasoning, language abilities appear to be more important than, but not exclusive of, cognitive abilities (Masterson, Evans, & Aloia, 1993). Children with LLD demonstrate difficulty with verbal analogies such as these (Kamhi, Gentry, Mauer, & Gholson, 1990; Nippold, Erskine, & Freed, 1988).

Some of the blame for the problems of children with dyslexia and dysgraphia must go to English itself. The rate of both disorders is twice as high in English-speaking countries as in those with less complex languages. Italian and Spanish, for example, have a one-to-one relationship between letters, or graphemes, and sounds, or phonemes. In English there are over 1,100 ways to combine the graphemes to represent the phonemes (Study: English language hard for dyslexics, 2001).

Possible Causal Factors

Several causal factors may contribute to LLD. Central nervous system dysfunction indicates a strong biological basis, but information processing, especially perception, is also important.

Biological Factors.   Learning disabilities occur more frequently in families with a history of the disorder and following premature or difficult birth. Children with a parent with dyslexia, especially those with a history of late talking, are at a higher risk for language impairment (Lyytinen et al., 2001). These facts, along with central nervous system dysfunction, demonstrate a biological link to the disorder. In addition, the use of neurostimulants, such as Ritalin, to enable children with hyperactivity to concentrate and attend further suggests a biological basis for some learning disabilities.

It has been suggested that a breakdown occurs along the neural pathways that connect the midbrain with the frontal cortex. This is the area of the brain responsible for attention, regulation, and planning (Bass, 1988). These biological factors alone are insufficient to explain the characteristics that accompany learning disability.

Social-Environmental Factors.   Although our definition of learning disability precluded any environmental causality, certain environmental factors are important. The language and, in turn, interactional difficulties of children with LLD certainly will influence the child's development.

Similarly, many of the acting-out behaviors of these children are in response to the very frustrating situations of their lives. Until the disorder is diagnosed, these children are accused of not trying or of being lazy or stupid. Many of the children with whom I have worked had extremely poor self-images. Many were afraid to try anything new; others would do anything for attention and recognition, even if such recognition was negative. The successes or failures that we have as we interact with others have a great influence on our future interactions.

Processing Factors.   Children with LLD do not appear to function in a manner appropriate for their intellectual level. They seem unable to use certain strategies or to access certain stored information.

Children with LLD exercise poor attentional selectivity, concentrating on inappropriate or unimportant stimuli (Levine, 1987). Appropriate and important information may be screened out along with other information. These children have difficulty deciding on the relevant information to which to attend in both oral and written communication.

As mentioned previously, discrimination is extremely difficult for children with LLD. The child has difficulty deciding on the relevant aspects of a stimulus that make it similar or dissimilar to another. Children with LLD do more poorly than mental-age-matched peers on rule extraction or identification from repeated exposures (Masterson, 1993b). Poor discrimination skills may also reflect deficits in working memory (Harris Wright & Newhoff, 2001).

Obviously, information that is poorly attended to and poorly discriminated will be poorly organized. These are children for whom the world often does not make sense, especially linguistically. Their storage categories reflect this confusion. Unlike children with MR, who do not organize spontaneously, children with LLD do organize information but too inefficiently for later use.

Memory is related to storage, or availability, and retrieval, or accessibility—distinct but related processes (Bjork & Bjork, 1992). Growth in word knowledge results in the creation of semantic networks in which words are related and organized. This growth occurs later and more slowly among children with LLD (Leonard, 1990; Reed, 1986; Wiig, 1990). One result is less accurate and slower retrieval by children with LLD (German, 1984; Wolf, Bally, & Morris, 1986).

Effective learners actively process, interpret, and synthesize information by using effective strategies to monitor and organize learning. Children with LLD often fail to access or use task-appropriate strategies spontaneously. These problems persist throughout adolescence and into adulthood. Strategies for working with children with LLD are presented in Table 2.6.

TABLE 2.6   Techniques to use with children with LLD

Attention

1. Reduce competing stimuli. Gradually reintroduce these stimuli as child becomes better able to tolerate them. Eventually intervention should move into the classroom with all the competing stimuli.
2. Highlight those aspects of a situation to which the child is to attend.
3. Use visual and physical cues to aid the child in attending to verbal ones.

Perception

1. Train initially with nonspeech environmental sounds, then speech sounds.
2. Use visual and physical cues to aid the child in interpreting verbal ones.
3. Use meaning-based tasks in which a sound change changes the meaning.
4. Visual or hand signals may be used to aid intonational interpretation and turn taking.

Organization

1. Help child to see underlying relationships. Use categorizational, associational, and word-class sorting tasks. Use "spreading" model so child realizes many possible associations.
2. Use same/different tasks and match to sample.
3. Be alert that the child's associations may not be the same as adult ones. Try to understand the relationships that may have validity for the child.

Memory and Generalization/Transfer

1. Practice serial recall, first visually (locomotive, touch), then auditorily.
2. Control for infrequent words, linguistic complexity, length, intonation, context, and semantic-logical relationship.
3. Use command following. Control for number of elements and steps.
4. Ask questions about things that happened immediately before. Next, ask questions about slightly distant events. Increase the time lapse. Finally, ask questions concerning what was just said.
5. Teach in the location where you want the feature to be recalled.

Similar Impairments: Prenatal Drug and Alcohol Exposure

I have decided to place children with fetal alcohol syndrome (FAS) and prenatal drug exposure in the learning disabilities section because of the similarities they present in their behavior and in their language. No doubt there will be objections to this placement.

FAS accounts for one in every 500 to 600 live births. A less severe form of the disorder, called fetal alcohol effects (FAE), is found in one in every 350. The incidence is probably much higher but underreported. At birth, infants with FAS have a low birth weight and short length often accompanied by central nervous system dysfunction as evidenced in microcephaly or a small head, hyperactivity, motor problems, attention deficits, and cognitive disabilities. Mean IQs are in the borderline retarded category with a range of 30 to 105. In general, these children are concrete learners with poor problem-solving abilities and difficulty generalizing. They are easily distractable, easily overstimulated, impulsive, and perseverative; they have poor memory, interpersonal skills, and judgment; and they exhibit language problems characterized by delayed development, echolalia, and language production that exceeds comprehension. Intervention suggestions are presented in Table 2.7. As infants, children with FAS are irritable and have weak sucking and delayed development. Language deficits

TABLE 2.7   Intervention strategies for child with fetal alcohol syndrome

Remove erroneous stimulation.

Provide preferential seating.

Use picture cues to strengthen verbal instructions.

Take care to describe and explain carefully and ask the child to repeat.

Use eye contact or the child's name prior to giving verbal instructions or directions.

"Hook" the child's attention with novel object, topics, and attention getters.

Be patient.

Challenge the child but remember that he or she may be easily frustrated.

Set definite behavioral limits.

Provide a tolerant and patient "buddy" to help the child with social interactions.

include problems with word order and word meaning and difficulties in the give-and-take of conversational discourse. Most often children with FAS are diagnosed as having a learning disability or ADHD.

Eleven to 35 percent of pregnant women ingest one or more illegal drugs. Although the percentages vary with race, ethnicity, age, socioeconomic status, and geographic location, the use of illegal drugs crosses all these boundaries. The effects on the infant vary with the amount and type of drugs, the method of ingestion, and the age of the fetus (MacDonald, 1992). Crack cocaine is especially destructive, with fetal death twice as common as among other noncocaine drug-dependent mothers and sudden infant death syndrome (SIDS) three times as high. Crack cocaine, a rapid-acting cerebrocortical stimulant, easily crosses the placental barrier, decreasing placental blood flow and fetal oxygen supply, reaching significant blood levels in the fetus, and altering the fetus's neurochemical functioning.

Like infants with FAS, those exposed to crack cocaine also exhibit low birth weight and small head circumference; they are jittery and irritable and spend the majority of their time sleeping or crying. An infant may still be unable to reach an alert state by one month of age (Lesar, 1992). Infants exposed to drugs also have hypertonia, rapid respiration, and feeding difficulties (Weston, Ivins, Zuckerman, Jones, & Lopez, 1989). Easily overstimulated, these hypersensitive infants actively avoid the human face, which, because of its complexity, may overload them cognitively (Griffith, 1988).

As might be expected, typical mother-child bonding is disrupted, with resultant delays in motor, social, and language development (Crites, Fischer, McNeish-Stengel, & Siegel, 1992). For her part, the addicted mother's primary commitment is to drugs, and she may fail to attend to the child. A cycle of infant passivity and parental rejection may be established.

The language characteristics of children exposed to drugs begin with few infant vocalizations, inappropriate use of gestures, and a lack of oral language. By preschool, these children are exhibiting word retrieval problems, short disorganized sentences, poor eye contact, turn-taking difficulties, few novel utterances, and inappropriate or off-topic responses (Mentis & Lundgren, 1995). In kindergarten, the child uses short, simple sentences and has a limited vocabulary, especially for abstract terms, multiple word meanings, and temporal/spatial terms. School-age years are characterized by problems with word retrieval and word order and by pragmatically inappropriate language (Rivers & Hedrick, 1992). Children with drug exposure are usually diagnosed as having a learning disability or ADHD.

Conclusion

LLD is an extremely complex concept. Although it is relatively easy to describe the outward behaviors of children with LLD, it is very difficult to explain the underlying processes. In short, biological or neurostructural differences and functional neuroprocessing differences in children with LLD affect their ability to attend to, discriminate, and remember linguistic and other stimuli, resulting in language that may be impaired in all aspects and in all modes of transmission and reception.

Specific Language Impairment

Specific language impairment (SLI) can be characterized as "significant limitations in language functioning that cannot be attributed to deficits in hearing, oral structure and function, or general intelligence" (Leonard, 1987, p. 1). In other words, this category of language impairment has no obvious cause and seems not to affect or be affected by anatomical, physical, or intellectual problems. Unlike some children with MR, but similar to most with LLD, children with SLI exhibit language performance scores significantly lower than their intellectual performance scores on nonverbal tasks. Children with SLI do not exhibit the perceptual difficulties seen in LLD nor the intellectual deficits of MR.

SLI is characterized more by the exclusion of other disorders than on some readily identifiable trait or behavior (Leonard, 1991). Clinical identification is difficult and is usually based on the absence of other contributing factors.

Even with a paucity of criteria for characterizing children with SLI, we can make certain definitive statements. Children with SLI may appear to be delayed in one aspect of language, although the language problem is not the result of delay, and children with SLI will not catch up to other children their age without intervention (Leonard, 1991). Even in their apparent delay, children with SLI are unlike children developing typically at any stage of development (J. Johnston, 1988b; Leonard, 1991).

The usual criteria for SLI are a performance IQ above 85 and a low verbal IQ. For most, expressive abilities are significantly below receptive (Kamhi, 1998). A reported auditory processing disorder may be a deficit in verbal working memory where the brain accumulates verbal information while language processing occurs (Friel-Patti, 1999; Montgomery, 2002b).

As many as 10 to 15 percent of children may be "late bloomers" who do not achieve 50 single words and two-word utterances by 24 months of age (Rescorla, 1989). Most of these children "outgrow" their delay, but approximately 20 to 25 percent of the problems with language persist into preschool and school age (Paul, 1989a, 1996; Rescorla, 1990; Thal, 1989). These children form the core of those with SLI.

As high as 7.4 percent of all kindergarten children have SLI (Tomblin, Records, Buckwalter, Zhang, Smith, & O'Brien, 1997). Although SLI is a changeable condition with maturity, two thirds of kindergartners with the impairment will still have difficulty with language as adolescents (Stothard et al., 1998). Even those with more typical language had lingering problems with phonological problems and literacy skills.

In general, children with SLI are perceived more negatively by teachers and peers (Segebert DeThorne & Watkins, 2001). Young children may have behavior problems; however, these decrease with age (Redmont & Rice, 2002). In elementary school, children with SLI take minor roles in cooperative learning, contribute little, and have fewer high-level negotiating strategies than their language-ability-matched peers developing typically (Brinton, Fujiki, & McKee, 1998; Brinton, Fujiki, & Higbee, 1998). By late elementary school or middle school, language problems take their toll on self-esteem and these children perceive themselves negatively in scholastic competence, social acceptance, and behavior conduct (Jerome, Fujiki, Brinton, & James, 2002).

Language Characteristics

As with other language impairments, significant language differences are seen across children. The language impairment may be primarily, but not exclusively, expressive or receptive, or a combination of the two, and affect different aspects of language, although language form seems to be affected more than other aspects (Aram, 1991; N. Nelson, 1993). In addition, the disorder changes within the individual child with age. Language difficulties of children with SLI extend across early language skills important for reading decoding and comprehension (Boudreau & Hedberg, 1999). Errors seen in speech may be present also in writing (Gillam & Johnston, 1992).

In general, children with SLI have difficulty (a) learning language rules, (b) registering different contexts for language, and (c) constructing word-referent associations for lexical growth (Connell & Stone, 1994; Ellis Weismer, 1991; Kiernan, Snow, Swisher, & Vance, 1997; Leonard, 1987). The result is difficulty in morphological and phonological rule learning and application and in vocabulary development (Bishop & Adams, 1992; Ellis Weismer, 1991; Rice, Buhr, & Oetting, 1992; van der Lely & Harris, 1990). Morphologic learning is more closely tied to overall language learning than other aspects of language (Dale & Cole, 1991). Pragmatic problems result from inability to use effective forms to accomplish language intentions. Specific language problems are listed in Table 2.8.

The conversational behaviors of children with SLI compared with those of mental-age-matched peers developing typically are marked by both qualitative and quantitative differences (Craig, 1993). Qualitative differences, such as difficulty initiating interaction and inappropriate responses, lead to increased interruptions by other children and other quantitative changes. The child with SLI is less likely to interact with other children over time as the child experiences repeated failure. As a result, children with SLI often are ignored by other children in the classroom and experience reduced interactional opportunities. Thus, children with SLI have poorer social skills and fewer peer relationships and report less satisfaction with these relationships than age-matched classmates (Fujiki, Brinton, & Todd, 1996).

As might be expected, given the auditory processing problems of children with SLI, morphological inflections are especially difficult (Dale & Cole, 1991; Leonard, McGregor, & Allen, 1992). Morphemes are small units of language that receive little stress in speech. Verb endings and auxiliary verbs pose a particular problem, as does use of pronouns (Frome Loeb & Leonard, 1991; Oetting & Morohov, 1997). The two problems are related because pronoun selection (*he* versus *they*) determines some verb endings (*walks* versus *walk*) (Connell, 1986a).

Verb morphology is a particular difficulty for young children with SLI. Auxiliary verbs, infinitives, verb endings, and irregular verbs offer persistent problems for both preschool and school-age children (Goffman & Leonard, 2000; Redmond & Rice, 2001). Although most tense markers are mastered at age 4 for children developing typically, children with SLI take an additional three years to achieve the same level of competence (Rice, Wexler, & Hershberger, 1998). Morphological problems found in English have also been reported for children with SLI learning Spanish and modern Hebrew as a native language (Bedore & Leonard, 2001; Dromi, Leonard, Adam, & Zadunaisky-Ehrlich, 1999).

Language comprehension and processing are active processes in which the listener infers the meaning from the auditory message, contextual information, and stored world and word knowledge. Children with SLI do not appear to employ actively all of this available information. In general, they

TABLE 2.8   Language characteristics of children with specific language impairment

Pragmatics	May act like younger children developing typically.
	Less flexibility in their language when tailoring the message to the listener or repairing communication breakdowns.
	Same pragmatic functions as chronological-age-matched peers developing typically, but expressed differently and less effectively.
	Less effective than chronological-age-matched peers in securing a conversational turn. Those with receptive difficulties most affected.
	Inappropriate responses to topic.
	Narratives less complete and more confusing than those of reading-ability-matched peers developing typically.
Semantics	First words and subsequent vocabulary development occurs at a slower rate, with occasional lexical errors seen in younger children developing typically.
	Naming difficulties may reflect less rich and less elaborate semantic storage than actual retrieval difficulties. Long-term memory storage problems are probable.
Syntax/Morphology	Co-occurrence of more mature and less mature forms.
	Similar developmental order to that seen in children developing typically.
	Fewer morphemes, especially verb endings, auxiliary verbs, and function words (articles, prepositions) than younger MLU-matched peers. Learning related to grammatical function as in children developing typically.
	Tend to make pronoun errors, as do younger MLU-matched peers, but tend to overuse one form rather than making random errors.
Phonology	Phonological processes similar to those of younger children developing typically, but in different patterns, i.e., occurring in units of varying word length rather than in one- or two-word utterances.
	As toddlers, vocalize less and have less varied and less mature syllable structures than age-matched peers developing typically.
Comprehension	Poor discrimination of units of short duration (bound morphemes).
	Reading miscues often unrelated to text graphophonemically, syntactically, semantically, or pragmatically.

Source: Based on Beastrom & Rice (1986); Bliss (1989); Brinton, Fujiki, Winkler, & Loeb (1986); Craig & Evans (1993); Craig & Washington (1993); Gillam & Carlile (1997); Kail & Leonard (1986); Leonard (1986, 1989); Leonard, McGregor, & Allen (1992); Liles (1985a, 1985b); Loeb & Leonard (1988); Merritt & Liles (1987); Rescorla & Ratner (1996); Rice & Oetting (1993); Rice, Oetting, Marquis, Bode, & Pae (1994); Rice & Wexler (1996); Watkins & Rice (1989).

have difficulty constructing an integrated representation of a series of events, whether the series is presented verbally or nonverbally (Bishop & Adams, 1992). Thus, vocabulary growth—which occurs typically as the result of inferring meaning from repeated exposure and without direct reference or prompting from adults—will be very difficult for the child with SLI using limited active processing strategies (Rice, Buhr, & Nemeth, 1990; Rice et al., 1992; Weismer & Hesketh, 1996).

Difficulty forming internal representations can also be seen in the play of children with SLI (Rescorla & Goossens, 1992). In general, toddlers and preschoolers with SLI exhibit less non-object play, less well-developed sequential play, and fewer occurrences of symbolic play than chronological-age-matched peers. The two groups exhibit equal engagement with toys and functional conversational play behavior. Overall, children with SLI develop play in the same manner as do children developing typically, but at a slower pace (Roth & Clark, 1987; Skarakis-Doyle & Prutting, 1988).

Possible Causal Factors

Causes of SLI are difficult to determine and may be as diverse as the children who have the impairment (J. Johnston, 1991; Tomblin, 1991). With such a diverse population, it is not surprising that several possible causal factors have been identified.

Biological Factors.   The language and learning problems of children with SLI suggest a neurological disorder (Aram & Eisele, 1994). Possible neurological factors include brain asymmetry, in which language functions are located in different areas from those found in the majority of individuals, and delayed myelination, the progressive process of nerve sheathing that results in more rapid transmission of impulses (Galaburda, 1989; Hynd, Marshall, & Gonzalez, 1991; Love & Webb, 1986). The reported adeptness of children with SLI in analyzing visual, spatial patterns is considered by some to be evidence of greater reliance on the right hemisphere of the brain. Language processing, at least linear or sequential processing, is concentrated in the left temporal lobe.

A biological cause is also suggested by a strong familial pattern. Sixty percent of children with SLI have an affected family member, 38 percent an affected parent. The relationship is particularly strong for children with SLI who exhibit expressive language problems (Lahey & Edwards, 1995). Further evidence of a biological factor can be found in preterm births. A sizable minority of infants born at 32 weeks or less are at considerable risk for SLI (Briscoe, Gathercole, & Marlow, 1998).

Social-Environmental Factors.   Although no one has suggested environmental causes, some differences do exist in the interactions of parents with children with SLI and those developing typically (Conti-Ramsden, 1990; Conti-Ramsden, Hutcheson, & Grove, 1995; K. Nelson, Welsh, Camarata, Butkovsky, & Camarata, 1995). Studies have reported conflicting data on the frequency of recast sentences by parents of children with SLI. Sentence **recasts** such as expansions are adult remixes or modifications in a child's utterance that maintain the focus of the original utterance and can be an effective language teaching technique. Even if parents of children with SLI recast as frequently as other parents, this effort may still not be enough for children who would appear to need even more of such input (Fey, Krulik, Frome Loeb, & Proctor-Williams, 1999).

When parents of children with SLI recast a child's utterance, they are most likely to recast the noun phrase, in contrast to parents of non-SLI children, who are most likely to recast the verb phrase. This is unfortunate because children with SLI have particular difficulty with the verb phrase.

Processing Factors.   Although children with SLI demonstrate typical nonverbal intelligence, they may also demonstrate cognitive impairments not exhibited on standard intelligence measures (Kamhi, Minor, & Mauer, 1990; Leonard, 1987). As mentioned previously, these children do not seem to employ active processing strategies that use contextual information and stored knowledge. Information-processing problems of children with SLI occur with incoming information, in memory, and in problem solving (Ellis Weismer, 1991; L. Nelson, Kamhi, & Apel, 1987). In addition, children with SLI demonstrate slower linguistic and nonlinguistic processing on both expressive and receptive tasks than age-matched children developing typically (Leonard, 1998; Miller, Kail, Leonard, & Tomblin, 2001; Windsor & Hwang, 1999a).

These characteristics suggest limitations in cognitive processing capacity in which tradeoffs exist between accuracy and speed of responding (Ellis Weismer & Evans, 2002). In the rapid give-and-take of conversation this tradeoff results in reduced processing and storage of phonological information, inefficient fast mapping and novel word learning, slow word recognition, and ineffective sentence comprehension (Bishop, North, & Donlan, 1996; Dollaghan & Campbell, 1998; Edwards & Lahey, 1998; Ellis Weismer & Hesketh, 1996; Ellis Weismer et al., 2000; Miller et al., 2001; Montgomery 2000a; Windsor & Hwang, 1999b).

Short-term auditory sequential memory, or memory for item order, and problem solving of complex reasoning tasks are also affected in children with SLI (J. Johnston & Smith, 1989; Kamhi, Gentry, et al., 1990; L. Nelson et al., 1987). Although poor recall of linguistic units suggests limits in verbal working memory, poor performance on nonlinguistic serial memory tasks suggests that the deficit may not be language specific (Ellis Weismer, Evans, & Hesketh, 1999; Fazio, 1998; Montgomery 2000a, 2000b). Some data suggest that the types of verbal tasks used may influence children's performance (McNamara, Carter, McIntosh, & Gerken, 1998; Montgomery & Leonard, 1998). In other words, the language performance of children with SLI may be indicative of overall problems in working memory. **Working memory** is an active process that allows for access to a small number of items in conscious awareness. Incoming linguistic and nonlinguistic information is held in working memory while processed. If the storage and processing demands on working memory exceed the resources available, comprehension suffers.

With inefficient allocation of mental resources to acoustic-phonetic processing, the child with SLI is easily overwhelmed by rapidly incoming information and cannot effectively employ lexical retrieval, recognition, and integration processes (Montgomery, 2002a).

Children with SLI orient more slowly to new information, have more limited capacity for sustained focus, and have greater difficulty refocusing and shifting focus than age-matched peers (Gillam, Cowan, & Day, 1995; Marler, 2000; Marler, Champlin, & Gillam, 2001; Riddle, 1992). Lack of attention contributes to inefficiency in forming representations of incoming acoustic information (Helzer, Champlin, & Gillam, 1996; Sussman, 1993). Temporal processing abilities are further slowed by simultaneous multiple linguistic operations. The result of storage/access memory deficits is lower rates of vocabulary learning (Swisher & Snow, 1994). Diminished phonological working memory for words also affects sentence comprehension (Montgomery, 1995).

Problem solving is also an active process that requires use of contextual information and prior knowledge. It should be noted, however, that when children with SLI are matched with younger children possessing the same language abilities, differences in short-term auditory memory seem to disappear (van der Lely & Howard, 1993).

Conclusion

Much discussion has taken place concerning the viability of SLI as a separate category of language impairment. It has been suggested that SLI is not a distinct disorder category, but merely represents children with limited language abilities as the result of genetic and/or environmental factors (Leonard, 1987, 1991; Tomblin, 1991). Some educators have suggested that SLI may not even be a useful concept, especially because clinical tools are unable to diagnose it easily and accurately (Aram, Morris, & Hall, 1993).

For now, the best diagnostic techniques appear to be rote memory tasks, such as counting or sequential digit recall, nonsense word repetition, rule induction (see dynamic assessment of children with LEP, page 111), story recall, grammatical completion, especially verb markers, number of different words in a speech sample, and memory plus interpretation tasks while listening or reading (Fazio, Naremore, & Connell, 1996; Montgomery, 1995; Rice & Wexler, 1996; Watkins, Kelly, Harbors, & Hollis, 1995). Memory and awareness tasks for intervention are presented in Table 2.9.

Pervasive Developmental Disorder/Autism Spectrum Disorder

The fourth edition of the American Psychiatric Association's *Diagnostic and Statistical Manual on Mental Disorders* (DSM-IV) (1996) lists autism along a continuum labeled Pervasive Developmental Disorder (PDD). Autism Spectrum Disorder (ASD) is at the more severe extreme, while a milder form of the disorder is called Pervasive Developmental Disorder—Not Otherwise Specified (PDD-NOS) (Bauer, 1995a, 1995b). In actual practice, children are labeled as ASD when the severe form of the disorder exists and as simply PDD when the milder form exists. Some children with PDD are labeled with Asperger's syndrome or are mislabeled as learning disabled or ADHD. If this is not confusing enough, other children with PDD are labeled hyperlexic and may exhibit some characteristics of ASD while others with this label appear more like children with learning disabilities. These labels are not assigned arbitrarily but are based on characteristics exhibited by the child. Don't be too confused by all these labels. We shall try to sort out these differences in the following discussion.

The American Psychiatric Association (1996) defines ASD as an impairment in reciprocal social interaction with a severely limited behavior, interest, and activity repertoire. The Autism Society of America further defines ASD as a disorder that has an onset prior to 30 months of age and that consists of *disturbances* in the following areas:

- Developmental rates and the sequence of motor, social-adaptive, and cognitive skills
- Responses to sensory stimuli—hyper- and hyposensitivity in audition, vision, tactile stimulation, motor, olfactory, and taste, including self-stimulatory behaviors

TABLE 2.9   Intervention for memory and awareness with children with SLI

Naming letters and objects	Repeating novel and nonsense ("funny") words
Recalling spoken sentences	Rhyming games
Using melody as a memory aid	Recalling of words that begin with specific phonemes
Listening to stories and nursery rhymes	Guessing games based on cumulative cues
Repeating nursery rhymes	Rehearsing verbally
Acting out pictures	Categorizing words and objects
Acting out rhymes	
Using gestures to aid recall	

Source: Adapted from Fazio (1996); Montgomery (1995).

- Speech and language, cognition, and nonverbal communication, including mutism, echolalia, and difficulty with abstract terms
- Capacity to appropriately relate to people, events, and objects, including lack of social behaviors, affection, and appropriate play

ASD is found in males four times more frequently than in females (Bauer, 1995a) and affects 1 in 500 children. Within the last few years there has been an explosion in the number of children in the United States diagnosed as PDD. Whether because of better diagnosis or a real increase, 1 in 150 children age 10 and younger are now classified as having some variety of PDD. In real numbers, that equals 300,000 children and over 1 million adults in the United States.

As in other language impairments discussed in this chapter, children with ASD are a diverse group. For example, to the best of our ability to measure, slightly more than half of the children with ASD have IQs below 50, with the remainder evenly split between 50–70 and 71 and above (Schreibman, 1988). The best prognostic or recovery indicators are a nonverbal IQ above 70 and meaningful speech by age 5 (Bauer, 1995b).

Although it is rare that the disorder is identified prior to 18 months of age, infants with ASD have been described as either lethargic, preferring solitude and making few demands, or highly irritable, with sleeping problems and screaming and crying (Coleman & Gillberg, 1985). Usually, between 18 and 36 months, the signs become more pronounced, including more frequent tantruming, repetitive movements and ritualistic play, extreme reactions to certain stimuli, lack of pretend and social play, and joint attention and communication difficulties including a lack of gestures.

In approximately 20 percent of the cases, parents report typical development until 24 months, especially among girls (Bauer, 1995a). Early identification is often difficult because of the lack of obvious medical problems and the early typical development of motor abilities. Infrequently, onset occurs in later childhood. Recent data suggests that young children with PDD exhibit clusters of impairment in joint or mutual attending, symbolic play, and social affective communication (Wetherby, Prizant, & Hutchinson, 1998).

Development often proceeds in spurts and plateaus, rather than smoothly. Most areas of development are affected by delay and disorder, although occasionally one area, such as mechanical or mathematical abilities, is typical or above. I have worked with children well above average in mathematics but unable to dress themselves or to participate in meaningful conversations. Motor behaviors may include toe walking, rocking, spinning, and, in extreme cases, self-injurious behaviors, such as biting, hitting, and head banging. One adolescent with whom I worked was covered with scars and scabs from self-inflicted scratches and bites. Another child pounded his head with his fist an average of more than 7,000 times in a five-hour school day.

Hyper- and hyposensitivity to stimuli may be found in the same child. For example, loud noises may get no response from the child, while whispering results in a catastrophic response. In general, children with ASD tend to prefer shiny objects, especially those that spin; things that can be twirled; and noises they produce themselves, such as teeth grinding. Children with ASD seem to prefer routines and may become extremely upset with change. Individual children may have very definite preferences in taste, touch, and smell. I worked with one child whose only food preference was dill pickles. Self-stimulatory behaviors may include rocking, spinning, and hand flapping.

Relational disorders may be the most distressful aspect of ASD, especially for parents (Bauer, 1995b; Bristol, 1988). In particular, children with ASD often avert their gaze or stare emptily and lack a social smile, responsiveness to sound, and anticipation of the approach of others. Parents often are treated as "things" or, at best, no different from other people. The effect on parents can be imagined.

As mentioned, children with a milder form of the disorder are labeled with Pervasive Developmental Disorder—Not Otherwise Specified, PDD-NOS, or simply PDD. Children with **PDD-NOS** exhibit many of the characteristics of ASD but to a lesser degree. For example, they may have difficulty with social behavior and exhibit poor eye contact and poor use of gestures and facial expressions. Their grammar may be disordered and they may use echolalia.

Other children may be labeled with **Asperger's syndrome,** characterized by an obvious lack of linguistic or cognitive disorders; by average or above-average intelligence, especially for abstract thinking tasks; by an inability to understand the rules of social behavior, including conversation; and by an intense interest in a limited range of one or two topics. Children with Asperger's syndrome may be poorly organized but perfectionist in their demands, with ability to concentrate deeply and difficulty transitioning.

Still other children may be labeled with **hyperlexia,** a disorder affecting boys and girls at a ratio of 7:1 and characterized by a spontaneous early ability to read—often at age 2½ or 3—but with little comprehension (Aram, 1997). Children with hyperlexia have an intense preoccupation with letters and words and extensive word recognition by age 5 but exhibit language and cognitive disorders in reasoning and in perceiving relationships. In addition to delayed language, these children experience difficulty with connected language in all modalities, especially integrating it with context in order to derive meaning (Snowling & Frith, 1986).

As with all the disorders discussed, there is a range of severity. Some children with mild forms of either semantic-pragmatic disorder or hyperlexia may be mislabeled as learning disabled depending on the characteristics present. This is not a science but a fine art.

Language Characteristics

Communication problems are often one of the first indicators of possible ASD. These may include a failure to begin gesturing or talking, a seeming noninterest in other people, or a lack of verbal responding.

Poor social interaction and poor language and communication skills are extremely characteristic of children with ASD. Speech does not seem to be difficult for those who speak, although speech is often wooden and robotlike, lacking a musical quality (Schuler & Prizant, 1987).

Between 25 and 60 percent of the population with ASD remains mute or nonspeaking. Until recently, this lack of speech also has meant that they remained noncommunicating. This situation is changing for some, but not all, children using augmentative and alternative communication (AAC).

Those children using speech and language may demonstrate immediate or delayed **echolalia,** a whole or partial repetition of previous utterances, often with the same intonation. Immediate echolalia is variable, increasing in highly directive situations, with unknown words, following an inability to comprehend, in the presence of an adult, in unfamiliar situations, in face-to-face communication with eye contact, and with longer, more complex utterances (Charlop, 1986; Violette & Swisher, 1992). Immediate echolalia also has been found to signal agreement in some children. No such data are available for delayed echolalia. One child with whom I worked would repeat many of the utterances directed to him during the day as he lay in bed prior to sleep.

In general, pragmatics and semantics are affected more than language form (Lord, 1988). The give-and-take of conversation seems to be particularly difficult. The range of communication functions is often very limited, and its development is sequential rather than synchronous, as seen in children developing typically. In addition, functions may be expressed in an individualistic or idiosyncratic manner, such as saying "Sesame Street is a production of the Children's Television Workshop" for "Good-bye."

Children with ASD also seem to have difficulty matching the content and form of language to the context (Swisher & Demetras, 1985). Occasionally, children will incorporate rote utterances, such as the child who says "Attention, K-Mart shoppers" to get attention. Even those individuals who have acquired language often have peculiarities and irregularities in their communication. Specific language characteristics are listed in Table 2.10.

Although errors in language form occur in children with ASD, these are not as severe as those for semantics and pragmatics. Syntactic errors that are present seem to represent lack of underlying semantic relationships. Phonological development appears to follow the same sequence as that of children developing typically and not to be delayed inordinately.

Possible Causal Factors

In the past, children with ASD have been classified as having an emotional-, physical-, environmental-, or health-related impairment. The cause may be any and all of these, although the primary causal

TABLE 2.10   Language characteristics of children with ASD

Pragmatics	Deficits in joint attending.
	Difficulty initiating and maintaining a conversation, resulting in much shorter conversational episodes.
	Limited range of communication functions.
	Difficulty matching form and content to context. May perseverate or introduce inappropriate topics.
	Immediate and delayed echolalia and routinized utterances.
	Few gestures used; misinterpretation of complex gestures.
	Overuse of questions, frequent repetition.
	Frequent asocial monologues.
	Difficulty with stylistic variations and speaker–listener roles.
	Gaze aversion, seeming use of peripheral vision.
Semantics	Word-retrieval difficulties, especially for visual referents.
	Underlying meaning not used as a memory aid.
	More inappropriate answers to questions than age-matched peers.
Syntax/Morphology	Morphological difficulties, especially with pronouns and verb endings.
	Construct sentences with superficial form, often disregarding underlying meaning.
	Less complex sentences than mental-age-matched peers developing typically.
	Overreliance on word order.
Phonology	Phonology variable within individual child, often disordered.
	Developmental order similar to children developing typically.
	Least affected aspect of language.
Comprehension	Impaired comprehension, especially in connected discourse such as conversations.

Source: Based on Alpert & Rogers-Warren (1984); Greenspan & Wieder (1997); Lewy & Dawson (1992); Lord (1988); Lord et al. (1989); Rumsey, Rapoport, & Sceery (1985); Swisher & Demetras (1985).

factors are probably biological (Schreibman, 1988). Even within this population, neuroanatomical and neurochemical features may differ.

Biological Factors.   Approximately 65 percent of all individuals with ASD have abnormal brain patterns. The incidence of autism accompanying prenatal complications, fragile X syndrome, and Ritt syndrome, a degenerative neurological condition, and among those with a family history of autism is higher (Schreibman, 1988). In addition, ASD is often accompanied by mental retardation and seizures. All of these suggest a biological basis but do not explain the actual disorder. Other studies have found unusually high levels of serotonin, a neurotransmitter and natural opiate; abnormal development of the cerebellum, the section of the brain that regulates incoming sensations; multifocal disorders of the brain; and impairment of the neural subcortical structures with accompanying impairment in cortical development (Courchesne, 1988; Schopler & Mesibov, 1987; Schreibman, 1988).

Recent studies have suggested a genetic link in ASD, although is seems doubtful that a solitary autism gene exists (Wentzel, 2000). It is more likely that several genes are involved and may be shared with other disorders.

Social-Environmental Factors.   Early studies blamed parents for ASD. No basis has been found for this conclusion. In general, parents interact with their children at the appropriate language level.

Processing Factors.   Children with ASD have difficulty analyzing and integrating information. When attending, they tend to fixate on one aspect of a complex stimulus, often some irrelevant, minor detail. In other words, responding is very overselective. This fixation, in turn, makes discrimination difficult.

Overall processing by these children has been characterized as a "gestalt" in which unanalyzed wholes are stored and later reproduced in identical fashion, as in echolalia. In this relatively inflexible system, input is examined in its entirety, rather than analyzed into its component parts. Information usually is reproduced in a context that is in some way similar to the initial context. This reliance on unanalyzed wholes could account for the tendency of children with ASD to repeat an agrammatical sentence, rather than to correct it as language-matched children with MR will do. It is possible that children with ASD depend more heavily on simultaneous language processing than on successive language processing.

The behavior of children with ASD suggests that very little of the world makes sense to them. They seem to overload quickly. Information "swallowed" whole could quickly "fill" the system.

Storage of unanalyzed wholes also might hinder memory. Children with autism reportedly are less able to use environmental cues to aid memory, possibly because those cues do not exist as separate entities in the child's memory. It is also difficult for these children to organize information on the basis of relationships between stimuli.

In addition, children with ASD have difficulty transferring or generalizing learned information from one context to another. This difficulty reflects the inability of these children to identify the relevant contextual information.

Conclusion

As with other disorders that have been discussed, PDD demonstrates heterogeneity. Great differences are found in severity, especially in communication abilities. In general, these differences affect the pragmatic and semantic aspects of language and may reflect processing difficulties such as stimulus overselectivity and storage of unanalyzed wholes.

Brain Injury

Children with brain injury are often confused with other children who have impairments, such as children with LLD, MR, or emotional disorders. Children with brain injury differ greatly as a result of the site and extent of lesion, the age at onset, and the age of the injury. In general, the smaller the damaged area, the better the **prognosis,** or chance of recovery.

Brain injury in children may result from trauma, cerebrovascular accident (CVA) or stroke, congenital malformation, convulsive disorders, or encephalopathy, such as infection or tumors. Each has different characteristics, although some similarities in language occur. Only the most prevalent types of injury are discussed here.

Traumatic Brain Injury (TBI)

Approximately 1 million children and adolescents in the United States have traumatic brain injury, or TBI, diffuse brain damage as the result of external physical force, such as a blow to the head received in an auto accident. TBIs are not congenital or degenerative. Individuals may range from nearly full recovery to a vegetative state in some very severe cases. Although the chances of survival have improved greatly in recent years, long-term disability is a continuing public health problem (Zitnay, 1995).

Deficits may be cognitive, physical, behavioral, academic, and linguistic (Ewing-Cobbs, Fletcher, & Levin, 1985; Rosen & Gerring, 1986; Savage, 1991; Savage & Wolcott, 1988; Ylvisaker, 1986). *Cognitive deficits* include perception, memory, reasoning, and problem-solving difficulties. Such deficits may be permanent or temporary and may partially or totally affect functioning ability. Psychological maladjustment or acting-out behaviors, called **social disinhibition,** may also occur. For example, I once evaluated a young man with TBI who kept insisting on kissing my hand. Other characteristics include lack of initiative, distractibility, inability to adapt quickly, perseveration, low frustration levels, passive-aggressiveness, anxiety, depression, fear of failure, and misperception.

Severity may range from a *mild concussion,* defined as a loss of consciousness for less than 30 seconds, through *moderate TBI,* a loss of consciousness or posttraumatic amnesia for 30 minutes to 24 hours, with or without skull fracture, to *severe TBI,* consisting of a coma for 6 hours or longer. Severity is not directly related to the deficits mentioned above (Russell, 1993).

Variables that affect recovery are extremely independent and are complicated by some of the characteristics of the population at risk for TBI (Lehr, 1989; Middleton, 1989; Savage, 1991). In general, this population has a lower IQ, higher social disadvantage, poorer schooling, and more behavioral and physical difficulties prior to injury than the general population (N. Nelson & Schwentor, 1990). Other variables include degree and length of unconsciousness, duration of posttraumatic amnesia, age at injury, age of injury, and posttraumatic ability (Dennis, 1992; Russell, 1993). In general, shorter, less severe unconsciousness, shorter amnesia, and better posttraumatic abilities indicate better recovery.

Age at the time of injury is a less definitive factor because the child is developing when the injury occurs. Younger children may exhibit more severe and more long-lasting problems. Although younger children have less to recover, they also do not have the benefit of as much past learning as older children.

Age of the injury also can be an inaccurate predictor. In general, the older the injury, the less chance of change, but this aspect is complicated by the delayed onset of some deficits (Russell, 1993). Neural recovery over time is often unpredictable and irregular.

Language Characteristics.   Language problems are usually evident even after mild injuries. Pragmatics seem to be the most disturbed aspect of the language of children with TBI. This fact can be noted in the narratives and in conversation of these children (Chapman, 1997; Liles, Coelho, Duffy, & Zalagens, 1989; Mentis & Prutting, 1987). Utterances are often lengthy, inappropriate, and off-topic, and fluency is disturbed (Ylvisaker, 1986). Language comprehension and higher functions such as figurative language and dual meanings also may be affected. The child may lose his or her train of thought in conversations, while in narratives the same child may not retain the central focus of the story, thus deleting important information (Chapman et al., 1997).

By comparison, language form is relatively unaffected. The majority of children with TBI regain the ability to manipulate language form and content (Chapman, Levin, Matejka, Harwood, & Kufera, 1995). Surface structure may seem relatively unimpaired. The child's language may be effective in school until the third or fourth grade, when students are required to use higher language abilities to analyze and synthesize (Russell, 1993). Semantics, especially concrete vocabulary, is also relatively undisturbed, although word retrieval, naming, and object description difficulties may be present (Ewing-Cobbs et al., 1987). Other characteristics are listed in Table 2.11.

Some deficits will remain long after the injury even when overall improvement is good (T. Campbell & Dollaghan, 1990; Ewing-Cobbs et al., 1987; Jordan, Ozanne, & Murdoch, 1988). Although there is considerable variability among children with TBI, many subtle deficits remain, especially in pragmatics (Dennis & Barnes, 1990).

TABLE 2.11   Language characteristics of children with traumatic brain injury (TBI)

Pragmatics	Difficulty with organization and expression of complex ideas. Off-topic comments. Ineffectual, inappropriate comments. Short narratives include story grammar and cohesion, as do those of typically developing peers.
Semantics	Word retrieval, naming, and object description difficulties, although vocabulary relatively intact. Automatized, overlearned language relatively unaffected.
Syntax/Morphology	Sentences may be lengthy and fragmented.
Phonology	Few phonological difficulties although there may be some dysarthria or apraxia due to injury.
Comprehension	Some problems due to inattention and speed of processing. Poor auditory and reading comprehension. Difficulty with sentence comprehension due to difficulty assigning meaning to syntactic structure. Most routinized, everyday comprehension unaffected. Vocabulary comprehension usually unaffected, except for abstract terms.

Source: Based on Butler-Hinz, Caplan, & Waters (1990); Ewing-Cobbs, Levin, Eisenberg, & Fletcher (1987); Jordan, Murdock, & Buttsworth (1991); Mentis & Prutting (1987); Sarno, Buonaguro, & Levita (1986); Savage & Wolcott (1988); Ylvisaker (1986).

Possible Causal Factors.   Obvious biological and physical factors are involved in TBI. More important is the manner in which informational processing is affected. As mentioned, children with TBI are often inattentive and easily distractible. Attention fluctuates, and they have difficulty focusing on a task.

All aspects of organization—categorizing, sequencing, abstracting, and generalization—are affected. Children with TBI seem stimulus-bound—unable to see relationships, make inferences, and solve problems (Cohen, 1991; Ylvisaker, 1986). They evidence difficulty formulating goals, planning, and achieving (Ylvisaker & Szekeres, 1989). This deficiency often is masked by intact vocabulary and general knowledge.

Finally, children with TBI exhibit memory deficits in both storage and retrieval. Long-term memory prior to the trauma is usually intact. Techniques presented in Table 2.6 might be helpful with these children.

Cerebrovascular Accident (CVA)

Cerebrovascular accidents occur when a portion of the brain is denied oxygen, usually because of a rupture in a blood vessel serving the brain. Most frequently, damage is specific and localized. Patterns of recovery suggest that adjoining portions of the cortex, the surface of the cerebrum, or upper brain, augment the functioning of the damaged portion (Papanicolaon, DiScenna, Gillespie, & Aram, 1990).

CVAs usually are found in children with congenital heart problems or arteriovenous (blood vessel) malformations in the brain. Prognosis is generally good (Aram & Ekelman, 1987; Aram, Ekelman, & Whitaker, 1986, 1987). Naturally, the variability will be great, depending on the site and extent of the lesion. Language problems often accompany left hemisphere damage, although any brain damage has the potential to disturb language functioning.

Language Characteristics.   Long-term subtle pragmatic difficulties are common. Language form usually returns quickly, although performance may deteriorate when demands increase. Word retrieval may be extremely difficult at first, with deficits in both speed and accuracy (Aram, 1988). Language comprehension also is affected initially. Children usually recover, although higher level academic and reading difficulties may persist (Aram & Ekelman, 1988).

Conclusion

The underlying relationship between cognition and language varies with age and with the aspect of language studied. At many points in development, we are not able to describe the exact relationship. It is not surprising that we cannot fully explain the mechanisms at work when the brain is injured. Still, we can predict that vocabulary and structural rules will return more easily than higher order functions, such as conversational skills that require complex synthesis of language form, content, and use. Even those children who seem to recover may continue to exhibit long-term subtle pragmatic difficulties.

Neglect and Abuse

Children who are neglected and abused constitute a large portion of the preschool and school-age population that, until recently, had not been identified as having distinct language problems. It is estimated that 1 million children are neglected or abused each year in the United States. Although these children do not constitute a clinically defined category, they do present language difficulties.

Table 2.12 presents the types of neglect and abuse that have been identified (Sparks, 1989). The effect of each type of abuse will vary with each child.

Neglect and abuse are extreme examples of a dysfunctional family and are a sign of the type of social environment in which the child learned language (Cicchetti, 1987; Cicchetti & Lynch, 1993; Salzinger, Feldman, Hammer, & Rosario, 1991). Although neglect and abuse are rarely the direct cause of the communication problem, the context in which they occur directly influences the child's development.

Neglect and abuse are not limited to any economic class, although incidence increases as income decreases. It is believed that the increased economic, social, and health problems and lower levels of education and employment of the poor increase the risk of maltreatment.

Language Characteristics

All aspects of language are affected, although it is in language use that children who are neglected and abused exhibit the greatest difficulties (Table 2.13). In general, children who are neglected and abused are less talkative and have fewer conversational skills than their peers. Utterances and conversations are shorter than those of their peers. They are less likely to volunteer information or to discuss emotions or feelings.

In school, these children have depressed verbal language performance. A high correlation is found between deficient verbal and reading ability and neglect and abuse (Burke et al., 1989).

Possible Causal Factors

Certainly, negative social-environment factors are important in the development of language by children who are neglected and abused, but biological factors should not be overlooked. Medical and health problems among the poor also can contribute. Direct effect is difficult to determine because of the multiplicity of overlapping factors, especially among the poor (Fox, Long, & Langlois, 1988; McCauley & Swisher, 1987; Sparks, 1989).

Biological Factors.   Neglect and abuse are not limited to poor families, but in these families or in cases of extreme neglect, biological factors also may contribute. Poor maternal health, substance abuse, poor or nonexistent pediatric services, and poor nutrition can all affect brain development and

TABLE 2.12   Types of neglect and abuse

Physical neglect	Abandonment with no arrangement for care, including inadequate supervision, nutrition, clothing, and/or personal hygiene, and/or failure to seek needed or recommended medical care.
Emotional neglect	Failure to provide a normal living experience, including attention and affection, and/or refusal of treatment or services recommended by professional personnel.
Physical abuse	Bodily injury, such as neurological damage, or death from shaking, beating, and/or burning.
Sexual abuse	Both nonphysical abuse, such as indecent exposure or verbal attack, and physical abuse, such as genital-oral stimulation, fondling, and/or sexual intercourse.
Emotional abuse	Excessive yelling, belittling, teasing/verbal attack, and/or overt rejection.

Source: Adapted from Sparks (1989).

TABLE 2.13   Language characteristics of children who are neglected and abused

Pragmatics	Poor conversational skills. Inability to discuss feelings. Shorter conversations. Fewer descriptive utterances. Language used to get things done with little social exchange or affect.
Semantics	Limited expressive vocabulary. Fewer decontextualized utterances, more talk about the here and now.
Syntax/Morphology	Shorter, less complex utterances.
Phonology	Similar to peers.
Comprehension	Receptive vocabulary similar to peers. Auditory and reading comprehension problems.

Source: Based on Coster & Cicchetti (1993); Coster, Gersten, Beeghly, & Cicchetti (1989); Culp, Watkins, Lawrence, Letts, Kelly, & Rice (1991); Fox, Long, & Langlois (1988).

maturation. Physical abuse also may cause lasting physical or neurological damage. We do not know the long-term effects on the brain of lack of environmental stimulation.

Social-Environmental Factors.   Either or both parents may be neglectful or abusing, but it is the mother's or caregiver's everyday responsiveness to the child that has the most effect on language development. The quality of the child–mother attachment is a more significant factor in language development than is maltreatment and can moderate or exacerbate the effects of neglect or abuse (Gersten et al., 1986; Mosisset et al., 1990).

Several factors, including childhood loss of a parent, death of a previous child, pregnancy complications, birth complications, current marital or financial problems, substance abuse, maternal age, and/or illness, can disturb maternal attachment. In turn, mothers may adopt two general patterns of interaction (Crittenden, 1988). Most abusive mothers are *controlling,* imposing their will on the child. As controllers, they tend to ignore the child's initiations, thus decreasing the amount of verbal stimulation received by the child. *Neglecting* mothers, however, are unresponsive to their infant's behaviors because they have low expectations of deriving satisfaction from the infant. Either situation includes a lack of support for the development of meaningful communication skills and little active interaction, such as playing games, hugging, patting, or nuzzling, and little nurturing maternal speech toward the baby (Allen & Wasserman, 1985).

The result is insecure attachment on the part of the child (Browne & Sagi, 1988; Carlson, Cicchetti, Barnett, & Braunwald, 1989; Crittenden, 1988). The child may be apprehensive in the presence of the parent and may avoid interaction to lessen the chance of hostile responses. Early stimulus–response bonds—the infant's notion that her or his behavior results in an adult reinforcing response—may be nonexistent, further depressing the child's behavior. Obviously, this is not an ideal language learning environment.

Conclusion

Only now are we beginning to understand the effect of caregiver behavior on the infant. Although it seems intuitive that neglect and abuse would cause language and communication problems, especially in language use, the data are only correlational, not cause and effect.

Conclusion

At this point, most likely, you are in need of a one-sentence summary statement that once and for all distinguishes each language impairment from the others. Unfortunately, I do not have one forthcoming. Still, one needs to make some sense from the wealth of information presented. At the risk of generalizing too much, let's try. At the beginning of the chapter, I cited six abilities needed for typical language development. It might be helpful to consider these in conceptualizing the language impairments discussed (Table 2.14).

Perceptual difficulties are reported for some of the disorders mentioned, but not all. Nor are they similar in type and severity. For children with SLI, perceptual difficulties seem to be limited to rapid, sequenced auditory stimuli, but perceptual difficulties are the essence of LLD and ASD. Even here the difference seems to be one of perception and sensory integration in LLD and threshold levels in ASD.

Attentional difficulties also accompany several of the language impairments discussed. Again the variability is great. Children with ASD are either seemingly inattentive or fixated on one, often irrelevant aspect of a stimulus. In contrast, children with TBI experience attentional fluctuations and seem to attend for only brief periods.

Although all children with language impairment have difficulty using symbols, this difficulty varies. Children with MR and ASD have great difficulty with symbol referent relationships, while those who are neglected and abused have little difficulty with language form and content.

Language is rarely taught formally. Instead, children acquire language by hypothesizing the rules from the give-and-take of conversational speech. This can be a difficult task if the child is inattentive or has difficulty perceiving language, as are children with LLD, ASD, and TBI.

The requirement of having enough mental energy is a tricky one. We shall broaden the concept somewhat. Children with MR may lack the mental abilities for some tasks, while those with SLI and TBI may use vital mental energy on lower level tasks, leaving little for language analysis and

TABLE 2.14   Language learning requirements and the difficulties of children with language impairment*

	Language Impairment					
Requirements	**MR**	**LLD**	**SLI**	**ASD**	**TBI**	**Neglect/ Abuse**
Ability to perceive sequenced acoustic events of short duration		X	X	X	X	
Ability to attend actively, to be responsive, and to anticipate stimuli		X		X	X	
Ability to use symbols	X	X	X	X	X	X
Ability to invent syntax from the language in the environment	X	X	X	X		
Enough mental energy to do all the above simultaneously	X		X		X	X
Ability to interact and communicate with others				X		X

*Xs represent problem areas in language learning and use.

synthesis. The frequently reported depression of children with TBI and children who are neglected and abused also limits the cognitive energy available for language learning.

Finally, the ability to interact and communicate with others probably is affected in each of the disorders discussed. The difficulty is in determining whether an inability to interact and communicate reflects a cause of the impairment, a result, both, or just an accompanying feature. Among at least two groups of children—those with ASD and those who are neglected and abused—inability to interact seems directly related to the language impairment exhibited.

Each impairment presents a somewhat different image. In a clinical sense, however, the important features to which a SLP attends are the individual characteristics of each child, not the diagnostic category. Naming and describing a language impairment does not necessarily explain it nor determine clinical intervention.

Implications

Language impairments are not outgrown. Even with intervention, they are rarely "cured." Typically, language impairments change and become more subtle (Wallach & Liebergott, 1984). Children with preschool LI may continue to have trouble with linguistic and academic tasks. Reading performance may be affected (Hill & Haynes, 1992). As adults, children with LI may continue to do poorly in speech and language, although nonlinguistic skills seem unaffected (Felsenfeld, Broen, & McCue, 1992). With or without intervention, certain ramifications of having an LI affect academic performance and social acceptance.

Poor oral language usually results in poor reading and writing ability. It has been hypothesized that poor reading reflects the child's lack of language awareness skills, called *metalinguistic abilities* (Menyuk et al., 1991). For example, a child may be unaware of syllable or phonetic segmentation of words. This awareness is crucial for reading. Lack of these higher level language skills may explain the poor reading performance of children with SLI.

Within the classroom, children with LI form a separate subgroup that interacts increasingly less with their peers developing typically (Guralnick, 1990; Hadley & Rice, 1991). One's relative communication skills influence participation. Because children with LI are poor communicators overall (Fey, 1986), they are increasingly ignored. As a result, children with LI are more likely to be overidentified as having a socioemotional disorder (Redmond, 2002). Teachers rate children with LI significantly below their peers in impulse control, likability, and social behaviors such as helping others, offering comfort, and sharing (Fujiki, Brinton, Morgan, & Hart, 1999). Increasing reticence to talk leads to withdrawal, especially among prepubescent and adolescent boys (Fujiki, Brinton, Isaacson, & Summers, 2001).

In general, a child's popularity is associated with her or his conversational skills (Hazen & Black, 1989). Children with LI initiate little verbal interaction, are less responsive, use more short and nonverbal responses, and are less able to maintain a conversation (Rice, Snell, & Hadley, 1991). The result is fewer interactions with others (Hadley & Rice, 1991).

Children with LI often continue to have poor vocabularies and poor higher level semantic skills. These include difficulties with abstract meanings, figurative language, dual meanings, ambiguity, and humor (Donahue & Bryan, 1984; Kamhi, 1987; Nippold, 1985; Spector, 1990; Wiig & Semel, 1984).

Syntax and morphology are usually characterized by the continued use of less mature forms (Curtiss, Kutz, & Tallal, 1992; Leonard, 1987, 1988). Word formation processes, consisting of a free morpheme plus one or more bound morphemes, are less mature (Clahsen, 1989; Leonard, Sabbadini,

Leonard, & Volterra, 1987; Leonard, Sabbadini, Volterra, & Leonard, 1988; Rom & Leonard, 1990). Similarly, phonological patterns usually reflect those of younger children (Ingram, 1991; Shriberg et al., 1986).

Finally, language comprehension difficulties, especially at higher levels such as detection of ambiguity, may persist. These difficulties reflect the underlying language difficulties evidenced in expressive language (Skarakis-Doyle & Mullin, 1990).

SLPs are responsible for intervening to correct some language difficulties, to modify others, and to teach compensation skills for still others. In the chapters that follow, we explore a model that proposes to do this in the most natural way possible.

Communication Assessment

3

Assessment of Children with Language Impairment

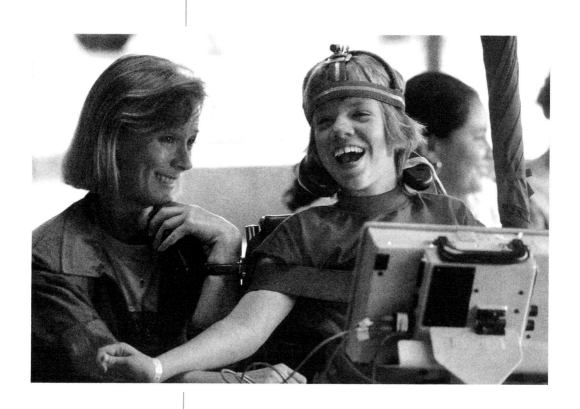

No clear line exists between assessment and intervention. Both are part of the intervention process, and portions of each are found in the other. Ideally, assessment and measurement are ongoing throughout intervention. No clinical goal should be determined or modified without first obtaining data on the communication performance of the affected child.

Adequate evaluation is one of the most difficult and demanding tasks faced by an SLP. The goal—much more complex than providing a score or a diagnostic label—is to describe the very complex language system of the child. Each child has a unique pattern of language rules and behaviors to be revealed and described.

The SLP should keep in mind the *why, what,* and *how* of assessment. Considering why the child is being assessed helps the SLP clarify the purpose. This clarity, in turn, enables the SLP to decide what specific behaviors to assess and the best evaluative methods to use. The reasons for assessment can be grouped as (a) identification of children with potential problems, (b) establishment of baseline functioning, and (c) measurement of change. Baseline functioning enables the SLP to determine the present level of performance, the extent of the language impairment, and the nature of the problem.

The data-gathering process is scientific in nature in that it must be unbiased and objective. This collection process should be precise and measurable, with very little intrusion by the SLP's conclusions. It is important, however, not to lose the child in the mass of data, and clinical intuition is an important factor in summarizing data and in determining which aspects of language to evaluate.

It is helpful to consider assessment procedures as existing along a continuum from formal, structured protocols to informal, less structured approaches. In general, the more structured the elicitation session, the less variety of structures and meanings expressed. Language elicited in more structured tasks is usually shorter and less complex, especially with younger children, than language sampled in less controlled situations (Fey, Leonard, & Wilcox, 1981).

Generally, the more specific the information desired, the more structured the approach. In this way, assessments can help the SLP sharpen and focus what was observed. Even formal tests or portions of tests can be used in an informal way as a probe of specific behavior. Naturally, normative data cannot be used when the test procedure is altered in any way.

In this chapter, we explore the differences between psychometric and descriptive assessment paradigms and describe a combined, or integrative, approach that attempts systematically to address the shortcomings of both approaches while describing the child's use of language in context. After discussing the integrated approach and applying it to more typical language impairment cases, we shall discuss the special assessment characteristics of early intervention and talk about some of the special needs of children with LI.

Psychometric versus Descriptive Procedures

The goals of communication assessment are to identify and describe each child's unique pattern of communication behaviors and, if that pattern signifies a language impairment, to recommend treatment, follow-up, or referral ("Preferred practice patterns," 1993). Through this process, the SLP determines (a) whether a problem exists, (b) the causal-related factors, and (c) the overall intervention plan.

There are two major philosophical approaches to this task. The *normalist* philosophy is based on a norm, or average performance level—usually a score—that society considers typical of normal functioning. In contrast, the *neutralist,* or *criterion-referenced,* approach compares the child's present performance to past performance and/or is descriptive in manner. The features of each are presented in Table 3.1.

The two approaches are really modes of interpreting measurable behavior and are not mutually exclusive (McCauley, 1996). For example, the results of testing can be reinterpreted to provide more descriptive information, including categories of behavior not included in the test and success with different formats (Olswang & Bain, 1996). Test items on which the child is unsuccessful can be probed to determine other methods that result in a correct response.

Tests are usually standardized and normed. **Standardized** means that there is a consistent manner in which test items are to be presented and child responses consequated. For example, the test manual may direct the SLP to give the following instructions:

I am going to read a sentence to you. When I'm finished, I want you to select the picture that best illustrates what I have said. Listen carefully, because I can only read each sentence once.

Most standardized tests are also **normed,** which means that the test has been given to a group of children that supposedly represent all children for whom the test was designed and scores determined for typical functioning. Ideally, the norming group has the same characteristics as the target population. In other words, gender, racial and ethnic, geographic, and socioeconomic differences present in the target population are also represented in the norming group in the same proportions. Even these constraints do not ensure that the test will be appropriate, especially with cultural- and linguistic-minority children. In addition, children with LI are rarely included in the norming group.

Traditional language assessment procedures heavily emphasize the use of standardized psychometric or norm-referenced tests. This situation is reflected in the fact that more than 100 norm-referenced language assessment tools are commercially available. Ideally, a standardized test has been given to a large number of children from various populations, has demonstrated reliability and validity, and has normative data that provide scale score, age equivalent, or numerical score comparisons.

Reliability is the repeatability of measurement. More precisely, reliability is the accuracy or precision with which a sample of language taken at one time represents performance of either a different but similar sample or the same sample at a different time. Factors that may affect reliability include individual change over time, sample differences, and the nature of the language sample in size or inclusiveness. Very limited samples of language usually result in unstable or undependable scores. Thus, the test must include enough language to be reliable yet not unwieldy. Add to these

TABLE 3.1 Comparison of norm-referencing and criterion-referencing

Norm-referencing	Criterion-referencing
Fundamental purpose is to rank individuals.	Fundamental purpose is to distinguish specific levels of performance.
Test planning addresses a broad content.	Test planning addresses a clearly specified domain.
Items are chosen to distinguish among individuals.	Items are chosen to cover content domain.
Performance can be summarized meaningfully using percentile or standard scores.	Performance can be summarized meaningfully using raw scores.

Source: McCauley, R. J. (1996). Familiar strangers: Criterion-referenced measures in communication disorders. *Language, Speech, and Hearing Services in Schools, 27,* 122–131. Reprinted with permission.

concerns the great difficulty reported in obtaining reliable performance from children, especially toddlers (Rescorla, 1991), and the chance of producing a reliable measure decreases.

Test makers and users are concerned with both internal consistency and various measures of reliability. **Internal consistency** is the degree of relationship among items and the overall test. If a test has high internal consistency, children who score well overall should tend to get the same items correct, whereas those who score low should tend to perform similarly among themselves.

Measures of reliability include *test-retest reliability, alternate form reliability,* and *split-half reliability.* In test-retest reliability, the child is administered the same test with a time interval between each administration. With alternate forms, the child is administered equivalent or parallel forms of a measure. Finally, a test may be divided into equivalent halves. In each case, the two test scores are compared and the consistency of scores measured. This value is expressed as a reliability or correlational coefficient or as a standard error of measure. The closer the reliability coefficient to a value of 1 and the lower the standard error or standard deviation of the error scores, the more reliable is the measure. In other words, a reliability coefficient of .84 indicates greater reliability than one of .62.

In addition, the SLP is concerned with the probability of two judges scoring the same behavior in the same manner. This value is called **interjudge reliability.** As a group, scoring procedures that use a definite criterion for correct-incorrect determination, such as accepting only specific responses as correct, are more reliable than those that use scaled scoring, such as grading responses by their degree of correctness. The latter can have increased reliability if each score has definite criteria or if the tester has received specific training.

Validity is the effectiveness of a test in representing, describing, or predicting an attribute of interest to the tester. In short, it is a measure of the test's ability to assess what it purports to assess. The tester is interested in measuring all of the attribute being tested but nothing other than that attribute. For example, some tests of receptive language abilities require the child to respond verbally. Clearly, this requirement goes beyond the stated domain of the attribute being tested.

Professionals should be cautious when choosing tests. Few language screening tests, for example, meet criteria for validity or provide information to enable SLPs to determine validity (Sturner, Layton, Evans, Heller, Funk, & Machon, 1994).

To test an abstract concept such as intelligence, test designers must select concrete tasks (Kamhi, 1993). These tasks, in turn, often become the defining features of the abstract entity supposedly measured. For example, intelligence becomes the sum of the test tasks.

Tests are not presentations of the overall attribute or behavior, but are merely samples. From the samples, testers make inferences about the overall attribute or behavior. If the samples are not valid measures, the inferences will be incorrect. Validity is not self-evident and must be proven. Three types of evidence are criterion validity, content validity, and construct validity.

Criterion validity is the effectiveness or accuracy with which a measure predicts success. This usually is calculated as the degree to which a measure correlates with some other suitable measures of success assumed to be valid.

Content validity is the faithfulness with which the sample or measure represents some attribute or behavior. In other words, the sum of the tasks involved should define or constitute the attribute or behavior being measured. Measures should reflect the professional literature, research, and expert opinion on the constitution of the attribute or behavior tested.

Finally, **construct validity** is the accuracy with which or the extent to which a measure describes or measures some trait or construct. Professionals are interested in the accuracy and significance of results and in how precisely the measure notes individual or group differences. Construct validity usually is determined by comparing the measure with other acceptable measures assumed to be valid. One study found that one-third of the kindergartners who failed one of two language screening tests passed the other, possibly indicating that the tests assessed different aspects of language (Summers, Larson, Miguel, & Terrell, 1996).

Tests, or measures, help the SLP determine how the child's performance, in the form of a score, compares with that of children who supposedly possess the same characteristics (McCauley & Swisher, 1984a, 1984b). Most frequently, tests are used to determine average and less-than-average performance for decisions about the need for intervention services (Lund & Duchan, 1993).

Unfortunately, many traditional assessment procedures do not reflect current definitions of the nature of language (Ray, 1989). Although normative tests may be good for measuring isolated skills, they provide very little information on overall language use.

More descriptive approaches, such as language sampling, highlight the individualistic nature of the child's communicative functioning noted in language development studies. In contrast, psychometric normative testing imposes group criteria on an individual, thereby obviating an assessment of the individual. Each method of assessment has its strengths and weaknesses, as well as possible applications within the clinical setting. These are described in the following sections.

Psychometric Assessment Protocols

Ideally, a test elicits a standard and representative sample of a behavior. A test is normed by using specified explicit procedures and administering the test to a sample from a specific population. As such, normed tests enable the SLP to compare individual performance with that of a larger population. In general, norm-referenced assessment tools have the advantages of objectivity, replicability, and elimination of unwanted or uncontrolled variation. Tests help focus and sharpen observational skills and are particularly helpful when deciding whether a problem exists (Longhurst, 1984).

Although normed tests are potentially valid, reliable, and precise in measurement, it is difficult to find a language test that is acceptable in all three areas. In addition, normed tests do not easily accommodate cultural and individual variation, nor do they begin to provide a true picture of the richness and complexity of the child's communication behavior. In other words, "at their best…tests provide an unclear picture of communication performance" (L. Miller, 1993, p. 13).

Tests are less complex than the language being assessed (Ray, 1989). Language is multidimensional and its use individualistic, making it difficult to measure (Damico, 1988). Most SLPs are either neutral or negative toward existing language tests. School-based SLPs are more negative. The main concerns seem to be the length of time needed for administration and interpretation and the inadequacy of most tests for use with multicultural populations (Huang, Hopkins, & Nippold, 1997).

Test Differences

Language assessment instruments differ widely even when purported to measure the same entity. Even tests that seem to be significantly correlated, suggesting an interrelationship of criterion validity, may seem less so when subtests or various portions of tests are compared. Nor does positive correlation mean that tests are acceptable substitutions for each other. (Friend & Channell, 1987). In addition, tests can differ in their levels of difficulty (Lieberman, Heffron, West, Hutchinson, &

Swem, 1987). Task variability is also a big factor and can affect test results, yielding different results for the same child (Fagundes, Haynes, Haak, & Moran, 1998).

All tests are not created equal and should be researched carefully by SLPs before being used. In the following section we explore some of these differences, specifically test content, and some of the common misuses of tests. Finally, the variables that should be considered in test selection are discussed.

Content

The major criticism of existing instruments is the inadequacy of the content covered in both breadth and depth. The degree of inequity varies with age of the child. In general, there are very few standardized measures for toddlers and adolescents and an abundance of measures for preschoolers and early-school-age children.

Two issues relative to content validity—relevance and coverage—must be addressed in test construction. Content relevance is the precision with which a certain aspect of language is delineated or defined. This is necessary to determine the dimensions of that aspect and its members. For example, tests of syntax may be organized on the basis of transformational grammar, R. Brown's (1973) fourteen morphemes, semantic-syntactic categories, or on no recognizable rationale. Without a framework, content items may be selected arbitrarily.

The issue of content relevance is made more complicated by our lack of an agreed definition of language (Lahey, 1990). In addition, the child's knowledge of language, called *competence,* is measurable only as behavior or *performance,* which are affected by contextual variables, such as speed and complexity. Thus, poor performance may indicate an underlying deficit, a difficulty accessing the underlying system, or a problem with the testing content.

Content coverage is the representativeness with which an aspect of language is sampled. Theoretically, coverage of language features should reflect general use. Some features may be more significant than others, although this fact can be verified only through statistical analysis. Otherwise, subtle language impairments may go undetected. A single test's rather limited sample of a child's skills is an inadequate base on which to build a sound remedial program (Lieberman & Michael, 1986).

The psychometric testing model produces data on minimal portions of behavior, thus reducing language to simple, often irrelevant dimensions that may not reflect the qualities of that language overall (Kamhi, 1993). By fragmenting language into observable and measurable features, tests may highlight skills only tangentially related to language ability. Tests tend to emphasize structural components of language because they are easy to observe. Although structured testing may reveal the child's ability to use language in one context, it reveals very little about the child's language as it is needed and used in everyday communication.

In addition, language use in isolation may bear little resemblance to language use in context (Newman, Lovett, & Dennis, 1986). For example, the child may use interrogatives throughout the day to obtain information, desired objects, and needed assistance but may be unable to form interrogatives in isolation when given a group of words to include. In addition, the process of the test situation may be so foreign to the child or the child's everyday communication environment that it influences the language the child produces. Performance may be affected also by factors as diverse as the child's state of health on the day the test is administered, attention level and comprehension of the instructions, and perception of the test administrator.

In short, norm-referenced approaches offer "canned" assessment with little consideration for the individual needs of the child with whom they are used. The tendency is for assessment procedures to take priority over the child, with test selection often based on commercial availability or clinical popularity (Duchan, 1982a; Kamhi, 1984). Tests are *a priori* and product oriented, offering little information on the appropriateness of the features being tested. The test results, in turn, offer little assistance in identifying individual problems and in planning intervention.

Misuse of Normative Testing

Norm-referenced tests should be used with caution. The best advice is to be an "informed clinician" and a wise consumer. SLPs should be mindful of the frequent misuse of these instruments (Lieberman & Michael, 1986; Stephens & Montgomery, 1985), among them (a) misuse of scores as a summary of a child's performance, (b) use of inappropriate norms, (c) inappropriate assumptions based on test results, (d) use of specific test items to plan intervention goals, and (e) use of tests to assess therapy progress.

Misuse of Scores

When does difference become disorder? We should remind ourselves that the 1 percent of the population who are blood type B-negative is not considered deviant, just different (L. Miller, 1993).

The most frequently used score on standardized measures is the mean, or average, score. Test makers assume that the average score for a sample population is the "normal" score for the larger population. Test scores that are extreme or that represent the performance of children whose ages are at the extremes for the norming population should not be considered as reliable as more central measures.

It is important to recall that a wide scoring area about the mean, called standard deviation, also is considered to fall within the normal range. When plotted, the total number of individuals receiving each score will form the familiar *bell-shaped curve,* represented in Figure 3.1. Approximately two-thirds of the population will score within 1 standard deviation on either side of the mean score. The

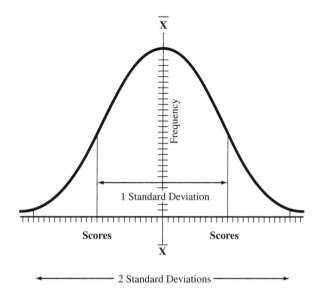

FIGURE 3.1   Parameters of the normal distribution.

SLP must decide where "non-normal" occurs. If she uses only 1 standard deviation for separating normal from non-normal, she will find that nearly one-third of the population, approximately 16 percent above and 16 percent below, fails to fall within this range. Two standard deviations is a better index of deviancy, leaving approximately 3 percent of the population above and 3 percent below those within the normal range. A second index is the 10th percentile, the lowest 10 percent of the norming sample. Children who score at or below the 10th percentile are often considered to be other-than-normal.

Scores at either end of the distribution represent a quantitative difference that can be called *disordered, exceptional, deviant,* or *impaired.* Obviously, our boundary of 2 standard deviations is relative. The SLP must decide when the difference is so great as to impair the individual.

The use of scores imposes some constraints that many professionals overlook. First, numbers establish equalities and inequalities. For example, 2 is twice 1 and half of 4. It would seem, therefore, that a child with a score of 4 correct has twice the skill of one with a score of 2, but this is a measure of the number of responses, not quality.

Second, all test items are assumed to be equal because each has the same weight (L. Miller, 1993). If there is one item each for the verb *to be* and past-tense *-ed,* they each receive the same score even though they are not of equal importance developmentally.

Beyond concerns about numerical equalities-inequalities, the SLP must consider the standards for comparison of children, such as chronological, mental, or language age. In addition, the exact relationship of cognition and language is unclear.

Age-equivalent scores—the average or projected age of children getting a certain number of items correct—seem to be even less reliable than are other indices, such as standard scores and percentile ranks, and less sensitive to individual differences (Lahey, 1990). Of course, all of these values are only as representative as the norming population. Often, specific age-equivalent scores are determined by test makers through interpolation from the scores achieved by children at various other ages.

These scores imply some standard of performance when in fact there is none, except the numerical score. Such scores are of little value in determining those who are language impaired. Often, differences of six months to two years between the age of the child and the age-equivalent score are used as evidence of an impairment. This issue is complicated for children whose mental age is below their chronological. It hardly seems fair to compare a 6-year-old child with mental retardation to a 6-year-old who is developing normally.

The use of age-equivalent scores also can lead to erroneous assumptions about children's behavior. The equality of scores does not translate to an equality of behavior and offers an inadequate description of that individualistic behavior. A child who achieves the same score as a younger child may not make the same kinds of errors (Lawrence, 1992). Two children with the same scores could have answered very different items correctly. In addition, all items are not of equal value even though the scores imply equality. Age-equivalent scores, if used, should be used with caution in a report and should be accompanied by some explanation of their value (Salvia & Ysseldyke, 1988).

Speech-language pathologists habitually should check the **standard error of measure (SEm)** for information about the confidence of test scores (J. Brown, 1989). Because tests are less than perfectly reliable, a certain amount of error is reflected in each score. The larger the SEm, the less confidence one can have in the test's results.

The SEm can be added to and subtracted from a test score to establish a band of confidence. For example, assume that a child received a score of 75 on two different tests with confidence intervals

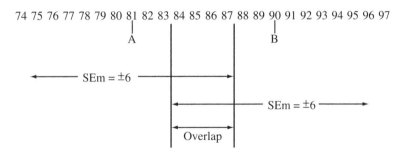

FIGURE 3.2   A comparison of scores using standard error of measure.

of 2 and 6, respectively. On the first test, the child's error-free, or true, score is most probably 73–77; on the second, it is 69–81. The SLP can have more confidence that the score of 75 on the first test is closer to the child's actual performance.

Larger SEm values also may mean that scores that seem very different actually overlap, as shown in Figure 3.2. Child A received a score of 81, and Child B received a score of 90. An SEm of 6 applied to each score results in an overlap. Therefore, the children's actual abilities may be much more similar than the test results indicate.

The SLP should check the test manual to obtain the SEm. Because this information is not always available, the SLP may wish to determine this value from Table 3.2 (J. Brown, 1989). The entering values of standard deviation and reliability coefficient usually are provided in the test manual.

Quantification of behaviors is not inherently bad. Measurement should be meaningful and functional and should reflect accurately the entity being evaluated (Kamhi, 1993). It is important that test designers define the entities being tested and provide a rationale in the test manual for the tasks selected.

SLPs should read, understand, and evaluate the manual accompanying the test and be knowledgeable about test construction and administration (Stephens & Montgomery, 1985). The literature about a certain test should be studied thoroughly before the test is used.

Inappropriate Norms

Often, the norming sample does not represent the population with which the SLP is using the assessment procedure (Lahey, 1990). In this situation, the norms are inappropriate and should not be used. This situation occurs most frequently with minority or rural children or with children from lower socioeconomic groups. In these cases, local norms should be prepared by following the norming procedure described in the test manual. Some tests, such as the Test of Language Development-Intermediate (TOLD-I) and the CELF, explain this process in detail.

Because test results are used to identify children appropriate for the norming group for subsequent renorming of that test, an interesting phenomenon can occur: Some low functioning but normally developing children will be identified as being language impaired (McFadden, 1996). In addition, because children with LI are routinely excluded from the norming group, this sample is truncated at the lower scoring end. As a result, the entire distribution (Figure 3.1) is shifted upward, leaving some of the nonimpaired children scoring below 2 standard deviations. Over time, there is a

TABLE 3.2   **Table of standard error of measure reliability and standard deviation values to estimate the standard error of measure (SEm)**

Standard Deviation	Reliability Coefficient								
	.95	.90	.85	.80	.75	.70	.65	.60	.55
30	6.7	9.5	11.6	13.4	15.0	16.4	17.7	19.0	20.1
28	6.3	8.9	10.8	12.5	14.0	15.3	16.6	17.7	18.8
26	5.8	8.2	10.1	11.6	13.0	14.2	15.4	16.4	17.4
24	5.4	7.6	9.3	10.7	12.0	13.1	14.2	15.2	16.1
22	4.9	7.0	8.5	9.8	11.0	12.0	13.0	13.9	14.8
20	4.5	6.3	7.7	8.9	10.0	11.0	11.8	12.7	13.4
18	4.0	5.7	7.0	8.0	9.0	9.9	10.6	11.4	12.1
16	3.6	5.1	6.2	7.2	8.0	8.8	9.5	10.1	10.7
14	3.1	4.4	5.4	6.3	7.0	7.7	8.3	8.9	9.4
12	2.7	3.8	4.6	5.4	6.0	6.6	7.1	7.6	8.0
10	2.2	3.2	3.9	4.5	5.0	5.5	5.9	6.3	6.7
8	1.8	2.5	3.1	3.6	4.0	4.4	4.7	5.1	5.4
6	1.3	1.9	2.3	2.7	3.0	3.3	3.6	3.8	4.0
4	.9	1.3	1.5	1.8	2.0	2.2	2.4	2.5	2.7
2	.4	.6	.8	.9	1.0	1.1	1.2	1.3	1.3

Note: This table of standard error of measurement is based on the formula SEm = $SD\sqrt{1 - r_{11}}$ where *SD* is the standard deviation of the test scores and r_{11} is the reliability coefficient for internal consistency of the test scores.

Source: Brown, J. (1989). The truth about scores children achieve on tests. *Language, Speech, and Hearing Services in Schools, 20,* 366–371. Reprinted with permission.

gradual increase in the language-impaired population. This problem arises, in part, because of our inaccurate criteria of what constitutes a language impairment.

Finally, we cannot assume that norms are stable. They change over time. In addition, changes in the format of the test, such as offering it on computer, also change the norms. Separate norms are needed when a test is offered in a computerized format (Wiig, Jones, & Wiig, 1996).

Incorrect Assumptions

Test scores may represent only scores and not actual differences in linguistic ability. Therefore, the SLP must analyze each child's performance on either different aspects or subtests in order to obtain descriptive information. Subtest scores should be interpreted independently from each other so as not to influence their interpretation.

The SLP also should be cautious in extrapolating global language development from scores on language tests, especially those that sample only one or two aspects of language. The Peabody Picture Vocabulary Test (PPVT) is an excellent receptive vocabulary test, but it does not address other aspects of language or indicate overall language use.

Identifying Intervention Goals

A thorough description of the child's behavior is needed before the SLP can identify areas needing intervention. Individual test items or subtests do not provide an adequate sample of that behavior. Because test items represent only a small portion of language, they do not provide enough information on which to base therapy goals. At the very least, more than one psychometric assessment procedure should be used because of the variability of some children across tests (Stephens & Montgomery, 1985). The more test scores available, the more reliable the assessment. Only through the use of a number of assessment protocols can the SLP hope to determine intervention objectives (Lahey, 1990). Psychometric tests are only a portion of the assessment process.

Measuring Therapy Progress

The continued use of a norm-referenced test to assess therapy progress may result in the child's learning the test, thus producing artificially high results. However, widely spaced testing or the use of different forms of the same test or of different but highly correlated tests can demonstrate changes in behavior over time (McCauley & Swisher, 1984b). Criterion-referenced tests are more appropriate for measuring individual progress.

Age-equivalent scores should not be used to measure change, however, because the scale units for items are not real values (Lawrence, 1992). All items are not equal. A child whose score has changed little may have made more progress than another child whose score has changed more.

Variables in Test Selection

The SLP should be a wise consumer of assessment materials and should base test selection on several factors. Of particular interest are test reliability and validity, discussed previously. Even language tests that meet very stringent psychometric or measurement criteria may not correlate highly or be very precise discriminators of impaired and nonimpaired language (Plante & Vance, 1994).

Other considerations in test selection include appropriateness of the test for a particular child, the manner of presentation and comprehensiveness, and the type and sensitivity of the test results. A test should be appropriate to the child's age or functioning level. In addition, the norming population should be sufficiently large and varied to include representatives of the child's racioethnic and socioeconomic background. If the child is from an identifiable minority, the SLP should check to see whether the norming information gives data by such groups.

Appropriateness may relate also to manner of presentation. The manner of presentation may reflect the overall theoretical basis of the test. A sentence imitation test, for example, relies on auditory processing of verbal stimuli, rather than on picture cues. Other practical issues related to presentation include the number of items and the content coverage discussed previously. Some children perform better under certain conditions than under others. For example, children with LLD can perform better if visual input accompanies the verbal.

Some tests offer a computerized version for children with motoric problems or those who may perform better on this format. Results of computerized test formats seem to be equivalent to those from the standard form of administration (Haaf, Duncan, Skarakis-Doyle, Carew, & Kapitan, 1999).

Too few or poorly discriminatory items can lead to less sensitive scoring, in which one question can change the child's performance score several percentage points. The type of result, whether percentage, percentile, or age equivalent, is also a practical consideration in test selection. Depending on the test, the interpretive value of such scores may be very limited.

When given a choice of different tests, SLPs display a remarkable similarity in the relative importance they attach to different measures (Records & Tomblin, 1994). Receptive measures, such as the Test of Auditory Comprehension of Language (TACL) and the PPVT are relied on heavily. Sentence imitation and grammatical closure tasks also are preferred. Familiarity with the test procedure, overall opinion of the measure, and clinical experience are all factors in test or task selection and in the relative importance attached to data obtained from different measures.

Summary

Perceptive professionals decry overdependence on and poor interpretation of the results of testing. Although standardized tests, especially those in language, frequently have been maligned (McCauley & Swisher, 1984a, 1984b), SLPs often are required to incorporate the results of these procedures into their overall assessments. It is important for SLPs to recognize that tests are informative, but not the be-all and end-all of evaluation. Awareness of a test's shortcomings can greatly aid the interpretation of a child's performance (Stephens & Montgomery, 1985).

The issue of testing is central to the purpose of assessment. Data gathered in an assessment should be relevant to the initial clinical complaint, to the determination that a problem exists, to individual differences and individual processing, to the nature of the problem, to prognosis, to intervention implications, and to accountability (Muma, 1986). Otherwise, it is just a *numbers game.* Although norm-referenced tests seem appropriate for determining if a language impairment exists, they are inconsistent in determining the specific area(s) of deficit (Merrell & Plante, 1997).

Descriptive Approaches

The descriptive approach, usually based on observation and a conversational sample of the child's language, is a widely taught method of defining children's communicative abilities. Unfortunately, because of time constraints, the method is not widely used, although it continues to gain favor. Descriptive approaches have the potential of allowing SLPs to regard the language process while maintaining contextual integrity and individual differences (Muma, 1986).

Spontaneous sampling alone is best used as an indicator of the child's overall language functioning, rather than as a device for noting specific language problems. More specific data can be obtained by probing the child's conversational behavior. In general, data from a language sample correlate significantly with results from elicited imitation and sentence completion tasks, although the syntactic structural patterns vary widely (Fujiki & Willbrand, 1982).

The advantages of the descriptive approach are that the SLP can apply his or her own theoretical model to the assessment process and can probe and assess areas that seem most handicapping to the child. For example, the SLP who follows a sociolinguistic model of language is free to explore the pragmatic and conversational aspects of the child's language. Thus, the clinical process can remain flexible and attuned to the client's needs (Kamhi, 1984). To do this, the SLP must understand the complex interaction of constitutional—biological, cognitive, psychological, and social—and environmental forces.

The continuous speech sample has several advantages over more formal structured-response testing, which reveals little about the use, content, and form of the child's language as needed and used in daily living. For example, single-word responses on a test may not be as adequate a database for analysis as a longer conversational response might be. Some language features are more sensitive to the linguistic and extralinguistic factors of continuous speech (McLeod, Hand, Rosenthal, & Hayes, 1994). Processes that affect individual sounds are less affected by the collection method.

The disadvantages of the descriptive approach are (a) the level of language expertise needed by the SLP in order to elicit and analyze the child's language, (b) the length of time needed to collect and analyze the child's language, and (c) the reliability and validity of the sample (Kelly & Rice, 1986). Although a number of descriptive protocols exist, the SLP may not feel sufficiently well versed in all aspects of language to choose those appropriate for each child. For many theoreticians, the communicative value of each language event lies in the pragmatic functions of each utterance. Yet, SLPs may not be comfortable with the pragmatic aspects of language. In addition, a large caseload may preclude the use of lengthy descriptive procedures. Finally, as in psychometric testing, the SLP may not elicit a valid sample of the child's usual language usage.

Reliability and Validity

Language samples are more susceptible than standardized measures to SLP bias, especially when used to assess intervention effectiveness (Nye et al., 1987). The SLP must attempt to analyze the language sample in the most objective manner possible. Descriptions of the actual behaviors observed are generally more reliable than subjective judgments of the causes or reasons for these behaviors. One way to increase reliability is to separate the actual events from inferences based on these events and to base decisions on the data from these events.

Reliability across observations can be increased by taking the following three precautions:

   1. *Define the behaviors to be observed as explicitly as possible and train observers to ensure good inter- and intraobserver reliability.* The selection of behavior categories to be observed will affect the validity of the observation. For example, it may be easier and more accurate to identify certain gestures than to record verbal intentions. Accuracy can be controlled by making comparisons between the ratings of two observers. This type of analysis helps sharpen definitions and to highlight possible areas of confusion.

   2. *Make judgments on only one type of behavior at a time.* This procedure may require the use of videotaping so that a language sample can be replayed often for additional judgments on other behaviors.

   3. *Do not make summation judgments while observing "on-line."* It is too easy for preconceived notions of the child to influence our interpretation. Judgments about overall behavior are best made after assessing the accumulated data. There is danger in attempting to fit the child into one of the language impairment categories mentioned in Chapter 2.

Some threats to validity are found within the sample itself. For example, preschool children vary in their attentiveness and disposition to talk moment by moment (Shriberg & Kwiatkowski, 1985). Given this condition, the possible threats to validity in a speech sample, even with older children, are *productivity,* or the amount produced; *intelligibility,* or the amount understood by the listener; *representativeness,* or the typicality of the sample; and *reactivity,* or the response of the child to differing stimuli (Shriberg & Kwiatkowski, 1985).

Productivity
The uncommunicative child or the child who produces only a few utterances will not give the SLP a productive sample from which to work even though such a sample may reflect accurately the

child's typical output. The child may have little language with which to talk. The key to greater production is for the SLP to plan a variety of elicitation tasks that serve the purpose of gathering the sample (Wren, 1985).

Intelligibility

Intelligibility is the amount of agreement between what the child intended to say and what the SLP interpreted from the sample. If much of the sample is unintelligible, few utterances will be suitable for analysis. In general, intelligibility can be increased with increased SLP control over the content of the child's utterances. In short, the SLP who knows the topic can determine more easily what the child said.

Representativeness

A sample may not represent the child's typical behavior. Language samples often are collected in an atypical context, for example, a clinical room with an unfamiliar SLP as the conversational partner. Much of the sample may be atypical when removed from the child's typical conversational context (Roth & Spekman, 1984b). Three issues are relative to the representativeness of the conversational sample: *spontaneity, variability of context,* and *stability of the structure/function sampled* (Muma, 1983).

Spontaneity is increased if the child is allowed to establish the topic and/or the activity. Interesting and varied stimulus materials can provide an excellent basis for spontaneous conversation and can elicit a variety of forms and functions.

Variability of the context and stimulus items will elicit a greater variety of child behaviors theoretically more representative of the child's everyday behavior. Data should be collected in a variety of settings, with a variety of partners, and on a variety of child-based conversational topics to ensure versatility. Because quantity and complexity vary with the task, no single task is likely to yield a representative sample of the child's language (Wren, 1985).

Unrepresentative samples may reflect other-than-normal usage by the child. In this situation, the structures or functions sampled may vary widely from one situation to another. Everyday situations are most likely to elicit typical use and thus provide some stability across situations.

Some discussion has concerned whether SLPs should try to elicit typical or maximum production from the child. This debate is fueled by the often-reported gaps between what children with LI are capable of doing with their language and what they typically do. The SLP must decide on the appropriate task to use. For example, storytelling tasks yield longer utterances, while picture interpretation tasks elicit greater language quantity.

Reactivity

The child's reaction to the techniques and the materials also will affect the overall validity of the sample produced. Sampling conditions and the nature of the content or stimuli available can greatly affect the sample. A directed condition, such as one in which the SLP uses a questioning technique, allows the examiner more control over the content being discussed and may, in turn, increase intelligibility. Unfortunately, this improved intelligibility may sacrifice productivity and representativeness. In general, too much control restricts the child's output. For example, sentence-building tasks in which the child is asked to "Make a sentence with the word *X*" elicit the least typical language and very short sentences (Wren, 1985).

Words or structures divorced from dialogue, as in the previous example, require high-level metalinguistic skills and thus are difficult for the child with LI. Other tasks, such as sentence repetition, sentence completion, and judgment of grammaticality, are unreliable and should not be used without a spontaneous conversational sample (Fujiki & Willbrand, 1982). Yet, even though the more open-ended conversation may be more representative, it is usually less intelligible and may be difficult for some children with LI. For example, children with LLD exhibit difficulty with conversations as with other assessment protocols (Donahue, 1984; Roth, 1986; Spekman, 1981).

Similarly, specific stimulus items may increase intelligibility by controlling the topics discussed. In addition, the use of these items may enable the SLP to repeat stimulus conditions in subsequent evaluations. Again, increased intelligibility may result in decreased productivity of a variety of forms and functions and limited content. Further, the child may develop or already have a stereotypic pattern of responding to the item. For example, a doll may elicit a "baby talk" style.

The items chosen and the directions given also may affect the validity of the sample. For example, pictures can be used to elicit language, but the instructions given to the child often affect the quantity of language produced. The typical directive "Tell me about this picture" elicits less language than a more directive style (Wren, 1985), such as the following:

I'd like you to make up a story from this picture. I want you to tell me a whole story that has a beginning and an end. Start with "Once upon a time" and tell me the whole story.

The best advice for any SLP is to remain flexible in order to shift between different contexts and different content and to elicit the kinds of language behavior desired. The SLP should have a variety of stimulus materials and be skillful in discussing a range of topics potentially interesting to the child (Shriberg & Kwiatkowski, 1985).

Summary

Descriptive approaches are not without problems. Although they are potentially more representative of the child's everyday performance than formal testing, this potential is not guaranteed. In addition, descriptive approaches require that the SLP have considerable knowledge of language and of the variables that affect children's language performance. Skillful manipulation of these variables by the SLP can enhance the potential intervention value of descriptive methods.

An Integrated Functional Assessment Strategy

Speech-language professionals usually suggest a combined assessment approach (Kelly & Rice, 1986; Klein, 1984; McCauley & Swisher, 1984b). The purpose of the assessment should influence its design. Almost universally, SLPs would agree that no single measure or session is adequate (Emerick & Haynes, 1986). This allows for multiple assessment of language features and behaviors in a variety of relevant contexts.

The SLP must consider the following seven variables in designing and implementing the assessment process (Kelly & Rice, 1986):

1. Child's chronological and functional age
2. State of child's sensory system (vision, hearing, etc.)

3. Caregiver concerns
4. Status of child's psychological functioning
5. Child's interests and materials available
6. Child's activity level
7. Child's attention span

Judicious manipulation of these variables facilitates elicitation of a representative sample. In general, alternation of structured and less structured tasks keeps the child's attention by providing variety. The SLP readily adapts the methods to the child and is mindful that the child will respond differently to different adults.

A combined or integrated assessment approach provides the most thorough evaluation and includes a questionnaire and/or caregiver interview, an environmental observation, an SLP-directed formal psychometric assessment, and a child-directed informal assessment consisting of a conversational sample from the child. The actual components will differ with each child. Each component is discussed in the remainder of this chapter.

At each diagnostic step, objectives should be derived from the information collected to this point. Thus, each step becomes more focused, and the possible language problems are highlighted. Figure 3.3 presents a possible stage process of collecting data. At each stage, the process becomes more focused. The following discussion deals with a number of assessment steps, both formal and informal, that are aspects of an overall integrated functional model.

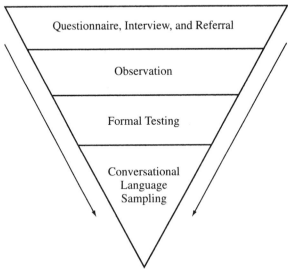

At each stage, data suggest a further delineation of
the possible language impairment. In the next stage,
the possible impairment can be more sharply defined.

FIGURE 3.3   A model of the assessment process.

Questionnaire, Interview, and Referral

Caregivers—parents, teachers, and others—are central to a functional assessment and intervention process (Kelly & Rice, 1986). Teachers can be a valuable referral source and should be encouraged to be alert for children with potential language problems. Initial caregiver involvement helps build rapport, increases the validity of the assessment results, and introduces the caregivers to the intervention process.

A caregiver interview or questionnaire can be a valuable source of initial information on client functioning and on the perceived problem from the caregiver's perspective. Caregiver expectations for the child also provide an indication of the caregiver's willingness and perceived need to work with the child. Caregivers should be encouraged to ask questions.

With very young children, caregivers can be a source of information for difficult-to-test behaviors. For example, vocabulary checklists completed by parents correlate well with other measures of vocabulary (Bates, Bretherton, & Snyder, 1988; Beeghly, Jernberg, & Burrows, 1989; Dale, 1991; Dale, Bates, Reznick, & Morisset, 1989). In fact, parental reports on the size of their 2-year-olds' vocabulary correlated well with the results of language screening tests (Klee, Carson, Gavin, Hall, Kent, & Reece, 1998). In other areas of oral language, such as intelligibility, parents are less accurate (Kwiatkowski & Shriberg, 1992).

It is best to ask questions of caregivers in a straightforward manner, with no hesitation that might signal embarrassment or discomfort. The SLP avoids tag questions (e.g., "You don't..., do you?") that seek agreement, rather than confirmation or information. Responses are treated matter-of-factly with little comment that might discourage the caregiver from talking. The SLP will be interested in the child's prenatal, perinatal, and postnatal medical history, family medical and educational history, the child's educational and social history, and descriptions of the child's behavior. A list of possible language questions is presented in Table 3.3.

Caregiver responses are analyzed and hypotheses are formed before deciding on the strategy for the remainder of the assessment. Potential language problems are researched thoroughly.

Observation

For the most natural interaction, the SLP will want to observe caregiver(s) and peer(s) with the child as conversational partners in such everyday settings as the home and the classroom. In the classroom, the SLP might observe the child participating in a number of activities. This situation is not always possible. Time may not permit observation alone. In this case, the SLP may wish to observe closely while collecting a language sample and may form tentative hypotheses for later confirmation from the analyzed sample.

If observation occurs in a more clinical setting, appropriate toys and both structured and nonstructured activities are provided for the child and conversational partner. Caregivers are encouraged to use familiar objects and the child's favorite toys or objects from home or the classroom. Ideally, the SLP would observe the child's behavior with various communication partners.

The SLP instructs caregivers to interact as typically as possible with the child. It is essential that caregivers not quiz or direct the child to perform during the observation. Optimum performance is attained if the SLP unobtrusively remains in the room or leaves and observes from outside via observation windows or video monitors.

TABLE 3.3   Interview or questionnaire format

Questions relative to language uses:

How does the child let you know items desired? What does the child request most frequently?
   What does the child do when requesting that you do something?
   When wanting you to pay attention?
   When wanting something?
   When wanting to direct your attention?
Does the child ask for information?
How does the child express emotion or tell about feelings?
   What emotions does the child express?
Does the child make noises when playing alone? Does the child engage in monologues while playing?
   Does the child prefer to play alone or with others?
Does the child describe things in the environment? How?
Does the child discuss events in the past, future, or outside of the immediate context?

Questions relative to conversational skill:

When does the child communicate best?
How does the child respond when you say something? How does the child respond to others? Does the
   child interact more readily with certain people and in certain situations, and if so, with whom and when?
With whom and when does the child communicate most frequently?
Does the child initiate conversations or activities with you and with others? What is the child's most fre-
   quent topic?
Does the child join in when others initiate conversations or activities?
Does the child get your attention before saying something to you?
   How does the child do this? Does the child maintain eye contact while talking to you?
Does the child take turns when talking? Does the child interrupt? Are there long gaps between your utter-
   ances and the child's responses? Will the child take a turn without being instructed to do so or without
   being asked a question?
When the child speaks to you, is there an expectation of a response? What does the child do if you do not
   respond?
When the child responds to you, does the response usually match or is it relevant to what you said?
How does the child ask for clarification? How frequently does this occur?
If you ask the child for more information or for clarification, what happens? Does the child demonstrate
   frustration when not understood?
When the child asks for or tells you something, is there usually enough information for you to understand?
When the child tells you more complex information or relates an event or a story, is it organized enough for
   you to follow the train of thought?
Does the child have different ways of talking to different people, such as adults and small children? Does
   the child phrase things in different ways with different listeners? Is the child more polite in some situa-
   tions?
Does the child seem confused at times? What does the child do if confused?

Questions relative to form and content:

Is the child able to understand simple directions?
Does the child know the names of common events, objects, and people in the environment? What types of
   information does the child provide about these (actions, objects, people, descriptions, locations, causa-
   tion, functions, etc.)?
Does the child seem to rely on gestures, sounds, or the immediate environment to be understood?
Does the child speak in single words, phrases, or sentences? How long is a typical utterance? Does the
   child leave out words? Are the child's sentences complex or simple? How does the child ask questions?
Does the child use pronouns and articles to distinguish old and new information?
Does the child use words for time, such as *tomorrow, yesterday,* or *last night*? Does the child use verb
   tenses?
Can the child put several sentences together to form complex descriptions and explanations?

Source: Compiled from Brinton & Fujiki (1989); Lund & Duchan (1993); and Spinelli & Terrell (1984).

The style of interaction is more than just the frequency of various forms of behavior. More important are the ways in which the child uses the various features of his or her linguistic interactional style. The key question is, How does the child interact with others?

Routinized situations may provide the child with a scaffold within which processing becomes automatized language (Lieven, 1984). The SLP needs to assess the child's familiarity with the situation and the degree to which that situation provides a prop for the child's language. Atypical situations will not elicit typical performance.

The INREAL/Outreach Program of the University of Colorado recommends an observation strategy called SOUL. The acronym stands for *silence, observation, understanding,* and *listening.* The adult remains *silent* for periods of time, assessing the situation before talking. *Observation* of the child's play and interactions with other people occurs prior to forming hypotheses. *Understanding* is the insight into the child that comes from the distillation of data collected during observation. Finally, *listening* requires total involvement by the adult and the use of responses appropriate to the functioning level of the child.

The SLP obtains from the caregiver interview some notion of what to observe. Reliability of observation is increased if the SLP's descriptions detail as closely as possible the actual observed behavior. Inferences and hypotheses come later. It is best if the observation is videotaped or audiotaped for later referral.

Table 3.4 is a list of some features that the SLP might observe. This list is not exhaustive. Each category is discussed in some detail in Chapters 6 and 7, where we consider the analysis of a conversational sample. The purpose of observation is to note within the larger scope of interaction the language characteristics to be tested, collected, and analyzed later in the assessment.

Reliability of observation is not fortuitous. SLPs should train together thoroughly so that their observations are as accurate and as objective as possible. This accuracy and objectivity can be accomplished by repeated observation and rating of videotaped samples by more than one SLP. Ratings then can be compared, discussed, and modified in light of reexamination of taped samples.

TABLE 3.4   Features to note while observing the child

Form of language. Does the child use single words, phrases, or sentences primarily? Are the sentences of the subject-verb-object form exclusively? Are there mature negatives, interrogatives, and passive sentences? Does the child elaborate the noun or verb phrase? Is there evidence of embedding and conjoining?

Understanding of semantic intent. Does the child respond appropriately to the various question forms (what, where, who, when, why, how)? Does the child confuse words from different semantic classes?

Language use. Does the child display a range of illocutionary functions, such as asking for information, help, and objects; replying; making statements; providing information? Does the child take conversational turns? Does the child introduce topics and maintain them through several turns? Does the child signal the status of the communication and make repairs?

Rate of speaking. Is the rate inordinately slow or fast? Are there noticeable or lengthy pauses between the caregiver and child's turn? Are there noticeable or lengthy pauses between the child's adjacent utterances? Does the child use fillers frequently or pause before producing certain words? Are there frequent word substitutions?

Sequencing. Does the child relate events in a sequential fashion based on the order of occurrence? Can the child discuss the recent past or recount stories?

Formal Testing

Within the evaluation, a change to more formal testing tasks might be accomplished through the use of a nonthreatening receptive task, possibly one requiring only a pointing response. Such a task allows the child to become accustomed to the SLP's direction.

Assessing All Aspects of Language

It is important that the SLP make a thorough assessment of all aspects of language. Only rarely is a language impairment limited to one aspect alone. Should this be the case, however, as with a high-functioning child with TBI who manifests only lingering pragmatic difficulties, testing of all aspects confirms the absence of problems and provides a holistic image of the child's language. This task may necessitate more than one session with the child and caregivers. Even when problems in a single area, such as vocabulary, are suspected, more than a single test should be used in order to best describe the language deficit (Grey, Plante, Vance, & Henrichsen, 1999). Issues relative to each aspect of language are discussed in the following section.

Pragmatics.   Very few tests are available that assess the child's conversational skills. In general, the tests are of two varieties—storytelling and topic discussion. In both test situations, the essential feature of conversational relevance is strained, and it is doubtful that a true description of the child's abilities is attained. For example, the topic discussion format makes it difficult to assess question comprehension (Moeller, Osberger, & Eccarius, 1986). In general, questioning is sampled inadequately, restricted in type, and lacking in variation of communicative contexts (Parnell & Amerman, 1983).

The nature of pragmatics makes formal testing difficult. It is also difficult to establish reliable norms, because such aspects of pragmatics as the amount of talking, the frequency of initiations, the type of discourse structure, and the register are situationally related. At present, it seems more appropriate to use a conversational sample to assess children's language use.

Semantics.   When does the SLP know that a child has learned a word? Tests typically assume an all-or-nothing phenomenon in which the child either does or does not know the meaning (Crais, 1990). In reality, acquisition of word knowledge is a gradual process that may continue through the lifetime of an individual. An individual child's success or failure on a test item may be dependent on several factors, such as the type of task or the manner of cuing. Testing tasks are often contrived, decontextualized, and highly literate (Nippold, Scott, Norris, & Johnson, 1993).

Testing of semantic abilities usually is confined to picture identification, word definitions, and word categories. Of interest are the child's comprehension and production vocabularies. Comprehension vocabulary usually is measured by having the child point to a picture that best represents the word produced by the test administrator. Such tests tell the SLP very little about the frequency of use or the depth or breadth of the child's understanding of the concept named. Comprehension of longer utterances usually is assessed by having the child follow simple commands or directives.

When a word is not fully understood by a child, he or she may rely on other comprehension strategies based on linguistic features, such as word order, or on nonlinguistic features, such as the position or size of the stimulus (Edmonston & Thane, 1992). These strategies are considered rarely in a formal assessment. During testing, the SLP should note behaviors such as locational preferences in pointing responses and verbal comments that accompany responding.

Expressive or productive vocabulary usually is tested by having the child name pictures or supply a definition. Scoring may be of a correct-incorrect or scaled type. The latter allows for partially correct responses. Descriptions by the SLP of the type of definition given by the child can be valuable in determining the maturity of the child's lexicon. Early definitions usually rely on use. These are followed in order by descriptions, use in context, synonyms and explanations, and finally, conventional definitions (Curtis, 1987).

Categorical understanding is assessed by asking the child to supply an antonym or a synonym or to name related words in a category. Between ages 5 and 9, the child undergoes a change in the organization of language, from a syntactic to a more categorical system. Thus, category membership and related words, not just simple word meaning, should be tested with all children in late elementary and high school.

Word-association tasks such as naming another member of a category may be ineffectual in differentiating children with LI and those without (Kail & Leonard, 1986). Responses are dependent more on the familiarity of the category and the number of responses possible (Crais, 1990).

Other semantic-related tasks include giving antonyms or synonyms, stating similarities and differences, telling all one knows about a word, detecting semantic absurdities, explaining figurative language, and noting multiple meanings. Each task requires different abilities, such as determining the task demands, focusing on critical semantic dimensions, and interpreting cues, that can be complicated by word-retrieval difficulties.

Children with LLD or TBI exhibit word-finding and word-substitution difficulties. Little is known about word-retrieval processes, especially among children. In children, the words substituted usually share some visual attributes with the target word referent, such as saying *sheet* for *cape* and *net* for *screen*. Late elementary school children with LLD exhibit more visually related word-substitution errors than do children developing typically (German, 1982). Additional word-finding substitutions found in children with LLD include functional descriptions, such as *book holder* for *shelf*.

Diagnostically, use of these word-finding strategies indicates that the child comprehends the word but has difficulty retrieving it. Although testing may reveal a deficit in naming skills, such tests rarely indicate the nature of the deficit. Identification of the word-retrieval strategies of these children may aid in the design of remediation techniques directly related to these strategies.

One method for attaining more information from tests is a double-naming technique (Fried-Oken, 1987). In this procedure, a standard naming test is administered twice. The results are examined to identify error response groups that occur once and twice. The double-error group or errors that occur on both administrations require further analysis.

The SLP administers a number of cues with the double-error words to determine whether the errors indicate word-finding difficulties and to identify naming strategies. In this procedure, cues are administered in the following order (Fried-Oken, 1987):

1. *General question.* The child is asked a general, open-ended question, such as, "Can you think of another word for this?" or "What is this again?" that provides no additional linguistic information.

2. *Semantic/phonemic facilitator.* Two cues, based on additional semantic and phonemic information, are administered. The order of presentation varies, but the SLP should record carefully the order and the response. The semantic cue describes the object's function, provides a categorical label or states the location. For example, if the picture shows a sofa, the SLP might say, "It's something you sit on," "It's a piece of furniture," or "You find it in the living room." The child's response and the type of semantic facilitator should be noted.

The phonemic cue includes the initial phoneme of the desired label ("The word starts with a /_/.") This type of cue requires certain metalinguistic skills in order for the child to use the information.

3. *Verification.* If the child is still incorrect, the SLP provides the correct label and asks whether the child has ever seen this object before in order to verify whether the word is in the child's repertoire.

The child's responses and the cues are analyzed to determine the qualitative nature of the errors and the child's naming strategy. Possible naming strategies of 4- to 9-year-old children are listed in Table 3.5.

Syntax.   Syntactic testing can be extremely complicated because of the complexity and diversity of the syntactic system. SLPs may wish to use entire test batteries or portions of several tests. The latter strategy is recommended for in-depth probing of potential problem areas. Naturally, when tests are used in a nonstandard manner or are combined with other subtests, the norms can no longer be used. Results must be described accurately and interpreted in light of the tasks involved.

There is considerable variability across tests in the length of individual syntactic items, the structures tested, and the type of testing tasks used. Test items are as diverse as highly unnatural tasks, such as word ordering or unscrambling and sentence assembling, and more natural tasks such as sentence combining (Nippold, Scott, Norris, & Johnson, 1993). Many mirror the highly decontextualized tasks found in school but do not reflect everyday language use.

In general, development of comprehension of syntactic forms typically precedes production. Thus, a thorough language assessment should include evaluation of both aspects. Although the receptive procedures used and the structures assessed vary widely across tests, the common element is that the child demonstrates understanding—usually by pointing to a picture or following directions—while producing only minimal language, if any.

TABLE 3.5   Naming strategy categories

Naming Strategy	Example
Phonological	foon/SPOON
Perceptual	lampshade/SKIRT
Semantic	tortoise/OCTOPUS
Semantic + perceptual	broom/MOP
	shirt/JACKET
Part/whole	shoelace/SHOE
Functional circumlocution	you can play songs/PIANO
Descriptive circumlocution	it has numbers and hands/CLOCK
Contextual circumlocution	in a band/TAMBOURINE
Superordinate	food/CRACKERS
Subordinate	Shetland pony/HORSE
Unrelated perseveration	canoe/HARMONICA
	canoe/MUSHROOM
Comment	I don't know/GLOVE
No answer	10+ seconds of silence/MITTEN
Gesture	"strumming"/GUITAR

Source: Fried-Oken, M. (1987). Qualitative examination of children's naming skills through test adaptations. *Language, Speech, and Hearing Services in Schools, 18,* 206–216. Reprinted with permission.

Syntactic production typically is tested by using either a structured elicitation or a sentence imitation format. In structured elicitation, the child might be asked to describe a picture, following a model by the test administrator. The model sentence establishes the sentence form to be used but differs from the desired sentence by the structure being tested.

In sentence imitation, the child gives an immediate repetition of the administrator's sentence. The underlying assumption of elicited imitation procedures is that sentences that exceed the child's short-term memory span will be reproduced according to the child's own linguistic rule system, which the child must use as a processing aid. Theoretically, the child's sentence should be very similar to the one the child would produce spontaneously. Thus, the child's imitated sentence should not contain any structures absent in the child's spontaneous language production.

Although elicited imitation serves as the basis of a number of diagnostic instruments and as a portion of several other tools, the validity of the procedure has been questioned frequently. The imitative procedure may underestimate, overestimate, or correctly estimate the child's actual language abilities. For example, although the performance of children with LI on elicited imitation tests can be enhanced by the addition of contextual cues, such as pictures or object manipulation, their imitations are still simpler than their spontaneous language production. Assumptions about the performance of nonimpaired children may not apply to children with LI.

Because the relationship between elicited imitation and spontaneously produced language is a very complex one, SLPs are advised to use elicited imitation results with caution and to rely on the data from spontaneous samples when the two differ (Fujiki & Brinton, 1987). Elicited imitation responses should be analyzed for the specific ways they differ from the model. Table 3.6 provides a method of scoring sentence imitation tasks that maximizes the available information for clinical use (Mattes, 1982). Each response is scored for grammatical acceptability, type of syntactic error, semantic equivalence, and quality of response.

Morphology.   Morphological testing usually focuses on bound inflectional morphemes. Most tests emphasize suffixes, such as tense markers, plurals, possessives, and comparators, because of their high usage and relatively early development. In general, children with good spoken and written language abilities have more morphological awareness and do better on such tests (R. C. Anderson & Davison, 1988; Bailet, 1990; Carlisle, 1987; Fisher, Shankweiler, & Liberman, 1985; Liberman, Rubin, Duques, & Carlisle, 1985; Nagy, Anderson, Schommer, Scott, & Stallman, 1989; Snow, 1990).

Suffixes can be divided into two types—inflectional and derivational. *Inflectional* suffixes indicate possession, gender, and number in nouns; tense, voice, person and number, and mood in verbs; and comparison in adjectives and do not change the part of speech of the base. For example, a noun can be made plural with the addition of the *-s* marker, but the noun remains a noun.

The second, larger category, derivational suffixes, is ignored in most tests. *Derivational* suffixes have a smaller range of application and many more constraints and irregularities than inflectional suffixes. Application may be unpredictable, as with *-tion,* which can be added to some but not all nouns, or may be somewhat unclear in meaning, as with *-ment* in *apart**ment**.* More than 80 percent of multimorpheme words do not mean what the constituent parts suggest (White, Power, & White, 1989). The development of derivational suffixes is not as clearly understood as that of inflectional suffixes but seems related to oral language production abilities, reading level and exposure, derivational complexity, and metalinguistic awareness (Carlisle, 1987, 1988; Fisher et al., 1985; Nagy, Anderson, & Herman, 1987; Nagy, Herman, & Anderson, 1985; Tyler & Nagy, 1987; Wysocki & Jenkins, 1987).

TABLE 3.6 Elicited language analysis procedures

			Format															

Student's Name:

Birthdate: _____ Examiner: _____ Test Date:

Test Item #	*Instructions:* Record the child's responses in the spaces below. Score responses in terms of grammatical acceptability, syntactic usage, vocabulary usage, and response quality by placing a check mark in the boxes that most accurately describe the response.	Grammatical Acceptability	Syntactic Usage on Structure Tested								Vocabulary			Response Quality			Comments
			Correct: Identical	Correct: Nonidentical	Substitution Error	Deletion Error	Insertion Error	Modification Error	Word Sequence Error	Non-Attempt Error	Equivalent in Meaning	Related in Meaning	Unrelated in Meaning	Delayed Response	Self-Corrected Response	Perseverative Response	

The child's elicited imitation is written in the appropriate column at the left. Omissions, substitutions, changes in meaning and the like are noted by marking the appropriate column. The errors and target structures can be recorded under the Comments column, such as "Omit past-tense -ed" or "Change passive voice to active." Such analysis may help delineate unlearned structures and the cognitive-linguistic knowledge base.

Response Categories

Grammatical acceptability. Child's response is a complete and grammatically correct sentence.

Syntactic usage on structure tested. The manner in which the grammatical structure tested is produced.

A. *Correct production: identical sentence frame.* Child's response is an identical word-for-word reproduction of the model.

B. *Correct production; nonidentical sentence frame.* The grammatical structure being tested is produced correctly, although the sentence frame differs from the model.

C. *Substitution error.* The child substitutes an inappropriate grammatical form for the structure being tested.

D. *Deletion error.* The child inappropriately omits the grammatical structure being tested.

E. *Insertion error.* The child inserts the grammatical structure being tested within a sentence frame where it is inappropriate.

F. *Modification error.* The child produces a modification of the grammatical structure being tested that is not acceptable in any context (e.g., *him's, ain't, it's is*).

G. *Word sequence error.* The child produces the grammatical structure being tested in an appropriate position within the response.

H. *Non-attempt error.* Performance cannot be evaluated (e.g., *I don't know*).

Vocabulary usage. Manner in which the child's response relates semantically to the stimulus sentence.

A. *Equivalent in meaning.* Although the specific vocabulary used by the child is not identical to the model, the response is identical in meaning.

B. *Related in meaning.* The child produces a response that is partially related to the meaning of the model. The child may omit essential elements or modify vocabulary.

C. *Unrelated in meaning.* The child produces a nonmeaningful response or one that is unrelated to the model.

Continued

TABLE 3.6 *Continued*

Response Categories
Response quality.   **A.** *Delayed correct response.* The child produces a correct response that is nonimmediate, requires a repetition of the model, or is produced after hesitation during response.   **B.** *Self-corrected response.* The child self-corrects an incorrect response without prompting by the examiner.   **C.** *Perseverative response.* The child produces a response that resembles that used on a previous test item but that is inappropriate for this item.

Source: Mattes, L. (1982). The elicited language analysis procedure: A method for scoring sentence imitation tasks. *Language, Speech, and Hearing Services in Schools, 13,* 37–41. Reprinted with permission.

The two most common expressive test formats for morphology are *cloze,* or sentence completion, and sentence imitation. Most cloze procedure test items give the root word and require the child to respond with the root plus a suffix, as in *teach-teacher.* Tests use either actual words or nonsense words. The rationale for nonsense words is that their use will not bias performance by previous exposure. In general, tests using nonsense words are more difficult for young children (Channell & Ford, 1991). Children with either MR or LLD have greater difficulty with nonsense word tests than children developing typically. Other testing tasks might include judgments of relatedness of words, such as *hospital* and *hospitable,* ability to deduce meaning from component parts, and ability to form words in different and changing linguistic contexts (Moats & Smith, 1992).

Although several tests have morphological portions or subtests, most have too few items and too narrow a scope to provide much valuable information (Moats & Smith, 1992). Prefixes and derivational suffixes are included on only a few tests.

Written Language.   A written sample should also be collected, especially if dyslexia or LLD is suspected. It should include first drafts of expository writing, narrative fiction, and nonfiction. The SLP can evaluate the sample for phonological and linguistic awareness; word boundaries; vocabulary and usage; ability to communicate thoughts precisely, sequentially, and systematically; generation and organization of ideas; morpheme usage; syntactic usage, semantic awareness, and word associations, such as opposites and synonyms; and handwriting (Greene, 1996). This area of assessment will be discussed in detail in Chapter 13.

Test Modification

As mentioned previously, tests can be modified to provide the information desired by the SLP. For example, the SLP may wish to test a child's pronoun use in depth. No test is available that adequately assesses only these structures. The SLP might construct his or her own assessment tool from portions of other tests. This type of locally prepared test may be very useful for thorough assessment. Obviously, individual test standards of administration have been violated and the norms would be invalid. Occasionally, published tests include subtest norms. In this case, a subtest on pronouns may be administered in its entirety as directed in the instructions, and the norming information would be applicable.

Test administration may be modified also for the child who cannot perform as required or for further investigation of the child's response strategies. For example, use of pictures or repetition of instructions may enhance the performance of some children. It is important to remember that nearly all tests are designed for children developing typically. The child with MR or cerebral palsy is at a very distinct disadvantage. In such cases, description of the child's ability when procedures are modified may be much more useful for intervention than a score or age equivalent. Adherence to prescribed test procedures is more likely to result in a measure of that child's limitations.

Testing procedures may be modified through the use of multiple sessions, increased time to respond, and increased trials. For children with attentional difficulties, the SLP might enlarge materials, use a penlight or pointer, highlight certain information, verbally remind the child to attend, or have the child repeat the test cue.

The performance of children with motor problems, ASD, or LLD might be affected also by visual or auditory distractions, placement of materials, temperature, lighting, light and dark contrasts, and positioning. Children who perseverate may need to be reminded that the correct answer is not always the same. Children with short-term memory problems may need to have cues repeated, to repeat cues aloud themselves, or to have cues broken into easily processible units.

Finally, children with TBI may need a longer time to respond. The SLP also should test beyond base and ceiling scores to identify "islands" of learning. Other modifications for children with TBI may include reduction of distractions, different response modes, enlarged print and reduction of print per page, simplified instructions, substituting multiple choice questions to facilitate recall, giving multiple examples, providing breaks when fatigue is evident, and darkening lines or print in visual displays (Russell, 1993).

Sampling

Conversational sampling has the potential for providing the most accurate description of the child's language as it is actually used in conversational exchange. Although sampling usually includes freeplay and unstructured conversation, it also may include structured conversation and probing of language features noted in observation and testing. In the next several chapters, we discuss the best ways to maximize the information from this source through design of collection situations and analysis methods.

Conclusion

It's important as you move through an assessment not to become too absorbed in the minutia of various isolated language features. This "forest for the trees" (N. W. Nelson, 1998) syndrome can result in missing the holistic nature of the child's communication system.

Early Intervention with Presymbolic and Minimally Symbolic Children

Children communicating at a level below 2 years of age have unique needs. Often, the goal of intervention is the *initiation* of effective communication. Such children may have rudimentary communication skills or use only single-symbol or short multisymbol communication.

Children who are *presymbolic* do not use conventional signs, words, or pictures for communication. They may possess no recognizable communication system or may use gestures, such as pointing or touching or moving objects. Children who are *minimally symbolic* use some visual, verbal, or tactile symbols alone or in combination.

Communication intervention will require both training of the child and adaptation by the child's environment (Cirrin & Rowland, 1985; Donnellan, Mirenda, Mesaros, & Fassbender, 1984; Prizant & Wetherby, 1988a; Simeonsson, Olley, & Rosenthal, 1987; Vicker, 1985). If children change their behavior but environmental expectations do not change accordingly, then the children may have little or no opportunity to use these new behaviors. Therefore, the SLP is interested in evaluating the child's abilities and needs and also the communication expectations and demands of the communication environment and the interaction of the child and the environment.

The Child's Abilities and Needs

The SLP is interested primarily in the child's current communication system, including the mode of communication, and in the level of presymbolic and/or symbolic functioning. A holistic description of the child's communication abilities and needs requires a variety of data collection methods. Of interest are the manner and content of both social and nonsocial communication.

Toddlers who are most at risk for language problems and poor likelihood of change have certain characteristics (Olswang, Rodriguez, & Timler, 1998):

- Small vocabularies for their age
- Few verbs except for all-purpose verbs such as *want, go, get, do, put, look, make,* or *got*
- More transitive than intransive verbs
- Six-month comprehension delay
- A large comprehension-production gap
- Few prelinguistic vocalizations and limited babbling structure
- Few consonants and glottal and back substitutions
- Vowel errors
- Restricted syllable structure
- Few spontaneous imitations
- Reliance on direct modeling and prompting during imitation tasks
- Little purposeful, combinatorial, or symbolic play
- Few gestures
- Behavior problems
- Few conversational initiations
- More interactions with adults than peers
- Difficulty gaining access to activities

Risk factors for developing useful communication skills include prolonged periods of untreated otitis media, a family member with persistent language and learning problems, low socioeconomic status, directive parents, and extreme parental concern (Olswang, Rodriguez, & Timler, 1998).

The child may have a rich and varied, albeit idiosyncratic, communication system. Several forms of presymbolic communication are listed in Table 3.7. Some forms may be situationally controlled. Only by using various methods to collect data from a number of sources can the SLP hope to gain a complete description.

TABLE 3.7 Examples of presymbolic communication

Generalized movements and changes in muscle tone
 Excitement in response to stimulation or in anticipation of an event
 Squirms and resists physical contact
 Changes in muscle tone in response to soothing touch or voice, in reaction to sudden stimuli, or in preparation to act

Vocalizations
 Calls to attract or direct another's attention
 Laughs or coos in response to pleasurable stimulation
 Cries in reaction to discomfort

Facial expressions
 Smiles in response to familiar person, object, or event
 Grimaces in reaction to unpleasant or unexpected sensation

Orientation
 Looks toward or points to person or object to seek or direct attention
 Looks away from person or object to indicate disinterest or refusal
 Looks toward suddenly appearing familiar or novel person, object, or event

Pause
 Ceases moving in anticipation of coming event
 Pauses to await service provider's instruction or to allow service provider to take turn

Touching, manipulating, or moving with another person
 Holds or grabs another for comfort
 Takes or directs another's hand to something
 Manipulates service provider into position to start an activity or interactive "game"
 Touches or pulls service provider to gain attention
 Pushes away or lets go to terminate an interaction
 Moves with or follows the movements of another person

Acting on objects and using objects to interact with others
 Reaches toward, leans toward, touches, gets, picks up, activates, drops, or pushes away object to indicate interest or disinterest
 Extends, touches, or places object to show to another or to request another's action
 Holds out hands to prepare to receive object

Assuming positions and going to places
 Holds up arms to be picked up, holds out hands to initiate "game," leans back on swing to be pushed
 Stands by sink to request drink, goes to cabinet to request material stored there

Conventional gestures
 Waves to greet
 Nods to indicate assent or refusal

Depictive actions
 Pantomimes throwing to indicate "throw ball"
 Sniffs to indicate smelling flowers
 Makes sounds similar to those made by animals and objects to make reference to them
 Draws picture to describe or request activity

Withdrawal
 Pulls away or moves away to avoid interaction or activity
 Curls up, lies on floor to avoid interaction or activity

Aggressive and self-injurious behavior
 Hits, scratches, bites, or spits at service provider to protest action or in response to frustration
 Throws or destroys objects to protest action or in response to frustration
 Hits, bites, or otherwise harms self or threatens to harm self to protest action, in response to frustration, or in reaction to pain or discomfort

Source: Stillman, R., & Siegel-Causey, E. (1989). Introduction. In E. Siegel-Causey & D. Guess (Eds.), *Enhancing Nonsymbolic Communication Interactions among Learners with Severe Disabilities* (p. 7). Baltimore, MD: Paul H. Brookes Publishing Co. Copyright 1989 by Paul H. Brookes Publishing Co. Reprinted by permission.

The child's presymbolic and/or symbolic functioning also should be fully described (Peck & Schuler, 1987). Table 3.8 presents presymbolic behaviors that a number of intervention specialists and programs consider important for assessment and training. Not all professionals agree on which presymbolic behaviors to target. Each SLP should add or delete presymbolic behaviors on the basis of literature review and personal experience with the presymbolic population.

TABLE 3.8   Possible presymbolic progressions for assessment

Means-end/tool use
* uses a tool that is contiguous with the goal as a means to obtain the goal (e.g., pulls string tied to object, pulls cloth under object)
* uses a tool that is noncontiguous with the goal as a means to obtain the goal (e.g., rakes in object with stick, moves chair in position and climbs on chair to obtain object on shelf)

Causality/communicative intent
* touches adult's hand or object to recreate spectacle
* uses gestural or vocal signal to regulate adult's behavior or to direct adult's attention
* discovers the source of an action (e.g., how to activate a mechanical toy, looks for the source of a thrown object)

Gestural/vocal imitation
* takes turns after adult imitates child's behavior or in familiar social routines
* imitates vocal or gestural behavior initiated by adult
* imitates a behavior at a much later time in the absence of the original model

Schemes for relating to objects/symbolic play
* explores the physical properties of objects
* uses recognitory gestures on realistic objects (e.g., combs own hair, brushes own teeth, eats from spoon)
* uses pretend schemes with miniature objects toward self (e.g., rolls toy car, drinks from doll's cup, pounds toy hammer)
* uses pretend schemes toward others (e.g., feeds doll with bottle, combs mother's hair)
* uses multiple pretend schemes in sequence (e.g., stirs pretend food in pan, pours food onto dish, and feeds doll)

Social relatedness/expression of emotion
* expresses emotions of joy, fear, and anger in appropriate situations or in response to adult's emotional expression
* responds differentially to strangers and caregivers
* uses gestural or vocal signals to establish closeness (e.g., pulls on adult's leg and reaches up to be picked up)
* knows how to get adult to react (e.g., to make adult laugh and make adult angry)
* expresses emotions of empathy, shame, guilt, affection, and defiance

Language comprehension
* uses nonlinguistic response strategies, including situational routines, contextual clues, intonation, gestures, and facial expression
* comprehends the meaning of single words (e.g., person names, object names, actions)
* comprehends multiword utterances based on semantic relations (e.g., action + object, agent + action, attribute + object)

Language production
* uses consistent preverbal forms tied to the context
* uses single-word approximations or intoned jargon to encode dynamic, changing states, or objects that can be acted upon by the child
* uses multiword utterances to encode semantic relations (e.g., action + object, attribute + object)

Source: Prizant, B. M., & Wetherby, A. M. (1988a). Providing services to children with autism (ages 0 to 2 years) and their families. *Topics in Language Disorders, 9*(1), 1–23. Reprinted with permission.

TABLE 3.9 **Semantic and illocutionary functions of early symbolic communication**

Semantic Functions	Illocutionary Functions
Nomination	Answer
This/that + nomination	Question or requesting information
Location	Reply
X + location	Elicitation
Negation	Continuant
Negation + X	Declaration
Modification (Types:	Practice or repeat
Attribution, possession, and recurrence)	Name or label
Modifier + X	Command, demand, request, protest
Notice	
Notice + X	
Action (signaled by agent, action, or object)	
Agent + action	
Action + object	

Source: Compiled from MacDonald (1978a); Owens (1982c).

Symbolic assessment should include more than a list of the symbols the child uses. Symbols are acquired initially to fulfill illocutionary functions already in children's repertoires. Children also treat symbols as representing various semantic functions that form building blocks for early multi-symbol utterances. The range of functions these symbols represents is important, regardless of the means or manner of communication. Table 3.9 presents some common semantic and illocutionary functions found in initial symbolic communication. Definitions are listed in Appendix A.

Questionnaire and Interview

The SLP can ascertain initially the manner and content of the child's communication and some indication of functioning level by questionnaire and/or interview with the child's caregivers and by observation. Responses can enhance the validity of later testing. Table 3.10 presents possible questions.

For children using symbols, the SLP will want to collect an initial lexicon. Caregivers can draw on their experience to provide a list of words or signs used. Checklists of possible symbols yield more responses from caregivers than do blank forms or even categorical inventories that give category names, such as nouns and personal names (Morrow, Mirenda, Beukelman, & Yorkston, 1993). Parental reports of their child's vocabulary can be as valid as other vocabulary measures if parents are given a preprinted list of possible words (J. Miller, Sedey, & Miolo, 1995).

Observation

Through structured observation, the SLP attempts to describe the communicative environment of the child. Descriptive factors include the amount of time the child spends in certain environments, the frequency of communication in these environments, and the partners, activities, and objects present. Both familiar routines and less structured contexts might be observed in order to note differing behaviors (Theadore et al., 1990).

One important aspect of evaluation is determining the communicative intention of the child's behaviors. It is not the behavior itself, but its relationship to the context, that indicates communica-

TABLE 3.10 Questionnaire or interview content for children who are presymbolic or minimally symbolic

How does the child communicate primarily?
    Does the child use vocalizations, gestures, postures, eye contact, or other means of communication?
    Who understands the child's communication efforts?
Does the child play alone or with others?
Does the child demonstrate any turn-taking behaviors?
Does the child enjoy making sounds? How often does the child make sounds?
Does the child ever initiate communication? How? In which situations?
Which situations seem to be high-communication contexts?
Which caregivers seem to engage in the most interaction with the child?
Does the child
    Make wants known?
    Request help?
    Point to objects or actions, name, or both?
    Request information?
    Seek attention?
    Demonstrate emotion?
    Protest?

Source: Compiled from Calculator (1988a); MacDonald (1978b); Owens & Rogerson (1988).

tion. Unlike symbols, signals, such as gestures, almost always require the context for interpretation (Ogletree, 1993). Of interest is the range of intentions exhibited.

Communication behaviors are consistent, identifiable responses associated with environmental events or with the child's physical or emotional state. Children with sensory, mental, and/or physiological impairments often do not use clearly recognizable communication. The child who turns away from another person or becomes self-abusive or increases self-stimulation when someone approaches is most likely communicating a desire not to communicate. Some communication may be unrecognizable as such and may be misinterpreted (Houghton, Bronicki, & Guess, 1987).

Communication behaviors may be message-specific, each communicating a single message, or may communicate a variety of messages. For example, loud vocalizations may signal several functions, such as attention getting, desire for an object, and/or need for assistance. Communication also may be intentional or unintentional, depending on whether the listener is considered by the child. The degree of intentionality and conventionality, as well as the sophistication of the signal itself, may vary with different functions and/or contexts.

Intentional or social communication is persistent, typically addressed to and modified for the receiver, and awaits a response. Such communication may be signaled by establishing eye contact, awaiting a turn, responding, interrupting, moving to a conspicuous position or toward the receiver, and/or stopping when the goal is reached. Even self-injurious behavior may signal a message, such as a desire to escape or to be left alone.

In contrast, unintentional or nonsocial communication, such as speaking when no one is present, does not consider the receiver. Situational responses, such as an eye blink following a loud noise, also are considered unintentional communication unless the child interacts in some way with the receiver.

Behaviors may be classified along several continuums. One continuum might begin with non-intentional behavior—the type of behavior-state communication, such as crying, seen in young infants—and progress through conventional communication (Dunst, Lowe, & Bartholomew, 1990). Another continuum might have gestural communication at one extreme and verbal at the other, noting stages of intentionality (Wetherby & Prizant, 1990). Gestural behavior may be dichotomized as contact/motoric and distal/signal (Atlas & Lapadis, 1988; McLean & Snyder-McLean, 1987; McLean, Snyder-McLean, Brady, & Etter, 1991). These continuums are summarized in Table 3.11.

Inappropriate, unconventional, idiosyncratic, or aberrant behavior may be used by some children to communicate intent (Carr & Durand, 1985; Donnellan et al., 1984; Wetherby & Prutting, 1984). Through systematic observation, the SLP can form initial tentative hypotheses regarding intentions. In turn, the SLP can confirm these hypotheses by systematic and meticulous manipulation of antecedent and/or consequent events during testing.

The SLP can record hypotheses regarding the child's intentions on a simple form similar to Figure 3.4 (Donnellan et al., 1984). Although designed for aberrant behavior, the form can be adapted and other child behaviors listed across the top. Hypotheses of intent are marked in the space corresponding to the behavior and to the possible intention. In the examples shown, tantruming is believed to signal an intention to attract attention, and touching an object may signal a desire for some item.

For children using conventional symbols, the SLP will want to observe turn taking, presupposition in the novelty of topics introduced by the child, and initiation and response. The SLP will also want to note perseverative behavior, echolalia, and reenactment (Wetherby & Prutting, 1984). In reenactment, the original event or part of it may be used to represent the event. Thus, the child might say, "Once upon a time," to mean, "I want you to read to me." This manner of representation is found in some children with autism.

Direct Testing

The purpose of direct testing is to determine the optimum input and output modes for communication, the desirability of an augmentative system of communication and the selection of type, and the presymbolic or symbolic functioning level of the child. This process is ongoing and may tax the creativity of even the best SLP because of the difficulty in testing some children.

If the child already has some type of rudimentary communication system, the SLP attempts to describe this system as accurately as possible. Initially, the SLP is interested in input and output means. The three primary expressive and receptive modes of communication are manual/visual, vocal/verbal/auditory, and tactile. Manual/visual means include gestures, signs, body movement, and/or visual contact or pointing. Vocal/verbal/auditory means include intonation, speech sounds, phonetically consistent forms, and/or spoken words. Tactile means include touch, signing in the hand, and physical manipulation, such as moving a partner's hand to a desired object.

For children who are presymbolic, the SLP assesses each of the three means for consistent responding and for focused behavior. The SLP should assess also the oral mechanism for motor development and control (Morris & Klein, 1987). Part of the evaluation may include a probe to determine the difficulty in establishing an initial communication system.

During testing, the SLP can confirm hypotheses about illocutionary function formed during observation. The SLP can manipulate events that precede and follow the behaviors in question and note the effect of these changes on the behavior's frequency and intensity. Changes in the behavior should indicate some relationship between the behavior and the environment.

Formal direct testing of age-related communication can be accomplished by using any number of infant communication or development measures. Many items are not appropriate for older children and may have little application to their experiences. Such instruments also may be difficult to

TABLE 3.11   **Stages in the development of intentionality**

Stage	Behavior	Example
Perlocutionary (Nonpurposeful)		
Preintentional	Reflexive behavior that expresses the inner state (wet, tired) and serves as signal for adult who interprets it. Not directed at others; no anticipation of outcome.	Cry, posture change, coo, facial expression (smile, frown)
Unintentional-intentional	Behavior is intentional or goal-oriented (reaching for a mobile) but is not intended to be communicative. Again, serve as signals that adults interpret. Not directed at others; no anticipation of outcome.	Reach for object, look at or regard object, fuss
Illocutionary (Purposeful)		
Nonconventional	Nonconventional gestures, usually *physical contact, used with intent* of affecting adult. Demonstrates intention to communicate by eliciting behavior, checking adult attending, and anticipating outcomes. Persistence or frustration if goal unmet.	Tug, push away, pull (proto-imperatives)
Conventional	Convention (standard) gestures and vocalization used with intention of affecting adult's behavior. Greater persistence.	Alternating gaze, hand object, point, wave, shake head, nod
Concrete	Limited use of iconic symbols *at some distance from the referent* to represent the environment. Range of intentions. May be accompanied by vocalization.	Point, reach, offer, request assistance, request information, sign
Symbolic/locutionary		
Abstract	Limited use of arbitrary symbols, used individually, to represent the environment. Some idiosyncratic symbols. Limited to the here and now. Still heavy reliance on gestures and vocalization.	Symbols
Formal	Rule-bound linear symbol combinations; referent need not be present. Language is primary means of communicating.	Combinations of symbols

Source: Adapted from McLean & Snyder-McLean (1988b); Prizant (1984).

Functions	Aggression	Bizarre Verbalizations	Inapp. Oral/Anal Behavior	Perseverative Rituals	Self-injurious Behavior	Self-stimulation	Tantrum	Facial Expression	Gaze Aversion	Gazing/Staring	Gesturing/Pointing	Hugging/Kissing	Masturbation	Object Manipulation	Proximity Positioning	Pushing/Pulling	Reaching/Grabbing	Running	Touching	Delayed Echolalia	Immediate Echolalia	Laughing/Giggling	Screaming/Yelling	Swearing	Verbal/Physical Threats	Whining/Crying	Complex Sign/Approx.	Complex Speech/Approx.	One Word Sign/Approx.	One Word Speech/Approx.	Picture/Written Word
I. Interactive																															
A. Requests for attention							X																								
Social interaction																															
Play interactions																															
Affection																															
Permission to engage in an activity																															
Action by receiver																															
Assistance																															
Information/classification																															
Objects																	X														
Food																															
B. Negations																															
Protest																															
Refusal																															
Cessation																															
C. Declarations/comments																															
About events/actions																															
About objects/persons																															
About errors/mistakes																															
Affirmation																															
Greeting																															
Humor																															
D. Declarations about feelings																															
Anticipation																															
Boredom																															
Confusion																															
Fear																															
Frustration																															
Hurt feelings																															
Pain																															
Pleasure																															
II. Non-interactive																															
A. Self-regulation																															
B. Rehearsal																															
C. Habitual																															
D. Relaxation/tension release																															

This form can be adapted to list the individual child's behaviors across the top. Hypotheses regarding the illocutionary functions of these behaviors can be recorded in the appropriate space.

FIGURE 3.4   Functions of children's behavior.

Source: Donnellan, A., Mirenda, P., Mesaros, R., & Fassbender, L. (1984). Analyzing the communicative functions of aberrant behavior. *Journal of the Association for Persons with Severe Handicaps, 9,* 210–222. Reprinted with permission.

use with children with multiple disabilities. Necessary modifications in testing procedures may preclude the outright use of a test's age norms. At best, these instruments provide only a gross estimate of the child's overall communication abilities.

Certain commercially available instruments assess varying numbers of presymbolic and symbolic behaviors. Most of these tools were created by modifying developmental scales to reflect more accurately the population being tested and the skills specifically needed for symbolic communication. Because the SLP is interested in not only the skill level of the child but also the ease of teaching presymbolic skills, a necessary portion of the assessment should include teaching.

No specific skills, such as the imitative behavior of clapping hands, will aid in the development of symbols. Hand clapping is one example of a larger behavioral class of imitation. The SLP is more interested in the presence or absence of these general classes of behavior and probes overall conceptual development of these classes.

The SLP should encourage caregivers to attend the evaluation and to assist by providing suggestions and actual test items from the child's environment, such as toys or grooming items. The presence of both the caregiver and familiar objects enhances the validity of the testing procedure. Often, children who are presymbolic and minimally symbolic have very concrete meanings for symbols or demonstrate very ritualized behavior. A cup may not be *cup* for the child unless it is the one used every day. This information would be unavailable without the caregiver's presence, and the SLP might assume incorrectly that the child does or does not know the symbol *cup*.

Sampling

Most measures of presymbolic or minimally symbolic communication emphasize language form, rather than communication (Wetherby & Prizant, 1991). Sampling is needed, therefore, as a supplement (Wetherby & Prizant, 1989). Structured situations may be used to elicit a variety of functions by enticing communication (Coggins, Olswang, & Guthrie, 1987; Prizant & Wetherby, 1988b; Wetherby & Rodriguez, 1992). Table 3.12 presents some possible structured situations. It may be best to intersperse different functions to keep the child's interest and reduce potential perseveration.

Assessment for AAC Use

Augmentative and alternative communication (AAC) is a method of transmitting information, ideas, and feelings that is other than speech. As such, AAC can be used to supplement or complement speech communication. Just as with speaking children, the SLP is concerned with the quantity and quality of language and with the ability of the child to communicate effectively in familiar contexts.

AAC systems can be divided into two categories: unaided and aided. *Unaided systems* consist of sign systems, such as American Sign Language or Signed English, and gesture systems, such as American Indian Signs (Amerind). *Aided systems* use a piece of equipment to assist communication. These usually are classified as nonelectronic and electronic. Nonelectronic devices include several types of communication boards as diverse as wallet foldouts, wheelchair-mounted trays, and Plexiglass windows containing pictures, photographs, and/or symbols. Textured shapes, such as corrugated cardboard, sponge, sandpaper, rubber stair treads, plastic mesh, needlepoint and cross-stitch, fur, carpet, and terrycloth toweling, have been used effectively with children with severe/profound MR, ASD, and multiple disabilities (Murray-Branch, Udavari-Solner, & Bailey, 1991). Electronic devices are as diverse as simple lights mounted above selected symbols and computer-assisted

TABLE 3.12   Structured situations for eliciting communication

Declaring

Adult looks through some books with the child.

Adult gives the child four blocks to drop into a can. Immediately on completion, adult hands the child a small doll.

Adult rolls a ball to the child. After a few returns, adult substitutes a different toy and rolls it.

Adult takes item from box, such as a marker, and offers one to child. Adult replaces marker after drawing and also places a strange object in the box, takes another marker, and hands the box to the child. A plastic spider has been used but might scare some children too much. A cotton ball could be placed in a food item.

Adult has a mechanical item move behind him or her that is visible to the child. Adult operates switch unknown to child.

Greeting

On meeting child, adult awaits greeting. If not forthcoming after 5 seconds, adult greets the child.

Adult waves hello and good-bye to objects as they are removed from or replaced in containers. After doing this three or four times, the adult removes or replaces without doing it.

Protesting

Adult holds a disliked food item near the child or hands it to the child.

Adult places the child's hands in a cold, wet, or sticky substance, such as pudding, glue, or Jell-O.

Adult offers child a choice of two items, then hands the wrong one.

Requesting action

Adult initiates a pleasurable game or action, then stops and waits.

Adult blows up a balloon and slowly deflates it, then holds it to his or her mouth and waits or hands it to the child and waits.

Adult plays Give-Me-Five, in which child slaps adult's hands. When tables turn, adult waits.

Requesting assistance

Adult activates a wind-up toy, lets it run down, then hands it to the child.

Adult opens a jar of bubbles, blows some, then closes the jar tightly and gives it to the child.

While the child is watching, adult places a desired food item in a clear jar that the child cannot open, and then places the container in front of the child.

Requesting item

Adult eats a desired food item without offering any to the child.

Adult places two glasses on the table and declares thirst, pours juice for self, and then places pitcher out of child's reach.

Source: Adapted from McLean, Snyder-McLean, Brady, & Etter (1991); Wetherby, Cain, Yonclas, & Walker (1988); Wetherby & Prizant (1990); Wetherby & Rodriguez (1992).

systems with simultaneous auditory and visual output. Even a portable transistor radio can be modified to produce an oscillating tone and serve as an attention-getting device (T. King, 1991).

One disclaimer before we begin this section. I have made a conscious choice to place AAC in the Early Intervention section. Issues related to AAC are fascinating and complex, too complex to be explored fully as a section of a chapter. I will address AAC topics in general and as they relate to young children. Where appropriate I will address issues for higher-functioning children. Remember, good decision making about intervention with speaking children, such as vocabulary selection, can be applied just as well with AAC users. We need not reinvent the entire profession of speech-language pathology because the means of communication has changed. Is there lots of new information? Yep! Is everything else irrelevant? Nope, good practices are good practices.

Assessing a child for AAC should be a team effort. At the very minimum, the team should include the child, her or his family, teacher, SLP, educational psychologist, and physical or occupational therapist.

There may be no single good assessment for augmentative communication use. Certain minimal presymbolic skills seem necessary, however, for use of some augmentative communication systems. The level of functioning necessary depends on the system selected. In short, the more symbolic the system, the higher cognitive skill involved. For example, some forms of gestural signaling may be accomplished at a relatively young developmental age when compared to speaking or signing.

With young children, initial systems will most likely be low technology systems, such as gesturing, signing, or use of pictures on a communication board. Initially, even complex computer systems will need to require simple input from a young child and be limited to pictures or photos.

Assessment/decision making is a three-tiered process in which the diagnostic team considers the appropriateness of AAC for the child, selects a system, and selects a code. Decisions about appropriateness are based on cognitive ability, communication motivation and abilities, and family acceptance of AAC.

Cognitive abilities are especially important for the size and quality of the augmentative repertoire that the child will develop (Silverman, 1989). Cognitive functioning alone, however, does not predict success, especially with gestural communication (McLean et al., 1991). Although Piagetian sensorimotor stages IV and early V are correlated with true symbol use, this correlation should not preclude augmentative instruction at a less than symbolic level that is useful to the child (Calculator, 1988c). Means-ends, pretend play, functional use of objects, and an awareness of symbols such as a stop sign seem important for symbol use (Mirenda & Schuler, 1988).

The SLP frequently assesses social skills, such as turn taking, eye contact, joint attending, receptive language, and gesturing when considering a child for an augmentative communication system. Receptive language skills seem necessary for AAC generalization.

AAC system selection is a complex process that may involve attempted use of one system or more. Usually, the child's communication system evolves over time as the child gains increasing competency.

AAC assessments should include a physical evaluation of manual dexterity, range and accuracy of movement, physical placement, oral-peripheral structure and functioning, and visual acuity. Observing hand movements in daily tasks may be more helpful than isolated movement tasks when evaluating manual dexterity. Various systems should be tried to determine those best suited to the child. It is not unusual to find children communicating via a number of AAC modes simultaneously.

Although the decision process involved in selecting or designing an AAC system for a child is a first step, the assessment does not need to be (Reichle & Karlan, 1985). A test-teach-retest model, in which the child attempts to learn various systems while being assessed, seems promising (Reichle, Piche-Cragoe, Sigafoos, & Doss, 1988).

In matching the child to an aided AAC device, the SLP considers characteristics of the device vis-à-vis the child, such as input and output, coding system, physical features of the device, language programming, and cost. For example, input can range from pointing or looking with a communication board to switch interfaces for electronic devices. Simple switches have a single function of starting or stopping an electronic scan that travels through the symbols until the child stops it on the desired symbol. These switches can be operated either by applying pressure from almost anywhere on the body or by sensing heat and movement near the switch. More complex switches allow for direct selection of symbols. Typing, a skill well beyond that of very young children, requires the most motor skill.

Unaided coding will be in the form of gestures, signs, or fingerspelling. The latter is inappropriate for a young child. Aided encoding for both communication boards and electronic devices may include, from least to most symbolic, pictures, photographs, miniatures, PICSYMS, Rebus symbols, Blissymbols, preprinted words and phrases, and/or letters. Examples are give in Figure 3.5.

Systems such as Macaw®, Voice Pal®, and DynaMo® use picture symbols and are primarily spoken output devices using digitized prerecorded speech. In contrast, other systems, such as Alpha Smart®, Link®, and LightWriter®, use letter coding and have visual output primarily, although the last two can also use synthesized speech. Finally, DynaVox/Myte®, Pathfinder®, and E-Z Keys® have both symbols and word input and have digitized or synthesized speech along with visual output. Obviously, some of these systems are beyond the abilities of very young children.

Assessment for Information Processing Deficits

As mention in Chapter 2, children with a variety of disorders exhibit difficulty processing verbal information. Although questions about cognitive functioning should be answered by a team that includes at least a neurologist, a psychologist, and an SLP, probing by the SLP can answer some questions and suggest alternative methods of intervention. Standardized testing will provide some insight but is no substitute for comprehension and production of language in real-life contexts.

Of most importance are changes in performance under varying task demands. The SLP can assess the child's performance by varying the speed of information using both familiar and unfamiliar words and structures (Ellis Weismer & Evans, 2002a). Usually there is a trade-off between accuracy and timing.

The SLP can assess memory with a variety of inputs, both verbal and nonverbal (Montgomery, 2002a). These may include digit and word tasks and nonword repetition. The length of the units to be repeated can be varied in both number and unit size, such as number of syllables.

In the classroom, the SLP can observe and assess note taking and expository writing (see Chapter 13). The SLP can read sentences to the child and have the child combine them or answer questions about the content. Longer units can be read and the child asked to identify content in the beginning, middle, and end.

Finally, the SLP should use the test-teach-retest form of dynamic assessment, the most ecologically sound manner for assessing cognitive functioning (Gillam, Hoffman, Marler, & Wynn-Dancy,

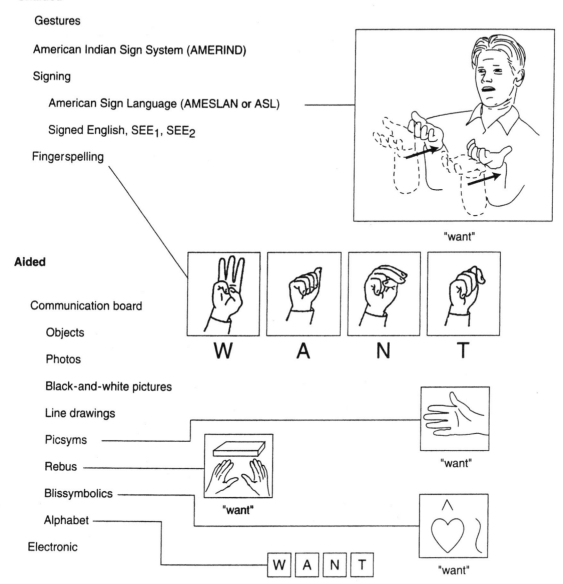

Unaided

  Gestures

  American Indian Sign System (AMERIND)

  Signing

    American Sign Language (AMESLAN or ASL)

    Signed English, SEE$_1$, SEE$_2$

  Fingerspelling

Aided

  Communication board

    Objects

    Photos

    Black-and-white pictures

    Line drawings

    Picsyms

    Rebus

    Blissymbolics

    Alphabet

  Electronic

FIGURE 3.5   Graphic and manual systems.

2002). Discussed in more detail in Chapter 4, dynamic assessment is concerned with the child's ability to learn rather than his or her level of past learning. For example, in the teaching phase, the child may be taught to identify the main idea in a paragraph or to interpret a comment, conversation, or narrative. In the retest phase, the SLP focuses on the kinds of change and the effort required. Of interest throughout are the child's ability to attend, perceive, and recall information, understand explanations, relate past information to new, infer, and generalize.

Conclusion

There is no one way to assess children with LI. A combination of interviewing, observation, testing, and sampling/probing offers a holistic approach that can incorporate not only the child but also significant others and familiar communication contexts.

4

Assessment of Children with Language Difference

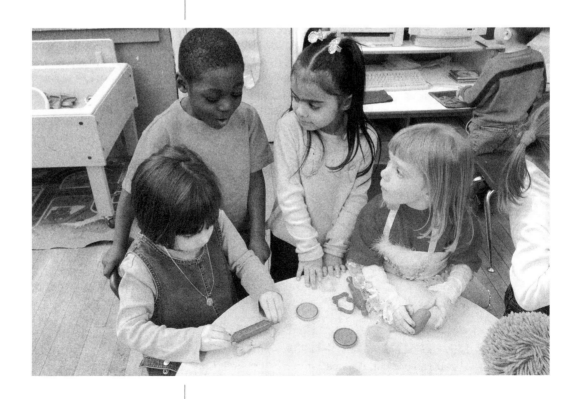

Language differences, such as dialects or the influence of a first language on a second, are not disorders. Such differences are valid rule-governed linguistic systems in and of themselves. A child learning a nonstandard dialect of American English or learning American English as a second language may also exhibit language disorders, such as LLD, SLI, or any of the others discussed in Chapter 2. The task for the SLP is to separate these natural differences from disorders.

An increasing proportion of children in U.S. schools are culturally and linguistically diverse. More than 35 million culturally linguistically diverse (CLD) speakers live in the United States. This number includes many Latino Americans and Asian Americans and some Native Americans for whom English is a second language. In addition, a portion of working-class African Americans use African American English, a dialect of American English. Nationally, approximately 7 million children speak English as a second language. In New York state, more than 130 languages are represented in the schools (Heberle, 1992).

In many large cities, more than 50 percent of the school population is CLD. Minority children have a greater dropout rate, are less successful in school, are overrepresented in programs for the disabled, and are underrepresented in programs for the gifted. The primary reason for children with limited English being referred for possible special education placement is difficulty with English (Damico, 1991b).

Unfortunately, in the United States, CLD children often live in poverty. This status can be related to a higher incidence of teen pregnancy, poor prenatal care, drug and alcohol abuse, low birth weight, poor nutrition, childhood illness and injury, and communication disorders. In addition, the demographics of immigration have changed recently to include many more immigrants from economically poor countries with poorer educations and few of the high literacy skills demanded by the changing U.S. economy (Heberle, 1992). The differences are both linguistic and cultural.

Within the CLD population is a continuum of proficiency in English (ASHA Position Paper, 1985), including bilingual English proficiency, limited English proficiency (LEP), and limited proficiency in both English and the minority language. It is important that the SLP be able to distinguish between a disorder and a difference that is the result of interaction of the native language and English. The SLP must appreciate the rule-governed nature of the native language and know its contrastive features. Elective speech and language services may be provided to individuals who are bilingual English proficient and who desire more standard production of English. It is important for the SLP to remember, however, that dialects of English that reflect the influence of the native language on English are not disorders.

Individuals who are **limited English proficient (LEP)** are proficient in their native language but not in English. Assessment and intervention should be conducted in the native language as mandated by federal law (PL 94-142 and PL 95-561), legal decisions (*Diana v. Board of Education*, 1970; *Lau v. Nichols*, 1974; and *Larry P. v. Riles*, 1972), and state educational regulations. Adequate service delivery by the SLP requires native or near-native fluency in both languages and ability to describe speech and language acquisition in both languages, to administer and interpret formal and informal assessment procedures, to apply intervention strategies in minority language, and to recognize cultural factors that affect service delivery to the CLD community (ASHA Position Paper, 1985). For the remainder of the text, we shall use the term *LEP* to refer to children learning English as their second language. Other children will be specified as needed.

Finally, those with limited proficiency in both English and the native language are truly communicatively handicapped. Language testing should establish language dominance and the most appropriate language for intervention (ASHA Position Paper, 1985). One error often made by inexperienced SLPs is to assume that the native language (L_1) is dominant. Young children may lose L_1 as they begin to acquire a second language (L_2), which in this case is American English.

State of Service Delivery

Although the demographics of the United States are changing, the overwhelming majority of SLPs will continue to belong to the majority culture for the foreseeable future (Shewan, 1988). Approximately one in three SLPs has some bilingual clients, but more than 80 percent of these professionals do not feel confident in their abilities to serve these clients (Shewan & Malm, 1989; Taylor, 1989). Inadequacies include a lack of academic preparation and experience, unfamiliarity with the language and/or culture, and a lack of appropriate assessment tools (Adler, 1991).

Lack of Preparation and Experience

Most academic programs offer little preparation for working with CLD children through either coursework or practicum. Until this deficiency changes, it is the responsibility of each SLP to educate him- or herself through continuing education. The following are some ways to interact more with culturally diverse populations:

Work alongside a bilingual speech-language pathologist as an assistant.

Take a foreign language course and/or a course in cultural diversity.

Join cultural organizations and attend cultural festivals.

Become a Big Brother or Big Sister or volunteer to work with culturally diverse youth.

Volunteer in organizations such as Habitat for Humanity.

Join organizations, such as National Coalition Builders Institute, that foster cooperation and understanding.

Join church groups that foster interactions with inner-city churches.

Go out of your way to introduce yourself to individuals from other cultures.

Each SLP should remember that when he or she enters the environment of another cultural group, he or she is a guest and should act accordingly. Members of the majority culture sometimes expect members of minority cultures to accept them with open arms. My experience has been that there is a period of adjustment in which mutual trust is built. Only then does acceptance begin to grow.

Unfamiliarity with Language and Culture

Becoming familiar with another culture and another language requires shedding many preconceived notions and becoming culturally aware. This requirement is followed by education about particular languages and cultures and about language development among CLD children. It is extremely difficult to become fluent in a second language as an adult or from classroom instruction. Therefore, one method for the SLP to use to overcome linguistic deficits is language interpreters. This alternative is discussed at the end of this section.

Growth of Awareness

All aspects of our lives are overlaid by culture. It affects our institutions and the way we act and think. **Culture** is a shared framework of meanings within which a population shapes its way of life. Culture is what one needs to know or believe to function in a manner acceptable to a particular group

(Campbell & Champion, 1996). It is neither static nor absolute, but has been shaped by the population's history and evolves as individuals constantly rework it and add new ideas and behaviors. It includes, but is not limited to, history and the explanation of natural phenomenon; societal roles; rules for interactions, decorum, and discipline; family structure; education; religious beliefs; standards of health, illness, hygiene, appearance, and dress; diet; perceptions of time and space; definitions of work and play; artistic and musical values, life expectations, and aspirations; and communication and language use. Culture interacts with language to influence cognitive and affective processes and the interpretation of behavior (Westby, 1995).

Each culture has a unique outlook. It is essential for SLPs to recognize that culture is pervasive and diffused throughout their own lives. Culture forms the basis for their values and worldviews. Therefore, culture influences the way individuals view other cultures.

SLPs from the majority culture in the United States typically have Euro-centered standards. These standards will influence each SLP's decisions about LI, although these standards may not apply to individuals from other cultures. For example, Vietnamese culture is much more tolerant of speech and language diversity than is U.S. majority culture. Likewise, the Navajo culture values a quiet, introspective persona, which may seem withdrawn by U.S. majority standards. Language differences affect much more than language form, including rules for appropriate interaction in specific contexts, awareness of content information required in different situations, appropriate structures for participation, and communication styles (Westby, 1995)

Words and concepts also are related culturally. For example, the word and the concept *crib* are not found in Korean. Table 4.1 offers other examples of cultural variants. Although SLPs cannot know all cultures, they can become increasingly culture sensitive. It is important to respect other cultures and to recognize that no one culture is the standard (N. Anderson, 1991).

Cultural sensitivity requires not only recognition of one's own culture but also examination of cultural notions held as "truths." Many traditional notions of the U.S. majority culture, especially those involving poverty and ethnicity or race, are inappropriate.

The following are guidelines for interacting with clients from different cultures (Taylor, Payne, & Anderson, 1987):

1. Each encounter is a socially situated communicative event subject to cultural rules governing such events by both participants.
2. Children perform differently under differing conditions because of their unique cultural and linguistic backgrounds.
3. Different modes, channels, and functions of communication may evidence differing levels of linguistic and communicative performance.
4. Ethnographic techniques and cultural norms should be used for evaluating behavior and making determinations of LI.
5. Possible sources of conflict in assumptions and norms should be identified prior to an interaction and action taken to prevent them from occurring.
6. Learning about culture is ongoing and should result in constant reevaluation and revision of ideas and in greater sensitivity.

This new awareness should lead to a recognition that "assessment is a subjective process that is highly influenced by the socio-political, cultural, and linguistic context" (Chamberlain & Medinos-Landurand, 1991, p. 112). In fact, to make sense of our behaviors, we must view them against the background of culture.

TABLE 4.1   Cultural variants that may influence assessment

Concept	Other Cultures*	Majority U.S. Culture
Achievement	Cooperation and group spirit. Accept status quo. Manual labor respected.	Emphasis on competition and success. Define self by accomplishments. *To the victor go the spoils.*
Age	Elders are revered. Growing old is desirable.	Youth is valued.
Communication	Respectful, avoid eye contact, loudness for anger. Silence means boredom. Nonlinguistic and paralinguistic important.	Casual, direct eye contact, loud voice acceptable. Silence means attentiveness. Emphasize verbal.
Control	Fate.	Free will.
Education	Formal for few. Entrance into mainstream society. Elders, peers, and siblings are teachers. Active, physical learning. Spontaneous, intuitive. Testing not integral.	Universal, formal, verbal. Key to social mobility. Teacher is authority. Classroom passivity rewarded. Reflective, analytical. Tests are part of learning.
Family	Extended, kinship important, more varied, elder or parent centered. Male or female dominated.	Nuclear, small, contractual partnership, child centered.
Gender/role	Males independent, pampered. Females have many home responsibilities.	Relative equality.
Individuality	Humility, anonymity, deference to group.	Individual makes own life. Stress self-reliance.
Materialism	Excessive accumulation is bad, status ascribed.	Acquisition, symbol of success and power.
Social interaction	Contact, physical closeness. Kinship more important than friends.	Noncontact, large interpartner distance. Large group of friends desired.
Time	Enjoy the present, can't change future. Little concept of wasting time. Flexible.	Governed by clock and calendar, punctual, value speed, future oriented. Time is money. Scheduled.

*No specific culture.

Source: Compiled from Chamberlain & Medinos-Landurand (1991); Goldman & McDermott (1987).

Education in Language, Culture, and Language Development

Sensitivity by SLPs is not enough. You must educate yourself about the dialects, languages, and cultures of the individuals you serve and about the process of dialect and second-language learning.

Typically, SLPs make two common errors in evaluating the language of CLD children. Either children are identified incorrectly as having a language disorder, or those with a disorder are missed. For example, African American children from rural Alabama who speak the African American English dialect common to that area continue to delete final consonants beyond the age at which middle-class European American children do (Haynes & Moran, 1989). The SLP who is unaware of this difference might conclude, incorrectly, that these children exhibit a disorder.

Cultures.   The breadth of cultural diversity is beyond the scope of this text. Suffice it to say that each SLP should become familiar with the cultures that he or she serves. Reading and observation are both essential methods of learning. The SLP must remember that cultures are not monolithic and that there is much heterogeneity, especially in the Latino American population.

Of particular importance are the child-rearing practices, family structure, attitudes toward LI and intervention, and communication style. Variants of communication style include nonlinguistic and paralinguistic characteristics, such as eye contact, facial expression, and gestures; intercommunicant space and the use of silence and laughter; pragmatic aspects, such as roles, politeness and forms of address, interruption rules, turn taking, greeting and salutations, the ordering of conversational events, and appropriate topics; and the use of humor (Fasold, 1990; Saville-Troike, 1986; Taylor, 1986b). It is best if the SLP is somewhat cautious at first, until he or she has a sense of cultural expectations.

Cultures differ in their beliefs about health, disability, and causation. A great deal of discomfort may surround disorder and intervention. Some families will be surprised by the extent of their expected role in intervention.

Dialects and Second-Language Learning.   It is not possible to learn all of the dialects or languages one might encounter, especially in large metropolitan areas. Therefore, each SLP should attempt to learn the contrastive influences between other languages and dialects and Standard American English. Common phonological, syntactic, and morphological contrasts are found in Appendix B. SLPs can learn high-usage words and forms of greeting in the language served.

Not all children with different dialects are the same. Each child's language will differ with the specific dialect spoken and the maturity of language and dialect development. Although data are limited, we know that children learning African American English, the dialect spoken by some inner-city and Southern rural African Americans, show only minimal evidences of their dialect by age 3. Earlier development is closer to the middle-class standard described in most development texts. By age 5, however, most African American English forms are being used, at least in part.

It is important for the SLP to remember that the range and frequency of dialectal forms will vary across children (Washington & Craig, 1994). Awareness and discrimination of dialects appear to increase slowly throughout elementary school while actual production gradually shifts to more standard use (Isaacs, 1996). Speaking a minority dialect does not influence the ability to comprehend the majority dialect.

Children in the United States who are bilingual Spanish-English or who use Spanish only may perform very differently even from each other (K. Wilcox & McGuinn-Aasby, 1988). These differences may reflect U.S. regional differences, country of origin, or dialectal or socioeconomic differences (M. Norris, Juarez, & Perkins, 1989).

In general, second-language learning is more difficult than first-language learning, which for most children is fairly effortless. A language assessment must distinguish between those errors that reflect this difficulty and those that represent a language impairment.

Most children are sequential bilingual learners: The first language (L_1) has reached a certain level of maturity before acquisition of the second language (L_2) begins. Sequential learning may maximize the interference between the two languages. **Interference** is the influence of one language on the learning of another. For example, the English /p/ is difficult for Arabic speakers but not for Spanish speakers. Interference in simultaneous bilingual acquisition seems to be minimal (Genesee, 1988). Children who learn L_1 at home and are not exposed to L_2 (English) until school move toward L_2 dominance in middle school, but the transition occurs earlier in comprehension than in production, suggesting interference in production (Kohnert & Bates, 2002).

The monolingual "age-stage" model of development is inappropriate when describing second-language learning (Roseberry & Connell, 1991). Likewise, rate of learning is a poor index because of the many variables that affect second-language learning.

Preschool children will have an immature L_1 when introduced to L_2 The result may be "semi-lingualism," in which the child fails to reach proficiency in either language. The child may be delayed in development of L_1 after exposure to L_2 if the second language is dominant in the culture. This situation is rarely considered in language assessments (Langdon, 1989). In general, competence in L_2 is related to the maturity of L_1. The more mature the child's use of L_1, the easier it is to learn L_2 (Jacobson, 1985).

Initially, the child in preschool may be silent for a while on exposure to L_2 and appear to have a language impairment. It takes time for the child to decipher the linguistic code (Schiff-Myers, Coury, & Perez, 1989). Older children possess metalinguistic skills that aid in this deciphering process.

School-age children exposed to L_2 may appear to have LLD. The decontextualized language of the classroom may be especially difficult. If exposure to L_2 does not occur until after age 6, it may take five to seven years to acquire age-appropriate cognitive and academic skills. The result is that in the United States many children have never fully developed L_1—often Spanish—and are deficient in academic use of English (L_2). L_1 may exhibit arrested development or be lost if it is not used, is not valued by the child, is discouraged by the parents, or is onsidered less prestigious, as in the United States.

Factors that affect L_2 competency are individual characteristics, such as intelligence; learning style; positive attitude about one's self, one's own native language, and the target language; extrovertism and a feeling of control; a lack of anxiety about L_2 learning; and home and community characteristics, such as parental and community attitudes and the level of literacy in the home. Low socioeconomic status alone is not a negative factor but may be paired with poor literacy or poor L_1 use in the home and/or little opportunity to converse one-on-one with mature L_2 users (K. Nelson, 1985).

When compared to adults learning L_2, children show a greater readiness to learn, are more perceptive of sounds, are less subject to interference from L_1, and learn through sensory activity within the immediate context (Hamayan & Damico, 1991). Adult learning is verbal and abstract, emphasizing rule learning; children form their own abstractions of the rules from context. Children tend to acquire "chunks" of language, usually high-usage phrases, with conscious rule learning becoming more important after age 9 (Hamayan & Damico, 1991). Although children usually do not learn L_2 faster or more easily than adults, they eventually outperform them (Genesee, 1987). Children are more likely to take risks.

In general, L_1 forms a foundation for the learning of L_2. What the child knows from one language is transferred to the other. This may be general knowledge about sentence construction and parts of speech or similar language processes if the languages are similar. Of course, interference also can occur, but its effects are usually minimal (Madrid & Garcia, 1985; Wolfram, 1985). A poor base in L_1 usually leads to difficulties in L_2.

Languages other than English are devalued in the United States. This is the result of racial and ethnic discrimination and has resulted in a bilingual educational policy that sends a very clear message on the relative value of English (Schiff-Myers, 1992). The result is weakened linguistic and ethnic ties. The most common educational paradigm is a transitional bilingual program in which the child receives two or three years of bilingual education prior to placement in a monolingual English classroom. The not-so-subtle message is that English is better. Long-term maintenance programs that attempt to continue use and development of L_1 are rare (Schiff-Myers, 1992). A period of even three years is insufficient for the child to attain academic proficiency in English.

It is important that the SLP recognize the process of sequential bilingual acquisition. This is a dynamic process; the child's language is changing. Performance may vary widely within and across children. Therefore, language assessments need to be tailored individually to each child (Hamayan & Damico, 1991; Hyltenstam, 1985).

Overcoming Bias in an Assessment

The goal of a communication assessment with children with LEP is to differentiate difficulties that result from experiential and cultural factors from those that are related to language impairment (Damico, 1991b). Both groups may have some language difficulties. Adolescents in need of intervention also exhibit greater difficulty expressing themselves, establishing greetings and opening and maintaining a conversation, listening to a speaker, and cueing a listener to a topic change (Brice & Montgomery, 1996).

Both cultural and linguistic factors influence performance in an assessment (Chamberlain & Medinos-Landurand, 1991). These may lead to misinterpretations and miscommunication. The SLP must be careful not to stereotype behavior and draw incorrect and unfair conclusions. For example, Latino American children may seem uncooperative and inattentive, when, in fact, their behavior signifies different concepts of time, body language, and achievement.

The SLP can avoid biasing data interpretation by asking the following questions (Damico, 1991b):

1. Are there other variables, such as limited exposure to English, infrequency of error, testing procedural mistakes, extreme test anxiety, or contextual factors, that might explain the difficulties exhibited with English?
2. Are similar problems exhibited in L_1?
3. Are the problems exhibited related to second language acquisition or dialectal differences?
4. Can the problems exhibited be explained by cross-cultural interference or related cultural phenomena?
5. Can the problems exhibited be explained by any bias effect related to personnel, materials, or procedures that occurred before, during, or after assessment?
6. Is there any systematicity or consistency to the linguistic problems exhibited that might suggest an underlying rule?

The SLP should interpret the child's performance in light of the intrinsic and extrinsic biases inherent in the assessment process. Intrinsic biases, such as knowledge needed and normative samples, are part of the test, while extrinsic biases, such as sociocultural values and attitude toward testing, reside in the child. When groups of minority children score similarly to the norming population—as on the *Communication and Symbolic Behavior Scales* (Wetherby & Prizant, 1993)—it suggests a less biased assessment device (Roberts, Medley, Swartzfager, & Neebe, 1997).

Language use patterns of both the child and the SLP and the language-learning history of the child also may influence the assessment. Communication and interactive style are culture bound.

Bias can be overcome by addressing cultural and linguistic influences in a four-step process (Chamberlain & Medinos-Landurand, 1991):

1. Recognize and identify variables that might affect the assessment.
2. Analyze tests and procedures for content and style. For example, the *Fluharty Speech and Language Screening Test* accepts an /f/ for /θ/ substitution on *teeth* as dialectal, but in New Orleans, African Americans substitute /t/ to produce *teet* (/tit/) (Campbell & Champion, 1996). In addition, simply asking children to repeat what the SLP says may go against the cultural norm. Some African American children are not expected to imitate adults.

3. Take variables into account and change procedures.
4. Teach test-taking strategies.

The SLP should be mindful that each child's level of acculturation will differ with the age of the child and the extent of exposure to both cultures.

Use of Interpreters

The accuracy of testing with children with LEP may be increased by using interpreters who speak the child's primary language (Watson, Omark, Gronell, & Heller, 1986). When an interpreter is not available, family members can aid the SLP.

CLD children—both bilingual and dialectally different—perform significantly better with familiar examiners (Fuchs & Fuchs, 1989). This finding suggests the use of interpreters familiar with both the language and the culture of the child and his or her caregivers. In addition, it suggests that consistency is important.

The SLP must recognize the limitations of the process and must select and train the interpreter carefully. They must work together as a team with mutual respect. Three factors seem critical in the use of interpreters—selection, training, and relationship to the family and community (N. Anderson, 1992; Chamberlain & Medinos-Landurand, 1991; Randall-David, 1989).

Selection

Selection should be based on the potential interpreter's linguistic competencies, ethical and professional competencies, and general knowledge and personality (Chamberlain & Medinos-Landurand, 1991). An interpreter should possess a high degree of proficiency in both L_1 and English, be able to paraphrase well, be flexible, and have a working knowledge of developmental, educational, and communication terminology.

Ethical and professional competencies should include an ability to maintain confidentiality, a respect for the feelings and beliefs of others and for the roles of professionals, and an ability to maintain impartiality. Confidentiality is especially important if the interpreter is a resident of the immediate geographic area served.

Finally, it is very desirable for the potential interpreter to have a knowledge of child development and educational procedures. Personal attributes include flexibility, trustworthiness, patience, an eye for detail, and a good memory.

Training

Training must include the critical factors of assessment and intervention, including procedures and instruments (N. Anderson, 1992). The interpreter must understand the importance of exact translation from L_1 to L_2 and the reverse.

Preassessment training includes the requirements of a thorough assessment and the specific test protocols, including technical language. Rapport-building strategies and questioning techniques also should be taught.

Prior to each evaluation of a child's language, the SLP and the interpreter should review each case and the assessment procedures; practice pronunciation of the name, introductions, questioning, and nonlinguistic aspects of the interaction; and discuss the topics to be introduced. During the evaluation, the interpreter can interact with the child and caregiver(s) while the SLP records the data and directs the process. In the postassessment interview with caregivers, the interpreter will convey the results of the evaluation as they are reported by the SLP.

Relationship with Family and Community
Prior to the assessment, the interpreter should try to get to know the caregiver(s) and child. It is very important that the interpreter convey the confidentiality of the proceedings, especially if the interpreter is from the community. During the assessment, the interpreter is to translate exactly. The SLP can aid this process by keeping interactional language simple and use of professional jargon to a minimum. It is the interpreter's responsibility to ensure that the caregivers thoroughly understand the process and the results and recommendations.

Conclusion
Working through interpreters is difficult and does not address some of the other problems in assessment with children with LEP. The following list contains suggestions for working successfully with an interpreter (Lynch & Hanson, 1992; Randall-David, 1989). The SLP should:

1. Meet regularly and keep communication open and the goals understood.
2. Have the interpreter meet with the child and caregiver(s) prior to an interview to establish rapport and to determine their educational level, attitudes, and feelings.
3. Learn proper protocols and forms of address in the native language.
4. Introduce himself or herself to the family, describe roles, and explain the purpose and process of the assessment.
5. Speak more slowly and in short units, but not more loudly.
6. Avoid colloquialisms, abstractions, idiomatic expressions, metaphors, slang, and professional jargon.
7. Look directly at the child and caregiver(s), not at the interpreter. Address remarks to the caregiver(s).
8. Listen to the child and caregivers to glean nonlinguistic and paralinguistic information. What is not said may be as important as what is said.
9. Avoid body language or gestures that may be misunderstood.
10. Use a positive tone that conveys respect and interest.
11. Avoid oversimplification and condescension.
12. Give simple clear instructions and periodically check the family's and child's understanding.
13. Instruct the interpreter to translate the client's words without paraphrasing.
14. Instruct the interpreter to avoid inserting her or his own word or ideas in the translation or omitting information.
15. Be patient with the longer process inherent in translation.

Although these suggestions will not ensure success, they may lessen some friction that potentially could disrupt effective delivery of services.

Lack of Appropriate Assessment Tools

We can expect the performance of CLD children on formal tests to be affected by cultural differences. Negative listener or tester attitudes also affect children, causing poor performance. The result is lower expectations and inappropriate referral or classification (Cummins, 1986).

Few nonbiased standardized language tests are available for evaluating CLD children (Bernstein, 1989). Tests are typically unique to one culture or language. Spanish versions of most tests fail to consider dialectal differences and are normed on monolingual children. In two judicial decisions regarding placement of Mexican American and African American children in classes for the retarded (*Diana v. State Board of Education,* 1991; *Larry P. v. Riles,* 1984), the courts ruled that judgments made on the basis of responses to tests whose norming populations are inappropriate for these children are discriminatory.

Many of the tests widely used in speech-language pathology are normed on population samples with a disproportionately high number of middle-class, European American, English-only children. Tests may yield lower scores for lower socioeconomic groups and for African American children. Some test items may be culturally biased against certain children. A critical need exists for nonbiased language testing for children of color, especially those from lower socioeconomic backgrounds (Rhyner, Kelly, Brantley, & Krueger, 1999).

In general, poor performance leads to lower expectations (Adler, 1990). It is inappropriate to compare children with LEP to native speakers of English. The use of chronological norms is especially questionable, given the great variety in developmental rate among CLD populations (Seymour, 1992). The child with LEP does not have language similar to a native speaker of English of a certain age. The problem becomes deciding what standard to use (Lahey, 1992).

The following five guidelines should be considered prior to using standardized tests with CLD children (Musselwhite, 1983):

1. What is the relationship of the norming population and the client? Are enough minority children included to give a fair representation? Are separate norms used for different minority groups?
2. What is the relationship of the child's experience and the content areas of the test? Items using farm content, for example, may have little relevance for children in the inner city.
3. What is the relationship of the language and/or dialect being tested and the child's language and/or dialect dominance? This issue is critical in determining language impairment. The determining factor should be the child's ability to function within her or his own linguistic or dialectal community (Iglesias, 1986).
4. Will the language of the test penalize a nonstandard child by use of idiomatic or metaphoric language?
5. Is the child penalized for a particular pattern of learning or style of problem solving?

All is not lost. American English standardized tests can be used with modified procedures to enhance performance. Modifications may aid the SLP in describing the child's language and communication skills. Obviously, the scores from such testing would be invalid. If reported, the scores must be qualified by a description of the modified procedures.

Dual sets of norms—those from the test and locally prepared ones—can be used to compare the performance of CLD children to that of the standard group and of their peer group (Musselwhite, 1983), but they must be used cautiously (Seymour, 1992). The test still may be in Standard American English. It seems more appropriate to measure the child's performance in his or her dialect and compare this performance to that of other children also using that dialect (Seymour, 1992). Unfortunately, we have very little data on this development and even fewer tests.

Parents, who presumably speak the same dialect, may be used as referents when very little normative data are available (Terrell, Arensberg, & Rosa, 1992). A language test can be given to both the parent and the child. Once enough data has been gathered, the SLP can compare the child's performance with that of the adult. Assuming the adult has no language impairment, child use that reflects parent use but that differs from Standard American English would represent a dialectal difference, not a disorder. For example, omission of final plosives found in African American English would result in omission of the regular past tense marker *-ed*. Just testing the child, the SLP might assume that the child does not have past tense. Parental omission would confirm a dialectal difference.

Some tests have been normed on population samples from different languages, such as children speaking English and Spanish, by using English and a Spanish translation. Results of translated tests must be used very cautiously because they assess structures important for speakers of English and ignore those of the other language. For example, *hitting* something with a stick in English is *sticking* in some Spanish dialects, but that verb is not used with other types of hitting.

The standardized norms from such translated tests could be used to identify children with language differences. Children who exhibit LI relative to their peer group, could be identified by use of the peer group norms.

Even this procedure may bias some results, given the diversity of some populations, such as Latinos. Norms for all speakers of a language fail to consider dialectal variations. Other variables, such as socioeconomic status, family grouping, length of time exposed to English, and quality of L_1 used at home, affect the child's performance. Locally prepared norms may be more appropriate.

The differences found between majority and minority children on knowledge-based tests are not found on process-based evaluations (Campbell, Dollaghan, Needleman & Janosky, 1997). Process-based tests can be useful in distinguishing LI from experiential difference. Processes are the mental operations required to manipulate linguistic material. Testing might include such tasks as nonword vocal repetition, completion of two language tasks simultaneously, and following directions. To ensure that past learning is minimized, tasks should be completely novel, and task-related vocabulary and grammar should be familiar or, if not, reviewed prior to testing.

An Integrated Model for Assessment

Current methodology in language assessment has been described as a "discrete point approach" (Acevedo, 1986; Mattes & Omark, 1984) in which language is treated as an autonomous cognitive ability divided into many components (Damico, 1991b). Language is not viewed as holistic; rather, it is separate from environmental variables and context. We addressed this issue in the previous chapter.

It is not surprising that several SLPs have suggested an integrated approach for CLD children, one that uses the child's natural environment and that depends on descriptive analysis, rather than on normative test scores. Language and communication are not static, divisible, and autonomous, but dynamic, synergistic, and integrative (Damico, 1991b). Such an assessment would focus on the functional aspects of language and on flexibility of use.

The overall question would be: "Is this child an effective communicator in his or her context?" The criterion is not norm referenced, but "communication referenced" (Bloom & Lahey, 1978), with the SLP determining the indices of proficiency. Data could be collected in natural settings (Iglesias, 1986) as the child converses with his or her natural conversational partners, parents, teachers, and peers.

Assessment would begin with data gathering. This collection process might include screening all children for other-than-English and for nonstandard dialectal use. This step could be followed by referral information from classroom teachers on children experiencing academic difficulty (Chamberlain & Medinos-Landurand, 1991). Early intervention may prevent difficulties or inappropriate classification later (Garcia & Ortiz, 1988). A teacher checklist of the child's language functions, a questionnaire, and/or caregiver interview might follow. Parents can also be a source of information. Not surprisingly, Spanish-speaking parents are as accurate in reporting the expressive vocabulary and grammar of their toddlers as monolingual English-speaking parents (Thal, Jackson-Maldonado, & Acosta, 2000). Parental reports of bilingual children's vocabulary and word combinations are consistent with sampling findings (Patterson, 2000).

In addition to verifying demographic information, the SLP should observe the child in the classroom and with peers and caregivers. Of interest is the child's language use, academic strengths and weaknesses, and learning style.

Data collection and observation would be followed by testing and language sampling. Sampling should include a wide variety of settings and activities to increase the accuracy of the language sample collected (Bernstein, 1989). Parents can be trained to listen to their child, observe language use, and discuss linguistic interactions. Appendix C provides a form for reporting the myriad data essential to a fair, unbiased evaluation of CLD children.

Children with LEP

The data collection stage is particularly important with children with LEP. Many variables affect second-language development and are of interest. In addition, seemingly simple information such as age—Is the child age 1 at birth or a year later?—is culturally dependent and can greatly affect determinations of impairment.

Considerations for children with LEP include the degree of exposure to English-speaking peers, self-esteem, personality (introverted vs. extraverted), motivation to learn English, family attitude toward English, ethnic community's view of education, the socioeconomic status of the family and of English-speaking peers, and the process of learning a second language (Roseberry-McKibben, 1994). The same child may appear very different depending on the stage of second-language development.

Four measures may be especially important in discriminating predominantly Spanish-speaking children with LI from those developing typically (Restrepo, 1998). These are parental reporting, a family history of speech and language problems, the number of errors per T-unit, and the mean length of T-units. A T-unit is a main clause and phrasal or clausal embedding attached to it. T-units will be discussed in more detail in Chapter 7.

Language assessments should occur where the child and the caregivers are most comfortable, such as the home. Parents, especially recent immigrants, may speak little or no English. A properly trained interpreter can be very helpful in obtaining needed information. Occasionally, older siblings have sufficient English skills to answer questions or to translate for their parents. Table 4.2 contains possible questions to be asked in an interview.

Observation should occur in several settings with different conversational partners, topics, and activities. This tactic will give the SLP some idea of the extent of bilingualism and possible language and communication difficulties.

The languages used in testing and the manner of their presentation differ with each child and the purpose of the evaluation. It is important to establish the primary language, language dominance, and language proficiency in both languages. Testing in both L_1 and English seems essential for assessment of language impairment. In fact, federal law requires bilingual testing before such determinations are made. Successive testing in the stronger language, followed by the weaker, results in the best performance, especially for young children with monolingual L_1 homes (Krashen & Biber, 1988), although simultaneous testing may be best for children who exhibit poor competence in both languages or who speak a combined L_1-L_2 language, such as "Spanglish" (Cummins, 1986).

TABLE 4.2   Interview questions for children with LEP or children with different dialects

Demographic
    How long has the family been in the United States?
    In which country were the parents born?
    From which country did the family immigrate?
    How much contact does the family have with their native country?
  * How long has the family been in this community?
    Is the family connected to a large community from their native country?
    Is there any plan to return to the native land to live?

Family
  * How old is the child?
  * Which family members live in the household? Number of siblings?
  * Are other individuals living in the household?
    In what cultural activities does the family participate?
  * Who is primarily responsible for the child? (Primary caregiver?)
  * Who else participates in caregiving?
  * Approximately how much time do the child and caregiver spend together on a typical day?
  * With whom does the child play at home?
  * How much education do family members have? In what language?

Childrearing
  * Are there scheduled meals?
  * What types of foods usually are eaten?
  * Is there an established bedtime?
  * Does the child misbehave? How? How is the child disciplined? Who disciplines?
    Are any television shows (radio shows, videos) in the native language? If so, how often does the child watch such shows?
  * Are stories read or told to the child? If so, in what language? How often?
  * Are there books, magazines, or newspapers in the home? In what language?
  * At what age did the child begin school?
  * Has the child attended school regularly?
  * How many schools has the child attended?
    What language has been used in the classroom?

Attitudes and perceptions
  * Is blame assigned for the child's problems or condition? To whom or what?
  * How does the family view intervention? Is there a feeling of helplessness?
    How does the family view Western medical practices and practitioners?
    Who is the primary provider of medical assistance and information?
  * From whom does the family seek assistance (organizations and individuals)?
  * What are the general feelings of the family when seeking assistance?
  * Does one family member act as the family spokesperson when seeking assistance?
  * How is the child expected to act toward parents, teachers, or other adults? Adults toward the child? Are there any restrictions or prohibitions, such as the child not making eye contact or not asking questions?
  * How important are English language skills?

Language and communication
    What language is spoken in the home? Between adults? Between caregivers and the child? Between the children? When playing with neighborhood friends? Other caregivers and the child?
    How much English is used in the home?
    What language is used in community activities, such as church, Girl Scouts, and team sports?
    At what age did the child begin to learn English? Where and how?
  * At what age did the child say the first word? Use two-word utterances?

*Applicable to both LEP and dialectally different children.

Source: Compiled from N. Anderson (1991); Chamberlain & Medinos-Landurand (1991); Mattes & Omark (1984); Schiff-Myers (1992); Wayman, Lynch, & Hanson (1990).

Normative testing should be supplemented by probing. CLD children score lower on knowledge-based testing, such as that found in normative procedures, but the same on process-based assessments, such as comprehension and production of real conversations (Campbell, Dollaghan, Needleman, & Janosky, 1997). **Dynamic assessment** tasks are more appropriate and de-emphasize grammar in favor of ability to communicate and learn (Butler, 1993; Damico, 1991b). Tasks are interactive, focused on learning, and yield information on learner responsiveness (Gillam, Peña, & Miller, 1999).

Within a dynamic assessment, the SLP is interested in the child's ability to respond to learning experiences and to change her or his behavior. The three primary methods are "testing the limits," graduated prompting, and test-teach-retest (Gutierrez-Clellan, & Peña, 2001). In testing the limits (Carlson & Wiedl, 1992), the SLP probes behind a child's response using elaborative feedback and verbal explanations by the child to determine his or her understanding of the task and the way in which he or she arrived at the response. For example, the child may have interpreted the word *buoyancy* as *boy-in-seat* (Peña, 2002).

Graduated prompting is a method of probing the child's readiness for learning. By subtly manipulating the prompts given to the child, the SLP determines the level of support needed by the child in order to be successful. In essence, the SLP is trying to bridge the gap between what the child knows and the requirements of the task.

In a test-teach-retest format, the SLP becomes an active agent of change. Focusing on "how" rather than "what" children learn, language-neutral dynamic tasks can provide a nonbiased assessment (Lidz & Pena, 1996). The initial test establishes a baseline measure, then during teaching the SLP supports learning and discovers how modifiable the child is and how the child responds to adult support. The method of teaching called *mediated learning experience* (MLE) is an individualized approach to the response and strategies used by the child and includes explaining the importance of the learning and giving evaluative feedback (Pena, 2002). An example of MLE is presented in Table 4.3. In retesting, or posttesting, children with LI usually demonstrate little change (Pena, Iglesias, & Lidz, 2001).

The SLP is also interested in the way in which a child thinks that results in the answers the child gives. This requires probing of the child's responses.

One method of testing or probing that circumvents the SLP's inability to speak the native language and the affects of delayed English acquisition is the *invented rule* (Connell, 1987c; Roseberry & Connell, 1991). For example, an invented rule might state that /i/ is added to a noun to mean a portion of that noun, as in book and book-/i/. This procedure can be taught through modeling and can be tested with novel objects. Modeling would be a two-step process:

"This is X, X," as the speech-language pathologist points.

"This is X-/i/, X-/i/," as the speech-pathologist points.

This would be repeated several times with a few items as the child repeats the SLP's production of the noun and the noun plus /i/. Testing would follow a cloze procedure:

"This is Y, Y. This is ___."

Again the SLP would point to pictures illustrating the meaning. Of interest is whether the child can abstract a language rule and then apply it to novel situations, certainly an important skill for language learning.

TABLE 4.3   Examples of Mediated Language Experiences (MLE)

Introduction

Today we're going to play with some special toys and use them in special ways. While we're using the toys, we'll think about the actions we do with each and the different names we use. Now, what are we going to be talking about? [Child response]

Um-hm, and why do you think it would be important to be able to name the different actions that we can do? [Child response]

Good, so we can explain our actions to other people. Can you think of anything else? [No response]

Do you ever ask for some help from your mother? [Child response]

And…[Child response]

Yes, of course, we can use actions to ask others to help us. Suppose I called your mother and said, "Dad!" [Child response]

You're right, it would be the wrong name. To help people understand us, we call things by their right name. I know that you have a dog. What's his name? [Child response]

Okay, if I called him something else, would he answer? [Child response]

No. So names are important. We call actions by their right name too. I have a whole box full of different objects. Some tell us what we do with them. Here's one your mother uses. It's called an iron. And what do we do with it? [Child response]

Right, we iron, we iron clothes. That was a hard one. How should we name the actions that go with each object? [No response] Would it help to name the object? [Child response]

Okay, let's begin that way. Suppose that you know the name of the object but not the name of the action? [Child response]

Well, I could tell you but can you think of a way to show me what you know? [Child response]

Good, you could show me by doing the action. Then together we can figure out the name of the action, maybe from the object used or their might be other ways to remember…. [Lesson continues]

Within lesson

Now we've named all the actions. Some objects have more than one. Let's try something else. You name the action and I'll name the object. Only one rule, you cannot repeat an action. If you can't think of the action, act it out and I'll try to help…. [Continues]

Do you know how to play Simon Says? [No response] Well, in this game you get to be the queen and you tell me what to do. Let's use your name: "Catalina says, 'Eat!'" [SLP pretends to eat in a very sloppy manner. Child laughs.] Now you try one…. [Continues]

Wow, that was fun. What a busy queen you are! Look at this. I have a book full of actions. Let's see if we can describe what's happening in the book…. [Continues]

Conclusion

You worked really hard today. Do you remember what we learned? [Child response]

Why are action names important? [Child response]

And what did you do when you couldn't think of the action word? [Child response]

Naturally, the same picture of objects would not be used for both testing and training to enable the SLP to assess learning and generalization. Possible pictures to be used for testing or training are presented in Figure 4.1. For example, the SLP says, "This is clock; this is ___ (clocky)."

Structured tasks designed by the insightful SLP can also provide more flexibility than standardized tests and may be effective assessment vehicles (R. T. Anderson, 1996). Table 4.4 is an example of a structured format that has been used effectively with Spanish-speaking 4-year-olds.

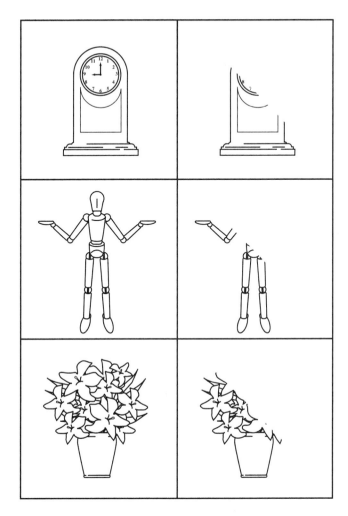

**FIGURE 4.1   Possible format for invented rule
assessment.**

Language samples are also useful but are not guaranteed to be nonbiased. All interactions are culturally based and have the potential of biasing results against the child. Members of the community or family should aid the SLP in analyzing the child's language sample.

Sampling should reflect an "authentic assessment" (Udvari & Thousand, 1995) that reflects the realistic demands of the CLD child's communication contexts, such as the classroom. In this setting, a sample should reflect the contextual, performance, and instructional constraints of the situation (Rosin & Gill, 1997). The child can then be measured against the minimal competency needed to function within that context (Stockman, 1996). Authentic assessment is a clear example of the functional assessment methods described in this text.

TABLE 4.4   Script for structures task

A. Negatives

Materials	Prompt
1. broken doll	**1.** Ask child to show body part that is missing. (¿Dónde está _____?)
2. car with wheels missing	**2.** ¿Qué le pasa al carro?
3. small box/large object	**3.** Pon (object) en la caja.
4. empty box	**4.** Busca _____ en la caja.
5. box that will not open	**5.** Abre la caja, por favor.

B. Verbs: third-person singular and plural—past and present progressive

Materials: family, house, and furniture

Perform the following actions with one family member (singular) and with more than one family member (plural).
   1. dormir
   2. comer
   3. cocinar
   4. saltar/brincar
   5. bañar(se)/lavar(se)

Verbal prompts:
   Ahora vamos a (action).
   1. past tense—Yo (action—past tense). ¿Qué hizo/hicieron?
   2. present progressive—A mí me gusta (action) y a él/ella/ellos también.

   ¿Qué está pasando?

C. Verbs: third-person present indicative

Materials: doll house and dolls

Prompts: While playing with the dolls, talk about different things that people do, such as "Las mamás cocinan; los niños corren." Then ask:
   1. ¿Qué hacen las mamás?
   2. ¿Qué hacen los niños?
   3. ¿Qué hacen las maestras?
   4. ¿Qué hacen los pájaros?
   5. ¿Qué hacen los perros?

D. Copula "ser"

Prompt: Provide incorrect information when identifying objects. Use the furniture and the dolls for prompting. For example, say that the mother doll is the father doll and insist on it. Repeat this with the following:
   1. mother/father
   2. table/chair
   3. bathroom/kitchen
   4. car/airplane
   5. cat/dog

E. Locatives (sobre/en/encima, debajo/abajo, detrás/atrás)

Prompt: Play hide and seek with a variety of objects (doll house) and ask the child where the objects are.

F. Plural, third-person subject pronouns and possessive constructions
Prompt: Game of Who has _____? Whose is _____? and What does _____ have?

Plural:
Prompt: Qué tienes/tengo?

/s/ morpheme	/es/ morpheme
carro	botón
plato	lápiz
taza/vaso	papel
mesa	avión
silla	tenedor

Third-person pronoun:
Prompt: Male and female dolls will participate as third-person referents in game: ¿Quién tiene (object)?

Possessive construction:
Prompt: Using male and female dolls, ask: ¿De quién es (object)?

Source: Anderson, R. T. (1996). Assessing the grammar of Spanish-speaking children: A comparison of two procedures. *Language, Speech, and Hearing Services in Schools, 27,* 333–344. Reprinted with permission.

Children with Different Dialects

Naturally, the SLP will want to gather similar data about the child with a minority dialect. Possible interview questions are contained in Table 4.2. Observation and testing are similarly important.

Family and community members can aid the SLP in assessing performance, especially in the language sample (Bleile & Wallach, 1992; T. Campbell & Dollaghan, 1992). In one study, African American Head Start teachers were asked to judge children with poor speech and those with typically developing speech (Bleile & Wallach, 1992). The poor-speech samples were analyzed and a set of community standards derived.

Similar but more stringent *social validation* has been accomplished by using direct magnitude estimates (DME) of subjective judgments. In DME, stimuli are scaled by assigning numerical values to them on the basis of their relative magnitude along some continuum. Each child's language speech sample is rated against a standard, the language of a child with no language impairment. If raters listen to several children and score them against a taped standard, they can begin to form a continuum of performance. For stability of scoring, at least ten listeners are required. Performance of a single child can be compared over time to measure improvements and can be compared with others by using the same dialect to assess overall performance.

Obviously, child-centered sampling has the potential of reducing the impact of biases found in testing. Performance will vary across different language tasks. For example, 4- to 6-year-old speakers of African American English (AAE) use more AAE forms on picture description tasks than in free play (Washington, Craig, & Kushmaul, 1998). Because even heavily dialectal speakers use dialectal forms on only about 20 percent of words, sample analysis should focus on nondialectal components (Craig & Washington, 2002). The shared features of AAE and Standard American English may be more diagnostically important in assessing language impairment among African American children speaking AAE (Seymour, Bland-Stewart, & Green, 1998).

Summary

Despite the incredible difficulties inherent in assessing CLD children, there is hope. The same integrated, functional methodology proposed for native speakers of English can be used with some modifications with these children as well. With sensitivity, unbiased administration of testing, and sampling within the everyday context of the child, a fair and meaningful assessment can be accomplished.

Conclusion

Unfortunately, sometimes a battery of readily available tests, given to every child regardless of possible language impairment, passes for thorough assessment. As with intervention, assessment procedures must be designed for the individual client. Standardized tests are only a portion of this process. Language tests are aids to the SLP and cannot substitute for the informed clinician.

A thorough assessment includes a variety of procedures designed to heighten awareness of the problem and enables the SLP to delineate more clearly the language abilities and impairments of the child. For training to be truly functional, a thorough description of the child and the child's language must be made.

5

Language Sampling

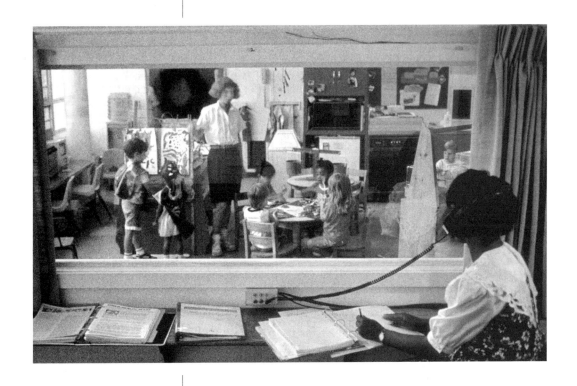

The testing context is a noncommunication one. Although tests are good for assessing global change, they miss many small or subtle behaviors. Language sampling provides more specific information for planning intervention because it includes both the content and context of language use. If the goal of language intervention is generalization to the language used by the child in everyday situations, it is essential that the SLP collect a language sample that is a good reflection of that language in actual use.

It is important that some portion of the sampling be accomplished in real communication situations (Olswang, Coggins, & Timler, 2001). In general, processing demands in contrived situations are fewer than in real-life interactions. With the increased demands and multiple cues of natural situations, the language performance of many children with LI will deteriorate. As demands increase, the cognitive and linguistic resources available to process them change. Within real communication, the variables include the structure of the interaction, the number of individuals involved, distractions, and the immediacy and complexity of the language being received and produced. If we are going to program for use within the child's natural communication contexts, then we must assess within those same contexts.

Good language samples do not just occur. They are the result of careful planning and execution. The SLP can design the assessment session so that the context fits the purpose of collecting the desired sample. The result is usually a combination of free conversation sampling and some evocative techniques.

The SLP must make several decisions before collecting the sample. After studying the interview, observational, and testing results, decisions must be made relative to the context, participants, materials, and conversational techniques to be used. It should be remembered that "there is no way to 'make' children talk…[the SLP] can only make them want to talk by creating a situation in which there is a reason to talk and an atmosphere that conveys the message that…[the SLP is] interested in what they have to say" (Lund & Duchan, 1993, p. 23). In this chapter, we cover the planning, collection, recording, and transcription of conversational samples.

Planning and Collecting a Representative Sample

Several issues are of importance when planning and collecting a language sample. Among the most prominent are the representativeness of the sample and the effect of conversational context. In addition, collection of several language forms and functions may require the use of evocative techniques. All of these issues are important for children with language impairments and also for CLD children.

Representativeness

Representativeness can be addressed by ensuring spontaneity and by collecting samples under a variety of conditions. Spontaneity can be achieved if the child and the conversational partner engage in real conversations on topics of interest to the child. To ensure spontaneity, the SLP can follow the (LCC)[3] formula for (a) *less clinician control,* (b) *less clinician contrivance,* and (c) *a less conscious child* (Cochrane, 1983).

The SLP's control of the context should be weak so as not to restrict the child's linguistic output in quantity or quality. Although there is some indication that SLP style has little effect on gross measures, such as MLU and Developmental Sentence scores, more subtle measures may be affected to a greater degree. Control devices, such as the use of questions and selection of topics, may cause the child to adopt a passive conversational role.

Not all children will participate freely in such exchanges and other, more structured approaches may be required. In general, the SLP can elicit longer and more complex language from young children with picture interpretation tasks than with imperatives or story recapitulation. In storytelling, the use of pictures can enhance the length and complexity of the sample, especially if the SLP gives cues, such as "Tell me a story about this picture. Begin with 'Once upon a time.'" The least spontaneous condition involves the specific linguistic tasks of answering questions or completing sentences. The effects of each technique will vary with each child. The SLP can relinquish some control by placing these tasks within a less formal or play format.

The sample will be less contrived if the SLP follows the child's lead and adopts the child's topics for conversation. More contrived situations, such as "Tell me about this picture" or "Explain the rules of Monopoly," do not elicit spontaneous everyday speech. The most contrived situation occurs when the SLP relies on a tried-and-true, never-fail list of standard questions.

Finally, if the child is less conscious of the process of producing language, the sample will be more spontaneous. Asking the child to produce sentences containing certain elements, for example, makes the linguistic process very conscious and may be very difficult, especially out of context. Although a child may not be able to produce a sentence with *has been* on demand, the same child may be able to relate the story of the three bears with "Someone *has been* sleeping in my bed." The former task requires metalinguistic or abstract linguistic skills that may be beyond the child's abilities.

The child's caregivers can offer suggestions to the SLP on contexts to help obtain a representative sample. It may be desirable for caregivers to serve as partners, especially with young children. After the sample has been collected, caregivers can review the data and comment on the typicality of the child's behavior.

A Variety of Language Contexts

The sampling environment can contribute to representativeness if there is a variety of contexts, including various settings, tasks, partners, and topics. Context is dynamic and complex, and the effects are very individualistic. One child may respond well to a certain toy and partner, while another child does not. Yet, the effect of context may be considered rarely in language assessment. Contextual variables include the task or purpose of the activity, the opportunities to use language, the extent of ritualization in the event, the amount of joint attending, and the responsivity of the partner (Coggins, 1991).

The task itself, as previously noted, can affect both the number and length of the conversational interactions (Conti-Ramsden & Friel-Patti, 1987). For example, young children are more referential, attempting to focus the listener's attention in free play and are more information seeking in book activities (Jones & Adamson, 1987). Similarly, parents are influenced by context and engage in more conversation when playing with dolls than they do with cars and trucks (O'Brien & Nagel, 1987).

The opportunities to use language will vary and may need to be provided. Although elicitation tasks may work for older children, they may not be effective with toddlers (Coggins, Olswang, & Guthrie, 1987).

Two aspects of context are structure and predictability (Bain, Olswang, & Johnson, 1992). *Structure* is the amount of adult manipulating of materials and evoking of particular utterances. *Predictability* is the familiarity of the overall task and materials. In general, children will produce a greater frequency and diversity of language features in low-structure situations and more new features in predictable ones (Bain et al., 1992). Free-play sampling contexts have both low structure and predictability. Possibly in such low-structure contexts, children assume that the adult knows very little about the situation. In restrictive, planned contexts, children may assume that the adult knows more, and thus the children say less.

Routinized events or routines provide mutually understood and conventionalized interactions. In routines, the partner provides order for the child, who, in turn, depends on the partner's cuing. This informal, predictable structuring allows for the child's maximum participation by providing scripts (Platt & Coggins, 1990). **Scripts** are linguistic and nonlinguistic patterns that accompany routines, such as "How are you?—Fine, thanks. How are you?" Scripts reduce the amount of cognitive energy required for the child to participate. In general, children produce fewer topics and fewer contingent utterances in "low-script" or unfamiliar contexts (Conti-Ramsden & Friel-Patti, 1987).

An attentive, responsive partner will elicit more language from the child. In joint, or shared, attention situations, children produce more extended conversation and are best able to determine the meanings and intentions of the partner (Snow, Perlman, & Nathan, 1987; Tomasello & Farrar, 1986). Similarly, timely responses by the partner increase the child's understanding. There may be as little as a one-second interval after a young child's utterance when he or she can perceive the contingency of the partner's following utterance.

As stated, the child's performance will vary with the amount of contextual support. This variability is important in considering intervention targets and methods (Coggins & Olswang, 1987; Olswang, Bain, & Johnson, 1990).

Variety ensures that the sample will not be gathered in one atypical situation. Instead, variety can reflect a sampling of the many interactional situations in which the child functions. Although variety is desirable, it is not always practical, especially in the public school setting. Audiotapes collected by the parent or teacher can provide an acceptable substitute.

Settings and Tasks

The best context is a meaningful activity containing a variety of elicitation tasks. In general, the child who is more familiar with the situation will give the most representative sample.

As mentioned, familiar routines provide a linguistic and/or nonlinguistic script that guides the child's behavior. For young children, play with familiar toys and partners is one of these routine situations. Language is a natural part of many routine events.

The SLP needs to decide whether the child's typical or optimal production is desired. For example, storytelling without picture cues yields a large MLU from preschoolers but does not elicit the quantity of language associated with picture interpretation or explanation tasks. This decision on type of production is critical because children with LI often perform below their linguistic knowledge level.

Settings should not be too contrived. Familiar, meaningful situations with a variety of age-appropriate and motivating activities provide greater variety and thus are more representative. Good settings for preschoolers include the free play mentioned earlier, snack time, and show-and-tell. School-age children can be sampled during group activities, class presentations, conversations with peers, and field trips. Generally, the child involved in some activity produces more language than the child who is watching others or conversing about pictures. It is better if the sample consists of two different settings in which different activities are occurring.

The challenge for the SLP is to find a collection technique that strikes a balance. Too highly structured methods often are not representative (Fujiki & Brinton, 1987). Free play, although low in structure, may be time-consuming and result in variable unreliable data. It has been suggested that for older children, an interview technique is an effective alternative (Dollaghan, Campbell, & Tomlin, 1990). For 8- to 9-year-old children with SLI the interview technique yields more and longer utterances, more complex language forms, more temporal adjacency and semantic contingency, and more reliable, less variable results than free play (Craig & Evans, 1992).

Conversational sampling should be authentic and functional (Damico, 1993). Authenticity comes from the use of real communication contexts in which the participants convey real information (Crystal, 1987; Damico, Secord, & Wiig, 1992; Douglas & Selinker, 1985). Functional sampling is most concerned with the success of the child as a communicator. Success can be measured by effectiveness in transmitting meanings, fluency or timeliness, and appropriateness of the message form and style in context (Damico, 1991a; Kovarsky, 1992).

The materials used should be interesting, age appropriate, and capable of eliciting the type of language desired. Interest can be piqued if the child is allowed to choose from a preselected group of toys or objects. Parents also can bring the child's toys from home in order to increase the validity of the sample.

If certain language features are desired, the SLP must increase the probability of their occurrence. With school-age children, discussion, rather than conversations based on pictures or toys in context, yields more mature language as measured by clause structure complexity, the ratio of hesitations to words, and grammatical and phonemic accuracy (Masterson & Kamhi, 1991).

The selection of clinical materials can affect the pragmatic performance of young children by modifying the physical context in which the sample is collected (Wanska, Bedrosian, & Pohlman, 1986). This selection is especially important, given the current emphasis on the use of play in pragmatic assessment and intervention. When no toys are present, children are more likely to initiate memory-related topics (Bedrosian & Willis, 1987).

In general, children around age 2 respond well to blocks, dishes, pull and wind-up toys, and dolls. Children around age 3 prefer books, clothes, puppets, and such toys as a barn with animals or a street with houses and stores. These toys encourage role-playing and language production. Kindergarten and early elementary school children respond best to toys with many pieces and to puppets and action figures. Finally, older children usually converse without the use of objects and can be encouraged to talk about themselves and their interests or to provide narratives. Narratives, a special type of language production, are discussed in Chapter 8.

The SLP should consider the nature of the toys to be used in a play assessment (Wanska et al., 1986). For example, toys with construction properties, such as Legos, Play Doh, or clay, might be used to determine whether the child can remove the conversation from the present. Such toys are more likely to elicit more displaced topics, especially as objects are being constructed (R. S. Chapman, 1981).

On the other hand, toys that encourage role-play might be used to elicit more verbalizations or vocalizations for objects, events, and actions. Compared with construction-type toys, a toy hospital elicits more discussion of the here and now and more fantasy topics and is more conducive to sociodramatic play and verbal representations of events and actions (Wanska et al., 1986).

Toys also may assist in eliciting specific linguistic structures. For example, children are more likely to produce spatial terms in play with objects than in conversation. Object movement and manipulation can serve as nonlinguistic cues for the child. Because children's cognitive knowledge and linguistic performance of spatial relationships may differ markedly, manipulation of toys can aid the SLP in assessing the child's comprehension (Cox & Richardson, 1985; Harris, Morris, & Terwogt, 1986). The toys and positions should be varied so as not to suggest answers to children (Messick, 1988).

Conversational Partners

Because the SLP is interested in the child's use of language, the unit of analysis becomes the conversational dyad of the partner and the child and their interactive behaviors in a given context (Prutting & Kirchner, 1983). The dyadic context enables the SLP to view the child's communication within the applied situation of the natural environment.

The importance of different partners is evident when we consider the conversations of adolescents. When teens talk to peers, they ask more questions, obtain more information, shift to more new topics, use more figurative expressions, and make more attempts to entertain than when they talk with their families (Nippold, 2000).

Conversational partners for young children are carefully selected and instructed in their role. It is especially important to use familiar conversational partners with children under age 3 because these children often respond poorly to strangers. Parents of young children or children with acknowledged disabilities may need special instruction to avoid having their children "perform." Uninstructed parents may feel compelled to quiz their child or to have their child recite stereotypic verbal routines such as nursery rhymes to enhance the child's linguistic output. The problem with such recitations is that they may have little to do with the conversational abilities of the child.

In general, it is best to involve the parent or caregiver and the child in some activity. Caregivers can be instructed to talk about what they and the child are doing. As mentioned, toys such as doll houses, action figure play sets, farms and towns, and puppets encourage interaction and role play.

Familiar conversational situations are chosen as well to attain the most typical spontaneous sample with the child conversing as naturally as possible. Interaction may involve one adult or child or a small group of children engaged in sharing, playing, or working in the home or the classroom.

The child should be assessed across several familiar persons with different interactive styles because of the effect that conversational partners—either individually or in small groups—have on the child's verbal output (Mirenda & Donnellan, 1986). For example, peer interaction usually involves more equal status between participants than do adult-child interactions. Adults tend to guide and control the topic when conversing with children, whereas child-child conversations are presumably more equal. As one might expect, these two conditions result in very different interactive styles for the child. If two children are talking, the adult should leave the room because children who are unsure of the situation will defer to the adult and thus skew the data.

The language performance of children below age 3, of minority children, and of children with LLD may deteriorate in the presence of an authority figure such as an unfamiliar adult. This does not mean that the SLP cannot act as a conversational partner. In many ways, the SLP may be the best conversational partner because of his or her knowledge of language and of interactions.

The SLP and all other participating adults need to be mindful of the inherent problems in adult-child conversations and act to reduce the authority figure persona. The adult can accomplish this by accepting the child's activity, agenda, and topics and by participating with the child. The best way to attain a semblance of equal authority is for the SLP and the child to engage in a play interaction. Instead of being directive, the SLP comments on and participates in their ongoing shared activity. With young children, participation may necessitate using the floor for play.

The SLP as the conversational partner can set the tone of the interaction by being nondirective, interest*ing,* interest*ed,* and responsive. The SLP should respond to the content of the child's language, not to the way it is said. At this point, the purpose is to collect data, not to change behavior. Our goal is *collecting, not correcting.*

By manipulating the situation skillfully the SLP can probe for a greater range of information. Initially, interaction may be dampened because the SLP is not the child's usual communication partner. Therefore, it is important for the SLP to get acquainted slowly and in a nonthreatening manner. This task is best accomplished by meeting the child on his or her terms through play and by following the child's lead.

The SLP possesses the clinical skill to elicit a variety of functions, introduce various topics, and ask questions about experiences. Role-play, dolls, and puppet play provide information about the child's event knowledge in a range of situations. There is the potential to elicit a greater variety of language than might be possible when the child and parent communicate.

Children who are reluctant to talk to adults may be more willing to interact with a puppet or a doll. I have found that small animals, such as guinea pigs, make excellent communication partners for children. For example, after explaining to the child that she must leave to run a short errand, the SLP introduces the guinea pig and asks the child to talk to it so that it will not get lonely. The child should be observed and his or her language recorded while the SLP is absent.

Despite conventional wisdom, neither the race of the conversational partner nor the race depicted in stimulus materials seems to affect language performance as measured by response length and response latency (H. Seymour, Ashton, & Wheeler, 1986). This is not to say that all children, particularly CLD children, will be unaffected. SLPs should be aware of potential difficulties and should approach each child with an open mind. Racial incompatibilities should not be expected, but the SLP should be conscious of this potential.

Topics

Children have a wide variety of interests, and the conversational partners must be careful to enable the child to talk about them. Children are more spontaneous and produce more language when they are allowed to initiate the topics of discussion.

The SLP should be prepared to shift topics as readily as activities. Therefore, the SLP must be conversant in topics of interest to children, such as school activities, holidays, movies, television programs, fads and fashions, videogames, and music.

Summary

Child variables, such as recent past experience and mood, can greatly affect language sampling, because the child is often the initiator in this protocol and because there are few performance constraints (Hess, Sefton, & Landry, 1986; Klee & Fitzgerald, 1985). To get the most representative sample possible, therefore, the SLP should use familiar situations, persons, and tasks or topics. Representativeness is enhanced if the conversational sample is collected in more than one setting, with different conversational partners and tasks or topics in each. Guidelines are summarized in Table 5.1.

It may be helpful to think of interactional situations along a continuum from relatively nondirected or free to more controlled or scripted (Coggins, 1991; Shriberg & Kwiatkowski, 1985). Such toys as a dollhouse, a farm, action figures, bubbles, or dress-up clothes are rather open-ended, especially when the partner has suggested, "Let's talk and play with these things." Books or Colorforms offer more control and can be used to elicit particular words, forms, and narratives. Familiar routines,

TABLE 5.1 **Ensuring representativeness in a conversational sample**

Keep it spontaneous	Variety
Less clinician control	Settings
Less clinician contrivance	Tasks
Less conscious child	Conversational partners
	Topics

such as doing the dishes, also can be used, along with such cues as "What are you going to do now?" to elicit more specific behavior. Interviews, picture labeling, and responding to questions offer the most control but at the sacrifice of spontaneity and representativeness. These latter techniques are more appropriately considered evocative techniques used to elicit specific behaviors.

Table 5.2 presents contextual variables that can be manipulated in an assessment to influence a child's performance. Each variable can be modified to offer minimal or maximal contextual support (Coggins, 1991).

Sampling should engage children in challenging interactions that stretch their language and reveal deficits (Hadley, 1998b). This requires a range of interactive situations and discourse types, including conversation, play, narration, and expository or factual/causal communication.

Evocative Conversational Techniques

Although the sample should represent everyday language use, free samples may have limitations, such as low frequency or nonappearance of certain linguistic features and conversational behaviors (F. Roth & Spekman, 1984b). Absence or low incidence does not mean the child does not possess these features or behaviors. Therefore, it may be necessary to supplement the sample with evocative procedures specifically designed to elicit them. Test protocols also might be modified to obtain more structured samples (Thomas, 1989).

The SLP may need to plan both the linguistic and nonlinguistic contexts for elicitation of various functions and forms. At first, some procedures may seem stiff and formal, even forced. Initially, the SLP may need to role-play the sampling situation and memorize conversational openers and

TABLE 5.2 **Continuum of contextual support**

Variable	Minimal Contextual Support	Maximal Contextual Support
Nonlinguistic		
Interaction	Naturalistic	Contrived tasks
Materials	No toys or props	Familiar and thematic
Interactor	Clinician	Mother/caregiver
Activities	Novel	Event routines
Linguistic		
Cuing	Indirect model	Elicited imitation

Source: Coggins, T. E. (1991). Bringing context back into assessment. *Topics in Language Disorders, 11*(4), 43–54. Reprinted with permission.

replies. Once familiar with the many ways of eliciting a variety of functions and forms, the SLP can relax and use the techniques more naturally as opportunities arise within the interaction.

Specific tasks that are within the child's experience also can be used to elicit specific language forms (F. Roth & Spekman, 1984b). This approach allows a broad range of pragmatic functions to occur. For example, a mock birthday party can be used to elicit plurals, past tense, and questions (Wren, 1985). The SLP might elicit plurals by saying the following:

> Today is X's birthday. Let's have a party. What are some things we'll need? (Or, Here are some things we need. What are these?)

The child's utterances are placed within context. Within the same situation, past tense might be elicited by dropping dishes and asking what happened or by reviewing whether you did everything to get ready ("Okay, now tell me what *you* did to get ready for the party. *I* washed the dishes"). Finally, questions can be elicited by a party game variation of Ask the Old Lady.

> Let's play a question game. This is X (puppet, doll, action figure). I want you to ask X some questions about his birthday party. I wonder how old he is. You ask him.

The child may need a demonstration before being able to complete the question task.

Specific procedures and activities can be used to elicit a variety of communication intentions, examples of presupposition, and the underlying social organization of discourse within a variety of situations. Table 5.3 lists examples of situations that each elicit a variety of language functions. In addition, the SLP is interested in ways to elicit various semantic and syntactic features. These elicitation techniques are presented in the following section.

Intentions or Illocutionary Functions

Illocutionary functions are the intentions of each utterance. Most utterances clearly demonstrate the speaker's intent. "What time is it?" demonstrates a desire for information. However, the relationship is not always so obvious. "What time is it?" might be used as an excuse. For example, the speaker who does not wish to do something and knows that time is limited might use this utterance to establish the time factor for other people.

> Well, I don't know…, it's getting late. What time is it? Oh, well, I really better be going.

Utterances also may express more than one intention. For example, the speaker might respond to a piece of art with "What do you call that *thing?*" Here, the speaker requests information and also makes an evaluation.

TABLE 5.3   Situations with the potential to elicit a variety of language functions

Dress-up	Role-playing
Playing house or farm	Playing school
Dolls, puppets, adventure or action figures	Acting out stories, television shows, movies
Farm set or street scene	Imaginary play
Simulated grocery store, gas station, fast-food restaurant, beauty parlor	Simulated TV talk show

A number of existing taxonomies of communication intentions can be applied to the language sample. Table 7.5 presents some illocutionary taxonomies that have been used clinically with child language samples. Guidance regarding the intentions expected at certain ages is presented in Table 7.6. The following are a broad range of intentions and accompanying activities that may elicit language functions or intentions within a conversational or situational context.

Answering/Responding
The SLP asks the child a variety of questions while engaged in play ("Where shall we put the houses?" "Who is that?" "What's in his hand?") and notes the type of question and the expected response.

Calling/Greeting
The SLP leaves and reenters the situation, role-plays people entering and leaving a business, calls on the telephone, or uses dolls, puppets, or action figures to elicit greetings. If the SLP turns away from the child with a favorite toy, the child also may call.

Continuance
Continuance is turn filling that lets the speaker know that the listener is attending to the conversation. Typical continuants include "uh-huh," "yeah," "okay," and "right." These can be observed throughout the session. The SLP notes when the child seems to rely on this function, rather than contribute anything new or relevant to the conversation.

Expressing Feelings
The SLP models feeling-type responses throughout the play interaction. Dolls, puppets, or action figures are described as having certain feelings and the child is asked to help. For example, the SLP could say, "Oh, Big Bird is sad. Can you talk to him and make him feel better?"

Hypothesizing
The SLP poses a physical problem for the child, such as, "How can we get everyone to the party on time?" or, "How can we get Leonardo out of the cage?" The child proposes solutions to the problem.

Making Choices
The SLP presents the child with alternatives, such as, "I don't know whether you'd rather have a peanut butter sandwich with jelly or fluff."

Predicting
In sequential activities, the SLP can ponder, "I wonder what will happen now" or, "I wonder what we'll do next."

Protesting
The SLP can elicit protesting by putting away toys or taking away snacks before the child is finished. The SLP can also hand the child something other than what was requested.

Reasoning
The SLP attempts to solve a problem, such as, "I wonder why the boy ran away" or, "I wonder what we did wrong."

Repeating

The SLP should note the amount of repetition of self and of the partner. This can take the form of empty comments in a conversation in which the child adds no new information, for example:

Adult: Did your class go to the zoo yesterday?

Child: Yeah, zoo.

Adult: What did you like best? The monkeys?

Child: Monkeys.

Adult: Monkeys are my favorite too. They're so funny.

Child: Monkeys funny.

Replying

The SLP should note occasions when the child responds to the content of what he or she has said without being required to do so. This behavior is one of the mainstays of conversation as each speaker builds on the comment of the previous speaker.

Reporting

Reporting can include several functions.

Declaring/Citing.   While engaged in an activity, the child spontaneously comments on the present action. The SLP models this behavior ("Car goes up the ramp") but does not attempt to cue a response because declaring/citing is a spontaneous function. The SLP also can engage in unexpected or unusual behavior and await the child's comment.

Detailing.   The SLP presents the child with two objects of different size or color. If the child takes one and says nothing, the SLP models ("I'll take the little one" or "Here's a green truck") and presents other objects later. The SLP does not attempt to cue a response because detailing is a spontaneous function.

Naming/Labeling.   The SLP presents a novel object or points to pictures in a book and remarks, "Oh, look." If the child does not label the object or picture, the SLP models the response ("Look. A clown.") and goes on. The child may do so on subsequent exposure to other novel objects. The SLP does not cue a response because labeling is a spontaneous function.

Requesting Assistance/Directing

The SLP presents interesting toys that require adult help to open or use. For example, she can place objects in clear plastic containers or drawstring bags that require help to open, give the child one portion of a toy while keeping the other on a shelf, or let windup toys run down. The SLP makes such comments as, "I wish we could play with this; it would be fun," "Oh, we could use more parts," or "Gee, we need to fix that." In another situation, the child helps two puppets or dolls solve a problem in which one will not share a special toy with the other. The SLP also can present the child with situations that require a solution, such as toys with missing pieces. During interactions the SLP should note self-directing or self-talk accompanying play. This behavior can be modeled.

Requesting Clarification
This intention can be elicited when the SLP mumbles or makes an inaccurate statement.

Requesting Information
The SLP places novel but unknown objects in front of the child. Naming the object correctly is labeling, and the SLP should confirm. If the child labels incorrectly, the SLP says, "No, it's not an X" or "No, can you guess what it is?" The responses "What's that?" or "What?" and those with rising intonation ("Frog?") should be considered requests for information.

The SLP also might direct the child to use an object not in the situation or not in the expected location. If modeling is required, the SLP can ask a question, such as, "Do you have the scissors?" When the child answers negatively, the SLP can direct the child by saying, "Ask Sally if she does."

Requesting Objects
The SLP exposes the child to enticing objects or edibles that are just out of reach.

Requesting Permission
The SLP hands an interesting object to the child and says, "Hold the X for me." The technique is more effective if the SLP uses a nonsense name for the object. The SLP then awaits a response from the child, such as, "Can I play with X?" or just, "Play X?"

An even more effective technique is to keep the object hidden in an opaque box. The SLP peeks into the box and tells the object that it can come out to play when someone wants to play with it. If necessary, a puppet can model the requesting behavior desired.

Creaghead (1984) has developed a scripted elicitation protocol that targets several communication intentions and conversational devices within two different structured activities. Table 5.4 presents an outline of the two protocols.

Some intentions are responsive in nature, for example, answering a question or following a directive or request for action. In addition to the child's production level of such requests, it is helpful to know the child's level of response (F. Roth & Spekman, 1984b).

With responsive functions, the SLP must not interpret noncompliance as noncomprehension. The child simply may not want to comply or may choose to ignore the request. My granddaughter is especially good at ignoring. The SLP first should be certain that the child can perform the behavior requested. The ages at which children comprehend different levels of requests are listed in Table 5.5.

It might be helpful for the SLP to use two children in an ask-and-tell situation so that each child can act as a model for the other. In a similar manner, the SLP and child can switch roles as questioner (or director) and respondent.

These are just a few suggestions for eliciting a variety of communication intentions. In summary, the SLP must consider the type of intentions displayed, their forms, the means of transmission, and the social conventions that affect these means. For example, some situations may call for the use of nonverbal means; others may not.

Presuppositional and Deictic Skills
Whereas intentions are noted at the individual level, other linguistic aspects, such as presupposition and deixis, underlie the entire conversational interaction. **Presupposition** is the speaker's assumption about the knowledge level of the listener and the tailoring of language to that supposed level.

TABLE 5.4   Elicitation protocol for communication intentions and conversational devices

Test Procedures—Format 1	Test Procedures—Format 2
As child enters the room—check GREETING	As child leaves the room—check CLOSING
Have cookies and crackers in jar within child's view but out of reach—check REQUEST FOR OBJECT	Give the child and yourself a piece of paper and tell the child to draw "mumble"—check REQUEST FOR CLARIFICATION
Hand child the tightly closed jar containing the cookies—check REQUEST FOR ACTION (help opening the jar)	After clarifying, do not give the child a crayon—check REQUESTING AN OBJECT
Ask child, "How do you think we can get the jar open?"—check HYPOTHESIZING	Ask the child if he or she wants a red or blue crayon—check MAKING CHOICES
Say "Do you want 'mumble'?"—check REQUEST FOR CLARIFICATION	Put on big glasses and then show the child a picture of a person and call it a dog—check COMMENTING ON OBJECT and DENIAL
Ask the child if he or she wants peanut butter or jelly on a cracker—check MAKING CHOICES	Ask the child, "Do you want to play with 'mumble'?"—check REQUEST FOR CLARIFICATION
Hand the child the opposite of what was chosen—check DENIAL	Tell the child to get the telephones, which are not in sight—check REQUEST FOR INFORMATION
Put the peanut butter and jelly on the table. Ask the child, "What are we going to do now?"—check PREDICTING	Ask the child, "What are we going to do?"—check PREDICTING
Tell the child to put peanut butter or jelly on the cracker—check REQUEST FOR OBJECT (knife)	The tester calls the child, then the child calls the tester on the telephone—check GREETING and CLOSING
Tell the child to get the knife, which is not in sight—check REQUEST FOR INFORMATION	Hold a conversation with the child. During this, make a remote-controlled toy move. The toy should be out of the sight of the tester and covered with a cloth—check COMMENT ON ACTION
Put the peanut butter and/or jelly on the cracker and eat it. Get out extra big toothbrush and pretend to brush teeth—check COMMENT ON OBJECT	Ask the child, "What happened?"—check DESCRIBING EVENT
Hold a conversation with the child. During this, pull invisible string so that rag doll falls off the table—check COMMENT ON ACTION	Ask the child, "What do you think is under the cloth?"—check HYPOTHESIZING
Ask the child, "What happened?"—check DESCRIBING EVENT	Ask the child, "Why did it move?"—check GIVING REASON
Ask the child, "Why did it fall?"—check GIVING REASON	Make the toy move briefly—check REQUEST FOR ACTION
During conversation—check ANSWERING, VOLUNTEERING TO COMMUNICATE, ATTENDING TO THE SPEAKER, TAKING TURNS, ACKNOWLEDGING, SPECIFYING A TOPIC, CHANGING A TOPIC, MAINTAINING A TOPIC, GIVING EXPANDED ANSWERS	During conversation—check ANSWERING, VOLUNTEERING TO COMMUNICATE, ATTENDING TO THE SPEAKER, TAKING TURNS, ACKNOWLEDGING, SPECIFYING A TOPIC, CHANGING TOPIC, MAINTAINING A TOPIC, GIVING EXPANDED ANSWERS
Stop leading the conversation and be silent—check ASKING CONVERSATIONAL QUESTIONS	Stop leading conversation and remain silent—check ASKING CONVERSATIONAL QUESTIONS
Request clarification—check CLARIFYING	

Note: These protocols may be used as suggested scripts for efficient elicitation of several communication intentions and conversational devices.

Source: Creaghead, N. (1984). Strategies for evaluating and targeting pragmatic behaviors in young children. *Seminars in Speech and Language, 5,* 241–251. Reprinted with permission.

TABLE 5.5   Age and comprehension of requests

Age in Years	Comprehension
2	I need a _____. Give me a _____.
3	Could you give me a _____? May I have a _____? Have you got a _____?
4	He hurt me. (Hint) The _____ is all gone. (Hint)
4½	Begin to comprehend indirect requests: Why don't you _____ or Don't forget to _____. Mastery takes several years.
5	Inferred requests in which the goal is totally masked are now comprehended. In this example, the speaker desires some juice: Now you make breakfast like you're the mommy.

Source: Adapted from Ervin-Tripp (1977).

Deixis is the interpretation of information from the perspective of the speaker. When a speaker says, "Come here," this must be interpreted as a point close to the speaker, not as a point with reference to the listener. Deictic terms include, but are not limited to, *here/there, this/that, come/go,* and *you/me.*

Presuppositional and deictic skills can be assessed in *referential communication tasks* (F. Roth & Spekman, 1984b). In referential tasks, one partner describes something or gives directions to the other partner, who is usually on the other side of an opaque barrier or unable to see the speaker (see Figure 5.1). Variations include blindfold games or telephone conversations. As a rule, preschoolers

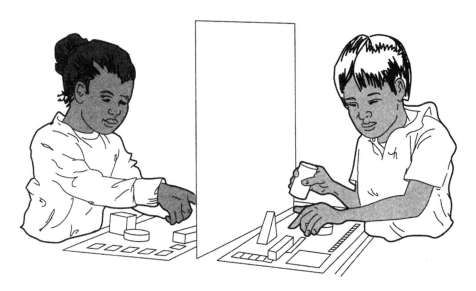

FIGURE 5.1   Barrier tasks.

perform better if describing real objects rather than abstract shapes. Deixis can be elicited by using object-finding tasks in which the child directs the conversational partner toward a hidden object.

In these tasks, the SLP must be alert to the use of direct/indirect reference. In direct reference, the speaker considers the audience and clearly identifies the entity being mentioned. Indirect reference typically follows direct reference and refers to entities through the use of pronouns or such terms as *that one*. The child with poor presuppositional skills may use indirect reference without prior direct reference.

Additional presuppositional information can be gathered by varying the roles, topics, partners, and communication channels available in the sampling situation. Roles can be varied so that the child has an opportunity to act as listener and speaker. Assessment of both roles is essential. For example, the child with LLD generally will ask few questions for clarification even when he or she has little understanding of what has been said. As speakers, these children make limited use of descriptors, provide very little specific information, and are less effective than children developing normally.

The choice of topics also can influence presuppositional behavior and provide for a variety of role taking. Children can be asked to describe events about which the SLP or partner is ignorant (e.g., a family outing). In this situation, the child must determine the amount of information necessary for the listener to understand the topic. The partner who asks the child to explain something that the partner already understands violates the principle that communication should make sense. There is no sense in explaining something that someone already understands.

As the number of communication channels decreases, the speaker is forced to rely more heavily on the remaining ones. For example, the use of a telephone requires the speaker to rely almost exclusively on the verbal communication channel. This situation is a challenge even for some nonimpaired language users.

While gathering the language sample, the SLP can manipulate channel availability systematically. During play, the SLP can look away and then ask the child to describe what he or she is doing. Barrier games or blindfold games with the child in charge also may elicit interesting information. Role-playing with the telephone is more realistic.

The use and nonuse of barriers will permit such verbal-only and verbal-plus communication. If the listener provides no feedback in verbal-only communication, the speaker must take an extremely active role in the conversation. In addition, barrier activities require listeners to adapt to the speaker's perspective.

Several other activities can be used to elicit presuppositional skills. Of interest is whether the child can encode the most informative or uncertain elements in a situation. In general, human beings tend to comment on entities and events that are new, changing, or unexpected. In the sampling situation, novel items can be introduced. The SLP must attend to the child's behavior to see whether the child refers to the novel stimulus.

I know of one clinic where a kitten is abruptly introduced into the sampling situation. The SLP says nothing but waits to see whether the child will comment and in what manner.

In general, young children with language impairment encode novel information less frequently than do children developing typically. Older school-age children with language impairment tend to use more pronouns with less identification of the referent than do children developing typically.

Pictures or objects, identical except for one element, can be used. The child can be asked to explain how the two differ. Hide-and-seek with objects can be used to assess comprehension and expression of deictic terms as the SLP and child direct each other to find the objects.

Games and stories can elicit indirect/direct reference. For example, a story can be told and then questions asked to elicit indefinite and definite articles and/or nouns and pronouns. The child also can retell a story to a second child who has not heard it. Any portion of extended discourse, such as describing a movie, explaining how to accomplish a task, or telling a story, will be valuable clinical data (F. Roth & Spekman, 1984b).

The SLP is interested in the lexical items used and also in the ambiguity of the referent. Of interest is the number of times the child mentions the referent by name or by the use of pronouns. Some children overuse the referent name, whereas others rely on the pronoun without sufficient return to the referent name to avoid confusion.

Finally, role-playing activities with very specific situations also can be helpful. The child in the following situation faces very definite behavioral constraints.

Imagine you and a friend are trying to find a drinking fountain. You see a man coming down the street. While your friend remains seated on a park bench, you try to find out about the fountain. I'll be the man. What would you say? (Child responds.) Now, I'm your friend. What would you tell me?

Discourse Organization

Discourse has internal organization. For example, a telephone conversation has a recognizable pattern, as does the telling of a personal event. The social organization of discourse can be assessed within familiar activities that provide a scaffolding for dialogue (F. Roth & Spekman, 1984b). The SLP may be interested in the amount of social and nonsocial speech. For example, preschool children frequently engage in nonsocial monologues in play, in contrast to older children, who participate more in dialogues or in social monologues. This change signals a growing awareness of the social nature of speech and language use.

The SLP can provide opportunities for the child to initiate conversation, to take turns, and to repair in response to self-feedback or the feedback of others in different situations. Turn taking may need to begin at a physical level with some reticent children. In conversation, the SLP might even say, "Now it's your turn," and point to the child initially. By failing to respond to the child or by responding inappropriately, mumbling, failing to establish a referent, misnaming, or providing insufficient information, the SLP may elicit requests for clarification from the child.

Semantic Terms

Relational terms, such as *in front of, more/less,* and *before/after,* are especially difficult for children with LLD and other language disorders. These children often use comprehension strategies that have several implications for assessment (Edmonston & Thane, 1992). For locational terms, these strategies may include probable location, physical properties of objects, and preferred location. Adjectival relational words, such as *big* and *little,* may be comprehended by using either a preference for amount or word synonymy. With temporal terms, strategies may include sequential probability and order-of-mention or main-clause-first. Each of these strategies is explained below.

It is easier for children to comprehend locational terms and to follow locational instructions when familiar objects are combined in familiar, predictable, or probable ways. Levels of comprehension can be determined by using the usual, or "normal," context or a "contextually neutral" context in which object placement is not so predictable (Lund & Duchan, 1993).

The physical properties of an object can influence responding. The child's rule may be, Containers are for *in,* and surfaces are for *on.* Containers can be turned on their sides by the SLP and used for both *in* and *on.* Other objects may be used with different terms (Edmonston & Thane, 1990).

Some objects are fronted or have an obvious front, while others are not. This characteristic affects comprehension and production of such terms as *in front of* and *behind.* In general, these terms are easier to use with fronted objects than with nonfronted objects. In addition, some young children interpret *behind* to mean *hidden from view by,* so they will place a small object correctly with large nonfronted objects (J. Johnston, 1984). Obviously, *in front of* and *behind* must be assessed with fronted and nonfronted and small and large objects (Edmonston & Thane, 1992).

With deictic terms, young children may employ a child-centered or speaker-centered strategy, preferring that location as the referent (Wales, 1986). Assessing contrastive terms, such as *here/there,* with different speakers may be useful.

Quantitative terms, such as *more/less, long/short,* and *big/little,* may be interpreted by using a preference for a greater-amount strategy in which the child usually chooses the largest one when in doubt. Assessing both words in different contexts and in different word order may help the SLP understand the child's errors.

Similarly, height of the objects used affects comprehension of such words as *big, tall, top, young,* and *old* (Coley & Gelman, 1989; Harris et al., 1986; Hobbs & Bacharach, 1990; Sena & Smith, 1990). Preschoolers often equate *big* with *tall* and *little* with *short height.* Objects can be placed so that their heights are similar by using stands of different heights.

Children also use a strategy in which they interpret contrastive terms such as *big* and *little* to be synonymous or assign the meanings to similar terms. In the latter, *big* becomes synonymous with *tall, wide,* and *thick.* Object dimensions can be controlled so that the widest objects are not always the biggest overall.

Finally, temporal sequential terms, such as *before* and *after,* may be interpreted by using a most probable, order-of-mention, or main-clause-first strategy. In the most probable strategy, the child trusts experience. Among preschoolers, this is the most widely used strategy with familiar, real-world sequences (Keller-Cohen, 1987). Order-of-mention, or the first-action-mentioned-occurred-before-the-second, is also popular among preschoolers, while children over age 5 often use the main-clause-first strategy in which the main clause of the sentence is assumed to have occurred first. Use of sequential terms as prepositions, as in *after school,* rather than as a conjunction, as in *she did X after she did Y,* also as in *after she painted,* may reduce the effect of these strategies on performance. Longer utterances may be used to demonstrate such strategy use.

Language Form

The SLP can manipulate the context to elicit particular forms. For example, the objects and the verbal routines chosen for play may facilitate the use of pronouns or prepositions. Specific syntactic forms, such as verbs, and morphological markers, such as the regular past-tense *-ed,* also can be elicited in creative ways. Some illocutionary functions or intentions discussed previously in this chapter, such as requesting information, have specific linguistic forms. A few elicitation methods for specific structures are listed in Table 5.6 (Crais & Roberts, 1991).

TABLE 5.6   Elicitation of some language features

Feature	Elicitation Technique
Prepositions	Hide objects and have the child try to guess their location.
Nouns, verbs, etc.	Ask specific *Wh-* type questions: *What's that?* for nouns. *Where's X?* for prepositions. *What's John doing?* or *What did (will) Mary do?* for verbs. *How does Carol feel?* or *How did Martin do X?* for adjectives and adverbs.
Plural *-s* marker	Play games with many parts, such as Mr. Potatohead or Colorforms and have the child request desired pieces (*I want the ears*).
Adjectives	Use similar objects of different sizes and colors. Ask child, *What do you want?*
Possessive pronouns	Play dress-up and ask, *Whose dress is this?*
Subjective pronouns	Play I Spy (*I spy something and he's big*).
Yes/no questions	Play Twenty Questions and I Spy.
Wh- questions	Play Hide-and-Seek and other guessing games (*What's in the bag? Where's the ball?*).

Source: Crais, E. R., & Roberts, J. (1991). Decision making in assessment and early intervention planning. *Language, Speech, and Hearing Services in Schools, 22,* 19–30. Reprinted with permission.

Language Sampling with CLD Children

It is even more important that the language of CLD children be collected in several different contexts (Damico, 1991b; Iglesias, 1986). Code switching and differing language and dialect use in context is extremely important information for determining the effectiveness of the child as a communicator.

Sampling should occur in monologue and dialogue situations in both languages or dialects. Monologue activities might include static, dynamic, and abstract tasks. Static tasks describe relationships among objects in the context and might include directing others to perform a task or describing entities by location, size, shape, or color. Dynamic tasks describe changes over time as in narration. Finally, abstract tasks might include opinion-expressing tasks, such as arguing or justifying.

Dialogue situations should include a variety of partners because of the special constraints that each imposes on the CLD child. The classroom is especially important because of the academic difficulties these children may encounter.

In each context, the conversational partner can pose communication problems for the child. Change and problem solving encourage communication and enable the SLP to determine the effectiveness of the child as a communicator. In addition, such situations can offer clues to the learning style of the child (Iglesias, 1986). Guidelines for collecting a language sample with CLD children are presented in Table 5.7.

Recording the Sample

There is no ideal length for a conversational sample. Length varies with the purpose of collection. For example, a 50-utterance sample may be adequate for lexical evaluation because it will contain

TABLE 5.7   Guidelines for language sampling with CLD children

Observe the child in various communication contexts, especially low-anxiety, natural communication environments.

Observe the child with speakers of both languages or dialects. Language mixing during collecting may confuse the child.

Record conversations with the child's family for comparison.

Explore with the family the child's communication in the home and community environment.

Use culturally relevant objects to stimulate conversation. Pictures should contain members of the child's racial/ethnic group.

Avoid the tendency to "fill in" for the child's communication gaps. Observe the child's strategies for getting the message through.

Note:
  Language uses and purposes. How flexible is the child's system?
  Success at communicating. Are certain content and situations more successful?
  Communication breakdowns. Where do they occur? With whom?
  Strengths and weaknesses. What strategies are used to compensate for weakness?
  Anxiety and frustration.

Source: Compiled from Battle (1993); Roseberry-McKibbin (1994); Stockman (1996).

73 to 83 percent of the lexical information found in a 100-utterance sample (K. Cole, Mills, & Dale, 1989).

In the light of the constraints of the clinical sample, 50 or 100 child utterances are considered adequate, providing there is some variety of setting, partners, tasks, or topics and that other data collection methods are used. At least two different samples should be included (K. Cole et al., 1989).

Occasionally, children fall into repetitive patterns of responding, such as naming pictures in a book. This kind of activity provides very little variation in the child's behavior. It is best either to limit this type of interaction or not to use it for analysis. If, on the other hand, the child frequently exhibits perseverative or stereotypic patterns, they should be recorded for analysis, saved for supporting data, or commented on in the assessment report.

The sample is recorded permanently by using videotape, audiotape, event transcription, or a combination of these (F. Roth & Spekman, 1984b). Taping is essential because the interaction must be reviewed repeatedly for information.

Although videotaping can be intrusive and expensive, especially the initial equipment purchase, it yields the best data for describing the verbal and nonverbal behaviors observed. The alternatives to videotaping are not as reliable and thus increase the variability in the behavior recorded. Even if videotape is used, the SLP may find a simultaneous audiotape helpful for transcribing the speech and language portion. The following recording methods are listed in order of decreasing desirability:

1. Simultaneous videotaping and audiotaping
2. Simultaneous audiotaping with pathologist descriptions of nonlinguistic behaviors recorded in one and the linguistic interaction in the other
3. Simultaneous audiotaping and written-data recording on time sheets (see Table 5.8). Having more than one observer may help ensure that no behaviors are overlooked and may increase the

TABLE 5.8 Time form for recording the nonlinguistic context

			Minute __2__
Time (sec.)	**Child's Behavior**	**Partner's Behavior**	**Other**
0			
.			
.			
.			
.			
10			
.	*Looks at partner*		
.			
.	*Points to truck*		
.			
20			
.			
.	*Reaches for truck*		
.		*Hands truck*	
.			
30			
.			
.			
.	*Pushes car*		
.			
40	*Looks at partner*		
.			
.	*Points to gas station*		
.			
.		*Moves car to gas station*	
50			
.		*Moves car to gas station*	
.			
.			
.			
60			

reliability of description of those that are observed. Writing data as the interaction progresses is extremely tedious but necessary.

It is important for later transcription that different data collection methods begin at the same time. This should be accomplished as unobtrusively as possible. A cough or some similar signal by the SLP can alert observers that recording has begun.

Transcribing the Sample

The conversational sample is transcribed as soon after recording as possible. This timeliness ensures that the SLP brings to the task as much memory of the situation as possible.

The format of the transcript varies with the purpose of the assessment. For most purposes, the type of format shown in Table 5.9 is suggested.

TABLE 5.9   Transcription format

			Minute __2__
Time (sec.)	**Child's Utterances**	**Partner's Utterances**	**Nonlinguistic**
0			
.			
.		*What do you need now?*	
.			
.			
.			
10			
.	*Can I have the truck?*		*C looks at partner*
.			
.			*C points to truck*
20		*Which one?*	
.	*That one*		
.			*C reaches for truck*
.		*Oh, the red one*	*P hands truck*
.		*Okay*	
30		*Now can we go on*	
.		*vacation?*	
.			
.	*Bro-o-om*		*C pushes car*
.			
40	*We need gas first*		*C looks at partner*
.			
.			*C points to gas station*
.		*Well then*	
.		*I'll drive my car*	*P moves car to gas station*
50		*over, too*	
.			*C moves car to gas station*
.			
.		*What else do we need?*	
.	*Gotta get soda and*		
60	*chips*		

The use of computerized analysis programs, such as the Systematic Analysis of Language Transcripts (SALT), requires a consistent transcription format (J. Miller & Chapman, 2003) (see Appendix D). This format will include not only the utterances but also the symbols for the program to aid it in identifying morphological markers and syntactic categories. Usually, multiple analyses can be performed without reentering the transcript or with only minor changes to accommodate different transcription conventions and analytic capabilities (Long, 1991).

The SLP transcribes the linguistic behavior of both the child and the conversational partner, along with the nonlinguistic behaviors of each. The timesheet format in Table 5.9 enables the SLP to evaluate delays or latencies on the part of the child.

All of the child's utterances, including false starts, nonfluencies, and fillers, are transcribed. Although these linguistic elements may not be used for calculation of utterance length, they are extremely important in determining language and communication difficulties.

All utterances of the conversational partner(s) also are transcribed. These are important in assessing the manner and style of the conversational partners. The SLP is interested in the amount of control and the amount of talking exhibited by the partner.

Determining utterance boundaries is often difficult. This is not an exact science, and the artistry of the SLP is needed at this point. An *utterance* is a complete thought that is divided from other utterances by sentence boundaries, pauses, and/or a drop in the voice. Table 5.10 contains examples of utterance boundaries.

Declaring sentences to be utterances is easy. Most of what is said, however, is not in complete sentence form. For example, the response to a question often omits shared information and might consist of such responses as "No," "Cookie," and "Okay." Each of these is a complete utterance. Longer responses, such as "No, later" or "No, let's go later," are also single utterances. This determination might change if the child were to respond with a pause and a drop in the voice after "No." "No (pause and drop voice). Let's go later." Now there are two utterances.

Partial sentences or phrases, nonfluent units, and run-on sentences are even more difficult. A partial sentence might consist of the child pointing to an object and saying, "Doggie." This would count as an utterance. In the following exchange, the child makes an internal repair:

> Partner: *I like to play mommy.*
>
> Child: *No, you not...me the...you baby.*

The entire unit is an utterance and will be analyzed in different ways by using all or part of what the child said.

For run-on sentences, the SLP can follow the general rule that allows two clauses to be joined together in a sentence with *and*. In the following example, sentence/utterance boundaries have been marked as they might be on a transcript:

> [I went to the party, and we ate pizza] [(and) We played games, and I won a prize] [(and) We had cake and ice cream.]

Division can be aided by the child's pauses and breath patterns. Children in the late preschool years often make long strings of clauses with *and* meaning *and then*. Counting these as a single utterance inflates the mean utterance length. Young children are less likely to form run-ons with other conjunctions. Once the sample is transcribed, it can be analyzed.

TABLE 5.10   Utterance boundaries

A sentence is an utterance.
  Mommy went to the doctor's tomor...yesterday.

Run-on sentences with *and* should contain no more than one *and* joining clauses.
  We went in a bus and we saw monkeys and we had a picnic and we petted the sheeps and one sheep
  sneezed on me and we had sodas and we came home.

  Utterances:
  1. We went in a bus and we saw monkeys.
  2. (And) we had a picnic and we petted the sheeps.
  3. (And) one sheep sneezed on me and we had sodas.
  4. (And) we came home.

Other complex or compound sentences should be treated as one utterance.
  He was mad because his mommy spanked him because he broke the lamp and spilled the doggie's water.

Imperative sentences are utterances.
  Go home.

Pauses, voice drops, and/or inhalations mark boundaries.
  Eat (pause and voice drop)...chocolate candy.
    Two utterances: Eat. Chocolate candy.
  Eat (momentary delay)...chocolate candy.
    One utterance: Eat chocolate candy.

Situational and nonlinguistic cues help to determine boundaries.
  Eat (hands plate to partner insistently)...chocolate candy (points to candy dish).
    Two utterances: Eat. Chocolate candy.
  Want (reaches unsuccessfully)...mommy (turns to look).
    Two utterances: Want. Mommy.
  Want mommy (reaches unsuccessfully).
    One utterance: Want, mommy.

The linguistic context also helps.
  Partner: Well, what do you want?
  Child: Candy (pause)...you get it.
    Two utterances: Candy. You get it.

Collecting Samples of Written Language

With school-age children and adolescents, the SLP also will want to collect samples of their written language. Underlying language processes make it imperative that the SLP sample all modalities. Collection and analysis of written samples is explained in more detail in Chapter 13.

If a teacher suspects that a child has a language impairment, he or she should contact the SLP, who can ask the teacher to compile a portfolio of the child's written work. It should include first drafts of both narrative and expository writing.

In addition the SLP should elicit a written sample as he or she observes the child. Of interest will be the child's general demeanor, the presence of frustration, the amount of help needed, and the look and quality of the finished product.

The child's written language can be compared to the spoken sample for similarities and differences. Of particular interest will be language features noted in the language of older children, such as cohesive devices, noun and verb phrase structure, illocutionary functions, vocabulary and word relationships, conjoining and embedding, along with spelling and penmanship.

Conclusion

Collecting a representative language sample that demonstrates the child's diverse abilities is a difficult task. Careful planning and execution are required, as are exacting methods of recording and transcription. Although these procedures may seem difficult and time-consuming initially, they can be accomplished easily and relatively quickly with practice. A properly planned and executed sampling and a thorough transcription will yield an abundance of linguistic and nonlinguistic information.

Guides for collecting a language sample include the following:

- Establish a positive relationship with the child before recording the language sample.
- Reduce your authority-figure persona to ensure more participation by the child. A child is more likely to respond naturally with someone who is an equal.
- Be unobtrusive while collecting the sample so that the child is less conscious of the process.
- The conversational partner should keep talking to a minimum. Although SLPs abhor a vacuum, when possible they should wait out the child.
- Avoid yes/no questions and constituent questions that require only a one-word response from the child. Ask process rather than product questions.
- Follow the child's lead in play and in the selection of topic. Determine the child's interests before beginning the collection process. Select those materials at the child's interest level that are likely to stimulate interest.
- If the child does not talk or responds in a very repetitive or stereotypic manner, model responses for the child or have another person model.

Only through sampling the child's linguistic abilities in a conversational context can the SLP gain insight into how the child's language works for the child. This is the first step in designing intervention that is relevant to the child and thus more likely to generalize to use environments.

6

Analysis across Utterances and Partners and by Communication Event

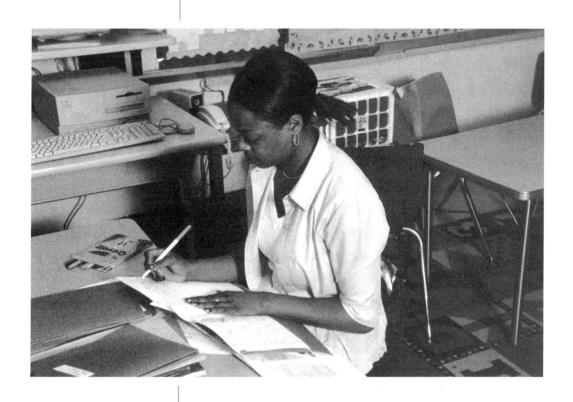

Language is complex and the analysis methods used with a conversational sample reflect this complexity. For this reason, analysis of a language sample should not be a fishing expedition for possible problems. Language analysis is best used to explore certain aspects of the child's behavior brought into question through other data collection methods. If a language disorder exists, it can be confirmed by descriptive analysis of a sample of the child's unique language pattern.

Traditional analysis has focused exclusively on the utterance or sentence as the unit of analysis. Although this type of analysis is appropriate for many language features, it may not be the best way to assess behaviors that transcend these units. To analyze language only at the utterance level is to miss many of the child's language skills, especially those aspects that govern cohesion and conversational manipulation. Only by going beyond individual utterances can the SLP gain an understanding of the child's use of the many language skills (Biber, 1986; Scott, 1987). For example, an analysis of a child's use of pronouns necessitates crossing utterance boundaries in order to describe the child's introduction of new information and reference to old or established information that may have been introduced by the child or the conversational partner.

TABLE 6.1   Types of analysis beyond the utterance

Across Utterances and Partners
Stylistic Variations
   Register
   Interlanguage and Code Switching
   Channel Availability
Referential Communication
   Presuppositional Skills: What Is Coded and How
   Linguistic Devices: Deictics, Definite and Indefinite Reference
Cohesive Devices
   Reference: Initial and Following Mention
   Ellipsis
   Conjunction
   Adverbial Conjuncts and Disjuncts
   Contrastive Stress

By Communication Event
Social versus Nonsocial
Conversational Initiation: Method, Frequency, and Success Rate
Topic Initiation: Method, Frequency, Success Rate, and Appropriateness
Conversation and Topic Maintenance: Frequency and Latency of Contingency
Duration of Topic: Number of Turns, Informativeness, and Sequencing
Topic Analysis Format: Topic Initiation; Type of Topic; Manner of Initiation, Subject Matter and Orientation;
   Outcome; Topic Maintenance; Type of Turn; and Conversational Information
Turn Taking: Density, Latency, and Duration
   Overlap: Type, Frequency, and Duration
   Signals
Conversation and Topic Termination
Conversational Breakdown
   Request for Repair: Frequency and Form
   Conversational Repair
      Spontaneous versus Listener-Initiated
      Strategy and Success Rate

In this chapter, we explore analysis across utterances and partners and by communication event, noting the adjustments the speaker must make to meet conversational demands. These analyses are suggested when the SLP suspects difficulties. Obviously, the many types of analysis mentioned in this chapter would be too numerous to examine and too time-consuming to perform with every child. Because little normative information is available on conversational skills, analysis at these levels is largely descriptive. Table 6.1 presents some types of analyses possible across utterances and partners and by communication event.

It is important for the SLP to remember that many of the language features discussed in this chapter are dependent on the behavior of the partner and vary with the situation and the culture of the child and the conversational partner (Crago & Eriks-Brophy, 1992). The stimuli and reinforcers and the child's response to each, the conversational roles of each partner, and the type and amount of communication are contingent on cultural values. Tasks should be culturally relevant with functional, meaningful, culturally appropriate language. Sampling results should be analyzed with cultural variability in mind.

Across Utterances and Partners

Analysis at the utterance level reveals much about the child's discrete, finite language skills but may obscure the child's knowledge of the "big picture," the cohesion that threads through conversations. Some linguistic devices serve this cohesive purpose, and larger units than the utterance must be analyzed to assess their development. Other devices vary across whole conversations, and one sample may be very different from another.

Stylistic Variations

The style of talking, whether formal, casual, or varied in other ways for the situation, usually does not change utterance by utterance. Rather, it is a manner of talking with a specific language partner or in a specific situation. Different styles also may be seen in role-play. The SLP is interested in the different styles used by the child in the various samples collected.

As early as age 4, children use a different style of talking when they address younger children learning language. This style resembles *motherese* or *parentese,* the stylistic changes made by parents when they address these same younger children. Mature language users have a variety of styles at their disposal and can switch styles with little effort. Such variation requires the speaker to consider the listener and the situation and the resultant requirements on the speaker.

Register
Style switching, the move from one style or register to another, must be judged against the age, gender, and language ability of the speaker and the listener. Styles differ according to role-taking characteristics, dialectal variations, amount of politeness, and conversational control.

Conversational roles can be established by the topics chosen, vocabulary (*dear, sir, honey*), pronunciation, and the discourse style selected. Usually, the more dominant partner takes longer turns and asks more questions. The degree of politeness also varies. In general, speakers are more polite when in the less dominant role or when requesting something that belongs to or is controlled by the other partner, who may be unlikely to grant the request.

Children with LLD often fail to use registers based on differing situational variables. Data suggest that these children do not adjust to different speakers or may adjust in different ways from children developing typically. Children with LLD may fail to recognize the characteristics of different settings. The child with LI may not be able to discriminate dominant from nondominant roles and the language form that goes with each. The most frequent problems with register include providing insufficient information for the listener, not knowing when to make a statement, asking inappropriate questions, giving insufficient reason for the cause and effect of a situation, and not adjusting register to the speaker (A. Johnson, Johnston, & Weinrich, 1984). It may be especially difficult for the child with LLD to express feelings and emotions. These expressions may be very direct.

The SLP studies the sample to determine the stylistic variations present. The value of collecting language samples in two very different but client-appropriate situations is apparent. The SLP should look for modifications in politeness, intimacy, and linguistic code based on the age, status, familiarity, cognitive level, linguistic level, and shared past experience of the listener (F. Roth & Spekman, 1984a). Of interest is the attention the child gives to the listener's characteristics. In addition to noting stylistic variations, the SLP looks for inappropriate styles—those that are too formal, too casual, or include excessive swearing.

The SLP might note features such as differing utterance length with various partners. Other variations include vocabulary and topic. More subjective indices include intonational patterns and the use of attention-getting and maintaining devices.

Interlanguage and Code Switching

With children with LEP, it is important to establish patterns of language use in both L_1 and L_2 (Hamayan & Damico, 1991). Two possible patterns are called interlanguage and code switching. **Interlanguage** is a combination of the L_1 and L_2 rules, plus ad hoc rules from neither or both languages. This "hybrid" language varies among children and within the individual child across situations (Tarone, 1988). Usually, interlanguages are transitional in nature, although some features may stabilize as a permanent form, especially if there is little motivation to change. Predictable patterns should be identified during observation and sampling. Of interest are the rules used by the child and any situational variables.

Linguistic **code switching** is the shifting from one language to another within and/or across different utterances. A complicated, rule-governed behavior, code switching does not signal poor language skills, although it may be used by children when they have inadequate L_2 skills. As with interlanguage, code switching is influenced heavily by contextual and situational variables (Sprott & Kemper, 1987). For example, the Spanish-speaking storyteller might use English when referring to Anglos and Spanish when referring to Latinos. Code switching usually occurs to enhance meaning, emphasize a change of topic, and convey humor, ethnic solidarity, and attitudes toward the listener (Hamayan & Damico, 1991).

The SLP should note uses of interlanguage and code switching, along with sampling variables such as the situation and the partner(s). It is especially important to identify patterns that may impede the transmission of meaning or interrupt communication.

Channel Availability

Most children below age 11 experience less communication success when they do not visually share the communication environment with the listener, as when on the phone (F. Roth & Spekman, 1984a). As the number of communication channels decreases, the child with LI should have increasing difficulty communicating. In fact, children with LLD often have great difficulty if forced to rely solely on the verbal channel. The SLP should note in the sample the relative success of the child's communication efforts as the number of channels varies.

Referential Communication

Referential communication is the ability of a speaker to select and verbally identify the attributes of an entity in such a way that the listener can identify the entity accurately (Bowman, 1984). To succeed, the speaker must be able to determine what information the listener needs, deliver that information in a specific manner, make comparisons, and use feedback on message adequacy and breakdown. While "He has brown hair" fails to communicate the referent, "The only boy in my history class has brown hair" succeeds.

Referential communication includes directions, explanations, and descriptions. These are three essential aspects of classroom discourse, and their impairment may contribute to the academic difficulties of children with LLD (Donahue, 1985).

Presuppositional Skills

Presupposition is the speaker's assumptions about the context and about the listener that modify the manner and content of the speaker's utterances (A. Johnson et al., 1984). The speaker must take the conversational perspective of the listener(s) and determine what information to communicate and its form.

From early on, informativeness is a characteristic of communication. Even toddlers tend to code information that is maximally informative, thus talking about things that are new, different, and changing. For most children, the receptive and expressive ability to consider a partner's perspective is well established by age 10. Although both comprehension and production require understanding of the critical features needed, production also requires knowing how and when to provide information. Children with LLD have poor referential skills and are less likely to adjust to the listener and more likely to provide ambiguous and insufficient information. In addition, although children with LLD seem to understand directions given by others, they take longer to comply than do age-matched children who are non-LLD (Feagans & Short, 1986) and have great difficulty giving adequate instructions.

The SLP should be alert to the informativeness of the child's utterances and to the social context. The following questions can be applied to the sample (F. Roth & Spekman, 1984a):

- What does the child choose to encode in the situation?
- Does the child encode what is novel or merely comment on what is already given?
- Does the child encode new information gesturally or linguistically?
- Are messages informative, vague, or ambiguous?
- Are different referents clearly established?
- Does the child talk differently about things present and things not?

What Is Coded and How.   Conversations usually contain information that is novel and informative. The SLP is interested in whether the child adds to the conversation or only comments on what is given. In the following exchange, the child takes a turn but adds nothing of substance to the conversation.

Partner: Wasn't that a great baseball game on TV last night?

Child: Yeah, great game.

Partner: What a great home run in the top of the ninth; I didn't expect Cincinnati to pull it out.

Child: Great home run.

Partner: I think they'll probably go on for the pennant. How about you?

Child: Pennant.

If this sounds like the conversation of someone who doesn't know the topic well enough to comment, that may be partially correct. The child may not be able to identify the topic. Frequent repetition may indicate a semantic (word retrieval), processing, or pragmatic (not sure of the contextual demands) problem.

Noninformative language can take several forms (Nicholas, Obler, Albert, & Helm-Estabrooks, 1985). Table 6.2 presents forms and examples seen in children with LI. These types of noninformative language may be especially useful when rating the language of children with TBI and LLD. The SLP can rate utterances to determine the strategy used by the child.

Linguistic Devices

Several linguistic devices are used to mark informativeness, including deictics and direct/indirect reference (F. Roth & Spekman, 1984a). Both of these devices can be used to note referents internal or external to the conversation; other cohesive devices, listed in Table 6.3, establish relations entirely within the discourse.

Deictics.   Deictic terms are linguistic elements that must be interpreted from the perspective of the speaker in order to be understood as the speaker intended. The use of deixis is based on the *speaker principle,* in which the referential point shifts as speakers change, and on the *distance principle,* in which referents are coded by their distance from the speaker.

Words with deictic meanings appear in several word classes, including personal pronouns (*I/me* and *you*), demonstrative adjectives (*this, that, these,* and *those*), adverbs of time (*before, after, now,* and *then*), adverbs of location (*here* and *there*), and verbs (*come* and *go*). The child's behavior, espe-

TABLE 6.2   Types of noninformative language

Empty phrases (common idioms, such as *and so on* and *et cetera excetera*)
Indefinite terms and highly nonspecific nouns (*one, thing, that*)
Deictic terms (*this, that, here, there*)
Pronouns used without antecedent nouns
Comments on task instead of stimulus
Neologisms (*Oh, you know the one that you fly in*)
Paraphrases
Repeated words or phrases
Personal value judgments about the stimulus (*That's pretty dumb*)
Use of *and* alone
Conjunctions *but, so, or,* and *because* alone

Source: Adapted from Nicholas, Obler, Albert, & Helm-Estabrooks (1985).

TABLE 6.3   Cohesive devices used in English

Relation	Explanation	Example
Reference	Initially, the entity is named and may use the indefinite article (*a/an*). Subsequent mention may use a pronoun, words such as *this, that,* and *one,* or use the definite article (*the*) with the noun.	*John* went looking for *a car. He* found *one* in the city. I want to buy *a coat,* but *that one* I saw last night is too expensive.
Ellipsis	Subsequent sentences omit redundant or shared information.	Who *ate all the cookies?* I did [eat all the cookies]. I would like to *make a phone call.* May I [make a phone call]?
Conjunction	Conjunctions join clauses to express additive, causal, and other relationships.	We went to the circus, *and* I saw elephants. John's angry *because* I drank his soda.

Source: Adapted from Halliday & Hasan (1976).

cially the errors, should be analyzed to determine confusion or overreliance on one principle or one aspect of a principle.

Definite and Indefinite Reference.   The mature language user is able to mark specific (definite) and nonspecific (indefinite) referents by manipulation of definite (*the*) and indefinite (*a/an*) articles. The speaker must consider what the listener knows about the topic under discussion.

Article use can be especially difficult for the child with LI. In part, this difficulty may reflect the use of articles in English to mark new and old information also. The tendency for children with LI is to overuse the definite article. Each article present in the sample can be analyzed for appropriate referential use. Asian American LEP speakers may omit articles reflecting nonuse in many Asian languages.

Cohesive Devices

Conversational *cohesion,* how language hangs together, can be a useful analysis tool. Cohesion can be expressed through syntax and vocabulary, for example, a pronoun or a demonstrative, such as *this* or *that,* to refer to the referent, which was identified previously in the conversation. *Conjoining,* the connection of phrases, clauses, and sentences through the use of such conjunctions as *and, because,* and *if,* also is used for cohesion. The major cohesive devices used in English are listed in Table 6.3.

The most frequent problems of cohesion relate to providing redundant information, deleting necessary information, using unclear and ambiguous reference, sequencing old and new information, and marking old and new information with articles and pronouns. In short, errors usually reflect including or excluding too much information or confusing new and old information.

Reference
Reference is a linguistic device used continuously in conversation to keep information flowing and to designate new and old information. In the process, new information is stated clearly and then

subsequently implied by the referral to it as old information, one utterance presupposing the other. Some children with language impairments, such as children with ASD, have difficulty marking new and old information (McCaleb & Prizant, 1985).

The SLP must note the method of introducing new information and the use of following mention. Speakers should ensure that listeners can easily determine noun–pronoun relationships. This investigation requires looking beyond traditional utterance-level analysis.

Initial Mention.   In initial mention, mature speakers establish mutual reference clearly, especially if the entity mentioned is not present. Generally, the referent name is stressed and preceded by the indefinite article (*a/an*). In English, the referent often is placed at the end of the sentence, the most salient position. The following are examples of the introduction of new information:

Did you see *John at the party?*

We went to a *circus* yesterday.

In addition, referents that are present may be pointed to or handled. Young children tend to rely more on these nonlinguistic behaviors to establish new referents.

Children with LLD or ASD have difficulty with new information (McCaleb & Prizant, 1985; Rees & Wollner, 1981). As speakers, they may not identify new information for the listener, assuming that the listener "just knows" what the speaker is thinking. As listeners, these children may have difficulty identifying the new information but will ask few questions to clarify. "These children often do not know what they do not know" and thus cannot inquire about it (J. Stark, 1985). With increasing language skills, the child is able to be more specific linguistically.

Children with word-finding difficulties or poor vocabularies may use empty words, such as *that, one,* or *thing,* that do not help clarify the referent. These children may rely on the immediate context and use pointing to specify the referent that their nonspecific vocabulary failed to identify.

Following Mention.   In following mention, previously identified referents often are moved to the initial position in English sentences and may be referred to by the use of the definite article (*the*) or a pronoun. "Did you see John at the party?" might be followed by "*He* was so thrilled." This referral to previously cited information is called **anaphoric reference.** Pronoun use is appropriate when the referent is unambiguous or clearly identified. The pronoun should be in close proximity so that there is no confusion as to which noun it refers.

The SLP is interested in the way the child introduces new information and refers to that information later. Also of interest is any confusion with article and pronoun use. Pronouns and a method of recording the child's use are included in Table 7.14. It is not uncommon for the preschool child or the child with LLD to introduce new information with "She did it," leaving the listener to determine who *she* is and what *it* is.

Ellipsis
Ellipsis is a process in which redundant information is omitted. For example, the response to "What do you want?" is "Cookie," which omits the shared information "I want."

Elliptical fragments are used frequently to keep the conversation moving smoothly and rapidly, but they are missed if linguistic analysis concentrates solely on full sentences. Children with LI may not realize that information is shared or may assume that it is shared when it is not. Either assumption interferes with the flow of conversation. For example, the child might repeat, "Cookies, Cookies, cookies," until someone asks, "What about cookies?" to which the child responds in surprise, "I want some," having assumed previously that the *I want* was shared.

Conjunction

Conjunctions, such as *and, then, so,* and *therefore,* are used to connect thoughts. Although preschool children have several conjunction-type words in their vocabularies, they rarely use them to join clauses. Even kindergarten children will overrely on *and,* which becomes an all-purpose conjunction. In addition, *and* often is used to mean *and then* when giving a sequence of events. A developmental progression for conjunctions is given in Table 7.16.

Just as conjunctions can be analyzed at the utterance level because of their use in linking clauses, conjunctions can be analyzed across utterances, as in the following exchange.

Parent: We had a great day at the zoo. I liked the monkeys best.

Child: And feeding the deer babies.

Analysis at the level of the child's utterance alone would miss the child's considerable skill.

Adverbial Conjuncts and Disjuncts

Adverbial conjuncts and disjuncts are conversational devices used for cohesion. *Conjuncts* are intersentential forms that express a logical relationship, such as the conjunctions *then* or *so.* Conjuncts are of two types: *concordant,* such as *similarly, consequently,* and *moreover;* and *discordant,* such as *nevertheless, rather,* and *in contrast. Disjuncts* are used to comment on or to convey the speaker's attitude toward the topic and include words and phrases such as *honestly, frankly, perhaps, however, yet, to my surprise, it's obvious to me that,* and the like.

Conjuncts and disjuncts develop rather late in childhood and, therefore, may be good measures of adolescent language. Growth is "slow and protracted" (Nippold, Schwarz, & Undlin, 1992, p. 108). By age 12, children use only an average of 4 conjuncts per 100 utterances (Scott, 1988a). In contrast, adults average 12 conjuncts per 100 utterances. Children between ages 6 and 12 use conjuncts infrequently and rely most frequently on *then, so,* and *though* (Scott, 1984a). Adolescents use the same conjuncts but also use *therefore, however, rather,* and *consequently* most accurately in both their reading and writing (Nippold, Schwarz, & Undlin, 1992). Comprehension seems to be better than production although similar (Nippold, Schwarz, & Undlin, 1992; Scott & Rush, 1985).

The conjunct *then* can be used to signal both continuity and discontinuity in adolescent and adult language (Segal, Duchan, & Scott, 1991). Initially, children use *then* to mean *next,* joining clausal information. Later, *then* is used to focus on ideas presented previously, in contrast to *now,* which signals that new ideas will be presented on some topic. In addition, *then* can signal discordance, as in "Then again, I believe..."

In mature narratives, *then* is used approximately 20 percent of the time to mark discontinuity by indicating a shift (Duchan & Waltzman, 1992). This shift might be to (1) a different discourse type, as in conversation to narration or the reverse, (2) a new scene or location, (3) a different character in a narrative, or (4) a new perspective. Use of *then* seems dependent on the use of other conjuncts, such as *anyway, meanwhile, whatever,* and *now.* Narratives, discussed in Chapter 8, offer insight into conjunct use.

Contrastive Stress

Contrastive stress or emphasis can be used to negate or correct the message of a conversational partner. For example, if one speaker said, "Jose brought the cookies," the other might correct, "*Mary* brought the cookies." Again, the SLP must transcend the traditional utterance-level analysis.

Communication Event

The term **communication event** can represent an entire conversation or a portion thereof that includes one topic. For purposes of our discussion, we use the larger definition and include within it a conversation that comprises one or more topics.

Usually, a shared or negotiated agenda(s) occurs within a conversation. Utterances within the event support this agenda. The teenager who wants to be granted a privilege, such as getting to use the family car, is polite, and each utterance supports this agenda.

Conversations may be too open-ended for some children unfamiliar with the process or unable to decipher the code. The child may be unclear about the purpose of conversation and his or her role in it. Much of this difficulty can be alleviated by using familiar conversational partners and situations and by following the child's lead. Younger children and those with LI may need events with more definite beginnings and ends, such as putting together a puzzle.

The social organization of discourse consists of the two roles of speaker and listener. The effective communicator has the ability to function in and contribute to the conversation by assuming responsibility for both roles. Assessment variables that might measure a child's ability to participate effectively are the amount of socialized speech and the child's adaptive style; conversation and topic initiation, maintenance, and termination; the completeness, relevance, and clarity of the child's behavior; on-topic exchanges and turn taking; and conversational repairs (James, 1989; Lund & Duchan, 1993; Prutting, 1983; F. Roth & Spekman, 1984a).

Analysis occurs at two levels: the molar and the molecular (Prutting, 1983). At the *molar level,* the SLP evaluates each behavior for appropriateness or inappropriateness within the conversational context. Inappropriate behaviors may indicate problem areas for further assessment. At the *molecular level,* the SLP is interested in the *frequency, latency, duration, density,* and *sequence* of the child's behaviors.

Frequency data will reveal inordinately high- or low-frequency features and information on the range of features. *Latency,* the span of time when an individual does not engage in behavior, is also important. Pauses and hesitations may reveal difficulty decoding the preceding utterance or forming a response. *Duration* is the length of time that the child and the partner are engaged in a certain behavior, such as conversational gaze or conversational turns by both partners. *Density* is the number of behaviors within a certain period of time. Of interest are the density of different conversational topics or specific linguistic structures, such as questions. *Sequence* includes the order of events within a topic or conversation. The child exhibiting difficulty with sequencing of a conversation may not understand the rules of conversational participation.

Decisions of appropriateness may be facilitated through the use of a modified ethnographic technique similar to that used in anthropological studies. Using an expository form of writing, the SLP attempts to describe each child utterance with reference to form, content, and use, discourse relations, code switching, learning and cognitive style, and the partner's arrangement and selection of nonlinguistic strategies, materials, and procedures (Constable, 1992). Thus, each utterance is given a reference frame in which to judge appropriateness. Table 6.4 provides a sample of a dialogue and the accompanying ethnographic analysis. Ethnographic techniques are especially important when assessing CLD children (Roseberry-McKibbin, 1994).

Social versus Nonsocial

Social speech is speech addressed explicitly to and adapted for a listener. It is characterized by explicitness and clarity, repairs of breakdowns, and an obligation for the listener to respond. Social communication includes dialogues and social monologues addressed to a listener or uttered for the mutual enjoyment of both the speaker and listener, such as rhyming and poetic nonsense. The speaker adapts the explicitness of the message for the listener and repairs breakdowns. The speaker's message is delivered as if the speaker expects a listener response.

In contrast, *nonsocial speech* is not addressed explicitly to a listener, and the listener has no obligation to respond. Nonsocial communication is usually for the speaker's own enjoyment and often consists of asocial monologues. An important measure of communication is the percentage of the child's utterances or the amount of total talk time that can be characterized as social (F. Roth & Spekman, 1984a).

Although preschoolers produce many asocial monologues, the amount of time spent in this type of production decreases with age. School-age children developing typically produce very little nonsocial speech. In general, children's communication becomes more interpersonal as they mature, with girls more likely to use language cooperatively (D. Cooper & Anderson-Inman, 1988). Boys are more likely to show domination and control, to interrupt and insult, and to play practical jokes. Older adolescents are more concerned for the wants and feelings of others, compromise and reach mutual agreement more, and are more concerned for long-term consequences in their communication than are younger adolescents or children (Selman, Beardslee, Schultz, Krupa, & Podorefsky, 1986).

TABLE 6.4   An example of ethnographic analysis

Language Sample	Ethnographic Analysis
Child: What's that? *Partner:* That's a "Thing-a-majibit." *Child:* What it do? *Partner:* What do you think it does? *Child:* On the table. *Partner:* YES, on the table. What about "On the table?" *Child:* On the table.	Child does not seem to know the identity of an object and inquires as to its name with an appropriate *wh-* question addressed to the partner. The partner supplies an appropriate answer but does not elaborate. The child seeks such elaboration by asking a second *wh-* question in which he omits the auxiliary verb. Other sentence elements are included in the proper adult word order. The partner does not answer the question but responds with a second *wh-* question in order to have the child guess at the function from its appearance. The child responds inappropriately to the partner's question, either ignoring the content of the question or miscomprehending the meaning of the *wh-* word. The partner does not pursue the question by restating or reformulating it. Instead, the partner confirms the child's utterance and asks a third *wh-* question incorporating the child's utterance. Again, the child does not respond to the content of the partner's question but repeats the previous utterance with no additional information to aid the partner's understanding.

Conversational Initiation

The most efficient way to initiate a conversation is to gain the listener's attention, greet the listener, and clearly state the topic of conversation or some opener, such as, "Guess what happened to me yesterday?" or "Where have you been? I haven't seen you in ages." Openers set the tone of the conversation and the subsequent turns. Opening and closing a conversation is one of the pragmatic problems most frequently encountered in children with LI (A. Johnson et al., 1984). Children with ASD initiate very little conversational behavior—even less than do other children with LI (Loveland, Landry, Hughes, Hall, & McEvoy, 1988). Of clinical interest is how the child initiates the conversation and how successful he or she is in having the conversation continue (F. Roth & Spekman, 1984a).

Method

It is best to get the listener's attention before initiating a conversation. This usually is accomplished by eye contact and a greeting. The child with LI may begin without any greeting or may interrupt an ongoing conversation with, "Hey." While in a classroom recently, I become aware that a preschooler was talking to my butt. He had neither sought my attention nor offered a greeting. Some children use the same opener repeatedly (e.g., "Guess what?"), whatever the conversational context. Data may need to be collected over a wide variety of situations to discern a pattern. Role-play can be used to determine the child's knowledge of conventional openers.

Frequency and Success Rate

Children who are withdrawn or unsure of the conversational expectations may initiate conversations only rarely. Instead, they adopt a more passive, responsive role. In contrast, other children may interrupt frequently and attempt to initiate conversation indiscriminately. Of interest to the SLP is the density of initiations, or the number of initiations over a given time. Obviously, this figure will change with the situation. For children, lunchtime, recess, and group projects may be appropriate forums in which to collect such data.

The success rate of children in initiating conversations is also significant. Although children may attempt to begin conversations frequently, they may be ignored or mocked, depending on the audiences they choose. Each of us has experienced the "cold shoulder" at least once. Children who are socially inappropriate may experience more than their share.

Topic Initiation

Once a conversation has been initiated, the participants negotiate the topics that will be discussed. **Topic** can be defined as "the proposition or set of propositions or subject matter about which the speaker is either providing or requesting new information" (Bedrosian, 1988, p. 270). This negotiation process begins with one partner introducing a topic; the other partner agrees to adopt that topic by commenting on it, disagrees by changing the topic, or ends the conversation. Mature speakers identify the topic clearly by name and, if in the immediate context, by pointing. Preschool children and those with LI rely more on nonlinguistic cues, such as pointing to and holding or shaking objects.

In general, children with LI are less adept than both their age-matched and language-age-matched peers in their ability to direct the conversation by introducing topics (Donahue, 1983). This lack of ability might reflect difficulty introducing topics clearly and/or these children's limited lists of potential topics (Bedrosian, 1985; Dollaghan & Miller, 1986).

Method

An effectively initiated topic is identified clearly in order to establish mutual regard. As mentioned, the speaker may point, look at, and/or state the topic. Generally, the speaker provides information the listener needs to identify referents and their relationships. Topics are negotiated between speakers, and even when explicitly stated, topics are based on the shared assumptions of each participant.

In general, the less sure the speaker is that the listener knows the topic, the longer the speaker will take to introduce it. The more mature speaker is adept at presupposing the prior knowledge of the listeners. In return for the introduction, listeners assure speakers that they understand, or they ask for clarification when they do not understand.

Topics typically are changed by stating a new one. Older elementary school children, adolescents, and adults increasingly use a conversational technique called *shading,* in which the conversation is steered from one topic to a closely related one. Adult conversations only occasionally contain very disparate topics. Although we don't possess much normative data, we know that between seventh and twelfth grade the number of abrupt topic shifts in an adolescent conversation decreases from 3.19 to 1.44 (Larson & McKinley, 1998).

The child with LI may not establish topics, preferring to adopt those of others. If the child does introduce topics, there may be little or no background information to aid the listener (Brinton & Fujiki, 1992). The child with LI may have a very restricted set of conversational or topic openers or may rely on a stereotypic utterance (e.g., "Guess what?"). Children with emotional difficulties may continue some internal conversation with the assumption that the listener has been privy to this information. As mentioned previously, children with word-finding difficulties or poor vocabularies may rely on nonspecific nouns, such as *one* or *thing.* Nonspecific verbs, such as *do* and *get,* also may be used frequently.

The child's responses to the openers of others may be nonexistent or noncontingent/off-topic. The child may not be able to identify the topic or to determine what response is required to the partner's opener.

Both the linguistic and nonlinguistic aspects of the sample should be analyzed. The nonlinguistic aspects regulate the linguistic ones and are significant in the regulation of turn initiation and termination, topic choice, and interruptions (Prutting, 1982).

Frequency and Success Rate

As with conversational initiation, the density and success rate of topic initiation are noteworthy. In general, less dominant speakers will introduce fewer topics and will be less successful in having their topics adopted by their partners. Lack of success also may indicate problems with topicalization, such as establishing and commenting on, marking changes in, and maintaining the topic for a sufficient length of time (A. Johnson et al., 1984). Related factors to be evaluated are the articulation clarity, degree of completeness, and form of the topic statement; social adaptation of the child's language style; degree of content relevance to the ongoing activity and to listener interests; use of eye contact; and physical proximity (F. Roth & Spekman, 1984a).

Appropriateness

The appropriateness of a topic is determined by the context. Some topics, such as the weather, are always appropriate, whereas others, such as age, income, or sexual behavior, are appropriate only in limited contexts. Each of us has favorite topics.

The SLP is interested in determining the child's favorite topics and in assessing their appropriateness in context. Although some topics will work in one context, they are inappropriate for others. Some children with LI have only limited topics or perseverate on a few regardless of the context. I worked with two brothers with ASD who seemingly could talk only about mathematics. A third child with severe LLD seemed limited to discussing throwing up.

Conversation and Topic Maintenance

Once a topic is introduced, speakers comment on that topic, each sentence reflecting the general discourse topic. In effective conversations, the participants seem to adhere to four principles: stay on topic, be truthful, be brief, and be relevant (F. Roth & Spekman, 1984a).

Each partner depends on a response's *contingency,* or relatedness to the preceding utterance. Each response adds new information on the topic. The topic is mentioned frequently enough to enable both participants to recall it as the conversation progresses, because the topic becomes less specific with each subsequent reference.

Topic continuance may be signaled by maintenance devices, such as *now, well, and then, in any case, next, so,* followed by *I (you, we, they)* (did something). Some devices, called *continuants,* maintain the conversation but add little if any new information. Examples of this behavior are *yeah, uh-huh,* and *okay* when used as a signal that the listener is paying attention. Other maintenance devices are repeating a portion or all of the previous utterance.

Children with LI tend to engage in fewer and shorter interactions than do children developing typically. The most frequent pragmatic problems for children with LI include terminating sentences, connecting discourse, listening and responding to the speaker, knowing when to take a turn, and knowing how to ask and answer questions (A. Johnson et al., 1984).

Although there is little difference between the turn-taking skills at the one-word level of children with LI and of those without, a disparity occurs and widens as language becomes increasingly more complex (Foster, 1985; Prelock, Messick, Schwartz, & Terrell, 1981; Reichle, Busch, & Doyle, 1986). Children with ASD may not respond to initiations, while other children with LI may overuse turn-fillers or acknowledgments ("Uh-huh") to keep the conversation going (Bedrosian, 1988; Brinton & Fujiki, 1989).

Frequency of Contingency

Semantically contingent utterances relate to or reflect the meaning of the prior utterance. One example of contingency is the topic of an utterance. Thus, a contingent utterance maintains the topic of the previous utterance and adds to it in some way. For example, in response to the utterance, "We went to Captain Jake's for dinner last night," a second speaker might make the contingent remark "Oh, did you enjoy the food?" A noncontingent remark would be "My uncle lives on a farm."

Assume for a moment that the name of the restaurant in the previous example was Uncle Jake's. In this situation, the child's remark, "My uncle lives on a farm," although off-topic, does have some link to the previous sentence. If these links can be identified, there may be a pattern that will reveal the child's processing strategy.

In general, children with LI are less responsive than are their age-matched peers developing language typically (Rosinski-McClendon & Newhoff, 1987). This low level of responsiveness may reflect a history of unsuccessful communication. Often, these children respond to questions with stereotypic acknowledgments (*uh-huh, yeh*) and with nonspecific requests for clarification (*what, huh*) (Rosinski-McClendon & Newhoff, 1987).

The frequency of contingent behaviors by the child and the caregiver also is of interest. The child who exhibits few contingent utterances may prefer to initiate new topics frequently (Prutting, 1983). The SLP notes the percentage of the child's utterances that are on-topic, the relevance of the child's questions, and the child's nonverbal responses, such as following directions or looking at something that was mentioned.

A large percentage of off-topic responses may indicate a semantic disorder characterized by difficulty in identifying the topic of discussion. A listener's ability to identify a topic subsequently affects comprehension of comments made about that topic.

The SLP should look for an underlying contingency that may not be readily obvious. Children with LLD may assume that their partners know the underlying relationship and, therefore, may only include unshared information.

Of particular interest are the child's responses to questions. Such responses should be appropriate to the question and factually correct. For example, the question "Why is he eating?" might elicit the following responses from different children:

1. Food.
2. Because.
3. He has to.
4. So he won't be hungry.
5. He's hungry.

The first answer is functionally inappropriate although functionally accurate. It does not answer the question, but tells what the man is eating. The second and third responses are appropriate but too brief to be accurate. The fourth and fifth answers fulfill appropriateness and accuracy criteria.

If an answer does not fulfill both requirements, it is in error and may indicate any number of possible breakdowns in the communication process. I have seen a child with severe emotional disorder who gave extremely inappropriate replies to emotional or personal questions, although her responses to factual questions were usually both appropriate and accurate.

A child with LI may not understand what the questioner desires or may not realize that a reply is required. The question form and the specific *wh-* question type also may be confusing.

In general, recognition and delivery of the general kind of information required develops prior to the ability to respond with the accurate information. Some *wh-* question forms seem easier than others. Three groupings, from easiest to most difficult, are as follows:

Easiest	What + be, which, where
	Who, whose, what + do
Most difficult	When, why, what happened, how

This order suggests a hierarchy for analysis and intervention. In addition, it is easier for children to respond to questions referring to objects, persons, or events within the immediate setting.

Various semantic question prompts can be used to facilitate production of the child's inadequate responses. The child's responses to these prompts can provide useful information for intervention.

Table 6.5 presents a procedure for comparing the efficacy of various prompts in eliciting appropriate and accurate responses from the child. A plus sign (+) indicates appropriate or accurate responses; a minus sign (–) indicates inappropriate or inaccurate ones.

Latency of Contingency

When the child makes contingent responses, there should be little delay or latency between his or her turn and the preceding speaker's turn. Gaps between the turns of mature speakers are brief or nonexistent. Research has indicated that the average amount of time needed for two adults to switch from one speaker to the next is half a second or less.

TABLE 6.5   Score form for the efficacy of various question prompts

Prompt Type	Strategy Description	Prompt Effectiveness (+, –)		Comments
		Appropriate	**Accurate**	
Standard focusing phrase with repetition	*Listen to the question* signals the student that a response was in error. Direct student's attention to the repetition; highlight content.			
Model example with related content	Use another adult or child in context to model correct response. Then ask child, same form, new content.			
Analogous examples	*What are alligators covered with?*—No response. *Seals are covered with fur. What are alligators covered with?*			
Visualization of relationships	*How are an apple and a cookie alike?* No response. Draw semantic feature chart: 		bakes	eat	grows on tree	 	apple	+	+	+	 	cookie	+	+	–				
Relevant comparison yes/no	*What does a hockey player need?* No response. *Does a hockey player need skates?* Yes. *Good. What does he need?*			

The child's inadequate responses can be modified by using question prompts. Successful responses following a prompt are recorded as a + under both the *appropriate* and *accurate* columns.

Source: Moeller, M., Osberger, M., & Eccarius, M. (1986). Cognitively based strategies for use with hearing-impaired students with comprehension deficits. *Topics in Language Disorders, 6*(4), 37–50. Reprinted with permission.

Preschoolers and children with LI may allow long gaps to develop without any of the apparent embarrassment found among adults when there are long unfilled pauses. A noticeable latency prior to the child's response may indicate word-finding difficulties. Frequently, the linguistically more mature partner will fill in for the child, an act that also violates the rules of turn taking.

Latency is an important measure for both contingent and noncontingent utterances, whether adjacent or nonadjacent. Delay may be evident in the adjacent utterances of a child with word-finding difficulties as well. Adjacent utterances are spoken as sequential behaviors by the same speaker. A nonadjacent utterance crosses conversational turns and is an utterance or turn of one partner followed by an utterance or turn of the other. Definitions and examples of these categories are presented in Table 6.6.

Duration of Topic

A topic is sustained as long as each conversational partner cares to continue and can contribute relevant information. The number of turns taken on a topic is a function of the particular topic and partners involved, the conversational context, and the conversational skill of each participant.

Number of Turns

The SLP is interested in the number of turns taken by the child and the partner on a given topic and in the manner of changing topic. In general, a greater number of turns will occur in an adult-child conversation if the child, rather than the adult, initiates the topic. Topics that are sustained longer than others may suggest the child's interest or knowledge or both.

Below age 3, children rarely maintain a topic for more than two turns. In general, preschoolers take very few turns on a single topic unless enacting scenarios, describing events, or solving problems (Schober-Peterson & Johnson, 1989). More turns generally will be produced when the preschool child is directing the partner through a task or when the child is telling a story. Although the

TABLE 6.6 Definitions and examples of utterance pairs

Types	Definitions	Examples
Contingent	The utterance of one speaker is based on the content, form, and/or intent of the other speaker.	S_1: What do you want for lunch? S_2: Peanut butter. S_1: I hope I don't miss my plane. S_2: Don't worry. Every flight is delayed.
Noncontingent	The utterance of one speaker is not based on that of the other.	S_1: What do you want for lunch? S_2: Gran'ma gots a new car.
Adjacent	Utterances spoken sequentially by the same speaker.	We went to the zoo. I saw monkeys and elephants. But my favorite part was petting the sheeps.
Nonadjacent	Utterances spoken sequentially by different speakers. The utterances may be contingent or noncontingent.	S_1: Here comes the school bus. S_2: Yukk, I was hoping he'd get a flat tire. (Contingent)

number of turns increases slightly with age, a great increase does not occur until mid-elementary school.

Informativeness

Each turn should add to the conversation by confirming the topic and contributing additional information. Children who have difficulty identifying the topic or determining what is expected of them conversationally may repeat or paraphrase old information, overuse continuants, or circumlocute. Circumlocution occurs when the child is unable to identify the topic or retrieve needed words and thus talks around the topic in a nonspecific manner. The SLP can rate each utterance for its contribution to the topic being discussed.

Sequencing

Once a topic is introduced, a sequence of conversational acts follows. In general, more specific information is introduced until a natural termination or a change in topic occurs. Answers or replies follow questions; comments or questions follow comments. New information is introduced and later referred to as old information. A lack of sequencing may indicate a semantic disorder or a pragmatic disorder characterized by a lack of presuppositional abilities.

Topic Analysis Format

Several topic analysis formats have been proposed (Bedrosian, 1982, 1988, 1993; Mentis & Prutting, 1991). Each addresses different aspects of topic initiation, maintenance, and change. These are presented in Table 6.7. Topic initiation analysis may include the type of topic, the manner of initiation, the subject matter and orientation, and the outcome. Topic maintenance analysis may consider the type of turn and the ability of the client to further the conversation with the addition of new conversational information.

Topic Initiation

Topic initiations occur when the topic of discussion is changed in some way. Utterances on that topic express concepts subsumed by that topic. Each new topic and directly related utterances can be identified on the transcript.

Type of Topic.   Each topic could be rated according to its novelty. Some children have a limited range of topics in their repertoire. Possible rating categories may include *new, related, reintroduced,* and *consecutive* (Bedrosian, 1982, 1988, 1993; Mentis & Prutting, 1991). New topics would be those appearing in the conversation for the first time and not linked to the immediate preceding topic.

TABLE 6.7   **Analysis aspects of topic**

Topic Initiation	**Topic Maintenance**
Type of topic	Type of turn
Manner of initiation	Conversational information
Subject matter and orientation	
Outcome	

Related topics would be linked directly to the previous topic. Reintroduced topics would have appeared in the conversation previously but prior to the immediate preceding turn. Finally, consecutive topics consist of two or more topics initiated in a turn with no opportunity for the listener to maintain the preceding topic or the first of the consecutive ones to be introduced. In addition, the SLP could check with the caregivers to determine whether any of the topics introduced by the child are habitual ones. Table 6.8 presents examples of different types of topic initiation.

Manner of Initiation.   The manner of topic initiation might include *coherent changing, noncoherent changing, shifting,* and *shading* (Bedrosian, 1982, 1988, 1993; Mentis & Prutting, 1991). Coherent changing occurs when one topic is terminated and a following topic's content is not derived from the immediate preceding topic. Noncoherent changing occurs with the absence of topic termination and/or an utterance signaling transition to a new topic. Shifting occurs when the topic being discussed serves as a source for a new topic. Shading differs from shifting in that shading is a change of focus on the same topic, rather than a discrete topic change. Table 6.9 presents the different manners of initiation.

Subject Matter and Orientation.   The *subject matter* is the content of the topic initiation. Two broad analyses might consist of judgments of appropriate versus inappropriate topics for the communication context. Orientation might include topics about self, a shared experience or interest with the listener, or a topic seemingly unrelated to the listener or a shared interest. If the topic is always the speaker or always unrelated, then serious communication problems may exist.

Outcome.   Outcomes may be rated as successful or unsuccessful (Calculator & Dollaghan, 1982). Success is dependent on the manner of initiation, the subject matter, and the form of the initiation. A command or demand form of topic initiation is probably not a good one to encourage conversational interaction. Success occurs when the conversational partner acknowledges the speaker's topic

TABLE 6.8   Types of topics initiated

Topic Type	Example
New	*Partner:* Uh-huh, and what else did you see at the zoo? *Child:* **Mommy got a new car.**
Related	*Partner:* I like monkeys too. What else? Were there any clowns at the circus? *Child:* **I don't like clowns. They're scary.** *Partner:* Clowns are scary? Why do you think clowns are scary?
Reintroduced	*Child:* And Ernie spilled s'ghetti all over Bert. *Partner:* Was Bert angry? *Child:* Uh-huh. And…and Ernie…And Ernie laughed. *Partner:* Poor Bert. That would be yukky. What else happened on *Sesame Street?* *Child:* Big Bird and Little Bird singed a song. *Partner:* Can you sing it for me? *Child:* Uh-huh. **I don't like s'ghetti on me.**
Consecutive	*Partner:* Oh, tell me the story. *Child:* Okay. This little girl… **Can you come to my birthday party? I got a new bike yesterday. Do you live here?**

TABLE 6.9   Manner of topic initiation

Manner of Initiation	Example
Coherent changing	*Child:* And he chased the dinosaur away. *Partner:* What a great story. Anything else to tell? *Child:* **I have a new baby.**
Noncoherent changing	*Child:* Let's have toast for breakfast. *Partner:* Let me fix it. *Child:* Those are supposed to go down. *Partner:* You do this one, and I'll do the other one. *Child:* **I'm gonna have a bowl of…What's that? I think it's a fireman hat. I wanta be a fireman.** *Partner:* May I wear it?
Shifting	*Partner:* There, I'm gonna make some eggs. *Child:* I don't like eggs. *Partner:* No, why don't you like eggs? *Child:* **I want some…some juice. I like juice.** *Partner:* What kind of juice do you want?
Shading	*Partner:* Let's have toast. *Child:* Where's the toaster? *Partner:* I'll cook the toast. *Child:* **I'll butter it. Where's the knife?** *Partner:* You have to find the knife. *Child:* It too sharp for toast.

in some way, responds, repeats, agrees or disagrees, or adds information to maintain the topic. Nonsuccess includes no response, an interruption, initiation of a new topic, or a request for repair.

Topic Maintenance.   Topic maintenance would be analyzed in all turns subsequent to topic initiation. Each turn can be analyzed in two ways on the basis of the continuous or discontinuous nature of the turn and on its informativeness.

Type of Turn.   Turns may be classified as continuous or discontinuous on the basis of their linkage or nonlinkage to the initiated topic (Table 6.10) (Bedrosian, 1985, 1993). Continuous turns include responses to requests or questions; acknowledgements, such as *uh-huh, okay,* and *yeah;* partial, whole, or expanded repetitions; appropriate emotional responses, including laughter and crying; topic incorporation, such as the addition of more information or a request for more; shading; agreement or disagreement; and a request for repair (Bedrosian, 1985). Discontinuous turns—ones not linked to the current topic—include topic initiations, off-topic responses, monologues, and evasion, including use of silence.

Analysis includes the frequency and range of each type of turn and the average number of turns per topic. The percentage of continuous versus discontinuous turns also would be valuable data (Bedrosian, 1993).

Conversational Information.   Turns might be analyzed for the extent to which they contribute to the development of the topic by adding relevant, novel information (Mentis & Prutting, 1991). Those

TABLE 6.10   Continuous and discontinuous turns

Type of Turn	Example
Continuous	*Partner:* What's that? *Child:* **A cowboy hat.**
	Partner: Put it on. *Child:* **No, it's too hot for a coat.**
	Partner: We have to make some bread for dinner. *Child:* **Okay, I'll help.**
Discontinuous	*Partner:* Do you want to hold the baby? *Child:* **I'll eat my cupcake now.**
	Partner: What else happened at school? *Child:* **I don't like my baby brother.**

adding new information include topic incorporation, such as unsolicited conversational replies that add more information or requests for new information, and answers and replies to questions that contain new information. Other turns—such as acknowledgments; requests for repair; partial, whole, or expanded repetitions; responses to requests or questions that do not contain new information; emotional responses; and agreement or disagreement—add no new information to the conversational exchange. Problematic turns include word searching, incoherent utterances, ambiguous utterances, and incomplete turns. Examples of conversational information rating are included in Table 6.11.

The SLP can calculate the percentage of turns contributing novel information and thus furthering the topic. Other types of turns may indicate possible problem areas. Specific strategies used by children should be investigated by analyzing the form of the utterances being used.

Summary

The topic analysis categories presented in this section overlap and are not always mutually exclusive. More than one turn type and informativeness category may be present in a turn. A possible analysis

TABLE 6.11   Informativeness of turns

Informativeness	Example
New information	*Partner:* Where's Mary? *Child:* **She's sick today.**
	Partner: We're going to the zoo tomorrow, *Child:* **Monkeys live in the zoo.**
No new information	*Partner:* And cowboys ride horsies too. *Child:* **Ride horsie.**
	Partner: Let's play with the stove. *Child:* **What?**
Problematic	*Partner:* What should we play now? *Child:* **A...a...with a...a...with a...you know.**
	Partner: Who's your teacher? *Child:* **At school.**

format is presented in Table 6.12. Each type of analysis gives the SLP an additional tool for sorting the child's language data.

Turn Taking

Turn taking is an excellent vehicle for evaluating the interactional framework of the listener and speaker. The unit of analysis is the dyad and the interaction, rather than the individual behaviors of the child (Prutting, 1982).

TABLE 6.12   Possible format for rating topics and turns

Categories	1	2	3	4	5	6	7	8	9	10	11	12	13	14	15	16	17	18	Total	% of Total
Topic Initiation																				
Type of topic																				
New																				
Related																				
Reintroduced																				
Consecutive																				
Manner of initiation																				
Coherent change																				
Noncoherent change																				
Shifting																				
Shading																				
Subject matter																				
Appropriate																				
Inappropriate																				
Orientation																				
Self																				
Shared																				
Unrelated																				
Outcome																				
Successful																				
Unsuccessful																				
Topic Maintenance																				
Type of turn																				
Continuous																				
Discontinuous																				
Conversational information																				
New information																				
No new information																				
Problematic																				

The rules of turn taking specify that if only two participants are involved, both have speaking turns. In general, children's conversations consist primarily of this nonsimultaneous talking pattern (Craig & Washington, 1986). If more than two are involved, however, no participant is guaranteed a speaking turn.

There is usually only one speaker at a time. If two or more speak simultaneously, all but one withdraw. Children with emotional disabilities may interrupt the speaker before the turn has ended, may ask and answer their own questions, and may take another speaker's turn (Rees & Wollner, 1981).

The listener pays attention to the speaker and demonstrates this behavior by turning toward or looking at the speaker, not interrupting, and/or acknowledging that he or she has heard and understood the speaker. Eye contact among children with LLD and emotional disturbances is often fleeting or nonexistent.

The minimum number of turns to complete an exchange is three. The person who begins the exchange must have a second turn before an interaction has occurred, for example:

Speaker 1: We just returned from Florida.

Speaker 2: Oh, did you go to Disney World?

Speaker 1: No, we were in Fort Lauderdale.

Each full conversational turn consists of three elements: an acknowledgment of the preceding utterance, a contribution by the present speaker, and an indication that the turn is to be shifted. In the preceding example, the previous turns are acknowledged by *oh* and *no*. Indications of turn allocation may consist of questions (as with Speaker 2), intonational markers, and pauses.

Transitions across speakers are orderly, occurring at transition points signaled by the participants. For example, the speaker will look at or address the listener when about to change a turn. The listener may look away, gesture, become restless, or emit an audible sigh when desiring a turn. A really anxious listener may cut off the last few syllables of the speaker's turn without disrupting the topic. Children with LI often do not use these subtle turn indicators and miss their signal value when used by others (Rees & Wollner, 1981).

Finally, the speaker who wishes to continue a turn may increase the speed or intensity of talking and continue through the transition point. If overlap occurs and interferes with understanding, the speaker "repairs" the misunderstood portion.

The SLP can mark on transcript turns 1, 2, and 3 for each exchange. In other words, the child should initiate, add to, and terminate exchanges. Of particular interest are eye contact, turn allocation signaling, and the location and cause of exchange breakdown. In addition, the frequency, variety or range, and consistency of the child's communication are noted. Within each turn, the SLP notes the presence or absence of the three aspects of a full turn and the average amount of time spent in a turn (F. Roth & Spekman, 1984a). The SLP also can examine the effects of adult behaviors on the child's conversational turns and later can help adults develop more facilitative styles.

Turns may be classified as *oblige, comment,* or *response* (Coelho, Liles, & Duffy, 1991). An oblige is initiated by the speaker and demands a response. In contrast, a comment is initiated by the speaker but does not require a response. A response is a reply to either an oblige or a comment. The percentage of each category may indicate active and passive speakers, those that initiate and those that respond.

All responses to obliges can be analyzed further as *adequate, adequate-plus, inadequate,* and *ambiguous* (Shadden, 1992). Adequate responses give only the information requested; they are appropriate for the request. Adequate-plus responses give more than requested, while inadequate do not give enough. Inadequate responses may be invalid, irrelevant, or insufficient. Ambiguous responses are unclear. Examples are given in Table 6.13.

Density

The SLP is interested in the density of turns within each conversation and on various topics. A low density may indicate that the child's conversational partner dominated the conversation by taking very long turns, relinquishing them to the child only occasionally, or that the child was very reticent. Children with ASD may take relatively few verbal turns, thus leaving the partner to fill the void (Loveland et al., 1988). In contrast, if the child talked for lengthy turns, the density also would be low because the listener would have little chance to reply.

Oddly enough, the rate of interrupting increases during the teen years, but the purpose changes. Increasingly, speakers interrupt not to disrupt or change the topic but to move the discussion forward to facilitate communication (Larson & McKinley, 1998).

Latency

The SLP can summarize the overall contingent and noncontingent latencies of the child. Whereas the average adult-to-adult turn changes within about half a second, the child may be slightly slower to react. Longer periods and/or the continual use of fillers and interjections may indicate difficulties with topic identification or word finding.

Duration of Turns

There is no ideal length for a turn, although most listeners know when a turn has continued for too long. We all know at least one incessant talker who does not know when enough has been said. A child who talks incessantly may be exhibiting a semantic disorder of not knowing what information

TABLE 6.13   Types of turns

Turn Type	Example
Oblige	Do you want some cookies? What time is it? What's that?
Comment	I really love to ski. I saw horses in the parade.
Response to comment	(Comment: This dessert is great!) It's an old family recipe.
Response to oblige	(Oblige: How old are you?)
Adequate	I'm 25.
Adequate-plus	I'm 25, and I have a master's degree.
Inadequate	I go to college.
Ambiguous	None of your business. Guess.

is needed to close the topic, a pragmatic disorder of not knowing the mechanisms for closing a topic, or a processing problem of not being certain what information was conveyed.

The SLP is interested in the average length of the child's and the partner's turns. Different situations, partners, and topics may yield clinically significant differences in the length of these turns.

Type of Overlap

Most turns will be nonsimultaneous (Craig & Evans, 1989). However, overlap or simultaneous speech can be very revealing. In general, overlap is of two types: *internal* and *initial*. Sentence internal overlaps are used to complete the other speaker's turn and secure a turn. This ability requires a high level of pragmatic-linguistic knowledge. The child with LI may interrupt internally, indicating a lack of understanding of the process. The child may add new information or change the topic, rather than completing the other speaker's utterance (Craig & Evans, 1989).

Sentence initial overlaps result when the listener interjects between sentences to secure a turn. This interjection may occur when the listener is unsure of the speaker's intention to continue or when the listener wants to gain a turn at speaking. Continual overlaps of this type may indicate a breakdown in turn taking as a result of the behavior of one or both partners. In contrast, a low incidence of interrupting, as noted among some children with SLI, may indicate passivity or an inability to initiate a "turn grab" (Craig & Evans, 1989).

Frequency of Overlap.   Although it may seem counterintuitive, data indicate that, as a group, children with LI exhibit less simultaneous speech in their conversations (Craig & Evans, 1989). Although children with LI may be responsive, many are passive in initiating interaction or turn taking (Fey & Leonard, 1983).

Duration of Overlap.   The adult rules for turn taking state that when an overlap in turns occurs (when two speakers speak at once), one speaker will withdraw. Young children or children with LI may continue to talk or try to outshout their partners. Some children withdraw habitually. The SLP must determine whether the child in question is more likely to withdraw or to continue talking.

How Signaled?   Changes in turn are signaled very subtly. The child with LI may miss such signals. Occasionally, such a child will respond only to questions, knowing that in this situation a response is required. Other children lack a basic understanding of the expectation to reply within a conversation. Still others cannot decipher the language code efficiently enough to respond.

Conversation and Topic Termination

Conversations or topics are ended when no new information is added. In the case of a conversational termination, the topic is not changed. As with the opening of a conversation, there are often adjacency pairs, such as "Bye, see ya"—"Have a nice day" or "Thank you"—"You're welcome."

Preschool children or those with LI may end the conversation abruptly when they decide it is over, occasionally just "turning tail" and exiting the conversational context. Children with LLD may not prepare the listener for the termination of the conversation by signaling with body language—for example, becoming restless, looking away, or looking at a watch. In the opposite extreme, children with LLD or emotional disorder may be unable or unwilling to end the conversation and may perseverate or continue to ask questions that have been answered previously.

Topics usually are terminated by shifting to another related topic. For more mature language users, this process is accomplished by *shading,* in which the speakers shift to another aspect of the topic or to a closely related topic, as in the following exchange:

Speaker 1: I biked along the canal path yesterday.

Speaker 2: Oh, I love to bike there at this time of year.

Speaker 1: I didn't know you bike. What sort of bike do you have?

Speaker 2: I have an inexpensive 12-speed.

Speaker 1: I have a 10-speed…

The original topic of the canal bike path slid into the topic of bicycles.

Whether topics are shaded or are changed abruptly, there is normally some continuity, and the new topic is stated clearly. When there is little left to discuss on a given topic, the conversation shifts. The SLP notes the method the child uses to terminate and change topics and to terminate conversations.

Conversational Breakdown

In essence, the entire analysis of the language of children with LI is an attempt to find where they are ineffectual, where they fail to communicate. It is important for the SLP to determine where these breakdowns occur and how the children attempt to repair them (Audet & Hummel, 1990). The SLP should try to determine the number of conversational breakdowns and describe the cause of breakdown, the repair attempt, the repair initiator, the repair strategy, and the outcome (F. Roth & Spekman, 1984b).

Requests for Repair

Requests for repair, called contingent queries, signal the listener's attentiveness or understanding and skill in addressing the point of conversational breakdown. Conversations may be maintained by use of contingent queries, such as *Huh?, What?,* and *I don't understand.* Such requests for repair maintain the conversation by indicating the point of breakdown, obligating the speaker to clarify, and specifying the appropriate form for that clarification.

The type of repair request varies with the linguistic maturity of the speaker and with the information sought. In general, young children use unspecific requests, such as *Huh?* and *What?* More mature speakers try to specify the information desired, as in the following exchange:

Speaker 1: "We went to the zoo and saw monkeys in big cages."

Speaker 2: "What was in the cages?" (Or "Where were the monkeys?" "Where did you go?")

Requests for repair may seek repetition of the preceding utterance, confirmation, or clarification.

Appropriate requests for repair and responses by the conversational partner demonstrate an awareness of the cooperative nature of conversation. Not only must the child attend to the partner's message, detect misunderstandings, and initiate an appropriate request, but he or she also must possess the knowledge and willingness to use clarification strategies to aid the partner's comprehension (Dollaghan, 1987a).

The child who continually responds with *Huh?* or *What?* may not be attending to the conversation or may have difficulty understanding. In the classroom, such children may rely on routines to make the world understandable. In this case, the child often may look around at the other children for assurance before performing the expected behavior.

The SLP is interested in the degree to which the child requests additional information toward maintaining the conversation and in the form of these requests. These conversational mechanisms can be triggered in conversation by the SLP's garbling or confusing the message. This can be accomplished by mumbling, failing to establish the topic, or providing insufficient information or confusing instructions.

The child with LI may be unaware that communication breakdown has occurred. The SLP can hypothesize about the child's awareness of misunderstanding and confirm the hypothesis through manipulation of utterances addressed to the child. In general, children first gain awareness of breakdowns caused by unintelligible words. The order of awareness to breakdown may be as follows (Dollaghan & Kaston, 1986):

Unintelligible word

Impossible command

Unrealistically long utterance

Unfamiliar word

Question or statement without an introduction and ambiguous, inexplicit, and open-ended statements

Frequency and Form.   In general, preschool children and those with LI, such as those with LLD, tend to blame themselves, rather than the speaker, for misunderstanding (Meline & Brackin, 1987). Thus, these children use fewer requests for repair than might be expected, especially given the greater likelihood of communication breakdown. The requests produced tend to be less specific, reflecting the difficulty encountered with these forms. In short, as listeners, children with LLD do not accept the responsibility to signal miscomprehension, even when taught the procedures for doing so. Instead, these children assume that the speaker will be unambiguous, informative, and clear.

Children's repair strategies can be assessed in different contexts, such as familiar topics, unfamiliar topics, and contrived pragmatic violations, by the SLP (Moeller et al., 1986). The child's attempts to repair can be recorded on a form such as that shown in Table 6.14. Checks in the appropriate spaces would signal the child's attempts to repair and clarify.

Although there are no norms for the frequency of repair requests, general guidelines do indicate a change in both the frequency and type of contingent query with age. The earliest requests for repair are repetitions of the partner's utterance with rising intonation (*Doggie go ride?*) or nonspecific requests for repetition (*What?*). With age, requests become more specific and increase in frequency, although both vary according to the conversational partner. With an adult partner, 24- to 36-month-olds use approximately 7 requests an hour, and 54- to 66-month-olds use approximately 14 (Fey & Leonard, 1984). When the partner is a familiar peer, the mean rate for 36- to 66-month-olds is 30 per hour (Fey & Leonard, 1984). Obviously, there is greater likelihood of misunderstanding when two preschool peers communicate.

TABLE 6.14   Record of requests for repair

Clarification Skills	Familiar Topic	New Topic	Contrived Pragmatic Violation
Fails to seek clarification			

Indicates nonunderstanding
—nonverbally
  puzzled expression
  shrugs shoulders
—verbally
  asks for repetition
  says/signs *What?*
  I don't understand
  I don't remember			

Indicates inability to answer
  I don't remember
  I don't know the word for it
  I can't explain it			

Requests specific clarification
  What did you say about the _____?
  What does _____ mean?			

A pattern of clarification requests may evolve as the speech-language pathologist records the number of requests by type and by conversational context of the familiar or new topic or the contrived violation. Contrived errors or violations can be used to elicit requests for clarification.

Source: Moeller, M., Osberger, M., & Eccarius, M. (1986). Cognitively based strategies for use with hearing-impaired students with comprehension deficits. *Topics in Language Disorders, 6*(4), 37–50. Reprinted with permission.

Conversational Repair

Conversational repair may be spontaneous or in response to a request for repair. Preschool children spontaneously repair very little. Even in first grade, children spontaneously repair only about one-third of their conversational breakdowns. Young children or children with LI often do not attempt to repair communication breakdowns. Children with unintelligible speech may find their repairs as unintelligible as their initial attempts.

Most 10-year-olds are able to determine communication breakdown and repair the damage. Although children with LLD at that age can identify faulty messages, they do not seem to understand when to use these skills. By age 2, most children respond consistently to neutral requests, such as "What?", although they are more likely to respond if the conversational partner is an adult rather than another child. Two-year-olds also tend to overuse "yes" and thus confirm interpretations even when incorrect, possibly because nonconfirmation requires clarification. By age 3 to 5, children respond correctly, even to specific requests, about 80 percent of the time regardless of the partner (Anselmi, Tomasello, & Acunzo, 1986).

Repair can provide valuable information about communication breakdowns. Breakdown can occur for a number of reasons, including lack of intelligibility, volume, completeness of information, degree of complexity, inappropriateness, irrelevance, and lack of mutual attention, visual regard, or mutual desire. In general, children with LI experience a greater number of breakdowns than do age-matched peers who are non-LLD (Fey, Warr-Leeper, Webber, & Disher, 1988; MacLachlan & Chapman, 1988).

Repairs usually focus on the linguistic structure or on the content or nature of the information conveyed. Extralinguistic signals, such as pointing, may be used to clarify. These strategies are not mutually exclusive. In general, successful outcome is related to the explicitness and appropriateness of the repair strategy chosen.

When the child repairs spontaneously, the nature of the original error and the repair attempts should be noted. The SLP scans the transcript for all fillers, repetitions, perseverations, and long pauses. All of these may indicate word-finding difficulties on the child's part. The original error or repair attempt may be based on any number of relationships with the intended word or phrase, as noted in Table 6.15.

Spontaneous versus Listener-Initiated.   The SLP is interested in the percentage of conversational repairs that are either self- or listener-initiated. Usually, listeners signal a breakdown with facial expression, body posture, and/or a contingent query.

Strategy.   Immature speakers usually respond to listener-initiated requests for repair by restating the previous utterance. First graders and younger children will repeat only once in response to a request before becoming irritated. By second grade, children usually are willing to repeat twice before becoming angry. Continued requests also may result in children providing additional information, although children with LI seem less flexible in the use of this strategy (Brinton, Fujiki, & Sonnenberg, 1988).

More mature speakers usually give additional information or reformulate, rather than repeat the utterance. Using their presuppositional skills, such speakers may hypothesize about the supposed point of breakdown and supply more information on this specific area. When requested to clarify, children with LI tend to respond less frequently and with less complex responses than do their peers developing typically (Brinton & Fujiki, 1982; Brinton et al., 1986). The responses of children with

TABLE 6.15   Relationship of word-finding errors and repair attempts to the intended word

Association	Example
Definition	*the thing you cook food on* for *stove*
Description	*the long skinny one with no legs* for *snake*
	book holder for *bookend*
	fuzzy for *peach*
Generic (less specific)	*do* for more specific verb
	hat for *cap, bonnet, scarf,* etc.
	thing or *one* for name of entity
Opposites	*sit* for *stand*
Partial	*ball...big ball...red ball* for *big red ball*
Semantic category	*stove* for *refrigerator* (both are *appliances*)
Sound	*toe* for *tie* (initial sound similar)
	goat for *coat* (rhyme)

LI lack flexibility and usually consist of repetition with little new information included to aid comprehension. Children developing typically seem to have a greater range of repair strategies at the same age (Brinton et al., 1988). The 10-year-old child with LLD is more likely to repeat, rather than reformulate, unsuccessful utterances (Feagans & Short, 1986).

The SLP should prepare a list of the various types of contingent queries and use them in conversation with the child. Of interest is the child's rate of responding to various requests and the nature of the child's response (Fey et al., 1988).

Frequency of Success.   The SLP is interested in how successfully the child identifies breakdowns, repairs them spontaneously, and follows listener requests. In general, children with LI make more inappropriate responses to listener requests than do age-matched peers (Brinton et al., 1988). The responses of the listener enable the SLP to determine the child's success.

Conversational Partner

Language does not occur in a vacuum. Children converse with many conversational partners, both at home and in school. Each partner helps form a dynamic context in which the child communicates and learns.

Parent-child interactions usually offer an example of a communication process finely attuned to the language skills of the child. Thus, the adult-child dyad represents a highly individualized learning exchange based on the interactional styles and skills of the two communicators.

Variables that affect language learning are complexity, semantic relatedness, redundancy, maternal responsiveness, and reciprocity. In general, maternal linguistic complexity seems to be related to the language learner's level of comprehension.

Semantically related utterances provide a contingency-based language-learning experience. The topic and subsequent content usually are derived from the child. Approximately 68 percent of a mother's speech is related directly to the child's verbal, vocal, and nonverbal behavior.

The mother's input tends to be highly redundant because it relates to ongoing contextual occurrences and attempts to explain, clarify, and comment on the child's experiences and behavior. In addition, the caregiver may repeat content several times in different forms.

Consistent maternal responsiveness teaches children that their responses and behavior have a predictable effect. One valuable lesson the child learns is that communication and communication partners are predictable.

These caregiver-child exchanges are reciprocal in that the child is treated as a full conversational partner and allowed to gain early conversational experience. Even infants are treated as full conversational partners by their mothers.

There is indication that some mothers of children with LI provide input that is not regulated by their children's level of understanding, and thus it is significantly longer and more complex than their children's level of comprehension. The MLU may be near that found in adult-adult communication and may include complex structures such as indirect directives, embedded constructions, and *how/ why* questions.

The proportion of utterances of mothers of children with LI that are related semantically is lower than that reported for mothers of children developing typically. In addition, the form of these utterances may be highly restricted, providing the child with a limited variety of input. Because few of the maternal utterances are related semantically, there is little redundancy. Instead, mothers discuss events in the past or future and objects or events not present within the immediate shared context.

Children with LI may have little effect on the conversational interaction, and their verbal and nonverbal behaviors may be ignored. Mothers may persist in introducing new topics, reflecting this non-child-centered approach. Mothers of children with LI may be more dominant in conversations than are mothers of children developing typically, and they may initiate conversation and use directives more frequently (Loveland et al., 1988). In short, these interactions often lack the qualities of language-learning conversational exchanges.

There is a wide range in parents' ability to interpret their children's utterances correctly (Kwiatkowski & Shriberg, 1992). When a child's utterances are unintelligible to a parent because of numerous phonological errors, the parent is more likely to use facilitative strategies, such as maintaining the topic or recasting the child's utterance (Conti-Ramsden, 1990; P. Yoder & Davies, 1990). Thus, the parent takes control of the topic, allowing little opportunity for the child to initiate (H. Gardner, 1989).

Especially when working with preschool children, the SLP should observe the conversational behavior of the primary caregiver and determine the language learning contributions. Utterances can be rated as to semantic relatedness, redundancy, and reciprocity. From these data, the SLP can comment on the overall teaching environment provided by the caregiver's utterances and behaviors.

Conclusion

A language sample is a rich source of information on the child and the conversational partner's language abilities. Analysis may be accomplished at the individual utterance level, across utterance and across partner, and by conversational event. Analysis should not be attempted unless the SLP has a good understanding of the child's language and of the caregivers' concerns. Then a language sample would be analyzed to examine the portion of language in question. A conversational sample can be the best example of a child's actual language use in context.

Utterance-level analysis is more appropriate for language form. Analysis of larger units, such as turns and topics, gives the SLP information on the use of language in context and answers questions about the efficacy of the child's use of language to communicate.

7

Analyzing a Language Sample at the Utterance Level

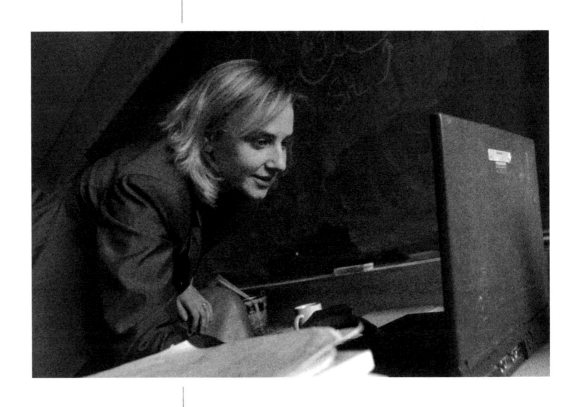

In this chapter, we consider a broad analysis of language that can be accomplished easily within utterances by noting significant aspects of use, content, and form. These aspects are outlined in Table 7.1. In Chapter 6, we discussed analysis across utterances and partners and by conversational event. This three-tiered—across utterances and partners, by conversational event, and within utterances—analysis method seems appropriate for describing the interactive qualities of language use within the context of conversation. Language is not a "unitary construct," but, rather, is multidimensional. It is the responsibility of the SLP to describe the unique character of each child's language.

Each utterance can be analyzed within use, content, and form categories following a variety of analysis formats (A. Johnson et al., 1984; Lund & Duchan, 1993). Individual utterances can yield the frequency and range of various features. Some data will be descriptive, whereas other data will be more normative. This situation reflects the research information available and the type of analysis desired.

A number of computer-assisted and unassisted language sample analysis methods are available. Several are listed in Table 7.2. Although each method yields different data, none presents a total picture of a child's language. In general, the more normative the results, the less descriptive and prescriptive, and vice versa. A few of the more widely used analysis methods are described in Appendix D. A generic analysis method might borrow useful portions from several of these.

Language Use

Much language use data can be gleaned from analysis with units larger than the individual utterance. Within conversations, topics, and turns, however, the SLP can analyze the breakdowns in communication noted in these larger units. The SLP also can analyze the functions or intentions of individual utterances.

Disruptions

Communication breakdown or disruption can occur for many reasons. The amount and type of disruption will vary with the language task, topic, and partner(s). In general, more breakdowns occur

TABLE 7.1   Analysis at the utterance level

Use	Form
Disruptions	Quantitative measures
Illocutionary functions and intentions	Mean length of utterance
Frequency and range	Mean syntactic length
Appropriateness	T-units and C-units
Encoding	Syntactic and morphological analysis
Content	Morphological analysis
Lexical items	Syntactical analysis
Type-token ratio	Noun phrase
Over-/underextensions and incorrect use	Verb phrase
Style and lexicon	Sentence types
Word relationships	Embedding and conjoining
Semantic categories	Computer-assisted language analysis
Intrasentence relationships	
Figurative language	
Word finding	

TABLE 7.2   Language sample analysis methods

Unassisted Methods

Pragmatics
  Adolescent Conversational Analysis (Larson & McKinley, 1987)
  Assessing Children's Language in Naturalistic Contexts (Lund & Duchan, 1993)
  Clinical Discourse Analysis using Grice's framework (Damico, 1991a)
  Language functions (Boyce & Larson, 1983; Gruenewald & Pollack, 1984; Prutting & Kirchner, 1983, 1987; Simon, 1984)

Syntax/Morphology
  Assessing Children's Language in Naturalistic Contexts (Lund & Duchan, 1993)
  Assessing Language Production in Children: Experimental Procedures (J. Miller, 1981)
  Developmental Sentence Analysis (L. Lee, 1974)
  Guide to Analysis of Language Transcripts (Stickler, 1987)
  Language Assessment, Remediation, and Screening Procedure (Crystal, Fletcher, & Garman, 1976, revised 1981)
  Language Sampling, Analysis, and Training: A Handbook for Teachers and Clinicians (Tyack & Gottsleben, 1977)

Narratives
  Narrative level (Larson & McKinley, 1987)
  Story grammar analysis (Garnett, 1986; Hedberg & Stoel-Gammon, 1986; F. Roth, 1986; Westby, 1984, 1992; Westby, VanDongen & Maggart, 1989)

Classroom-based
  Classroom Script Analysis (Creaghead, 1992)
  Curriculum-Based Language Assessment (N. Nelson, 1989, 1992)
  Descriptive Assessment of Writing (Scott & Erwin, 1992)

Computer-Assisted Methods

Syntax/Morphology
  Automated LARSP (Bishop, 1985)
  Computerized Profiling (Long & Fey, 1988, 1989)
  DSS Computer Program (Hixson, 1985)
  Lingquest 1 (Mordecai, Palin, & Palmer, 1985)
  Parrot Easy Language Sample Analysis (PELSA) (F. Weiner, 1988)
  Pye Analysis of Language (PAL) (Pye, 1987)
  Systematic Analysis of Language Transcripts (SALT) (J. Miller & Chapman, 2003)

in narration than in conversation. In addition, the longer the utterance, the more breakdowns present (MacLachlan & Chapman, 1988). Disruptions tend to occur at the developing edge of the child's language where production capacity is "stretched" and there's increased risk of processing difficulty. These utterances are of particular diagnostic significance (Rispoli & Hadley, 2001). Children with LI experience more disruptions than children without.

The frequency of disruptions is inversely related to subjective impressions of communicative competence (Damico, 1985a). More disruptions are equated with less competence. In addition, disruptions can be a valuable clue to a child's process of forming an utterance and to the level of cognitive and linguistic demands made on the speaker (Dollaghan & Campbell, 1992). Obviously, this type of analysis is not needed for all children with LI but may be helpful for those with word-finding problems or with "tangled," slow, or too long utterances.

Analysis requires that the SLP transcribe all words and word portions and all speechlike vocalizations. Pauses of 2 seconds or more also should be noted. Pauses should be obvious on a timed transcript format, as suggested in Chapter 5. All **mazes** should be identified. Mazes are language segments that, like physical mazes, disrupt, confuse, and slow movement—movement of the conversation in this case. Mazes may consist of silent pauses, fillers, repetitions, and revisions. Typical syntactic analysis occurs after most mazes are eliminated.

Analysis steps may consist of the following (Dollaghan & Campbell, 1992):

1. Identify disruptions by the categories in Table 7.3.
2. Determine the overall frequency of disruption and the frequency for each category. Each occurrence counts as one disruption. Frequency can be calculated per 100 unmazed words. Examples are included in Table 7.4.
3. Compare the frequencies to the rough normative data for school-age children and adolescents that follows:

   Mean performance per 100 unmazed words: fewer than two pauses of 2 or more seconds duration; fewer than two repetitions; fewer than one revision; fewer than one orphan (see Table 7.3); fewer than six disruptions overall

4. Note variation in different communication situations.

Scoring and analysis will require training and practice. Reliability can be attained with repeated practice by two or more SLPs working side by side and comparing their analyses.

Illocutionary Functions or Intentions

At the individual utterance level, pragmatic analysis can describe the illocutionary functions or intentions expressed and understood. The frequency and range of these intentions can be compared with those of other children of the same age. The appropriateness and form of these intentions are also of interest. Although there is little normative data on the sophistication of intention form, each intention can be analyzed for its form and means of transmission.

In adolescence, language is extremely important in peer group identification and personal self-worth (Cooper & Anderson-Inman, 1988). The underlying language difficulties of many children with LI result in pragmatic deficits (Donahue & Bryan, 1984; Lapadat, 1991).

Frequency and Range

Very little normative data are available on the frequency and range of intentions (F. Roth & Spekman, 1984a). This paucity reflects the contextual variability of intentions and the lack of agreement by professionals on the intentions expressed at various ages. Intentions are heavily influenced by and heavily influence the conversational context.

A number of taxonomies of illocutionary functions are available, reflecting different ages and contextual situations. I have attempted, in Tables 7.5 and 7.6, to equate these functions and to demonstrate possible changes over time. The SLP may wish to develop a taxonomy based on one or a combination of the taxonomies presented.

The range of intentions becomes wider and more complex with increasing age. In addition, with maturity, the child may express multiple intentions within a single utterance. Thus, the more mature

TABLE 7.3 Disruption analysis categories

Categories	Transcription	Definition and Example
Pauses		
Filled	Place in ( )	Conventional, but nonlexical, one-syllable filler vocalizations. Example: *(um), (er), (ah)*
Silent	Colon & seconds	Silent interval of 2 seconds or more.* Example: *Then we :3 Then we went home.*
Pause strings	( ) & silent marker	Silent and filled pauses in succession. Example: *So he (a-a-a-) :4 he (a-a-a-) :3 he*
Repetitions		
Forward	[RPF]	Repetition of incomplete linguistic unit that is then completed. Example: *Mom said we, **Mom said we could go too.** [RPF]*
Partial	[RPP]	Repetition of incomplete unit with no completion. Example: *So we did eat fast, **did eat.** [RPP]*
Exact	[RPE]	Repetition of previously complete unit. Example: *Mom said you have to go home, **you have to go home.** [RPE]*
Backward	[RPB]	Repetition with additional word(s) inserted prior to repetition. Example: *We went to, **I mean, we went to school.** [RPB]*
Revisions		
Purposes		
Correct error	[RVE]	Revision to correct overt incorrect information. Example: *We saw monk…**horses.** [RVE]*
Add information	[RVA]	Revision to add more information for better comprehension. Example: *And this man he gonna cut…**he was a doctor** [RVA]…cut open…*
Delete information	[RVD]	Revision to delete information for better comprehension. Example: *She had cows and horses on…**no, just cows** [RVD] on her…*
Unknown	[RVM]	Revision for unknown or mysterious reason. Example: *She gave the cookies to the kids, **to them kids.** [RVM]*
Domain affected		
Lexical	[L]	Change in vocabulary. Example: *She love my puppies, **kitties.** [L]*
Grammatical	[G]	Change in syntax or morphology. Example: *She love, **loves** [G] my puppies.*
Phonological	[P]	Change in phonology or articulation. Example: *She woves, **loves** [P] my puppies.*
Multiple	[M]	Change in more than one domain. Example: *She wove, **loves** [M] my puppies.*
Orphans		
Single phoneme or string	[OP]	Seemingly unrelated stray sound(s). Example: *Then man **b-b-b** [OP] go to…*
Word(s)	[OW]	Seemingly unrelated stray word(s). Example: *He take, **eat,** dog for a walk.*
Word(s) and phoneme(s)	[OS]	Seemingly unrelated stray word(s) and phoneme(s). Example: *I **b-b-boy** [OS] walk every day.*

*2 seconds is an arbitrary length. Adult pauses are much shorter.

Source: Adapted from Dollaghan & Campbell (1992).

TABLE 7.4   Sample of disruption analysis

Partner: Do you help your parents at home?
Child: My daddy, my daddy **[RPE]**...**:03** I help my daddy with, my daddy to work **[RVE][G]**.
Partner: Oh, you help your dad? What do you do?
Child: He work in, outside **[RVA][L]** in a garden.
Partner: What do you do in the garden?
Child: Pull weeds and pick **(um)** matoes, tomatoes **[RVA][P]**.
Partner: Um-m, I love tomatoes. I have tomato plants in my garden, too. What else do you do?
Child: I do the leave stuff, the leave stuff with the **[RPP]**...**:02** oh, you know **[RPB]**...**:03** the thing that go
   like this and the leaves.
Partner: You rake the leaves.
Child: Yeah, and I sit, no, jump **[RVE][L]** and my sister.
Partner: You jump on your sister?
Child: Yeah, in the leaves, in the pile of leaves **[RVA][G]**.

TABLE 7.5   Illocutionary functions of children

Early Symbolic (Below age 2)	Symbolic (Age 2–7 years)
Dore (1974), Owens (1978)	R. Chapman (1981), Dore (1986), Folger & Chapman (1978)
Requesting action	Requests (for)
	Action/assistance/objects
Form: Command, demand	Form: Question, command, embedded command, indirect request, suggestion
	Permission
Regulation	Regulation
Protesting	Protesting
	Rule setting
Requesting information	Requesting information
	Form: Choice (yes/no), product (what, which, who...)
	Process (how, why...)
Replying	Replying
Continuants	Acknowledgments
	Qualifications
	Agreements
Comments	Comments
	Assertives
Naming	Identifications
	Descriptions
Personal feelings	Personal feelings
	Statements
	Reports
	Evaluations
	Attributions/details
	Explanations
	Hypotheses
	Reasons
	Predictions

Continued

TABLE 7.5   *Continued*

Early Symbolic (Below age 2)	Symbolic (Age 2–7 years)
Declarations	Declarations
	Procedurals
Choice making	Choice making
	Claims
Answers	Answers
	Providing information
	Form: Choice, product process
	Clarification
	Compliance
	Conversational organization
Calling/Greeting	Attention getters
	Speaker selection
	Rhetorical questions
	Clarification requests
	Boundary markers
	Politeness
	Exclamations
Repeating	Repetitions
Practicing	Elicited imitations
As children become older, they add new functions and continue to diversify those they already possess.	

TABLE 7.6   Intentions and age of mastery

Within Brown's Stage I (MLU 1.0-1.99) (Usually prior to 24 months)	Answering/Responding Continuance Declaring/Citing Making choices Naming/Labeling Protesting/Denying Repeating
Emerging within Brown's Stages II and III (MLU 2.0-3.0) (Usually at 24–36 months)	Calling/Greeting Detailing Predicting Replying Requesting assistance/Directing Requesting clarification Requesting information Requesting objects
After Brown's Stage III (MLU 3.0 +) (Usually after 36 months)	Expressing feelings Giving reasons Hypothesizing

Sources: Compiled from Carpenter & Strong (1988); Owens (1978).

speaker's ability to express different functions is more flexible. With maturity, the speaker discusses more emotions and feelings, including such phrases as "I think…," and provides justifications.

After selecting the most comfortable taxonomy or combination of taxonomies, the SLP rates each utterance of the child and conversational partner for the intentions expressed. Of interest are the conditions under which each intention occurred, possible environmental cues, and the discourse demands, such as the type of discourse (dyad, group) and nature of the task (motor, verbal, visual, or tactile) (Audet & Hummel, 1990).

The normative data available, though only limited, do demonstrate that within a conversation, partners use a wide range of intentions; no intention predominates unless warranted by the situation. The child developing typically will initiate conversation and reply to the initiations of the partner, seek information and provide it, ask for assistance, and volunteer information. In contrast, some children, such as those with ASD, may initiate communication only rarely and respond with minimal replies (Loveland et al., 1988).

Occasionally, adults or children fall into perseverative patterns of communicating, for example, the parent who constantly quizzes her or his child to name the pictures in a book or the child who keeps repeating a pleasing or tantrum phrase. Such behavior can skew the data or allow one type of intention, such as answers, to predominate. These patterns should be noted during conversational sample collection, and the situations gently changed. The use of different situations and different partners may ensure a better distribution of intentions.

Some children, such as the incessant questioner, use only a limited range of illocutionary functions. If this behavior persists across a number of situations and partners, the SLP can be reasonably certain that this narrow range of functions represents the child's typical behavior.

Appropriateness

A very narrow intentional range may indicate inappropriate use of language. The question of appropriateness must be judged against other factors, such as age, race or ethnicity, region of the country, socioeconomic status, gender, and, most important, the communication context.

The language sample can confirm the caregiver's observation that "John seems to ask questions all of the time, even when he knows the answers." Although the observation may not be unfounded, only data from the language sample can offer concrete proof.

The child who responds inappropriately may not know the linguistic context and may need more contextual cues. For example, children with LI have more difficulty responding to *wh-* questions than do children developing typically (Parnell, Amerman, & Harting, 1986). These children have more difficulty with both the accuracy and the functional appropriateness of their answers. Analysis of both of these types of errors is discussed in the section on contingency in Chapter 6. In general, children with LI fail to recognize the request for information inherent in questions. Even relatively simple *What + be* questions, such as "*What is* your favorite TV show?" are difficult when they concern nonimmediate or noncontextual referential sources. Thus, analysis of the context within which questions are asked is as important diagnostically as the analysis of the variety of *wh-* questions produced and comprehended.

Encoding

Intentions can be analyzed by using a means of transmission format, such as verbal/vocal/nonverbal (F. Roth & Spekman, 1984a). The transition from linguistic through paralinguistic to nonlinguistic can be used to describe a hierarchy of competency or effectiveness based on the child's developmental level. The nonlinguistic context and behaviors of the conversational partners must be transcribed to make this information available.

In general, the child with poor linguistic skills will rely on other means of communicating intentions. Although some very sophisticated information can be communicated nonlinguistically, as in the popularly named *pregnant pause,* less mature language users tend to depend on nonlinguistic and paralinguistic means more than do mature users. As with the various intentions expressed, a range of transmission means should be exhibited by the child and partner.

If the child uses an augmentative form of communication, that form should be specified even more and might include physical manipulation of an object, physical manipulation of a partner, gestures, and a sign or other augmentative device. Two children described as nonverbal may have very different means of communicating their intentions.

Content

The understanding of word meanings and word relationships is affected by many factors, such as age, gender, and regional and racial/ethnic differences. To know a word is to know more than just a definition. It means the child understands that word's relationship to similar words of meaning and sound and to words of an opposite meaning and understands the semantic class into which the word can be placed.

Meaning extends beyond the word, however, and larger units of analysis, such as the phrase or the sentence, also must be considered. What is said—for example, "Don't hit me"—may be very different from the intended message, which might be "Go away, I don't understand what you want."

Obviously, all of this information cannot be ascertained from a brief language sample. Word understanding can be assessed by playing games like Simon Says or by directing the child through a series of tasks. The SLP can make statements in which words obviously are used incorrectly in order to judge the child's reactions. Word games that solicit definitions or antonyms also can provide valuable information. Sorting and categorization tasks can be part of a play situation and can provide information on the child's ability to categorize and classify. The child can be asked to name the members of a category or to deduce the category name from a list of members. The SLP can play the "fool" and make ridiculous comparisons ("A mouse is bigger than an elephant") or silly pairings ("The comb goes between his toes") to gauge the child's reactions.

Vocabulary abilities are strongly related to reading comprehension (Curtis, 1987; Nagy & Herman, 1987). Reading and writing analysis is discussed in Chapter 13. The child with semantic difficulties also may exhibit academic failure.

Children with LI and with LLD usually do not have difficulty with referent-symbol tasks, such as those represented by the Peabody Picture Vocabulary Test. These children may have difficulties, however, with double meanings, abstract terms, synonyms, and nonliteral interpretation (Seidenberg & Bernstein, 1986). In addition, the physical setting can be especially important for children with LI because they depend much more on the context for support than do children developing typically. The child may understand a word only given certain physical situations.

Initially, word meanings are learned by a process called *fast mapping,* in which a hypothesized meaning is assigned to a word on first meeting. In general, children learn new words after only one exposure by forming an initial, albeit partial, understanding based on the linguistic and nonlinguistic contexts (G. Miller & Gildea, 1987; R. Sternberg, 1987). This meaning gradually is refined or replaced over time.

Children with LI and those who are developing typically seem to learn word meanings in this fashion, although some children with LI, such as those with TBI, may require more subsequent exposures than do children developing typically (Keefe, Feldman, & Holland, 1989; Rice, Snell, & Hadley, 1990). Another difficulty for children with LI is related to recall of the phonological shape or pattern of new words (Dollaghan, 1987b). This problem also may reflect the generally slower recall rate reported for children with LI (Sininger, Klatzky, & Kirchner, 1989).

It may be best to assess definitions in formal decontextualized activities, such as testing, but word use in conversations can also indicate correct usage. Between ages 5 and 10, the nature of definitions changes from functional to categorical and more elements are added. By second grade, 49 percent of definitions include categorical membership, such as *an apple is a fruit,* increasing to 76 percent by fifth grade (Nippold, 1995).

Multiple definitions are more difficult to interpret in a decontextualized or isolated format because of the use of content to disambiguate (C. Johnson, Ionson, & Torreiter, 1997). In general, a sentence format aids performance but this varies with word type. Words with multiple definitions appear frequently. For example, 72 percent of the 9,000 most frequent words in one elementary reading series had multiple meanings.

Lexical Items

Obviously, there are several levels of semantic analysis relative to individual words and relations between words and larger units. At the word level, the child demonstrates individual word meanings and word classes. Several questions arise relative to word use and the range of meanings and relationships.

Norms are difficult to establish, especially for older school-age children and adolescents because of the individualistic nature of lexical growth. In addition, increases in vocabulary occur at a slow and steady pace into adulthood. School-age children and adolescents exhibit semantic development in the following areas (Scott, Nippold, Norris, & Johnson, 1992):

Comprehension of literate verbs, such as *interpret* and *predict*

Comprehension of textbook terms, such as *invertebrate* and *antecedent*

Comprehension of adverbs of magnitude, such as *slightly* and *unusually*

Comprehension of adverbial conjuncts, such as *meanwhile* and *conversely*

Comprehension of sarcasm based on its linguistic aspects, as well as intonation

Comprehension of slang terms used by peers, such as *phat*

Comprehension of complex proverbs

Comprehension of complex metaphors

Explanation of infrequently occurring idioms, such as *to vote with one's feet*

Explanation of ambiguous messages

Definition of abstract concept words, such as *courage* and *justice*

Type-Token Ratio
The **type-token ratio (TTR)** is the ratio of the number of different words to the total number of words. The number of different words (NDW) in a sample of fixed length is strongly correlated with

age and measures of semantic diversity (J. Miller, 1991). Significantly lower values than those in Table 7.9 on page 190 might suggest retrieval problems or poor vocabulary.

The total number of words (TNW) also increases steadily with age and is a general measure of verbal productivity (J. Miller, 1991). For example, 3-year-olds use 205 words in 50 utterances, while 8-year-olds use 379. Although a general measure of ease of language use, TNW also is affected by other factors, such as motor ability and word retrieval. For these reasons, the validity of TNW as a measure of preschool language development has been questioned by some professionals (Gavin & Giles, 1996). Values of TNW are listed for a 20-minute sample in Table 7.9.

As a quantitative measure, TTR has had a checkered past of professional acceptance. This uncertainty reflects recognition that the value may vary widely with the language sample size. In general, less variability is found across larger samples of 350 words or more (Hess et al., 1986). Multiple settings and more representative samples would yield theoretically more stable values, although there may be great situational variability for an individual child (Hess, Haug, & Landry, 1989).

Children between ages 2 and 8 demonstrate TTRs of 0.42 to 0.50 (Klee, 1992). Children who receive values greater than 0.50 have greater variability and flexibility in their language, whereas those below 0.42 tend to use the same words over and over again. Very low values may indicate perseverative or stereotypic behavior, word-retrieval problems, or restricted vocabulary. Children with LEP also may score lower because of their lack of English vocabulary.

A low value may indicate overreliance on words with broad application but unspecified meaning (empty words), such as *thing* and *one*. Children with poor vocabularies or word-finding difficulties may use empty words, rather than more specific words that are not at their disposal.

Two spontaneous language profiles emerge from the samples of children with word-finding problems (German, 1987). Some children exhibit word-finding difficulties both on structured naming tasks and in spontaneous samples. They exhibit reformulations, time fillers, empty words, repetitions, starters, and grammatical errors. Other children with LI exhibit these behaviors only on structured naming tasks, although they produce relatively less language in spontaneous samples than do children developing typically.

Mature speakers should possess a variety of words for describing sensory experiences, such as sight (*clearly*), sound (*loud*), smell (*stunk*), and feelings (*happy, tired*). They should be able to describe the environment in terms of time (*at five o'clock*) and location (*in front of*). Entities should possess physical qualities, such as shape (*sort of round*), size (*big*), number (*two, many, few*), substance (*metal, wood*), and condition (*new, ragged*). There should be terms for relationships, such as comparisons (*bigger than, as big as*) and qualifications (*nearly, not quite, only, enough*); and verbs for describing actions (*run, jump, eat*), states (*am, is, are*), and sensory processes (*feel, hear, see*). Finally, the speakers should be able to describe causation (*because...*) and motivation. As noted previously, these terms develop slowly. The full range is characteristic of the mature speaker.

Deictic terms, or terms that must be interpreted from the perspective of the speaker (e.g., *here, there, this, that, come, go*), offer a special problem for the child with LI. The shifting reference that occurs with each speaker change contributes to the child's difficulty. Children with LLD, ASD, or emotional disturbances may lack either the listener or speaker perspective. These children also may refer to themselves by name and may echo the utterances of others.

Over-/Underextensions and Incorrect Usage

The SLP should note all inaccurate uses of words that indicate some variation between the child's meaning and the conventional one. In general, meanings mature from the personal experiential ones found in preschool children to the shared conventional ones of adults.

Some children use words incorrectly because they do not know the shared conventional definition. Others use word substitutions that are incorrect. For example, a recent letter from a young adult with LLD included the following:

> I wish I could write as good as you. You know where to put paragraphs and how to use *punctuality* [my italics] right.

Because I am usually late, I assume he meant *punctuation.* Further testing by the SLP can reveal the basis of the child's substitutions. The child may miss the target word slightly, as in the above example, or may have word-finding difficulties, resulting in word substitutions.

Children with LEP may use L_2 words in either very restricted or overextended ways. Restricted use may be limited to specific features of a word or to word-for-word transfer in which the word has only the meaning of its L_1 equivalent. In the latter—for example, the English *for,* which is *pour* in French and has slightly different syntactic uses—might be used only where *pour* would be used.

Style and Lexicon

Children begin to use different styles of talking relatively early. Analysis across utterances and partners might highlight a conversational style shift. These changes can be analyzed further for the vocabulary used in different styles.

Slang is a casual manner of spontaneous conversation among peers and is important for adolescents. Used appropriately, slang separates adolescents from children and adults and establishes group identity and solidarity (Cooper & Anderson-Inman, 1988). Certain vocabulary—*rad, phat, bad*—is characteristic of adolescent slang. Word meanings change quickly and are invented often by youth (R. L. Chapman, 1987). Knowledge of slang vocabulary increases with age, with boys knowing more terms for vehicles and money and girls for clothing, boys, and unpopular individuals.

The adolescent with LI may seem odd in peer situations because he or she underuses or overuses adolescent slang or uses it inappropriately. Although difficult to assess because of its changing nature and subgroup use, slang is, nonetheless, extremely important. In brainstorming sessions, teens developing typically can suggest vocabulary targets for assessment and training.

The child's literate vocabulary, consisting of words primarily used in common academic contexts, is also important. A good, literate lexicon is needed to achieve academic success, especially among adolescents (Nippold, 1993). Possible lexical items are *analyze, criticize, deduce, define, infer, interpret, predict, remember,* and *understand.* Classroom teachers can suggest other useful literate terms.

Word Relationships

Each word in a language is related to other words in ways that account for the richness of language. These relationships consist of word associations (e.g., *salt and pepper* or *king and queen*), synonyms, antonyms, and homonyms. Some of these associations are expressed in the conversational sample, whereas others need to be probed by the SLP. These associations reflect underlying cognitive organizational strategies.

Semantic Categories

Semantic categories, such as agent, action, and location, are the earliest word classes children use. Indeed, most of the early language development of toddlers is concerned with semantic units.

Several categorization schemata attempt to describe the semantic classes of young children and adults. Table 7.7 is a composite of these semantic category schemata. The SLP is interested in the range of semantic categories expressed by the child.

Semantic knowledge, or the underlying concepts about properties of entities, may be a better framework than linguistic form for the assessment of children with "nonstandard" dialects, including African, Latino, and Asian American English and Appalachian English.* The adequacy of the semantic knowledge of these children is often questioned on the basis of the form of their language. It is assumed, incorrectly, that nonstandard speakers acquire concepts later than do speakers of dialects closer to Standard American English (SAE).

The developmental trends are very similar and suggest guidelines for assessment of the semantic features of nonstandard speakers (Stockman & Vaughn-Cooke, 1986). By age 30 months, working-class, nonstandard speakers use mostly two-word combinations and encode several semantic categories, such as existence, action, location, state, negation, attribution, notice, intention, and recurrence. These guidelines can be used to help identify nonstandard-speaking children who may need clinical intervention.

Intrasentence Relationships

In addition to an interest in the child's word meanings and relationships, the SLP investigates other relationships expressed in the sentence through the use of conjunctions, negatives, and prepositions (Lund & Duchan, 1993) and various sentence forms, such as passive voice.

Four types of conjunctive relations are expressed in conjoined sentences (Bloom, Lahey, Hood, Lifter, & Fiess, 1980): additive, temporal, causal, and adversative.

In the *additive* form, two clauses with no dependent relationship simply are joined to one another. In the sentence "Julio ate pie, and Brigid drank coffee," neither event depends on the other for its existence.

In the *temporal* form, one clause depends on the other to precede or follow or occur at the same time, as in "I'm going to the store before I go to the party" or "I'll rake the leaves while you finish painting the trim."

Causal conjoining implies a dependency in which one clause is the result of the other, for example, "I went to the party because I was invited." The preschool child may use *because* alone or at the beginning of a clause, as in "Cause I want to," although true causal conjoining occurs much later (see Table 7.16 on page 198).

Finally, in *adversative* conjoining, one clause contrasts with information in the other, as in "I read the article, but I was unimpressed." One clause opposes or negates the other.

Negatives may be expressed in several ways and develop at different stages. The four mature negative forms include (a) *not* and *-n't,* (b) negative words, such as *nobody* and *nothing,* (c) the determiner *no* used with nouns, and (d) negative adverbs, such as *never* and *nowhere.* Again, the more mature language user should have a variety of forms. Those used by the child can be compared with the developmental data available in Table 7.16.

Prepositions are some of the hardest working and most versatile English words. They can be used to mark location (*in the box*), time (*in a minute*), or manner (*in a hurry*) and to fill adjectival and adverbial functions. These small, often unstressed words may be misinterpreted or misunder-

---

*The somewhat objectionable term "nonstandard" merely denotes degree of difference. Nonstandard dialects differ more from the ideal Standard American English—which none of us use—than other dialects, such as Eastern New England American.

TABLE 7.7 Semantic categories

Semantic Function	Description	Example
Action	The predicate expresses action with a transitive or intransitive clause.	We *grew* pumpkins and squash. (Transitive) She *gave* us a dollar. (Transitive) He *swims* daily. (Intransitive)
State	The predicate makes a statement about the way things are with a transitive, intransitive, or equative clause.	I *want* a hot fudge sundae. (Transitive) Tigers *look* fierce. (Intransitive) She *is* tall. (Equative) My sister *is* now at Harvard. (Equative)
Agent or actor	Animate instigator of action. Sometimes inanimate, especially if natural force. Usually the subject but may also be passive complement.	*Mike* threw the ball. *Termites* destroyed our cabin. *Wind* blew down the trees. The *cat* chased the dog. The *dog* was chased by the cat.
Instrument	Usually refers to the inanimate object used by the actor to effect the action stated in the verb. The actor is usually not stated but may be. The instrument function may also be adverbial, as in *on his drum*.	The *axe* split the wood. The building was erected by a *crane*. She used the *baseball bat* with great skill. The shaman kept rhythm on his *drum*.
Patient	The entity on which an action is performed. The patient may be a direct object in transitive clauses or the subject in intransitive clauses.	Mike threw the *ball*. The *lighthouse* withstood the hurricane.
Dative	The animate recipient of action. Usually the indirect object but may also be the direct object if it does not undergo any action but receives something.	Father bought *mother* a bouquet of roses. Our mascot brought *us* good luck. He built a treehouse for his *daughter*. I loved that *movie*.
Temporal	Fulfills the adverbial function of time in response to a *when* question. May also be the subject of a sentence or a complement.	I'll see you *later*. We'll meet at *four o'clock. Then,* I'll know. *Tomorrow* is a holiday. *Tuesday* will be our first meeting. It is *time to leave*.
Locative	Fulfills the adverbial function of place in response to a *where* question. May also be the subject of a sentence or a complement.	Some of us looked *in the old log*. I knew it was right *here*. *Chicago* is indeed a windy city. *Our house* has three bedrooms.
Manner	Fulfills the adverbial function of manner in response to a *how* question.	We stalked the big cat *carefully*. He worked *with great skill*.
Accompaniment	Fulfills the adverbial function of *with* X in response to *with whom* or *with what* questions.	He swam *with his sister*. She left *with Jim*. He hunted *with his dogs*.
Empty subjects	Serve a grammatical function.	*It* was sunny. *There* may be some rain.

Source: Adapted from Chafe (1970); Fillmore (1968).

stood by children with both LI and LEP. A strategy they use is overreliance on one form. As mentioned previously, the SLP examines the sample for the breadth of use.

In general, children with LI exhibit difficulty interpreting sentences in which the information might be interpreted in a reverse manner (van der Lely & Harris, 1990). For example, a passive sentence, such as "The cat is chased by the dog" might be interpreted incorrectly as "The cat chased the dog" by using a agent-action-object interpretation strategy. Children with LI have difficulty interpreting the grammatical functions of words and integrating grammatical and semantic information.

Figurative Language

Nonliteral meanings used for effect are more characteristic of school-age and adult language than of preschool language (Nippold, 1988a; Nippold & Martin, 1989). Examples include metaphors, similes, idioms, and proverbs. For the purposes of analysis, jokes and puns also can be considered figurative language. Figurative language occurs frequently in oral conversation and written texts. Interpretation of idioms is highly correlated with reading ability.

Children as young as 3½ are able to comprehend some idioms, especially the more literal ones (Abkarian, Jones, & West, 1992). In general, figurative interpretation increases with increasing age. Individual interpretive ability is related to each person's world knowledge (Winner, 1988). For example, *smooth sailing* has more meaning for the child who has some boating experience.

Idioms occur frequently in the classroom. There may be as many as four figures of speech per speaking minute. Teachers use idioms in approximately 11 percent of their utterances, while third- to eighth-grade reading programs contain idioms in approximately 6.7 percent of their sentences (Lazar, Warr-Leeper, Nicholson, & Johnson, 1989).

Idioms differ greatly in their difficulty of interpretation. In general, more familiar and more transparent or guessable idioms are easier. The child's world and word experience appear to be a key factor in interpretation (Nippold & Rudzinski, 1993).

The SLP considers the range of figurative language used. Some children overrely on well-worn phrases and expressions, with little knowledge of their actual meaning. Such expressions as these can be probed by the SLP to determine the child's actual knowledge.

Comprehension and production of idioms might be analyzed on the basis of *decomposability* of the idiom. Decomposable or analyzable idioms can be broken easily into their component parts. For example, *pop the question* or *let off steam* can be broken into components that each contribute to the overall meaning, as follows:

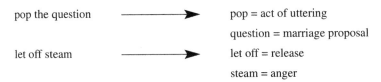

Nondecomposable idioms, such as *kick the bucket,* are difficult to break into components.

Comprehension depends on the child's intuition about the internal semantics of the idiom. In general, young children are better able to interpret decomposable idioms than nondecomposable. Third and fourth graders do equally well on both types in context. If no contextual information is available, these children also are better able to comprehend decomposable idioms (Gibbs, 1991).

Analysis of figurative language is especially important for children with LEP. Idiomatic expressions may be interpreted literally and/or based on cultural interpretation.

Word Finding

Word-finding difficulties are an impaired ability to generate a specific word that is evoked by a situation, stimulus, sentence context, or conversation. In Chapter 3 we discussed a method of probing for word-finding difficulties and strategies. In Chapter 6 we noted that latency may signal such difficulties. Other symptoms include frequent pauses, repetitions, circumlocutions, fillers, nonspecific words, frequent pronouns, and high usage of cliches and routinized expressions, such as *you know* (Bates et al., 1988; Snyder & Godley, 1992). Inaccurate naming may be analyzed using the strategies presented in Table 3.7.

Several intrinsic and extrinsic variables affect word-retrieval skills. Intrinsic variables include the frequency of occurrence of the word, familiarity with the word, age of acquisition, category, and degree of abstractness. In general, more frequently used, more familiar, earlier learned, and less abstract words are easier to retrieve (Stowe, 1988). Words from large prototype categories, such as fruits and vegetables, are easier to retrieve than those from well-defined categories, such as months, based on a small set of specific features. In actual use, categories overlap and relative importance for naming will vary.

Extrinsic variables include the context, syntactic requirements, type of stimulus and manner of presentation, priming, and use of categories. In general, sentence contexts are easier than picture ones, which, in turn, are easier than definitions. Formulation of more difficult sentences, however, interferes with word recall, probably because of the greater cognitive energy needed to form the sentence. Priming results when preceding words aid recall (Balota & Duchek, 1989; Glass & Holyoak, 1986). Finally, use of subordinate categories can aid word recall (Kail, Hale, Leonard, & Nippold, 1984).

The effect of these variables can be very important and difficult to assess in a language sample. It is important, therefore, to use familiar partners, topics, and situations to facilitate retrieval.

Form

Language form includes syntax, morphology, and phonology, or the means used to encode the intentions of the speaker. Even though most language analysis methods concentrate on this aspect of language, very few normative data are available. The task is partially normative and partially descriptive, involving both quantitative and qualitative analysis. Several available analysis methods are described in Appendix D. A discussion of phonological analysis is beyond the scope of this text.

Quantitative Measures

Quantitative measures include mean length of utterance (MLU), mean syntactic length (MSL), T-units and C-units, and the density of sentence forms. Each is discussed in some detail.

The SLP must be cautious with all word and morpheme counts. Careful editing of utterances is required so that interjections, false starts, and the like are not included in the count. Circumlocutions, or talking around an unretrievable word, actually may increase the length of the child's utterances. It is recommended that the SLP follow consistent rules for counting. For example, incomplete words, nonessential repetitions, revisions not containing a complete thought, unintelligible words and phrases, and fillers might be offset in brackets and not counted. These structures are retained, however, for disruption analysis.

Quantitative measures may present some problems (Scott & Stokes, 1995). In general, there can be wide variability across children and situations. In addition, many values change only slowly with age. Still, average words per sentence values increase from 7 to 14 between third and twelfth grade.

Combinations of quantitative data may yield better information than individual bits of information. For example, MLU, percentage of utterances containing one or more errors of morphology or syntax, and chronological age seem to be optimal for predicting clinical diagnosis of SLI (Dunn, Flax, Sliwinski, & Aram, 1996). Structural errors might include word misordering; omission or incorrect use of a morpheme; omission of articles, auxiliary verbs, or contractions; use of telegraphic speech; or incorrectly selected negatives. Children between the ages of 49 and 53 months may have MLU values of 4.1 compared to 3.12 for those with SLI. The percentage of utterances with structural errors is 10.97 and 23.56 respectively.

Mean Length of Utterance

Mean length of utterance is the average length in morphemes of the speaker's utterances. Up to an average of 4.0, MLU is considered a good measure of language complexity. Not all linguists agree (J. Johnston & Kamhi, 1984; Klee & Fitzgerald, 1985; Lahey, 1994). In general, there is less variability in MLU below 4.0 (Rondal, Ghiotto, Bredart, & Bachelet, 1987). This mean is reached by the nonimpaired child at around age 4, but MLU continues to increase with age. At lower MLUs, new structures added to the child's utterances increase the complexity of those sentences. After this level of development, much of the growth in complexity is the result of internal reorganization of utterance form, rather than addition of new structures. This explanation of the relationship between length and complexity is extremely simplified, and there are many related factors.

To calculate MLU, the SLP divides the language sample into utterances. It is best not to include in analysis the portions of conversation that occurred while the child was adjusting to the partner or to the situation. The number of morphemes in each utterance is counted and totaled for the entire sample. Rules for counting morphemes on the basis of the order of development with nonimpaired children are included in Table 7.8. Brief rationales for these rules are included where appropriate.

The total number of morphemes for the entire sample is divided by the number of utterances from which it was derived to determine the MLU. This value then can be compared to the age data in Table 7.9. It is obvious from the table that a wide variability and a wide range of ages are considered within the normal range. Even so, the need to collect a typical sample is very important. If data have been collected in two or more settings, the MLUs from each can be compared to assess the stability of the overall data.

Although age and MLU are correlated as shown in Table 7.9, some interesting data suggest cautious acceptance of this correlation. First, the relationship of rate of MLU change and age is not a constant, as seen in Table 7.9. Second, some language impairments are not evidenced by delays in MLU as might be expected (Klee, Schaffer, May, Membrino, & Mougey, 1989).

As with any single measure, MLU alone is a poor diagnostic tool and the validity and reliability of results will vary with the sample size (Eisenberg, McGovern Fersko, & Lundgren, 2001). Standard errors of measure may differ .19 at 18 months to .71 at 60 months based on a 50-utterance sample. Values are less for 100 utterance samples.

TABLE 7.8   Rules for counting morphemes relative to preschool children

Structure	Example	Count	Rationale
Each recurrence of a word for emphasis	No, no, no.	1 each	
Compound words (2 or more free morphemes)	Railroad, birthday	1	Compound words learned as a unit by preschoolers
Proper names	Bugs Bunny, Uncle Fred	1	Proper names, even those with titles, learned as a unit by preschoolers
Ritualized reduplications	Choo-choo, Night-night	1	
Irregular past tense verbs	Went, ate, got, came	1	Verb tense learned as new word by preschoolers, not as *verb +ed*
Diminutives	Doggie, horsie	1	Phonological form CVCV easier than CVC for preschoolers and does not denote smallness
Auxiliary verbs and catenatives	Is, have, do; gonna, wanna, gotta	1	Preschoolers do not know that such words as *gonna* are *going to*
Contracted negatives	Don't, can't, won't	1–2	Because negatives *don't, can't* and *won't* develop before *do, can,* and *will,* count as one until the positive form appears. Then count the negative forms as two morphemes. All other negatives—*couldn't*—count as two.
Possessive marker (-'s)	Tom's, mom's	1	
Plural marker (-s)	Cats, dogs	1	
Third-person singular present tense marker (-s)	Walks, eats	1	
Regular past tense marker (-ed)	Walked, jumped	1	
Present progressive marker (-ing)	Walking, eating	1	
Dysfluencies	C-c-candy, b-b-baby	1	Count only the final complete form.*
Fillers	Um-m, ah-h	0	

*In the example "I want can … I want can … I want candy," only the last full reduction is counted, being three morphemes.

Nor is a low MLU necessarily indicative of language impairment. Utterance length may vary with the situation, and some children with LI, especially those with circumlocution or empty words, may have inflated MLUs.

An alternative MLU has been proposed that includes no elliptical utterances, no imitative ones, and no single-word yes/no responses (Johnston, 2001). Alternative MLU values are presented in Table 7.9. This "conversational MLU" may be closer to actual discourse properties of the child's language.

TABLE 7.9   Quantitative measures of language

Age in Months	MLU	*Range of Mean MLU	**MSL	**TNW (20 min.)	**NDW (50 utt.)
18	1.1	1.0–1.2			
21	1.6	1.1–1.8	2.7	240	36
24	1.9	1.6–2.2	2.9	286	41
27	2.1	1.9–2.3	3.1	332	46
30	2.5	2.4–2.6	3.4	378	51
33	2.8	2.7–2.9	3.7	424	56
36	3.1	3.0–3.3	3.9	470	61
39	3.3	3.2–3.5	4.2	516	66
42	3.6	3.3–3.9	4.4	562	71
45	3.8	3.4–4.3	4.7	608	76
48	3.9	3.6–4.7	4.9	654	81
51	4.1	3.7–5.1	5.2	700	86
54	4.3	3.9–5.8			
60	4.4	4.0–6.0			
108	8.8	7.2–10.4***			

TTR (type-token ratio) changes little with age but is in the range .42–.5 for 2- to 9-year-olds.

*Combined data from four different studies (Klee, Schaffer, May, Membrino, & Mougey, 1989; J. Miller, 1981; Scarborough, Wyckoff, & Davidson, 1986; Wells, 1985)

**MSL (mean syntactic length), TNW (total number of words), and NDW (number of different words) extrapolated from tables in Klee (1992).

***From J. Miller, Freiberg, Rolland, & Reves, 1992.

Mean Syntactic Length

Mean syntactic length (MSL) is the mean length in words of all utterances of two words or more—those utterances with some internal grammar. This measure eliminates all one-word responses, such as yes/no answers. MSL seems to correlate more strongly than MLU with age (Klee & Fitzgerald, 1985). Values for MSL are listed in Table 7.9 (Klee, 1992).

T-units and C-units

Expressive language syntax of older children and adolescents can be measured in **T-units** (minimal terminal units), consisting of one main clause plus any attached or embedded subordinate clause or nonclausal structure (discussed in the following section). Thus, the unit has shifted from the utterance to the sentence in its shortest allowable form. Any simple or complex sentence would be one T-unit, but a compound sentence would be two or more. For example, the sentences "I want ice cream" and "I want the one that is hidden in the blue box" each constitute one T-unit with varying numbers of words and clauses. "I want the ice cream in the picture, and he wants a shake" consists of two main clauses and thus two T-units. Examples of T-units are given in Table 7.10.

TABLE 7.10 Examples of T-units and C-units

Sentence Structure	Example	Number of T-units and C-units
Simple—one clause	They watched the parade on TV.	1 T-unit, 1 C-unit
Complex—embedded clause	Washington has the horse I want.	1 T-unit, 1 C-unit
Compound—conjoining of two or more clauses	*They went to the movie,* but *I stayed home.*	2 T-units, 2 C-units
	Mom went to work, I went to school, and *my sister stayed home.*	3 T-units, 3 C-units
Partial sentences		
Elliptical answers	(Who went with you?) Marshon.	1 C-unit
Exclamations	Oh, wow!	1 C-unit
Aphorisms	A penny saved.	1 C-unit

The T-unit is more sensitive than MLU to the types of language differences seen after age 5, such as phrasal embedding and various types of subordinate clauses. Throughout the school years, a slow but regular increase occurs in sentence length in both oral and written contexts.

Children's language can be described in words per T-unit, clauses per T-unit, and words per clause. A gradual and progressive increase in words and clauses per T-unit and in words per clause in spontaneous speech occurs with increased age throughout childhood and adolescence, although the values change only gradually during early school years (Table 7.11) (Klecan-Aker, 1985; Scott et al., 1992). The values for spoken words/T-unit and clauses/T-unit are similar for Spanish.

To calculate these values, the SLP divides the sample into sentences, each equaling one T-unit. The number of words and clauses then can be determined for each and divided by the number of T-units to calculate an average. The words per clause can be determined similarly.

It should be noted that the type of conversational task will influence some T-unit measures. Information-giving tasks increase the words and clauses per T-unit. In addition, at this level of development, T-unit values can be misleading because complexity and length are not directly related. For example, among adolescents, phrases may be used in place of subordinate clauses for conciseness, suggesting greater syntactic sophistication (Nippold, 1993). These include participial phrases (***Working until midnight,*** *John missed his bus*), infinitive phrases (*Candace was not afraid **to use the computer for typing her assignment***), and gerund phrases (***Seeing your photos*** *convinced us that we should go to Puerto Rico*) (Scott, 1988b).

A variance of the T-unit is the **C-unit.** C-units are similar to T-units but also include incomplete sentences in answer to questions (Table 7.10). C-unit values are given in Table 7.11.

The length increase in C-units is primarily through the increased use of low-frequency structures. These include post-noun modifiers, such as apposition structures (*Mary **my instructor** showed us*...) and prepositional phrases (*The man **in front** is*...), complex nominals (***Dogs and cats** can*...or ***Rules such as stop on red** are*...), and elaborated verb tensing, such as modal auxiliaries (***could** have been*), perfect aspect (***had been** working*), and passive voice (*The window **was broken by** a fly ball*). Analysis of these structures might accompany calculation of C-unit values.

Although data are not complete, some values for T-units and C-units have been calculated for children speaking primarily African American English and Spanish. These are presented in Table 7.11. Children speaking AAE demonstrate infinitive phrase embedding and clausal embedding at an early age. Three-year-olds have one or more complex syntactic forms in 6.2 percent of their utterances, while

TABLE 7.11   T-units and C-units by age and grade

Units	Age 4	Age 6	Grades 3–4	Grades 6–7	Grade 9	Grades 10–12
Words/T-unit						
Spoken			7.8	9.7		11.4
Oral Spanish		5.64				
Written			9.5	9.4–11.8		10.6–14.3
Words/C-unit						
Oral				9.82	10.96	11.7
Oral AAE	3.14	3.81				
Written				9.04	10.05	13.27
Clauses/T-unit						
Spoken		1.26	1.31	1.5		1.5
Written			1.3	1.6		1.6–1.8
Subordinate Clauses/C-unit						
Spoken				.37	.43	.58
Written				.29	.47	.6
Words/clause						
Spoken		7.14	7.75			
Written				7.26		8.82

Source: Adapted from Crowhurst & Piche (1979); Scott, Nippold, Norris, & Johnson (1992).

4-years-olds increase that to 11.7 percent (Jackson & Roberts, 2001). Additional values include mean number of morphemes per C-unit for AAE speakers (Craig, Washington, & Thompson-Porter, 1998):

Age	Mean Morphemes/C-Unit
4	3.48
5	3.76
6	4.24
Preschool	3.55
Kindergarten	3.98

Number of errors per T-unit was also found to be a significant value for predominately Spanish-speaking children (Restrepo, 1998). Five- to 7-year-old Spanish-speaking children developing typically made only .09 (S.D. = .05) errors, while those with LI made .39 (S.D. = .21).

Syntactic and Morphological Analysis

Many children with LI experience difficulty with syntax and morphology. For example, children who are mildly to moderately behaviorally disordered seem to have word-order difficulties (Camarata, Hughes, & Ruhl, 1988).

It should be noted that some utterances defy analysis, such as those containing contrasting stress used to negate. For example, one speaker might say, "Penny went," only to be corrected by the other speaker with "*Mary* went." At a syntactic level, these two sentences would appear to be similar.

Morphological Analysis

The SLP is interested in intraword development, as well as in sentence development. With preschool children, he or she will want to analyze Brown's fourteen morphemes as suggested by J. Miller (1981). These are listed in Table 7.12. Other morphemes, such as pronouns, also may be of interest. Older children may use a variety of morphological prefixes and suffixes. A list of the more common prefixes and suffixes is included in Appendix E.

TABLE 7.12   Brown's fourteen morphemes and age of mastery

Stage of Mastery	Morpheme	Example	Age Range of Mastery* (in months)
II	Present progressive -*ing*, (no auxiliary verb)	Mommy driv*ing*.	19–28
	In	Ball *in* cup	27–30
	On	Doggie *on* sofa	27–30
	Regular plural -*s*	Kitties eat my ice cream. Forms: /s/, /z/, and /Iz/ *Cats* (/kæts/) *Dogs* (/dɔgZ/) *Classes* (klæsIz/), *wishes* (/wIʃIz/)	24–33
III	Irregular past	*Came, fell, broke, sat, went*	25–46
	Possessive *'s*	Mommy*'s* balloon broke. Forms: /s/, /z/, and /Iz/ as in regular plural	26–40
IV	Uncontractible copula (verb *to be* as main verb)	He *is*. (response to "Who's sick?")	27–39
	Articles	I see *a* kitty. I throw *the* ball to daddy.	28–46
	Regular past -*ed*	Mommy pull*ed* the wagon. Forms: /d/, /t/, and /Id/ *Pulled* (/pʊld/) *Walked* (/wɔkt/) *Glided* (/g l aI d Id/)	26–48
	Regular third person -*s*	Kathy hit*s*. Forms: /s/, /z/, and /Iz/ as in regular plural	26–46
V+	Irregular third person	*Does, has*	28–50
	Uncontractible auxiliary	He *is*. (response to "Who's wearing your hat?")	29–48
	Contractible copula	Man*'s* big. Man *is* big.	29–49
	Contractible auxiliary	Daddy*'s* drinking juice. Daddy *is* drinking juice.	30–50

*Used correctly 90% of the time in obligatory contexts.

Source: Adapted from R. Brown (1973); J. Miller (1981).

Correct usage of Brown's fourteen grammatical morphemes can be a clinical aid for establishing the developmental stage of preschool children (J. Miller, 1981). Table 7.12 presents the morphemes by stage of mastery, the stage in which each morpheme is produced correctly by children in 90 percent of the obligatory contexts.

The percentage correct value is determined by dividing the number of correct appearances by the total number of obligatory contexts. In obligatory contexts, the child might use the morpheme correctly, make an error substitution, or omit the morpheme. Table 7.13 presents selected portions of a language sample and the calculation of percentage correct for the regular plural marker.

The percentage correct yields only limited data. More descriptive information can be gained. For example, the SLP who calculated only the percentage correct for past-tense *-ed* still would not know whether errors were related to nonuse of *-ed* where required or to use of *-ed* on irregular past tense verbs. The pronoun error analysis format in Table 7.14 offers guidance for analysis with other forms.

After calculating percentage correct, the SLP can attempt to describe the child's stage of language development. This process is not an exact science. Rarely is the determination clear-cut or is one and only one stage identified.

Morphological markers are applied to word classes. For example, the past tense marker *-ed* is confined to verbs. Therefore, the SLP should also note word classes in which errors occur. Occasionally, errors are confined to only one word class, such as verbs. Nouns would be affected by such markers as plural regular and irregular, possessive, and articles. Verb markers include third-person singular, past tense regular and irregular, present progressive, modals, *do* + verb, copula (*am, are, is, was, were*), and perfective (*have* + *be* + verb). Finally, adjective and adverb markers include, but are not limited to, comparative (*-er*) and superlative (*-est*) and adverbial *-ly.*

Pronouns offer a special case of morphological analysis because of the complex nature of the underlying semantic and pragmatic functions. If the child's strategy is "when in doubt, use the noun," then it will be difficult to find errors in pronoun substitution (Haas & Owens, 1985). More in-depth

TABLE 7.13   Calculating percentage correct for plural

Utterance	Correct	Incorrect	Type of Error
2. Want more cookies.	x		
3. Three cookie.		x	Not marked
4. No, one big cookies.		x	Marked singular
22. Dogs.	x		
27. Give the pencils to me.	x		
28. I want two pencils.	x		
31. You color the foots.		x	Marked irregular
40. What blue crayons?	x		
TOTAL	5	3	

$$\text{Percentage correct} = \frac{\text{Total of correct}}{\text{Total of correct} + \text{incorrect}} = \frac{5}{8} = 62.5\%$$

TABLE 7.14 Possible pronoun analysis method

Stage	Pronoun	Correct	Incorrect	Total	Percent Correct	Substitution				Omission	Ambiguous Reference	Overuse of Nominal
						Case	Gender	Person	Number			
I (MLU: 1.0–2.0)	I											
II (MLU: 2.0–2.5)	me											
	my											
	it (subj.)											
	it (obj.)											
III (MLU: 2.5–3.0)	you (subj.)											
	your											
	she											
	them											
	he											
	we											
	her (poss.)											
IV (MLU: 3.0–3.75)	his											
	him											
	you (obj.)											
	us											
	they											
	our											
V (MLU: 3.75–4.5)	its											
	myself											
	yourself											
	her (obj.)											
	their											
Post V (MLU: 4.5+)	herself											
	himself											
	ourselves											
	themselves											
	TOTAL											

Comments:

Note: Pronouns, arranged by stage of acquisition, are scored as correct or incorrect, although the total and percent columns are initially left blank. Incorrect pronoun use is then analyzed as a substitution or omission error. Substitution may be multiple, as when *she* is used for *his*, demonstrating substitutions of case and gender. When this step is completed, the sample is checked to ensure that the referent has been clearly identified for each pronoun and that the child has not overused the referent name in place of a pronoun. These are also errors, and once noted, they should be added to the incorrect total on the left. When this step is completed, the total and percent correct columns can be completed.

analysis is required, possibly similar to that presented in Table 7.14. The types of errors made reveal the underlying rules that the child is using.

When analyzing the oral and written language of school-age children and adolescents, the SLP will want to note the scope of prefix and suffix use. In addition to inflectional suffixes, such as plural -*s* and past-tense -*ed,* derivational suffixes also should be analyzed. These suffixes, more common in written than in oral language, are used to change word classes, as in adding -*er* to a verb such as *teach* to create the noun *teacher.* The two most common derivational changes are from verbs to nouns and from verbs to adjectives (Scott, 1984a, 1988b).

CLD Children. The SLP should be mindful of dialectal and bilingual variations. Even though a child omits a morphological ending, it cannot be assumed that the child does not understand or is not able to produce the morpheme. For example, children who speak African American English may omit some word endings for phonological reasons. Others are omitted because they are redundant, such as the plural -*s* when the noun is preceded by a number as in *ten cent.* The CLD child's abilities must be established by the testing of both the marker and the concept associated with it.

The standard for comparison of children's performance is the communication community of each child. A child's language is impaired to the extent that he or she is unable to communicate effectively in that community. Two errors that occur in language assessment are (a) mistaking dialectal variations for disorders and (b) overlooking disorders mistakenly assumed to be dialectal variations. In general, dialectal variations develop by age 5, with a few noticeable at age 3 (Battle, 1990).

Language sampling analysis of bilingual Spanish-English children should consider code switching, dialectal differences, English proficiency, and the effects of context on the child's language performance (Gutierrez-Clellen, Restrepo, Bedore, Pena, & Anderson, 2000).

The most frequent morphological errors of speakers with LEP are presented in Table 7.15. Morphological markers often are omitted or overgeneralized. Some Spanish speakers lump English syllables together, decreasing intelligibility. A Cuban American friend calls me "Bobowens." This chunking may cause small units such as morphemes to be de-emphasized.

Syntactic Analysis

Analysis also is accomplished at the intraclausal and clausal levels. For this type of analysis, it is best to exclude imitations, short answers to questions, and stereotypic or rote responses because these types of utterances are not usually clinically significant.

For analysis purposes, it is helpful to separate sentences and nonsentences. Sentences are grouped as declarative, negative declarative, imperative, negative imperative, interrogative, and negative interrogative. Sentences can be grouped for further analysis by length or structure. For example, declarative sentences can be categorized as subject-verb, subject-verb-object, subject-verb-complement, and multiple clauses, either embedded or conjoined. The form of the preschool child's sentences can be compared with normative data, such as those in Table 7.16, to best determine the child's stage of development, although descriptive data are also valuable. The SLP should note intrasentential noun and verb phrase development, sentence types, and embedding and conjoining. These and other sentence analyses are especially important for school-age children and adolescents.

The SLP can use Table 7.16 in a comparative fashion. For example, let us assume that the child said, "I want a big doggie." The noun *doggie* has been expanded by the addition of an article and an adjective. This noun phrase occurs in the object position of the sentence. Expansion of the noun

TABLE 7.15 **Frequent morphological errors of speakers with LEP**

Morpheme	Type of Error	Possible Explanation
Articles	Omission or overgeneralization of *the*	Articles are used infrequently in many languages.
Auxiliaries and modals	Omission	Many languages do not have auxiliary verbs and rely on verb markers.
Contractions	Omission	Unstressed forms often omitted; a phonological error.
Copula	Omission	Unstressed forms often omitted.
Gerund	Omission of *-ing* ending	Many languages do not have this form.
Plural *-s*	Omission or error in agreement, as in *many tree*	Unstressed forms often omitted; used when other languages mark by adjective.
Possessive *-'s*	Omission or overgeneralization	Many languages use the *possession of possessor* form.
Prepositions	Substitution errors	Very complex system in English; multiple meanings of words.
Pronouns	Substitution errors, noun-pronoun agreement errors	Most languages do not have as many pronouns as English.
Regular past *-ed*	Omission or overgeneralization	Unstressed forms often omitted.
Third-person *-s*	Omission or overgeneralization	Exception to English rule of no person or number markers.

TABLE 7.16 **Preschool language development and Brown's stages**

Stage	Approx. Age	Sentence Types	Intrasentential/Morphology
Early I (MLU 1–1.5)	12–21 mos.	Single words. *Yes/no* questions use rising intonation. *What* and *where*. *Negative* + X. Semantic word-order rules.	Pronouns *I* & *mine*. Isolated nouns elaborated as *art./adj.* + *noun*. Serial naming without *and*.
Late I (MLU 1.5–2.0)	21–26 mos.	*S + V + O* appears. Negative *no* and *not* used interchangeably. *Yes/no* question form is *This/that + X?*	*And* appears. *In* & *on* appear.
Early II (MLU 2.0–2.25)	27–28 mos.	*Wh-* question form is *What/where* + *noun?* *To be* appears as main verb.*	Present progressive (*-ing*), no aux. verb mastered by 90%. Pronouns *me, my* & *it, this* & *that*. Nouns elaborated in object position only [(*art./adj./dem./poss.*) + *noun*].

Continued

TABLE 7.16 *Continued*

Stage	Approx. Age	Sentence Types	Intrasentential/Morphology
Late II (MLU 2.25–2.5)	28–29 mos.	Basic *SVO* used by most. Negative element (*no, not, don't, can't* interchangeable) placed between noun and verb.	*In/on* & plural *-s* mastered by 90%. *Gonna, wanna, gotta, hafta* appear.
Early III (MLU 2.5–2.75)	30–32 mos.	*What/where + N + V?* Inversion in *What/where + be + N?** *S + aux. verb + V + O* appears. Aux. verbs include *can, do, have, will*.	Pronouns *she, he, her, we, you, your, yours,* & *them*. Noun elaboration in the subject & object position [*art. + (modifier) + noun*]. Modifiers include *a lot, some* & *two*. Select irregular past (*came, fell, broke, sat, went*) & possessive (*-'s*) mastered by 90%.
Late III (MLU 2.75–3.0)	33–34 mos.	*S + aux. verb + be + X* appears. Negative *won't* appears. Aux. verbs appear in interrogatives; inverted with subject in *yes/no* type.	*But, so, or,* & *if* appear.
Early IV (MLU 3.0–3.5)	35–39 mos.	Negative appears with aux. verb + *not* (*cannot, do not*). Inversion of aux. verb and subject in *Wh-* questions.	Uncontractible copula (verb *to be* as main verb) mastered by 90%. Pronouns *his, him, hers, us,* & *they*. Noun phrase elaboration includes *art./dem. + adj/poss./mod. + noun*. Clausal conjoining with *and* appears. Clausal embedding as object with *think, guess, show, remember,* etc.
Late IV (MLU 3.5–3.75)	39–42 mos.	Double aux. verbs in declaratives. Add *isn't, aren't, doesn't,* and *didn't*. Inversion of *be* and subj. in *yes/no* interrogatives. Add *when* and *how* interrogatives.	Articles (*the, a*), regular past (*-ed*), & third person regular (*-s*) mastered by 90%. Infinitive phrases appear at end of sentence.
Stage V (MLU 3.75–4.5)	42–56 mos.	Indirect objects appear in declaratives. Add *wasn't, wouldn't, couldn't, shouldn't*. Negative appears with other forms of *be*. Some simple tag questions appear.	Pronouns *our, ours, its, their, theirs, myself,* & *yourself*. Relative clauses appear attached to object. Infinitive phrases with same subj. as main verb.
Post-V (MLU 4.5+)	56+ mos.	Add indefinite negatives (*nobody, no one, nothing*), creating double negatives. *Why* appears in more-than-one-word interrogatives. Negative interrogatives after 60 mos.	Irregular past (*does, has*), uncontractible auxiliary *to be*, and contractible auxiliary *to be* and copula (*to be* as main verb) mastered by 90%. Remaining reflexive pronouns added. Multiple embedding; embedding + conjoining. Relative clauses attached to subj. appear.

*Copula

phrase in the object position is an example of structure occurring at Stage II and above, according to the intrasentential column of Table 7.16. The verb is unelaborated, as is the subject noun. These represent structures at the Stage I level or above. No further analysis is needed for sentence type.

The child with LEP may not exhibit difficulty in a sentence-by-sentence analysis. Analysis of connected speech beyond the sentence may provide more insight. Word-order errors and cohesive difficulties become evident in analysis of units larger than the individual sentence.

Noun Phrase. Noun phrase elaboration is assessed by describing the number and variety of noun phrase elements. Analysis of noun phrases is especially appropriate for children in late childhood or adolescence. The order of the elements within the noun phrase is relatively fixed, although the order of development is not. The noun function is obligatory, and the other modifiers are nonobligatory. Some or all of these elements may be present in the noun phrase, as shown in Table 7.17. Some elements may be used in combination, whereas the use of others is more exclusive.

Initiators consist of a small core of words that limit or quantify the phrase that follows. Examples are *only, a few of,* and *merely.* Most of these words can serve also as adverbs. The SLP must be careful to identify the accompanying noun phrase.

Determiners come in many varieties and include, in order of mention, quantifiers; articles, possessive pronouns, and demonstratives; and numerical terms, such as *two, twenty,* or *one hundred.* *Quantifiers* include such words as *all, both, half, twice,* and *triple.* In combination with initiators, determiners can yield *nearly all, at least half,* and *less than one-third. Articles* include common

TABLE 7.17 Elements of the noun phrase

Initiator	+ Determiner	+ Adjectival	+ Noun	+ Post-Noun Modifier
Only, a few of, just, at least, less than, nearly, especially, partially, even, merely, almost	**Quantifier:** All, both, half, no, one-tenth, some, any, either, twice, triple **Article:** The, a, an **Possessive:** My, your, his, her, its, our, your, their **Demonstratives:** This, that, these, those **Numerical Terms:** One, two, thirty, one thousand	**Possessive Nouns:** Mommy's, children's **Ordinal:** First, next, next to last, last, final, second **Adjective:** Blue, big, little, fat, old, fast, circular, challenging **Descriptor:** *Shopping* (center), *baseball* (game), *hot dog* (stand)	**Pronoun:** I, you, he, she, it, we, you, they, mine, yours, his, hers, its, ours, theirs **Noun:** Boys, dog, feet, sheep, men and women, city of New York, Port of Chicago, leap of faith, matter of conscience	**Prepositional Phrase:** On the car, in the box, in the gray flannel suit **Adjectival:** Next door, pictured by Renoir, eaten by Martians, loved by her friends **Adverb:** Here, there (embedded) **Clause:** Who went with you, that you saw
Examples				
Nearly	all the one hundred	old college	alumni	attending the event
Almost all of	her thirty	former	clients	
Just	half of your	brother's old baseball	uniforms	in the closet

forms such as *the, a,* and *an.* Possessive pronouns include *my, your,* and *their. Demonstratives* serve as articles but are interpreted from the perspective of the speaker as in *this, that, these,* and *those.*

Adjectivals consist of nouns marking possession, as in *mommy's sock,* ordinals, such as *first, next,* and *final;* adjectives, such as *little, big,* and *blond;* and nouns used as descriptors, as in *hot dog* stand and *cowboy* hat. Thus, a speaker might say, "Brother's first little cowboy hat." The exact order of adjectivals in a noun phrase is more complex, requiring more explanation than space allows.

The *noun* function can be filled by subjective pronouns, such as *I, you,* and *they;* objective pronouns, such as *me, you,* and *them;* genitive pronouns, such as *mine, yours,* and *theirs;* simple singular and plural nouns, such as *boy, girls,* and *women;* and mass nouns that have no distinction between singular and plural, as in *sand, water,* and *police.* When a pronoun is used, the noun to which it refers usually has already been identified. Therefore, few noun modifiers are used, and the noun phrase is relatively simple. The noun function also may be complex or may consist of a phrase, as in *Statue of Liberty, need to succeed,* and *city of Los Angeles,* or a compound, as in *Tom and Bob* and *duty and responsibility.* Finally, if the noun is understood by both the speaker and the listener, it may be omitted, as in the following exchange:

"What did you and Barb do last night?"

"(We) Went to that movie at the mall."

Post-noun modifiers may take many forms, including prepositional phrases (*in the gray flannel suit*), embedded clauses (*who lives next door*), adjectivals (*next door* and *driven by my mother*), and adverbs (*here* and *there*). Post-noun modifiers may be used singly or in combination—for example, "The man *who lives in the green house on the next block* bought all of the candy *that I was selling.*"

The development of elements of the noun phrase takes most typically developing children many years and continues into adolescence. As noted in Table 7.16, elaboration begins in isolation and then moves to the object position in the sentence before appearing in the subject position. This pattern is only the beginning of the development process; with increasing age, the child should use more and more noun elaborations. Adjectives and determiners appear at the two-word stage for both children with LI and those without. Initiators and post-noun modifiers appear later, with children with LI exhibiting a marked delay. For children developing typically, clausal post-noun modifiers appear in late Stage IV and V (Table 7.16).

Most 5-year-olds use no more than one modifier with each noun. Thus, most internal development of the noun phrase occurs in later childhood and adolescence. Both elaborated pre-noun and post-noun modification, using relative clauses and prepositional phrases, develop during this period (Nippold, 1993; Perera, 1986a, 1986b; Scott, 1988a, 1988b). The most elaborated forms usually are produced in written language.

The SLP is interested in the distribution of these elaborations in these positions and the average number of morphemes within noun phrases. It may be helpful for the SLP to use a format of analysis similar to that in Table 7.17.

Children with LI can be expected to have simpler, less elaborated noun phrases. Pronouns offer a special problem. Children with LEP may exhibit confusion with modifier order and pronoun use.

Verb Phrase.   As mentioned in Chapter 2, verb morphology is particularly difficult for children with SLI. Analysis of verb phrase construction and inflected morphology can be a useful measure for identifying 3½- to 6-year-olds with SLI (Bedore & Leonard, 1998).

Verb phrase elaboration consists of the verb and associated words, including noun phrases used as complements or as direct or indirect objects. The SLP is concerned with the verbs used and those that are missing or incomplete. Other elements of the verb phrase that are present or absent are also important and reflect the maturity of the speaker's language system.

Predicate relationships take three forms: intransitive, in which the verb cannot take an object; transitive, in which the verb can take an object; and equative, which consists of the copula (*to be*) plus a complement of a noun, adjective, or adverb. Verb phrases can be described by the length and range of types, as demonstrated in Table 7.18.

Simple transitive (*Mommy throw*) and equative verb phrases (*Doggie big*) appear at an MLU of about 1.5 (Kamhi & Nelson, 1988). At this stage, the verbs are unmarked for tense or person, and the copula is omitted. As language becomes more complex, verbs become marked, the copula appears, and intransitive verb phrases appear. By Stage II, the progressive *-ing* marker and catenatives (*gonna, wanna, gotta, hafta*) appear. The perfective form (*have* + *verb-en*) and the passive voice begin to be used by Stage IV. Adverbial phrases also appear in Stage IV. Late childhood and adolescent language development is characterized by increasing verb complexity with the use of auxiliaries, modals, and perfective forms, such as *have been going*. There is also increasing use of adverbs and adverbial phrases, such as prepositional phrases of manner (*in silence*), place (*in the city*), and time (*in a week*) (Scott, 1984a). In general, children with LI who exhibit these more complex structures tend to use them less frequently than do children developing typically.

Tense markers are used to describe the temporal relationships between events. For example, if the event being described is taking place while the speaker mentions it, the speaker uses the present

TABLE 7.18 **Elements of the verb phrase**

Modal Auxiliary	+ Perfective Auxiliary	+ Verb to be	+ Negative*	+ Passive	+ Verb	+ Prepositional Phrase, Noun Phrase, Noun Complement, Adverbial Phrase
May, can, shall, will, must, might, should, would, could	Have, has, had	Am, is, are, was, were, be, been	Not	Been, being	Run, walk, eat, throw, see, write	On the floor, the ball, our old friend, a doctor, on time, late

Examples:

Transitive (May have direct object)

May	have				wanted	a cookie
Should			not		throw	the ball in the house

Intransitive (Does not take direct object)

Might	have	been			walking	to the inn
Could			not		talk	with you

Equative (Verb *to be* as main verb)

		is	not			a doctor
		was				late
		were				on the sofa
May		be				ill

*When modal auxiliaries are used, the negative is placed between the modal and other auxiliary forms, for example, "Might not have been going."

progressive verb form (auxiliary + verb-*ing*) to indicate an ongoing activity (*walking, eating*). In contrast, the perfect form of the verb (have + verb-*en*) indicates that the action is being described in relation to the present. Thus, "I have been working here for two years" implies that this action is still occurring, whereas "I *have eaten* my dinner" implies that the action is now complete. Verb tense analysis can be accomplished in a form similar to that presented in Table 7.18. Table 7.16 identifies the ages at which most preschool children acquire auxiliary and modal auxiliary verbs.

Irregular past tense verbs are a special problem (Shipley, Maddox, & Driver, 1991). English contains approximately 200 irregular verbs. Many are archaic and used infrequently, but the rest, such as *went, saw, sat,* and *ate,* are among the most frequently used verbs. Development begins in the preschool years and extends into adolescence. Their irregular nature precludes rule learning and generalization, and most acquisition is by rote (Shipley & Banis, 1989). Some morphophonemic regularities do occur, however, and may influence the relative ease of learning (Shipley et al., 1991). The least difficult verbs to learn are those that exhibit no change from present to past, such as *cut/cut* and *hurt/hurt.* The most difficult seem to be those with a final consonant change from /d/ to /t/, as in *build/built* (Shipley et al., 1991). Other morphophonemic changes include internal vowel change (*fall/fell, come/came*), vowel change with added final consonant (*sweep/swept*), total change (*go/ went*), and vowel change with a final dental consonant (*ride/rode, stand/stood*). Obviously, other factors, such as the concept expressed (semantics) and the sounds involved (phonology), also affect learning. Table 7.19 presents the ages at which 80 percent of children are able to use different irregular verbs in a sentence completion task.

Adverbs also mark temporal relations, in addition to manner and result. Temporal relations can be expressed between two events (*before, next, during, meanwhile*), with the continuation of an event (*for the past year, all week*), in the recent past (*recently, just a minute ago*), and with repetition (*many times, again*).

Verb aspect indicates temporal notions, such as momentary actions, duration, and repetition. Momentary actions are of short duration (*fall, break, hit*). In contrast, duration is marked by verbs

TABLE 7.19   Irregular verbs and age of acquisition

Age in Years	Irregular Verbs
3:0 to 3:5	Hit, hurt
3:6 to 3:11	Went
4:0 to 4:5	Saw
4:6 to 4:11	Ate, gave
5:0 to 5:5	Broke, fell, found, took
5:6 to 5:11	Came, made, sat, threw
6:0 to 6:5	Bit, cut, drove, fed, flew, ran, wore, wrote
6:6 to 6:11	Blew, read, rode, shot
7:0 to 7:5	Drank
7:6 to 7:11	Drew, dug, hid, rang, slept, swam
8:0 to 8:5	Caught, hung, left, slid
8:6 to 8:11	Built, sent, shook

Source: Adapted from Shipley, Maddox, & Driver (1991).

of longer action with definite beginnings and ends (*sleep, build, make*). Phrases also may be used to convey a definite act (*sing a song*) and an act without a well-defined terminal point (*sing for your own enjoyment*). Still other verbs describe repetitive actions (*tap, knock, hammer*).

The development of tense markers seems to be related to the temporal aspect of each verb. The SLP should investigate the relationship between tenses the child uses and the verbs to which these tenses are applied. No doubt, this analysis will require something larger than a 50- to 100-utterance sample.

Modal auxiliary verbs, such as *can, could, will, should, shall, may, might,* and *must,* are used to express the speaker's attitude (Bliss, 1987). Syntactically, modals function in the formation of questions and negatives. They are used also in such statements as "I *will* do it tomorrow."

As with the pronoun system, modals represent a complex interaction of form, content, and use that is reflected in the slow rate of acquisition, which usually lasts from age 2 to age 8. Semantic categories of modals include wish or intention (*will, would*), necessity or obligation (*must, should*), ability or permission (*can*), certainty (*will*), and probability or possibility (*may, might*) (Bliss, 1987).

Those modals associated with action, such as *can* and *will* (ability, intention, and permission request), are acquired first. During the third year, the number of modals and the categories increases. After age 4, the child clarifies the different forms and their uses.

Children with LI rarely use modal auxiliaries, possibly because of the linguistic subtleties expressed. In general, children with LI have more difficulty with catenatives (*gonna, wanna*), modals, and auxiliary verbs than their language level would suggest. The SLP is interested in the range and frequency of modals the child exhibits.

CLD children may experience difficulty with verb tense and with auxiliary verbs. Irregular past tense verbs may exhibit substitutions. Verb endings may be omitted as a general phonological rule pattern. Verb-subject agreement is also difficult.

When analyzing a sample, the SLP pays particular attention to the level of development, the range of semantic concepts, the variety of usage, and the types of errors (Bliss, 1987). Variety of usage is noted with different pronouns, verb tenses, negative and positive statements, and sentence types.

Sentence Types.   A single event may be described by the agent that originates the action, the action or state changes, and/or the recipient or object of that action (Duchan, 1986b). The agent as a noun or a noun phrase is usually first, followed by the action word or verb, which in turn is followed by the recipient or object of that action in the form of a noun or a noun phrase ("John threw the ball" or "Mother ate the cookie").

If the agent performs the action for the benefit of some other person, that beneficiary—the indirect object—either precedes or follows the noun phrase describing the object of the action. For example, in "He painted the picture for mother," *for mother* follows the object of the sentence. Likewise, we could say, "He painted *mother* a picture." Instruments used to complete the action usually are placed after the action and follow the preposition *with,* as in "He painted *with a brush.*"

Sentences that differ from the predominant subject-verb-object format may be difficult for the child with LI to decipher and form. Often, overreliance on the S-V-O strategy is not noted until the child begins school. The child with LI may resist rearrangement or interruption of this form and may attach other structures only at the beginning or the end. Yes/no questions may be asked with rising intonation, rather than through transformation of the subject and verb elements. Passive sentences, which use an object-verb-subject form, may be misinterpreted.

The SLP is interested in the range of internal sentence forms and in the different sentence types. Sentence types include positive and negative forms of the declarative, interrogative, and imperative. Declarative sentences are statements ("He likes ice cream" or "She does not want to go").

Interrogatives include three types of questions, including yes/no, *wh-* or constituent, and tag. The form of yes/no questions may vary from a statement with rising intonation ("You went to the store?") to a transformation using the copula or an auxiliary verb ("Is he happy?" or "Did she eat her pie?").

Wh- questions begin with such words as *what, where, who, why, when,* and *how.* Either the copula or auxiliary verb and the subject are transformed from their order in a statement ("What is her age?" or "Why did he go?"). A less mature form that can be used with some *wh-* questions places the *wh-* word at the end of the sentence ("She likes *what?*"). These types typically are used for clarification, however, and are discussed later in the chapter.

Tag questions are statements with question tags attached ("She's lovely, isn't she?").

The preschool development of questions is given in Table 7.16. Mature tag questions, because of their complex nature and infrequent use in American English, are acquired much later than are yes/no and *wh-* interrogatives. Some children do not master the mature tag form until mid-elementary school (Reich, 1986). A less complex form using *okay* or *all right* (or the Canadian *eh*) may appear in preschool ("I do this, okay?"). The statement portion is negative or positive, while the question portion is the reverse.

The range of sentence types and the maturity of form are of interest. These are listed in Table 7.16.

With more mature speakers, the SLP must consider the use of emphasis, pauses, and intonation to mark different meanings for the same form. Pauses mark the end of conceptual units and direct the listener in the type of response required. For example, "Do you like football (pause) or baseball?" requires a very different response from "Do you like football or baseball?" Rising intonation is used on an entire word for unexpected or surprise events and falling intonation for the expected. As mentioned previously, rising intonation at the end of a word or a sentence signifies a question, and falling intonation signifies a statement.

Imperatives are commands ("Eat your dinner" or "Stop that"). The subject, *you,* is understood. SLPs must be careful not to confuse these sentence types with utterances in which the child omits the subject. The child who repeatedly omits the subject in other sentences probably should not be credited with imperative forms.

The behavior of other people may be influenced also by requests. These are discussed in Chapter 5 and in the illocutionary functions section of this chapter because of the pragmatic aspects of this form.

Negative sentences, whether declarative, interrogative, or imperative also possess characteristic developmental forms (Table 7.16). The child's first negatives are marked by *no* and slightly later by *not.* Initially, these two forms are used interchangeably. To these are added *don't* and *can't,* also used interchangeably, followed by *won't.* Positive forms of *do, can, will,* and *would* develop later, followed by negative forms for the verb *to be* and for other auxiliaries. By school age, the child develops indefinite forms (e.g., *no one, nothing*) and indirect negative imperatives ("Watch out for the hole"). These do not require syntactic negative transformations. During the school-age years, the child masters such negative prefixes as *un-, non-,* and *ir-.*

Embedding and Conjoining.   Both embedding and conjoining involve relationships between clauses. In addition, embedding involves the relationships between phrases and clauses.

A *clause* consists of a noun phrase and a verb phrase. A clause that can stand alone is an independent clause, or sentence, even though it contains only the noun and the verb ("John ran"). Some clauses contain both elements but are not independent. These clauses, such as "that you want," must be attached to an independent clause or sentence in a process called *embedding.* In this manner, *"that you want"* can be embedded in "The toy is on sale" to form "The toy that you want is on sale." Two or more independent clauses can be joined together by a conjunction, such as *and* or *but,* in a process called *conjoining.*

Clausal embedding initially develops in the object position at the end of the sentence (Table 7.16). Called *object noun complements,* these dependent clauses take the place of the object following such words as *know, think,* and *feel* ("I know *that you can do it*"). Object noun complements using *that* ("I think *that I like it*") appear at an MLU of 4.0, most frequently following the verb *think* (Tyack & Gottsleben, 1986). By an MLU of 5.0–5.9, this type of embedding accounts for only 6 percent of children's two-clause sentences. Object noun complements using *what* ("I know *what you did*") account for 8 percent of these sentences.

Relative clauses attached to nouns develop next, beginning in the object position, as in "I want the dog *that I saw last night*." Finally, the relative clause moves to the center of the sentence, describing the subject, as in "The one *that you ate* was my favorite." During late childhood and adolescence, an increase occurs in relative clauses either attached to the subject or serving as the subject, as in ***Whoever wishes to go*** *should come to the office.* This type of clausal embedding is more common in written language than in oral (Perera, 1986a, 1986b; Scott, 1988a, 1988b).

Relative clauses appear less frequently among preschoolers than other forms of clausal embedding, although by school age, 20 to 30 percent of two-clause sentences may be of this type. Relative clauses appear at about 48 months initially as post-noun modifiers for empty nouns, such as *one* or *thing* (Wells, 1985). The most common relative pronouns for preschoolers are *that* and *what.* During the school years, pronouns expand with the addition of *whose, whom,* and *in which.*

Phrases also may be embedded in clauses. As in clausal embedding, phrasal embedding usually develops initially at the end of the sentence. A *phrase* is a group of related words that does not contain a subject and a verb and are of several types, including prepositional, participial, infinitive, and gerund phrases. Such phrases take the place of nouns or modify nouns. Prepositional phrases also may be adverbial in nature, as in "She will arrive *in a minute.*" During late childhood and adolescence, an increase occurs in both the number and length of adverbial phrases (Scott et al., 1992).

Infinitive phrases first appear in the object position, most frequently following *want* ("I want *drink pop*"). This form with the *to* omitted emerges at a median age of 30 months (Wells, 1985). Infinitives with a different subject from the main verb ("Mommy, I want you to *eat it*") appear somewhat later.

The SLP is interested in the number and type of embeddings. Some developmental data are included in Table 7.16. The position of these embeddings within the sentence is also important, given the developmental significance of position.

Clausal conjoining appears relatively late in preschool development, although some conjunctions appear much earlier. Usually, *and* is the first conjunction learned; it is used to join objects in a group. Throughout the preschool period, *and* continues to be the most frequently used conjunction, being five to twenty times more common than *but* (Scott, 1988a). Around 30 months of age, children begin to sequence clauses, using *and* as the initial word in each sentence. As noted in Table 7.16, *and* is also the first conjunction used to join clauses. At this point, *and* is used for sequential events and is interpreted as *and then.* Even among school-age children, 50 to 80 percent of all narrative sentences begin with *and* (Scott, 1987). With age and an increase in written communication, use of *and* decreases. Between ages 11 and 14, only 20 percent of spoken narrative sentences begin with *and.*

In written narratives, the rate is only about 5 percent (Scott, 1987). Other conjunctions may express a causal relationship (*because*), simultaneity (*while*), a contrasting relationship (*but*), and exclusion (*except*). Conjunctions develop in the following order: *and, because, when, if, so, but, until, before, after, since, although,* and *as* (Scott, 1987; Tyack & Gottsleben, 1986; Wells, 1985). The most frequently used conjunctions through age 12 are *and, because,* and *when.*

Early strategies that rely on the order of mention for interpretation may persist with the child with LI. Thus, the child ignores the conjunctions and their intended meanings. The sentences "Go to the market before you go to the movie" and "Go to the market after you go to the movie" are interpreted as having the same meaning.

The SLP is interested in the range and frequency of the conjunctions used and in the amount of conjoining present in the sample. This information is especially important with more mature speakers and is discussed in the following chapter on narratives.

The SLP also should note multiple embeddings and embedding and conjoining that occur within the same sentence. Again, this usage is much more characteristic of school-age language than of preschool language. The narratives of children ages 10 to 12 years are easily distinguishable from those of preschoolers by the presence of multiple embedding and conjoining within the same sentence (Perera, 1986a, 1986b; Scott, 1988a, 1988b).

TABLE 7.20   Computer-assisted language sample analysis software

Software	Description
Syntax/Morphology	
Automated LARSP (Bishop, 1985)	Based on Language Assessment, Remediation, and Sampling Procedure (LARSP) (Crystal, Fletcher, & Garman, 1976) Calculates MLU Uncoded transcript
Computerized Profiling (Long & Fey, 1988, 1989)	Based on Conversational Act Profile (Fey, 1986), Developmental Sentence Analysis (DSS) (L. Lee, 1974), Profile in Semantics-Lexical (PRISM-L) (Crystal, 1982), Profile of Prosody (PROP) (Crystal, 1982), Profile of Phonology (PROPH) (Crystal, 1982) Calculates MLU and type-token ratio Uncoded transcript
DSS Computer Program (Hixson, 1985)	Based on Developmental Sentence Analysis (DSS) (L. Lee, 1974) Coded transcript
Lingquest 1 (Mordecai, Palin, & Palmer, 1985)	Calculates MLU and type-token ratio Coded transcript
Parrot Easy Language Sample Analysis (PELSA) (F. Weiner, 1988)	Calculates MLU Coded transcript
Pye Analysis of Language (PAL) (Pye, 1987)	Flexible analysis categories Coded transcript
Systematic Analysis of Language Transcripts (SALT) (J. Miller & Chapman, 1985)	Based on Brown's Stages of Development Flexible analysis categories Calculates MLU, NDW, TNW Coded transcript

Source: Adapted from Long (1991).

Computer-Assisted Language Analysis

Several computer-assisted language analysis (CLA) methods are available, each based on some particular model of language structure. CLAs provide the SLP with a quick, efficient, standard analysis routine.

Most CLA formats have three common features (Long, 1991). First, all utterances must be coded to assist the computer in identifying structures. This time-consuming step may be shortened for the SLP by having an assistant make an initial transcription on a disk (J. Miller et al., 1992). The resultant disk can be corrected and readied for analysis by the SLP. Second, the computer recognizes, analyses, and tabulates the identified structures from the transcript. Third, the program displays the results in an interpretable format. A list of available CLA syntactic and phonological software is provided in Table 7.20.

Once mastered, CLA is more efficient than analysis by hand; this efficiency increases as the complexity of analysis increases (Long & Masterson, 1993). Although CLAs may quicken the analysis phase of sampling, they cannot replace the clinical intuition of the trained SLP. Nor can CLAs fill the deficiency caused by a poorly collected sample. In addition, only the SLP can use the data generated to make clinical decisions.

Early Intervention with Presymbolic and Minimally Symbolic Children

At a symbolic level, whether collected verbally or through some augmentative and alternative communication (AAC) means, the sample is analyzed for the number of symbols in the child's lexicon and in the variety of semantic and illocutionary functions the child displays.

The SLP collects a conversational sample and rates each utterance for the semantic and illocutionary functions found in early child language (Owens, 1982b). Although such categories may be inappropriate for older children with retardation, they do suggest a standard set of functions with which to begin. Normative distributions are not available for these functions, which are usually situationally related. Of greater interest is the range of functions the child uses.

The SLP collects samples by observing everyday activities or routines with the child's primary caregivers, such as teachers, parents, and classroom aides. Children engaged in familiar, meaningful activities with age-appropriate materials are likely to interact more and to produce more language than do children in other situations.

Analysis can be accomplished at the utterance level. For children who speak, an *utterance* consists of one or more symbols separated from other symbols by a pause, a drop in the voice, or an inhalation. Children using AAC may look at their partner or pause between utterances. Whatever the mode of transmission, the SLP records and rates each utterance for both semantic and illocutionary function and for the number of symbols used. Appendix A provides definitions of the most common functions listed in Table 7.21. A form such as Figure 7.1 may be helpful for recording and analyzing the data. The SLP records the number of symbols per utterance under the appropriate functions demonstrated by the utterance. The process of AAC symbol acquisition and combination is similar to typical early language development. It is imperative, therefore, that symbol assessment and vocabulary selection enable clients to form symbol contributions (Wilkinson, Romski, & Sevcik, 1994).

Repetitive utterances, such as "baby baby," and certain combinations, such as "all gone," may function as single-symbol utterances. The child may repeatedly produce "dog here" yet not use

TABLE 7.21 **Semantic and illocutionary functions of early symbolic communication**

Semantic Functions	Illocutionary Functions
Nomination	Answer
This/that + nomination	Question or requesting information
Location	Reply
X + location	Elicitation
Negation	Continuant
Negation + X	Declaration
Modification	Practice or repeat
(Types: Attribution, possession, and recurrence)	Name or label
Modifier + X	Command, demand, request, protest
Notice	
Notice + X	
State	
Experience + state	
Action (signaled by agent, action, or object)	
Agent + action	
Action + object	

Source: Compiled from Dore (1975); MacDonald (1978a); Owens (1982c).

either symbol independently or in combination with other symbols. If this is suspected, it can be confirmed by the caregivers or through observation, and the utterance rated as a single word.

The SLP then uses the total number of symbols and the total number of utterances within each function from Figure 7.1 to compute the MLU of each function. Of interest are the range of semantic and illocutionary functions and the length and means of communicating each (Caro & Snell, 1989; Owens, 1982a). The SLP can use the results as follows to select training objectives (Owens, 1982d):

Teach relevant functions that do not occur.

Provide opportunities for low-frequency functions to occur.

Teach longer forms for functions with low MLUs.

Reduce or modify stereotypic, perseverative, or echolalic utterances that seem nonfunctional.

Although much individual variation exists, we can assign some values to the behaviors of children developing typically. By 24 months, 85 to 95 percent of English-speaking children have 50 single words in their expressive vocabularies and are combining words. Spanish-speaking children have very similar development and 90 percent have 50 single words by 25 months. Bilingual Spanish-English children are only slightly slower, but by 26 to 27 months, they have 82 single words. At 23 to 25 months, 84 percent of bilingual children are combining words (Patterson, 1998).

Especially important for children with LI is the number of unique two-word combinations that could fit into the structure of an adult sentence (Hadley, 1999). These constructions indicate a growing area of language development and compare well with other measures, such as MLU.

Utterances	Nom.	L.	Neg.	P.	Att.	R.	Not.	O.	Act.	Ag+	+Ob	A.	Q.	R.	D.	P.	N.	S.	O.	Ges.	Sig.	Voc.	Ver.	Init.	Resp.
	SEMANTIC FUNCTIONS											**ILLOCUTIONARY FUNCTIONS**								**FORM**				**TYPE**	
1. *BALL*	1																1			1			1	1	
2. *(WANT) BALL*									2		2							2		1			1	2	
3. *(THROW) BALL*									2		2							2		1			1	2	
4. *THROW ME*		2											2					2		1			2		2
5. *WANT THAT?*	2												2										2	2	
6. *NO THAT*			2															2			2		2		2
7. *MORE THROW*						2			2									2		2			2	2	
8. *BALL?*	1												1										2	2	
9. *THROW BALL ME*		3							3		3							3		3			3	3	
44.																									
45.																									
46.																									
47.																									
48.																									
49.																									
50.																									
OVERALL TOTAL (Words)	4	5	2	0	0	2	0	0	9	0	7	0	3	0	0	0	1	13	0	9	2	0	16	14	4
TOTAL NO. OF UTT.	3	2	1	0	0	1	0	0	4	0	3	0	2	0	0	0	1	6	0	6	1	0	9	7	2
MLU by functions (Divide total words by total utterances)	13	25	2	0	0	2	0	0	23	0	23	0	15	0	0	0	1	22	0	15	2	0	18	19	2

Nom. = Nomination
L. = Location
Neg. = Negation
P. = Possession
Att. = Attribution

R. = Recurrence
Not. = Notice
O. = Other
Act. = Action
Ag+ = Agent + Action

+Ob = Action + Object
A. = Answer
Q. = Question
R. = Reply
D. = Declaration

P. = Practice
N. = Name
S. = Suggestion, Command, Demand, Request
O. = Other

Ges. = Gesture
Sig. = Sign
Voc. = Vocalization
Ver. = Verbalization
Init. = Initiate

Resp. = Respond

In the first utterance, the child pointed at the object and said one symbol ("Ball"), clearly a semantic *Nominative* and an illocutionary *Name*. Utterances 4 ("Throw me"), 6 ("No that"), and 7 ("More throw") are two-symbol examples of the semantic rules *X + Locative*, *Negative + X* and *Recurrent + X*, respectively. At the two-symbol level, these semantic functions are expanded by adding another symbol. This format applies to the first seven semantic functions. In contrast, utterance 3 ("Throw ball") is an example of a different type. The *Agent*, *Action*, and *Object* categories are expanded by combining categories. Thus, utterance 3 is an example of a two-symbol *Action* and a two-symbol *Object*. Utterance 2 is similar. Utterance 9 represents a combination of *X + Locative* and *Action + Object* to form *Action + Object + Locative*, a three-category combination scored under each appropriate category. In all utterances, gestures support the communication but language is the primary form of communication. Gestured portions of an utterance are in parentheses. If more than one form is used, the verbal symbol is underlined.

FIGURE 7.1 Functional analysis of a language sample of a child who is minimally symbolic.

Although this type of analysis is inappropriate for nonspeaking children, other measures are more useful. For example, five or more nonimitative words in a sample indicate a good prognosis for developing speech as a primary means of communication (Yoder, Warren, & McCathren, 1998). Other good predictors are

- Number of intentions expressed through a vocalization with at least one true consonant
- Rate of proto-declaratives, utterances that share affect or experience without requesting
- Close match between the words child says and those the child comprehends

The Communication Environment

The SLP is interested in more than just the functioning of the child. Of interest are the situations, activities, and locations that are high-communication contexts and the child's communication behavior in each. The SLP is interested also in identifying caregivers who evoke the most communication from the child and in describing their behaviors, especially the communication demands they place on the child (Mahoney & Weller, 1980). The ideal environment is one that nurtures development and enhances generalization (Haring, Roger, Lee, Breen, & Gaylord-Ross, 1986). The child should have ample opportunities to express him- or herself and to make choices (Falvey, McLean, & Rosenberg, 1988).

The SLP may wish to conduct a four-step survey of the child's communication needs and uses (D. Yoder, 1985). First, the SLP describes the functionally most relevant and least restrictive communication environments, at present and in the foreseeable future. These might include the classroom or the home. Second, the SLP divides these environments into subenvironments by the most relevant and functional activities in each, such as snack time or bathing. Third, the SLP determines the skills needed to participate in each activity. Fourth, the SLP describes how each activity and/or environment may be adapted to allow or enhance the child's participation. This process provides the data needed to design intervention programs to teach interactional skills and environmental adaptation.

The Interaction of Child and Environment

Although the child and the environment are important in themselves, the data gathered from each are most meaningful when we consider how each affects the other. Communication is an interaction between the child and the caregivers, and learning can be measured only by the effect the child's newly acquired behaviors have on the environment of which these caregivers are a part. For maximum generalization, the child's caregivers must become language facilitators.

In determining the language facilitator potential of each caregiver, the SLP first must determine the quality of the interaction between the child and the caregiver. The SLP then can, when appropriate, suggest modifications in the caregiver's behavior that may, in turn, change the child's communicative behavior.

Several observational tools are available, including the Observation of Communication Interactions (OCI) Scale (Klein & Briggs, 1987), the Parent-Infant Interaction Scale (G. Clark & Seifer, 1982), and the Diagnostic Interactional Survey (DIS) (Owens, 1982c). If the child is presymbolic, the SLP is interested in the manner in which partners perceive the child's behavior (Ogletree, 1993). For children using symbols, the SLP would want to note caregiver responsiveness and consistency and the adjustments caregivers make for the child's developmental level and emotional state (Greenspan, 1988; Ogletree, 1993). The appropriateness of caregiver verbal models is also important.

Qualitative judgments of child-caregiver interaction might be based on the presence or absence of certain behaviors by both individuals, such as child strategies for engagement, termination, and reengagement and the primary modes of signaling.

In general, children who are presymbolic engage in a greater frequency and higher level of communication when they initiate interactions. The child's level of responding in both adult-initiated and child-initiated interactions might be described, noting vocalizations, limb movements, and facial and body postures (J. Norris & Hoffman, 1990a).

One rating system, ECOmaps, evaluates social play, turn taking, nonverbal communication, language, and conversation within the interaction by using a 1–9 scale (MacDonald & Carroll, 1992a; MacDonald & Gillette, 1982). These areas are evaluated in three contexts: play with objects, play with people alone, and spontaneous interactions during caregiving. In addition, the SLP engages the child in interaction and notes differences between this interaction and that with the caregiver. The scales rate actual behavior or an approximate percentage of the time that each interactant engages in the specific behaviors listed. Results allow for an estimate of communication match for that behavior; severe inequities signal a potential mismatch that requires intervention. A progressive match in which the caregiver is monitoring the child's performance and modeling slightly above that level is more desirable. The Teaching Strategies ECOmap rates the caregiver's use of events and strategies the child needs to communicate at a higher level. Finally, the Problems ECOmap identifies specific potential interactional problems.

Conclusion

The conversational sample is a rich source of data about children's language. Within utterances both qualitative and quantitative measures are possible. Obviously, such analysis is time-consuming. SLPs should analyze only areas of suspected difficulty rather than attempt a blanket analysis. Of interest is the child's present communication system and the communication characteristics of the child's communication partners. Unlike the larger-unit analyses discussed in Chapter 6, within-utterance measures can be compared more readily to similar data from children developing typically.

Narrative Analysis

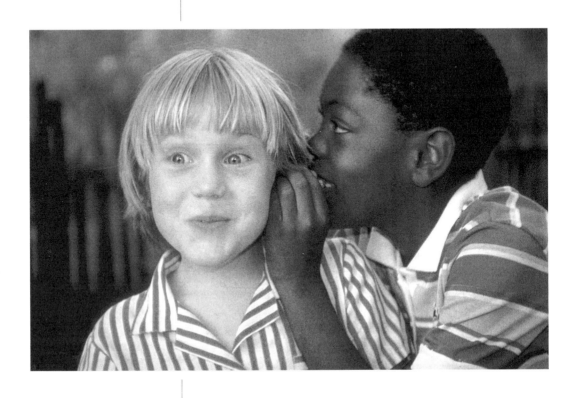

Narratives are a self-initiated, self-controlled, decontextualized form of discourse. As such, narratives are an important part of the language assessment of older school-age children and adolescents because they provide an uninterrupted sample of language that the child or adolescent modifies to capture and hold the listener's interest (Crais & Chapman, 1987; Hewitt & Duchan, 1995; Liles, 1985a, 1985b, 1987; Scott, 1988b).

The narrative speaker is responsible for ordering and providing all of the information in an organized whole (F. Roth & Spekman, 1985). Narratives, therefore, are found more frequently in the communication of more mature speakers. The clinical importance of narratives can be summarized as follows:

> Narrative analysis is one of the most valuable skills a language clinician can possess. People of all ages from all cultures experience stories daily…in representing events in their own lives and in participating in the happenings, both real and imaginary, in the lives of others. Knowledge of story structure contributes to people's understanding of how the world functions, facilitating predictions of actions and consequences, causes and effects. (Hedberg & Stoel-Gammon, 1986, p. 58)

Although narration and conversation share many qualities, they differ in very significant ways. First, narratives are extended units of text. Second, events within narratives are linked with one another temporally or causally in predictable ways. Narratives are organized in a cohesive, predictable, rule-governed manner representing temporal and causal patterns not found in conversation. Third, the speaker maintains a social monologue throughout. The speaker must produce language that is relevant to the overall narrative while remaining mindful of the information needed by the listener.

In most narratives, the language does not center on some ongoing activity, but usually communicates some experience not directly shared by the speaker and the listener. To share the experience, the speaker must present an explicit, topic-centered discussion that clearly states sequential and causal relationships.

The major characteristics found in narratives but not in conversation are the agentive focus and the temporal contingent structure. In other words, narratives are about agents—people, animals, or imaginary characters—engaged in events over time. Other differences include the narrative use of extended units of text, introduction and organizing sequences that lead to a narrative conclusion, and the relatively passive listener role that provides only minimal informational support to narratives (F. Roth, 1986).

Narratives are not limited to fictional storytelling. Narrative evaluation should not consist solely of the child or adolescent recounting fairy tales or formulating stories from pictures. For the purposes of language analysis, we consider *oral narration* to include the telling of self-generated stories, storytelling of familiar tales, retelling of movies or television shows, and recounting of personal experiences. Most conversations include narratives of this latter type. How often we begin conversations with "You'll never believe what happened to me coming to work today," or "Let me tell you what it means to get into a hassle."

Diagnostically, narratives are good for eliciting a variety of complex syntactic structures (Gummersall & Strong, 1999). The narratives of children with LI such as LLD and TBI are shorter and less mature and have less mature episode and sentence structure than those of age-matched peers developing typically (S. Chapman, 1997; Merritt & Liles, 1987, 1989; F. Roth & Spekman, 1986). Students with LLD demonstrate knowledge and use of story grammars but convey and recall less information. In addition, children with LLD retrieve less information and make fewer inferences than do children who are non-LLD. Although the stories of children with LLD contain all of the elements in the generally appropriate order, they are substantially shorter and contain fewer and more poorly organized complete episodes (Liles, 1990). Episodes are also less likely to be related linguistically (F. Roth & Spekman, 1985). In addition, more statements of children with LI are not integrated into the episode structure (Liles, 1990). This paucity of information may reflect a lack of presuppositional skills (F. Roth, 1986). Possibly because of the communication demands placed on the child in narration, the narratives of children with LLD exhibit a greater rate of communication breakdown in the form of stalls, repairs, and abandoned utterances (MacLachlan & Chapman, 1988). Although children with LLD and those without display similar patterns of cohesion, such as the use of conjunctions and unambiguous reference, children with LLD are less efficient in their use (Liles, 1985a). In general, children with LLD use fewer conjunctions and exhibit more ambiguous reference, often failing to consider the needs of their audience (Liles, 1987). The internal story organization of children with LI is also less complete than that of age-matched peers (Merritt & Liles, 1987). The narratives of children with LI contain more statements that are not integrated into the episode structure than do those of children without impairment. Usually, such children have difficulty describing and manipulating props and activities (Sleight & Prinz, 1985).

As only one linguistic form used in communication, oral and written narratives should form only a portion of any child's language analysis. The results should be compared with the child's other linguistic abilities prior to making judgments on the adequacy of the child's language system.

Development of Narratives

Children speaking American English begin to tell self-generated, fictional narratives between ages 2 and 3 (Sutton-Smith, 1986). These stories may have a vague plot and usually center on certain highlights in the child's life. There is little recognition of the need to introduce, to explore with, or to orient the listener to the story, and these stories usually lack easily identifiable beginnings, middles, and ends. Disquieting events are the theme, and children repeat phenomena that they find disruptive or extraordinary in their own lives.

Two-year-olds usually construct additive chains in which one sentence is added to another, as in "This is kittie. This doggie bowl." There is no story line, no sequencing, and no cause and effect. The sentences may be moved anywhere in the text without changing the meaning of the entire text.

In these early stories is a dominance of performance and textual qualities over text (Sutton-Smith, 1986). Sound production and prosody may be used to move the story along. Between ages 3 and 7, children's narratives gradually change from prosody to prose with plots (Sutton-Smith, 1986). It is not until age 8 that children can tell narratives really well.

Temporal event sequences emerge between ages 3 and 5. Events follow a logical sequence. Although there is sequencing, there is no plot and no cause and effect or causality.

Causal chains are infrequent until ages 5 to 7. Causality involves descriptions of intentions and unobservable states, such as emotions and thoughts, and the use of causal connectives. This development can be seen among children speaking both Spanish and English (Gutierrez-Clellan & Iglesias, 1992).

"To tell a story, a child must be able to relate the chain of events in such a way as to explain what happened and why" (Kemper & Edwards, 1986, p. 14). The elements of event knowledge are seen in the narratives of 4-year-olds. Underlying every story is an event chain, a chronology of events. Events include actions, physical states (e.g., possession, attribution), and mental states (e.g., emotions, dispositions, thoughts, intentions) that are linked causally as motivations, enablements, initiations, and resultants in the chain. Causal explanations are a repetitive cycle of these events. Children gradually learn to link events serially and only later with causal connectives. Connectives are acquired in the following order: *and, and then, when, because, so, then, if,* and *but* (Bloom et al., 1980). The fuller adult range of connectives (*therefore, as a result of, however*) is acquired gradually during the school years.

Between ages 2 and 10, the child's stories begin to contain more mental states and more initiation and motivation as causal links (Kemper & Edwards, 1986). Around age 4, children's stories begin to contain more explicit physical and mental states. Agentive actions or natural or social processes influence characters' thoughts and emotions. By age 6, children's stories describe motives for actions.

Generally, it is not until age 6 that children's narratives are causally coherent. Narratives require the skill to manipulate content, plot, and causal structure. Between ages 5 and 7, plots emerge consisting of a problem and some resolution of that problem. Gradually, these simple plots are elaborated into a series of problems and solutions or are embellished from within.

Narratives of 7-year-olds typically involve a beginning, a problem, a plan to overcome the problem, and a resolution. Both adults and children prefer goal-directed stories, such as the overcoming of an obstacle, to non-goal-directed stories. The plot usually centers around the past actions of a clearly fictional main character, allowing the storyteller greater flexibility. The presentation is manipulated dramatically by performance.

Causal chains may go through stages of development before they emerge as full goal-directed narratives. The narrative may be truncated. The problem may be solved, but the method is unclear. Similarly, the problem may be resolved but not because of the intervention of the principals in the story.

By second grade, the child may use not only beginning and ending markers (*once, last week, once upon a time, lived happily ever after, the end*), but also evaluative markers, such as *that was a good one.* Story length increases, greatly aided by syntactic devices such as conjunctions (*and, then*), locatives (*in, on, under, next to, in front of*), dialogue, comparatives (*bigger than, almost as big as, littlest*), adjectives, and causal statements. Although disquieting events are still central to the theme, there has been a change from inconsistent to consistent characters and from distinct but similar episodes to a chronology (as yet there is no fully developed plot).

The sense of plot in fictional narratives is increasingly clear after age 8 (Sutton-Smith, 1986). Now there is definite resolution of the central problem. The child's presentation relies primarily on language, rather than on his or her performance. The child manipulates the text and the audience to maintain attention.

In general, the narratives of older children are characterized by the following (J. Johnston, 1982b):

Fewer unresolved problems and unprepared resolutions
Less extraneous detail
More overt marking of changes in time and place
More introduction including setting and character information
Greater concern for motivation and internal reactions

More complex episode structure
Closer adherence to the story grammar model

Narratives are more cohesive and coherent.

Children learn to recognize, anticipate, respond to, tell, and read narratives within their homes and their language community. Because different sociocultural groups provide different learning situations for children, various types of narratives emerge (Heath, 1986b). Although every society allows children to hear and produce at least four basic narrative types, the distribution, frequency, and degree of elaboration of these types vary greatly. The four genres include three factual types, called *recounts, eventcasts,* and *accounts,* and fictionalized *stories* of animate beings who attempt to realize some goal (Stein, 1982).

The recount, common in school performance, brings to present attention those past experiences the child participated in, read about, or observed. Someone in authority usually asks the child to verbalize this shared experience. This form occurs infrequently outside of middle- and upper-class school-oriented families.

The eventcast is a verbal replay or explanation about some current or future event. A child often uses eventcasts to direct the actions of others in imaginative play or to try to influence others' behavior. Use of eventcasts enables the child to consider and analyze the effect of language on others.

Accounts seem to be the preferred form for children's spontaneous narratives. Within accounts, children share their experience ("You know what?"). Children initiate this narrative form, rather than report information requested by adults. Therefore, accounts are highly individualized.

In contrast, stories have a known and anticipated pattern or structure. Language is used to create the story form, and the listener plays a necessary interpretive function.

In middle- and upper-class school-oriented families, the earliest types of narratives are eventcasts that occur during nurturing activities, play, and reading with children. Caregivers share many accounts and stories, and by age 3, children are expected to appreciate and use all forms of narration. Invitations to give recounts decrease with age.

By the time most children begin school, they are usually familiar with all four forms of narration. This is not true for all children. In a white, working-class Southern community referred to as Roadville, recounts, tightly controlled by the interrogator, are the predominant form throughout the preschool years. Accounts do not begin until children attend school. Children and young adults also tell few stories, which seem to be the province of older, higher status adults.

In contrast, working-class, African American Southern children produce mostly accounts or eventcasts and have only minimal experience with recounts because of the difficulty in gaining adult attention. These children are at a disadvantage when they encounter the differing expectations of educational institutions (Heath, 1986a). Likewise, Chinese American children are encouraged to give accounts within, but not beyond, their families.

Narrative Breakdown

Narratives are an expression of the organization and interconnection of data in the brain. The storyteller must construct a context within which to relate events, both real and imaginary. Narratives consist of two frameworks, scripts and story frames (Naremore, 2001). Scripts consist of typical, predictable event sequences formed on the basis of experience, either real or vicarious. Scripts are not about any one experience but are generalized, organized hierarchically and causally, inhabited by characters, and contain a predictable sequence of events. Each event is represented in the brain and becomes part of a generalized event sequence.

Narrative frames are mental models of story structures. We use them to facilitate production and comprehension of narratives. In short, narrative frames are mental organizers that reduce processing demands.

The narrative of children with LI may breakdown because of linguistic difficulties or because the child doesn't know the script or the narrative frame. If too much mental capacity is used for linguistic processing, the narrative frame and/or the script may collapse. In similar fashion, poor script knowledge or poorly formed narrative frames may require too much mental "energy," leaving the child little capacity for linguistic processing.

Prior to collecting a narrative, the SLP should attempt to determine if the child has script and narrative frame knowledge. Script knowledge can be assessed by inquiring about they child's experiences, routines, and event knowledge (Naremore, 2001). Assessment of the retrieval of script knowledge can be accomplished by asking the child to act out the script with toys, pictures, or other items. If the child is successful, the SLP attempts to have the child recite an event account with a cue such as "Tell me what you do when you do X" or "Tell me what happened one time when you did X." If the child needs more help, the SLP can ask a few questions to determine the setting, then begin as follows:

You ride the bus to school every day. Last week on the way to school, you…

Note that the focus is the child and the tense is present. The SLP can assist the child with the event recount by saying, "And the…" or "Tell me what happened next." The recount should have some logical organization.

Knowledge of narrative frames can be determined by discussing with the child the purpose of narratives and determining the child's experience with narrative frames, either at home or in school. The SLP is interested in the use of narratives at home and in story reading. Narrative frames will be analyzed in more detail after a few narratives have been collected.

Children will not possess scripts for all possible events. Nor will all children possess narrative frames. Cultural variations are to be expected and will be discussed at the end of this chapter. The SLP should be reasonably positive that the child possesses event and script knowledge and a notion of narrative frames prior to beginning a narrative collection and analysis.

Collecting Narratives

The quality of the narrative is influenced by the selection of appropriate stimuli and topics based on the age, verbal ability, interests, and gender of the child or adolescent (Hedberg & Stoel-Gammon, 1986). Stimuli may include objects or pictures used for original constructions and heard or read stories used for retelling. In general, the task used to elicit the narrative influences the speaker's adaptation to the listener.

There are many different types of stories and many different contexts within which to tell them. The story type and context affect the eventual narrative form produced (Scott, 1988b). In general, maximally naturalistic topics and contexts elicit the most representative narratives. Other variables that may affect the narrative form are the story genre, the child's experiential base, the task in which the narrative is told, the source of the narrative, the topic, the formal or informal atmosphere of the context, and the audiovisual support available (Scott, 1988b).

Because the unit of analysis is the entire narrative, several oral and written narratives should be collected. The wide variation in narratives that can be produced by a single child within different contexts supports this notion. Prior to collecting, the SLP decides on the type of narratives desired and the stimuli to be used in their collection.

In general, fictionalized narratives with a vicarious experiential base may result in incomplete narratives with little emphasis on goals, characters' feelings or motivations, and endings. The pace, action orientation, and frequent commercial interruption found in television form a very different base for narratives than does experience or even traditional fables or fairy tales.

The type of elicitation task will affect the child's performance (Gibbons, Anderson, Smith, Field, & Fischer, 1986; Griffith, Ripich, & Dastoli, 1986). Books elicit descriptive information, whereas films elicit action sequences (Gibbons et al., 1986). Films also elicit more causal sequences in retelling than do oral stories. Pictures tend to constrain the form of the narrative and may lead to the production of additive chains, although children with Down syndrome express more verbal content in narratives to wordless picture books than would be expected from formal test results (Miles & Chapman, 2002). Stories in response to pictures tend to exclude character information, internal responses, or intentions (Griffith et al., 1986). Shared information may be omitted and new information treated as old even when the listener has not viewed the picture. In contrast, individual photographs or discussions of familiar events foster temporal chains.

Narrative retelling and recall can be used to determine the child's memory organization (Lovett, Dennis, & Newman, 1986). In narrative retelling, the child listens to a well-formed story and then reconstructs the story orally or in writing. Retelling of short narratives even may serve as a screening tool with young elementary school children. At this age, children should be able to retell the story without deviating significantly from the original in sequence or content.

In general, children with LI produce longer and more complete story grammars in retold narratives than in self-generated ones (Merritt & Liles, 1989). Clause length is also greater in retold narratives. Comprehension can be assessed within retold narratives by questioning the child when the retelling is complete. In general, children with LLD perform much like younger children, recalling less of the stimulus story (Crais & Chapman, 1987).

It is important to consider the amount of structure inherent in the stimulus and its effect on retold story construction. For example, nondescript dolls or puppets or sets of vehicles provide no structure. In contrast, a sequence of related pictures provides maximal structure. In general, the more structure found in the stimuli, the less structure the child must provide. The best stories, measured by the most complete episodes and the amount of information, occur when children retell a story without picture cues (Schneider, 1996). Although pictures provide additional input, thus reducing the memory load, they provide no linguistic structure. The task then becomes one of story generation rather than retelling. Pictures may distract children with LI.

In story retelling tasks, the SLP must consider the comprehension skills needed to understand the story, the mode of presentation (oral or written), story length, the child's past experience with the story genre (e.g., fairy tale, mystery), the child's interest in the content, and the degree of story structure (Hedberg & Stoel-Gammon, 1986). In general, more familiar, more interesting, and more structured stories result in more complete, better organized retellings.

Well-formed stories should be chosen for retelling, and these should be modified to enhance clarity and organization (Gordon & Braun, 1985). Stories should be rewritten to reduce complexity in their oral form and to summarize important sections. Subparts and transitions between parts of the narrative may need to be highlighted. Good narrative models often have repetitive elements.

Independent, self-generated narrative production requires the child to use her or his own organizational structure and narrative formulation. Narratives can be classified as fictional, personal-factual, or a combination of the two. Fictional or make-believe stories are good vehicles for preschoolers and may be stimulated by objects or pictures (F. Roth & Spekman, 1986; Westby, 1984, 1985). The SLP should provide a model narrative, begin the story for the child, or ask the child to relate a story about the object or picture, beginning with, "Once upon a time…" This initial structure usually results in a more literate style.

Personal-factual narratives may be collected from conversation or prompted. This type of narrative is very common in preschool and early elementary school, especially in show-and-tell activities. Preschoolers naturally create these types of narratives in conversation with each other (Preece, 1987).

The SLP should not try to elicit these narratives with open-ended prompts, such as "What did you do yesterday?" It may be helpful for the SLP to establish some common experience with the child and to share a narrative about this experience as an example for the child. To get a narrative, the SLP has to give one. Using a combination of narration and probing questions, the SLP can tell a personal story related to a common event, such as going to the doctor, and prompt the child with leading questions to stir the child's memory of past events ("Have you ever been to the doctor?"). Experiential topics prompted in this fashion usually result in the longest and most complex narratives.

Topics such as a new sibling or a death usually result in very truncated narratives. The child can be prompted to relate the scariest or funniest thing that ever happened (Garnett, 1986). In addition, the child might be asked to relate a favorite movie, television show, or story, although these prompts may elicit a sequential list of events (McCabe & Rollins, 1994).

The SLP should add nothing to the child's narrative other than feedback in the form of "uh-huh," "okay," "yeah," "wow," or a repetition of the child's previous utterance. These neutral but enthusiastic responses will not influence the course of the story as others might. The narrative can be resumed or the child prompted to continue by such utterances as, "And then what happened?"

Stories are enhanced also by familiarity with the physical setting and with the listener. The SLP should decide ahead of time on strategies for terminating rambling stories and for probing to elicit longer ones. A suggested guideline is not to expect children to engage in storytelling unless their MLU is 3.0 or more (Hedberg & Stoel-Gammon, 1986).

Narrative Analysis

Narrative analysis is a portion of an overall language analysis. As with dialogues, narratives can be analyzed in several ways, such as narrative levels, high points, story grammars, and cohesive devices (Lahey & Silliman, 1987). *Narrative levels* are concerned with the structural relationship of the narrative parts to the narrative as a whole. Events may be seemingly unorganized or organized sequentially or by causality.

Narrative levels do not have a goal-based organization, whereas story grammars (what happens in the story) do. Narrative level analysis is most appropriate for the stories of 2- to 5-year-olds (Applebee, 1978) and for school-age children with limited verbal abilities; story grammar analysis is best for those over age 5 (Glenn & Stein, 1980). The narratives of preschool children may be evaluated also by using high-point analysis to determine the type of narrative structure (McCabe & Rollins, 1994).

Story grammars describe the internal structure of a story, including its components and the rules underlying the relationships of these components (Stein & Glenn, 1979). By serving as a framework, story grammars may facilitate narrative comprehension. Ideally, components of a story are told in a way that increases understanding. Story grammars may be used to remember and interpret stories and to anticipate content.

Cohesion analysis describes the linguistic devices used to connect the elements of the text. In narratives, coherence, or making sense, is conveyed through cohesion. Inappropriate or inadequate use of cohesive devices results in a disjointed text that is difficult to comprehend.

From the analysis, the SLP should address the following questions (J. Johnston, 1982b):

- Does the narrative contain chains? If so, what type?
- Does the narrative follow the typical story grammar model? Is the story organized maturely?
- What are the guiding scripts of the narrator, and what do they reveal about the storyteller's knowledge of events and expectations?
- What linguistic means are used to create a cohesive unit?

In addition, the SLP is interested in the sensitivity of the narrator to the perceived needs of the listener.

Narrative Levels

Children use two strategies for organizing their stories: centering and chaining. *Centering* is the linking of attributes or objects to form a story nucleus. The links may be based on similarity or complementarity of features. Similarity links are formed by perceptually observed attributes, such as actions, characteristics, and scenes or situations. Causal links are not present, although sequential ones may be. Complementary links consist of conceptual bonds based on abstract, logical attributes, such as members of a class or events linked by cause-and-effect bonds. *Chaining* consists of a sequence of events that share attributes and leads directly from one to another.

Most stories of 2-year-olds are organized by centering. By age 3, however, nearly half of the children use both centering and chaining. This percentage increases, and by age 5, nearly three-fourths of the children use both strategies.

These organizational strategies can result in six basic developmental stages of story organization (Applebee, 1978), presented here in developmental order:

Heaps are sets of unrelated statements about a central stimulus. The statements identify aspects of the stimulus or provide additional information. The common element may be the similarity of the grammatical structure, for there is no overall organizational pattern.

Dogs wag their tails and bark. Dogs sleep all day. A dog chased a cat.

Sequences include events linked on the basis of similar attributes or events that create a simple but meaningful focus for a story. The organization is additive, and sentences may be moved without altering the narrative.

I *ate* a hamburger. And Johnny *too*. Mommy *ate* a chicken nuggets. Daddy *ate* a fries and coke.

Primitive temporal narratives are organized around a center with complementary events.

I go outside and swing. Bobby push swing. I go high and try to stop. I fall. And I start to cry. Bobby pick me up.

Unfocused temporal chains lead directly from one event to another, while linking attributes, such as characters, settings, or actions, shift. This is the first level of chaining, and the links are concrete. As a result of the shifting focus, unfocused chains have no centers.

The man got in his boat. He rowed and fished. He ate his sandwich. (Shift) The fishes swimmed and play. Fishes jump over the water. Fishes go to a big hole in the bottom. (Shift) There's a dog in the boat. He's thirsty. He jump in the water.

Focused temporal or causal chains generally center on a main character who goes through a series of perceptually linked, concrete events.

This boy, he found a jellybean. And his mother said not to eat it. And he did. And a tree growed out of his head.

Narratives develop the center as the story progresses. Each incident complements the center, develops from the previous incident, forms a chain, and adds some new aspect to the theme. Causal relationships may be concrete or abstract and move forward toward the ending of the initial situation. There is usually a climax.

There was a boy named Juan. And he got lost in the woods. He ate plants and trees. And he was friends with all the animals. He builded a tent to live in. One day, he builded a fire, and the policemen found him. They took Juan home to his mommy and daddy.

Each narrative is divided into episodes that are analyzed according to this scheme. Table 8.1 contains examples of narratives and their analysis by narrative level.

High-Point Analysis

High-point analysis is a method for identifying narrative macrostructure. The high point, or most significant point of a narrative, is revealed not in the past events recalled, but in an event's meaning to the narrator. The accompanying structure has developmental significance.

It is best to use narratives that describe events in which the narrator is present (McCabe & Rollins, 1994). The SLP should separate the narratives and select the longest personal event narratives for analysis. Length and complexity have been shown to be related (McCabe & Peterson, 1990). The narratives of some children with LI may have very poorly defined boundaries that make this demarcation difficult.

The evaluated high point is marked by children in many ways. These markings include paralinguistic features, such as emphasis, elongation, and use of environmental noises ("It went BOOM!"); and linguistic features, such as exclamations ("Wow!"), repetition, attention getters ("Here's the best part."), exaggeration, judgments or evaluative statements ("It was my favorite."), emotional statements, and explanations (McCabe & Rollins, 1994).

TABLE 8.1   Narrative level analysis

Example	Classification
Simple frames	
Granma lives on a farm. There are horsies and piggies. The cows moo. I can ride on the tire swing in a tree. And the calf licked me. That's all.	Sequence
Once there was two kids, Cassidy and…and Fred. Fred's a funny name. And they was fighting. Their mother said, "Why are you fighting?" Cassidy and Fred doesn't know why. They stop and be friends.	Focused chain
Complex narrative frame with episodic development	
The kids all went to Burger King on Halloween. Super Zhiming—that's me—got a cheeseburger. My sister got a Whopper. Mommy and Daddy got nuggets and salad bar. They were eating when a big ghost came out of my milkshake. He threw milkshake on everyone and got them mad. Super Zhiming stuck the ghost with a fork. The ghost got flat. All the air came out. Daddy was so happy that he buyed ice cream cones for all the kids.	Sequence Narrative

Once he or she has identified the high point of the narrative, the SLP can analyze for narrative structure. Different types of structures are presented in Table 8.2. Next to each is the age at which these structures are most common for Caucasian, English-speaking, North American children. The SLP can use this table to determine whether the child is using narrative structures typical of his age group.

After age 5, fewer than 10 percent of children produce one-event, two-event, leapfrog, and miscellaneous narratives. No children over age 6 produce leapfrog narratives. The chronological narra-

TABLE 8.2   High-point narrative structure

Narrative Structure	Characteristics	Expected Age in Years
One-event narrative	Contains one event.	Below 3.5
Two-event narrative	Contains 2 past events but no logical or causal relationship in the real world or in the narrative.	3.5
Miscellaneous narrative	Contains 2 or more past events that in the real world are logically or causally related.	Very low frequency at all ages (3.5–9)
Leapfrog narrative	Contains 2 or more related past events, but the order does not mirror the real-world relationship.	4
Chronological narrative	Contains 2 or more related past events in a logical or causal sequence without a high point.	Present at all ages (3.5–9)
End-at-high-point narrative	Contains 2 or more related past events in a logical or causal sequence with a high point but no following events (resolution).	5
Classic narrative	Contains 2 or more related past events in a logical or causal sequence with both a high point and a resolution.	6+

Source: Adapted from McCabe & Rollins (1994).

tive type, common at all ages, is of little diagnostic value (McCabe & Rollins, 1994). Obviously, a small sample of a few narratives will be needed for an adequate evaluation.

Normal variations are to be expected within and across children. Many young children will "test the waters" by stating the high point first ("I got stung by a bee") and then, if it is accepted, will proceed with the narrative. This is not an example of impaired narration and can be analyzed by using the suggested narrative structures.

Cultural differences must be considered too. African American children often tell topic-associating narratives in which events that happened at different times and places may be combined around a central theme. The narratives of Japanese children may be succinct collections of experiences, rather than single detailed sequential events (Minami & McCabe, 1991). Children from Latino cultures often do not relate sequential events (Rodino, Gimbert, Perez, Craddock-Willis, & McCabe, 1992).

Story Grammars

Story grammars provide an organizational pattern that can aid information processing (J. Johnston, 1982b). The competent storyteller constructs the story and the flow of information in such a way as to maximize comprehension. The SLP notes the story grammar elements present and produces a model of the child's story grammar (S. Chapman, 1997; F. Roth, 1986).

A *story* consists of the setting plus the episode structure (story = setting + episode structure) (J. Johnston, 1982b). Each story begins with an introduction contained in the setting, as in "Once upon a time in a far-off kingdom, there lived a prince who was very sad…" or "On the way to work this morning, I was crossing Main Street…," or simply "we went to the zoo today."

An *episode* consists of an initiating event, an internal response, a plan, an attempt, a consequence, and a reaction. An episode is considered to be complete if it contains an initiating event or response to provide a purpose, an attempt, and a direct consequence (Stein & Glenn, 1979). Episodes may be linked additively, temporally, causally, or in a mixed fashion. A story may consist of one or more interrelated episodes.

The seven elements of story grammars occur in the following order (Stein & Glenn, 1979):

1. Setting statements (S) that introduce the characters and describe their habitual actions, along with the social, physical, and/or temporal contexts that introduce the protagonist.
2. Initiating events (IE) that induce the character(s) to act through some natural act (e.g., an earthquake), a notion to seek something (e.g., treasure), or the action of one of the characters (e.g., arresting someone).
3. Internal responses (IR) that describe the characters' reactions, such as emotional responses, thoughts, or intentions, to the initiating events. Internal responses provide some motivation for the characters.
4. Internal plans (IP) that indicate the characters' strategies for attaining their goal(s). Children rarely include this element.
5. Attempts (A) that describe the overt actions of the characters to bring about some consequence, such as attain their goal(s).
6. Direct consequences (DC) that describe the characters' success or failure at attaining their goal(s) as a result of the attempt.
7. Reactions (R) that describe the characters' emotional responses, thoughts, or actions to the outcome or preceding chain of events.

The two very different stories in Table 8.3 present examples of story grammars.

There is a sequence of stages in the development of story grammars (Glenn & Stein, 1980). Certain structural patterns appear early and persist, whereas others are rather late in developing. The overall developmental sequence is as follows, although much individual variation exists:

Descriptive sequences consist of descriptions of characters, surroundings, and habitual actions. There are no causal or temporal links. The entire story consists of setting statements.

This is a story about my rabbit. He lives in a cage. He likes to hop around my yard. He eats carrots and grass. The end.

Action sequences have a chronological order for actions but no causal relations. The story consists of a setting statement and various action attempts.

I had a birthday party. (S) We played games and winned prizes. (A) I opened presents. (A) I got balloons. (A) I blowed out the candles. (A) We ate cake and ice cream. (A) We had fun.

Reaction sequences consist of a series of events in which changes cause other changes, with no goal-directed behaviors. The sequence consists of a setting, an initiating event, and action attempts.

There was a lady petting her cow. (S) And the cow kicked the light. (IE) Then the police came. (A) Then a fire truck came. (A) Then a hook-and-ladder came. (A) And that's the end. (S)

TABLE 8.3   Story grammar examples

Narrative	Story Grammar Elements
I. Single Episode	
There was this girl, and she got kidnapped by these pirates.	Setting statement (S)
	Initiating event (IE)
So when they were eating, she cut the ropes and got away.	Attempt (A)
	Direct consequence (DC)
And she lived on a island and ate parrots.	Reactions (R)
II. Multiple episode	
Once there was this big dog on a farm.	Setting statement (S)
And he got hungry 'cause there wasn't enough food.	Initiating event$_1$ (IE$_1$)
The dog...his name was Max...was sad with no food, so his owner went to find some.	Internal response$_1$ (IR$_1$)
	Attempt$_1$ (A$_1$)
He met a witch, but she wouldn't give him food 'til he killed a yukky toad.	Initiating event$_2$ (IE$_2$)
	Internal response$_2$ (IR$_2$)
He was scared but he decided to build a trap.	Internal plan$_2$ (IP$_2$)
	Attempt$_2$ (A$_2$)
He dug a hole and filled it with frog food.	Direct consequences$_2$
The frog wanted to eat the man but got caught.	(DC$_2$)
The man went back to the witch and she got some hamburgers for the man and the dog.	Direct consequence$_1$ (DC$_1$)
And the man and Max ate hamburgers and were happy.	Reaction$_1$ (R$_1$)

Abbreviated episodes contain an implicit or explicit goal. At this level, the story may contain either an event statement and a consequence or an internal response and a consequence. Although the characters' behavior is purposeful, it is usually not premeditated.

> There was a mommy and two kids. (S) And the kids baked a cake for the mommy's birthday. (S) They forgot to turn on…off the stove and burned the cake. (IE) The kids went to the store and buyed a cake. (C) The end. (S)

Complete episodes contain an entire goal-oriented behavioral sequence consisting of a consequence statement and two of the following: initiating event, internal response, and attempt.

> This man was a doctor. (S) He made a monster. (IE) And it chase him around his house. (IE) He run in his bedroom. (A) He push the monster in the closet. (A) And the monster go away. (C) That's all. (S)

Complex episodes are expansions of the complete episode or contain multiple episodes.

> Once there was this Luke Skywalker. (S) And he had to fight Darf Invader. (S/IE) They fought with swords. (A) And he killed him. (C) And he got in his rocket to blow up these kind of horse robots. (IE) And he shot them. (A) Then all the bad soldiers were killed. (C)

Interactive episodes contain two characters who have separate goals and actions that influence each other's behavior.

> Sally never helped her mom with the dishes. (S) She got mad and said that Sally had to do it. (IE) So, Sally washed the dishes but she was mad. (IR) Then Sally dropped some dishes. (A) Then she dropped more. (A) And her mom said that she didn't have to do any more dishes. (C) And Sally watched TV every night after dinner. (S)

Specific structural properties associated with each structural pattern are listed in Table 8.4.

Children with LLD produce fewer mature episodes than do their age-matched peers who are non-LLD. In addition, children with LLD make fewer complete setting statements and are less likely to include response, attempt, and plan statements in their narratives (F. Roth & Spekman, 1986). Inter-episodic relations are also weaker in the narratives of children with LLD.

Story grammar analysis alone may lack the sensitivity to differentiate children with LI from those without (Hewitt & Duchan, 1995; Merritt & Liles, 1987; Ripich & Griffith, 1988). The portrayal of subjective states—*think, remember, feel, know*—as in the internal response element of story grammars is especially difficult for children with LI and may be central to narratives (Astington, 1990).

Unfortunately, there are few normative data for clinical use. In general, children developing typically produce all of the elements of story grammar by age 9. Children's narratives can be used, however, to approximate their functioning level and to determine which structural elements are present (Hedberg & Stoel-Gammon, 1986). Table 8.5 contains several narratives analyzed by story grammar structural pattern and narrative level.

Cohesive Devices

Text consists of the linguistic properties of a narrative, not the form of individual sentences (J. Johnston, 1982b). Ratings of good-to-poor narratives are related most closely to textual measures

TABLE 8.4   Structural properties of narratives

Structural Patterns	Structural Properties	Structural Patterns	Structural Properties
Descriptive sequence	Setting statements (S)(S)(S)	Complex episode	Multiple episodes Setting statement (S) Two of the following: Initiating event (IE$_1$) Internal response (IR$_1$) Attempt (A$_1$) Direct consequence (DC$_1$) Two of the following: Initiating event (IE$_2$) Internal response (IR$_2$) Attempt (A$_2$) Direct consequence (DC$_2$)
Action sequence	Setting statement (S) Attempts (A)(A)(A)		
Reaction sequence	Setting statement (S) Initiating event (IE) Attempts (A)(A)(A)		
Abbreviated episode	Setting statement (S) Initiating event (IE) or Internal response (IR) Direct consequence (DC)		
Complete episode	Setting statement (S) Two of the following: Initiating event (IE) Internal response (IR) Attempt (A) Direct consequence (DC)	Expanded complete episode	Setting statement (S) Initiating event (IE) Internal response (IR) Internal plan (IP) Attempt (A) Direct consequence (DC) Reaction (R)
		Interactive episode	Two separate but parallel episodes that influence each other

TABLE 8.5   Story grammar analysis

Narrative	Story Grammar Elements	Structural Pattern	Narrative Level
I. We went to a farm. I got to feed chickens. Then I saw cows in the barn. Cows give milk. Cows stay in the field all day and eat grass. At night they come in.	(S) (S) (S) (S) (S) (S)	Descriptive sequence	Unfocused temporal chain
II. There was this boy who lived in a city. And one day a giant bug got out of this place where they keep bugs. And the boy got in an airplane and shot it.	(S) (IE) (A)	Reaction sequence	Focused temporal chain

III.
Once there was two boys.
One boy fell into a big hole
  with rats and he was scared.
His brother got a ladder
  but the rats ate it.
So, he threw his lunch in the hole.
The rats ate it, too, and the
  boy climbed up a rope and was safe.
	(S)
	(IE$_1$)
	(IR$_1$)
	(A$_1$)
	(DC$_1$/IE$_2$)
	(A$_2$)
	(DC$_2$)
	(R)
		Complex episodes	Narrative

Even though the third narrative possesses advanced structural properties, it demonstrates some pronoun confusion. The relationship of the boys is not established until the third utterance.

than to sentence-level ones (McFadden & Gillam, 1996). Textual level measures may include the following:

Number of T-units per narrative

Number of connectives (*because, so, then*) per T-unit

Number of plot units or thematic elements (participants, location, plan, attack or action, emotion or feelings) per narrative

Percentage of plot units expressed as problem-resolution pairs (*And they were starving, so they… And they **ate all the food they could.***)

Children with LI and those with poor reading abilities exhibit some difficulty communicating well-organized, coherent narratives (Norris & Bruning, 1988). In general, they produce event and sentential relationships more poorly than do their age-matched peers (J. Johnston, 1982b; Liles, 1985a, 1985b, 1990; Merritt & Liles, 1985). The most common cohesive errors among children with LI are an *incomplete tie,* in which the child references an entity or event not introduced previously, and an *ambiguous reference,* in which the child does not identify to which of two or more referents she or he is referring (Liles, 1990).

Cohesion repairs require particular organizational strategies not found in conversation. Older children, aged 8.5 to 12.5, most often make meaning repairs in narratives and in conversation, recognizing the importance of being comprehended successfully (MacLachlan & Chapman, 1988; Purcell & Liles, 1992). Cohesion repairs are made frequently by both children developing typically and those with LI, but with different levels of success (Purcell & Liles, 1992). In general, both types of children are equally successful with repairs within T-units, usually consisting of single-word repair. In repairs across T-units, requiring reorganization of several sentences, however, children with LI are less successful. This difference may reflect underlying language skills and processes (Butler, 1986; L. Miller, 1984; Van Kleeck, 1984; Wallach & Liebergott, 1984).

Of interest in the text are cohesive devices that linguistically connect the components. In short, any sentence element that sends the listener outside of the sentence for a referent is a cohesive device. For example, a pronoun may require referral to the previous sentence in order to determine the referent. The five types of cohesive relations are reference, substitution, ellipsis, conjunction, and lexical items. Of these, lexical cohesion may be the most difficult to assess reliably (Liles, 1990).

Because there is little normative data on the development of these relations, descriptive analysis is the best diagnostic approach. In general, mature story grammar develops prior to mature use of cohesive devices. It is possible, therefore, to have good episodes but poor cohesion. The two are related but not dependent. The cohesion within and between episodes becomes important as children develop complex and interactive episodes. There is a metalinguistic quality about cohesion in that the speaker must pay attention to the text apart from the story itself. Cohesive relations are discussed in Chapter 6 and are reviewed only briefly in this section.

Reference

Reference devices, which refer to something else in the text for their interpretation, consist of pronouns, definite articles, demonstratives, and comparatives. The link with the referent should be clear and unambiguous. Clarity is often a problem when the child changes the story narrator frequently, uses dialogue, or includes several characters. Pronouns and definite articles are used to refer to referents previously identified in the narrative.

In contrast, demonstratives locate referents on a continuum of proximity. Nominals, such as *this, that, these,* and *those,* refer to a person or a thing; adverbs, such as *here, there, now,* and *then,* refer to a place or a time. Use of *now* and *then* usually is restricted to referring to the time just mentioned. In addition, *now* and *then* can serve as conjunctions.

Finally, comparatives are both general, referring to similarities and differences without reference to a particular property, and specific, referring to some specific quantity or quality. General comparatives include such words as *another, same, different(ly), equal(ly), unequal, identical, similar(ly),* and *else.* Specific quantity words include *more, less, so many, as few as, second, further,* and *fewer than.* Quality words and terms consist of *worse than, as good as, equally bad, better, better than, happier than,* and *most happy/happiest.*

Substitution and Ellipsis

Substitution and ellipsis both refer to information within the narrative that supposedly is shared by the listener and the speaker. In substitution, another word is used in place of the shared information. The words *one(s)* and *same* can be substituted for nouns, as in "Make mine the *same*" or "I'll take *one,* too." Such words as *do* can be substituted for main verbs, as when we emphasize, "I *did* already." Finally, such words as *that, so,* and *not* can be substituted for whole phrases or clauses, as in "I think *not*" or "Mother won't like *that.*"

Ellipsis differs from substitution in that shared information simply is omitted. Whole phrases and clauses may experience ellipsis. Any portion of the noun phrase may be omitted, as in the following examples:

> I have *four of her brightly wrapped red gifts.* Which is *yours*? Would you like *two*? Do you have *green*?

Verbal material also may be omitted, as in the response "He can't" to the question "Will John attend the concert tonight?" Clausal ellipsis may be demonstrated with the same question when the answer is "Probably."

Conjunction

The four types of conjunctive relations are additive, temporal, causal, and adversative. Whereas additive relationships usually are represented by *and,* temporal ones may be signaled with a variety of words, such as *then, next, after, before, at the same time, finally, first, secondly,* and *an hour later.* Causal conjunctive relationships may be expressed with a variety of terms, such as *because, as a result of, in that case, for,* and *so.* Finally, adversative conjunctions include *but* and others, such as *however, although, on the other hand, on the contrary, except,* and *nevertheless.*

Conjunction use may be independent of the specific clausal structure linked. In other words, conjunctions link the underlying semantic concepts and thus represent the relationship of these units, which may differ from the syntactic units. The way episode parts are linked may reflect the child's underlying episodic organization. We would expect, therefore, that conjunctive relationships between episodic elements would be more complex and difficult than those between sentences. This increase seems to be true for both children with LI and those without (Liles, 1987). This may account for the fewer conjunctions found in the narratives of children with LI (Greenhalgh & Strong, 2001).

Lexical Items

Words themselves express relationships by the morphological endings used. For example, the present progressive -*ing* ending is used to express actions taking place at the present time. The following example demonstrates a clear understanding of the relationship of the process to the product:

> He *had been writing* for several months. After the book was finally *written,* he celebrated for days. He swore never *to write* another novel.

Categorical relationships can be expressed and demonstrate convergent and divergent organizational patterns. Convergent thought goes from the members to the category, as in "She had *petunias, dahlias, roses, and pansies* in her garden, but she could never have enough *flowers.*" Divergent thought goes from the category to the members, as in "She liked several kinds of *sports* but was best at *soccer, rugby, and lacrosse.*"

Finally, words can express relationships, such as opposition or part-to-whole. In a narrative, the SLP can look for antonyms, synonyms, ordered series, and part-whole or part-part relationships. Ordered series include memorized sequences, such as the days of the week, or hierarchies, such as instructor, assistant professor, associate professor, and full professor. Part-whole relationships are expressed by entities that form a portion of the whole, as in rudder-boat, pedal-bike, and January-year. Finally, part-part relations contain parts of the same whole, as in nose-chin, finger-thumb, and rudder-sail.

Conclusion

Narratives require the manipulation of extended units of language. Cohesive devices are indirectly assessed by certain quantitative measures. Those measures that differentiate between children with LI and those without are presented in Table 8.6 (S. Chapman, 1997; Liles, Duffy, Merritt, & Purcell, 1995).

Reliability and Validity

Narrative analysis is not without its detractors. The reliability and validity of narrative analysis as a clinical tool has been questioned (Klecan-Aker & Carrow-Woolfolk, 1987). Naturally, reliability and validity will vary with the aspects of narratives measured.

Establishing developmental level by the number of story grammar components present appears to have very high inter- and intrajudge reliability (Klecan-Aker & Hamburg, 1991; Klecan-Aker, Swank, & Johnson, 1991). This developmental level and other quantitative measures, such as words per T-unit and words per clause, also correlate strongly with language test scores, suggesting that narrative analysis has strong construct validity.

TABLE 8.6   Quantitative measure of narrative structure

	Age 8 yr. 7 mo.	Age 10 yr. 3 mo.
Words/main clause	7.2	8.5
Words/subordinate clause	6.7	7.4
Subordinate clauses/T-unit	.24	.25
% grammatically correct T-units	.94	.94

CLD Children

Children entering school with good narrative abilities are better prepared to comprehend and produce the decontextualized language of reading and writing (Gee, 1989; Westby, 1984). Other children are at greater risk of academic failure (Orum, 1986; U.S. Bureau of the Census, 1990). To tell, retell, or comprehend the literate narratives found in English, a child must have a concept of story grammar and a cultural script for the story. An evaluative technique such as "Tell me a story" may be irrelevant to children not exposed to bedtime or other similar storytelling situations.

Narrative performance among various cultural, ethnic, and linguistic groups may differ greatly. These differences reflect both cultural and individual differences in storytelling. Storytelling is never context or culture free (Gutierrez-Clellan & Quinn, 1993). Rather, it is the product of the contextual interaction of the narrator and the audience and of the sociocultural norms of each, which shape each person's presuppositions and expectations. Even the purpose and context for narratives varies across cultures.

Telling narratives is a social event governed by cultural norms and values. Not every culture expects the narrative monologues seen in American English. Among some Latinos, Native Americans, African Americans, Jewish Americans, and Hawaiian Americans, stories are produced conversationally with audience cooperation. The story is built by the storyteller acting out the parts as the audience challenges and contradicts.

Narrative completeness will reflect also each child's experience and world knowledge (Ross & Berg, 1990). Pictures and topics that are used to elicit the child's narrative may be beyond the child's experiential base and result in diminished performance. It is difficult for children to tell stories with unfamiliar scripts. A child unfamiliar with a farm, for example, may use the word *truck* for *tractor* and *garage* for *barn*.

Even the temporal qualities of narratives reflect the temporal realities of different cultures. The importance of seconds, minutes, and hours in Western culture is not found in others. A good friend once told me of his grandfather, a Cherokee elder, who measured time by the slow, purposeful movement of the earth and moon. A Bolivian American friend laughingly confided that her parents usually arrived at a wedding in time to throw the rice.

Narratives in Standard American English dialects tend to be linear and temporal-causal. This is not true of all dialectal speakers. The narratives of Athabaskans, a native Alaskan people, are spatially or circularly organized (Silliman, Diehl, Aurillo, Wilkinson, & Hammargren, 1995). Many Native American narratives stress community, harmony, and tribe rather than individual actions to overcome some challenge (Westby & Roman, 1995). Although the narratives of speakers of African American English are linear, they meander more than those of majority speakers and, thus, are longer, with more shifts of time, place, and characters.

Many of the aspects of narrative analysis discussed previously are based on American English forms and cultural expectations, such as the narrative organization and the use of linguistic devices. The analysis in this chapter assumes that all narratives are composed of an elaborated story grammar. Episodic structure and content vary with culture (Kay-Raining Bird & Vetter, 1994). The narratives of the Athabaskan people characteristically include four actors, four major instruments of action, and four sections: introduction, scene 1, scene 2, and closing (Silliman et al., 1995). In contrast, the narratives of Japanese children are very sparse, consisting of two-unit episodes: a challenge and a consequence.

Likewise, the narratives of African American children have less formal beginnings and endings and less chronology while containing more judgments on characters and their actions (Heath, 1983).

In addition, the stories of African American and Puerto Rican children embed such evaluations within the narrative and are less likely than European American children to state the point of the story explicitly at the end (Iglesias, Gutierrez-Clellan, & Marcano, 1986).

Grammatical contrasts offer further examples. In Spanish, referential cohesion is demonstrated in the introduction of and the later referral to different entities in the story. Characters, props, and places may be referenced by the nominal (*un nene/a boy*), elliptical (*El fue a la tienda, cogio un poco de comida/He went to the store, got some food*) (Gutierrez-Clellan & Heinrichs-Ramos, 1993, p. 560), or the demonstrative (*este/this*). In addition, characters and props may be referenced by the pronominal *(elle/she)*. With increasing age, Spanish-speaking and English-speaking children use ellipsis more for place (Gutierrez-Clellan & Heinrichs-Ramos, 1993). Once the setting has been introduced, it is not named again unless changed.

Whereas the use of ellipsis in English requires previous nominal reference, speakers of Spanish may omit referential information because verb endings mark this information (*tuvo/I had; tuviste/ you had*). Children speaking Spanish who are familiar with this practice may omit nominal reference in English too, giving the impression that they do not understand cohesion.

Still, there is much similarity in narrative development. By age 4, children speaking Spanish have a wide range of referential strategies. The nominal and elliptical forms are used for characters in the subject position, while pronominals are used for those in the object (Gutierrez-Clellan & Heinrichs-Ramos, 1993).

As children speaking Spanish get older, a greater number of props and places are introduced, and their narratives become more detailed, though not necessarily much longer (Gutierrez-Clellan & McGrath, 1991). More and more information is embedded, decreasing the number of sentences needed to express the same information. Redundant information is omitted. The number of characters changes little, however, from ages 4.5 to 8 years.

Children speaking Spanish develop causal sequences at about the same age as children speaking American English. From ages 4 to 9, there is a decrease in two-clause causal sequences and in the proportion of unrelated statements and an increase in three-clause causal sequences (Gutierrez-Clellan & Iglesias, 1992). Action sequences predominate as a means of moving the story forward. Physical and emotional states as the cause of change tend to remain stable from ages 4 to 9.

Other devices, such as paralinguistics, may be used by other cultures more than by the majority American culture, which tends to rely on rising and falling intonation (Gee, 1986; Michaels, 1986). For example, African American and Puerto Rican children use more loudness, pitch, rate, stress, rhythm, and intonation along with exclamations and repetitions than do majority children to move the story forward and to make evaluative or emotional comments (Iglesias et al., 1986). In other cultures, false starts and hesitations function as internal organizers, while slower pace through repetition, redundancy, and silence may signal the point of the story or its conclusion (Gee, 1986, 1989).

Narrative Collection and Analysis

The cultural variability of narratives requires the SLP to assess narrative development in a wide variety of culturally relevant contexts approaching the natural environment of the child (Gutierrez-Clellan & Quinn, 1993). If the child does not consider the task "worthy," he or she may give less than an optimum or even typical performance (Iglesias et al., 1986).

The SLP may err on the overly cautious side by assuming that all differences are cultural or that the child can only produce narratives of a familiar type in familiar contexts. A third option, discussed previously, is a dynamic assessment that evaluates the child's learning potential or teachability (Feuerstein, Rand, Jensen, Kaniel, & Tzuriel, 1987).

A dynamic assessment of narrations consists of a collection and analysis, mediated instruction, and collection and analysis (Gutierrez-Clellan, Peña & Quinn, 1995; Gutierrez-Clellan & Quinn, 1993; Peña, 2002). With school-age children, the SLP first collects narratives in response to wordless picture books and analyzes each for the number of words, C-units, clauses, clauses/C-unit, episodic structure, story components, and story idea and language. Wordless picture books include *Bird and His Ring* (Miller, 1999b), *Frog, Where Are You?* (Mayer, 1969), *One Frog Too Many* (Mayer & Mayer, 1975), and *Two Friends* (Miller, 1999a).

In the second step, the SLP chooses one or two areas of the narrative for a mediated language experience (MLE). The SLP helps the child explore the goals of a story, the importance of these goals, the consequences of omitting these goals, plans for using this information, and developing strategies.

The second collection and analysis is similar to the first but attempts to answer five questions (Peña, 2002):

> Was the child able to form a more complete and coherent narrative?
> How difficult was it for the SLP to achieve positive change?
> Did the child pay attention and include more elements in the second narrative?
> Was the child able to transfer the learning without SLP support?
> Was learning quick and efficient?

Children developing typically usually make rapid change and are very responsive.

For more-mature children and adolescents, several narratives can be collected in various contexts and analyzed as above and for the "rules" appropriate for each type of narration. The characteristics of each type of narration based on temporal, referential, causal, and spatial coherence are included in Table 8.7 (Gutierrez-Clellan & Quinn, 1993). The SLP must remember that the "rules" for certain types of narration may be unfamiliar to some children and may be a difference, rather than a deficit. The types of cohesion used by the child should reveal his or her narrative style.

In the second step, the different types of narratives are explained to the child by using cues, such as "Talk like a book in school" or "Talk like you would to a friend," and examples. Within the training, the child is given different types of narratives to produce. Feedback is used by the SLP to seek clarification, additional information, relevant comments, and reference. After some intervention, the SLP attempts to determine whether the child can learn different types of narration, can transfer the types of cohesion across contexts, and can tell narratives without cuing and feedback.

Two measures that seem particularly important are the length of causal sequences and the number of unrelated statements. Among children speaking Spanish, an increase in the length of causal sequences and a decrease in the number of unrelated statements are indicators of greater causal cohesion (Gutierrez-Clellan & Iglesias, 1992).

Dynamic procedures work well with children from different sociocultural backgrounds (Lidz, 1987; Peña & Iglesias, 1989; Sewell, 1987). The procedures require that the task be explained, that the reasons for certain responses be stated adequately, and that the child respond differentially to the SLP's cues (Gutierrez-Clellan & Quinn, 1993).

TABLE 8.7   Types of narration and cohesion

Temporal Coherence
  Is there a temporal order of events?
  Are temporal connectives necessary? If so, are they used?
  Are shifts in time marked?

Causal Coherence
  Are physical and mental states used to interconnect actions? (*He was very tired, so he went to sleep.*)
  If not, can connectives be inferred easily?
  Are causal connectives necessary? If so, are they used?

Referential Coherence
  Participants
    Is adequate reference to the participants made?
    Are new characters introduced clearly? If not, are they referred to as if introduced elsewhere in the text?
    Are characters reintroduced in an unambiguous manner?
    Can the referent be inferred from general world knowledge?

  Props
    Is identification of specific objects necessary? If so, are props mentioned adequately? If not, are props
      introduced by gestures or deictics, such as "that thing"?
    Can the identity of props be inferred from descriptions or functions?

Spatial Coherence
  Is information about location necessary? If so, are locations identified?
  Are shifts in location clearly marked?

Source: Adapted from Gutierrez-Clellan & Quinn (1993).

Conclusion

The near universal use of some form of narrative suggests its importance in communication. As in dialogue analysis, it is important to analyze narratives simultaneously at several levels. Although there are few normative data on narrative development against which to compare a child's or adolescent's performance in any culture, the SLP can use the model described in this chapter to analyze and describe performance.

In general, the more mature the narrative, the more complete the structure and the story grammar. In addition to causal chains, more mature narratives contain greater cohesion to aid the listener in interpretation. Mature narratives are structurally cohesive and proceed from one event to another in a logical fashion that demonstrates the narrator's attempt to guide the listener.

More mature narratives also include more insight into the thoughts and feelings of the central characters and greater use of devices for expressing time and place. There are fewer extraneous details and loose ends.

The SLP should be cautious when evaluating children from cultures whose narratives do not closely follow the literary pattern described in this chapter. Children from some Spanish-speaking and some Native American cultures may have less experience with story narratives. To varying degrees, these cultures make extensive use of more descriptive narratives. The use of pictures and elicitation techniques, such as "Tell me a story about this picture," may evoke a very different narrative from what is sought.

Intervention

CHAPTER 9

A Functional Intervention Model

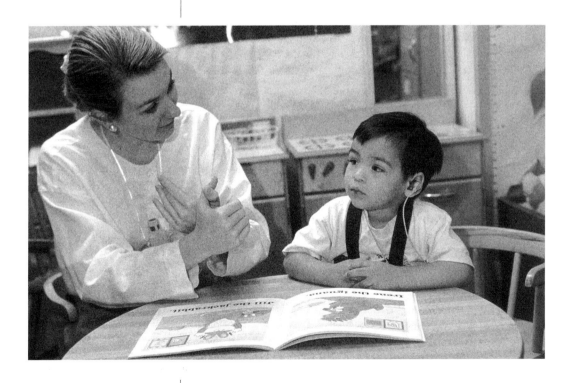

Traditional language intervention does not consider either the integrated nature of language or the context of language use (Duchan, 1997). Language is viewed as a hierarchically organized set of rules, rather than as a holistic set of variable context-sensitive rules (Rice, 1986). Although the focus may include form, content, and use, the overall design is usually additive, rather than integrative. Often, the stated goal is to learn specific language units, not enhance communication. Language methods that emphasize very specific skills seem to have very specific, limited effects. There is little evidence that newly acquired forms will generalize to everyday conversational use (Olswang & Bain, 1991).

Clinical intervention should be a well-integrated whole in which the various aspects of language combine to enhance communication. The purposes of intervention should be (a) to teach a generative repertoire of linguistic features that can be used to communicate in socially appropriate ways in various contexts and (b) to stimulate overall language development (Duchan, 1997; Russell, 1993; Warren & Kaiser, 1986a).

A functional language intervention model attempts to target language features that the child uses in the everyday context, such as the home or the classroom, and to adapt that context so that it facilitates the learning of language. Table 9.1 presents a comparison of the traditional language intervention model with a functional integrated approach.

The functional approach recognizes a need to orient language training toward the inclusion of family members and teachers as language facilitators and toward the use of everyday activities for encouraging functional communication. Therefore, routines within the home, school, and community are used with an array of language facilitators. In this way, aspects of language can be trained as they relate to one another within the context of a meaningful experience. As a result, the intervention experience more closely approximates patterns of nonimpaired language development. Content is based on common experiences.

This functional approach, with its integrative and interactive aspects, changes the nature of the clinical interaction and the role of the SLP. The SLP becomes a consultant for the other language

TABLE 9.1 Comparison of traditional and functional intervention models

Traditional Model	Functional Model
Individual or small group setting using artificial situations.	Individual or small or large group setting within contextually appropriate setting.
Isolated linguistic constructs with little attention to the interrelationship of linguistic skills.	Relationship of aspects of communication stressed through spontaneous conversational paradigm.
Intervention stresses modeling imitation, practice, and drill.	Conversational techniques stress message transmission and communication.
Little attention to the use of language as a social tool during intervention sessions.	The use of language to communicate is optimized during intervention sessions.
Little chance or opportunity to develop linguistic constructs not targeted for intervention.	Increased opportunity to develop a wide range of language structures and communication skills through spontaneous conversation and social interaction.
Little opportunity to interact verbally with others during intervention.	Increased opportunity to develop communication skills by interacting with a wide variety of partners.

Source: Adapted from Gullo & Gullo (1984).

facilitators, who interact more frequently with the child, training them to modify the contexts within which language can occur and to elicit and modify the child's language. The SLP and caregivers collaborate in the child's language intervention.

Concern for generalization is foremost and governs the overall intervention approach. Planning by the SLP, along with the language facilitators, is essential. Implementation and generalization may be hampered or impeded by any number of factors, such as the targets selected, the intervention setting, the training methods used, and caseload and scheduling considerations.

Intervention should begin with a generalization plan (Stremel-Campbell & Campbell, 1985) that identifies features of the child's communication environment relevant to generalization. All too often, generalization is the last step in the intervention planning process, rather than the overall organizing aspect.

Once the appropriate generalization variables have been identified, the SLP can begin to design intervention strategies. The relevant features of the communication environment that have been identified can now be enlisted. Ideally, such intervention enables the SLP to (a) develop linguistic constructs at the child's developmental functioning level, taking into account the strategies children normally use when acquiring language, (b) integrate all linguistic areas within the communication framework, and (c) provide meaningful and age-appropriate contexts (Gullo & Gullo, 1984).

In this chapter we discuss principles of intervention in a functional approach and an overall model for intervention, focusing on the variables that affect generalization.

Principles

Use of a functional approach to language intervention requires the SLP to change some methods and to be mindful of certain principles that aid communication with and learning for the child. It is important to engage the child in a meaningful dialogue or in some other communication event, and this event becomes the vehicle for learning and generalization.

The following section includes some of the most important principles of the functional approach. Undoubtedly, some important ones have been omitted that the reader will want to include in her or his repertoire.

The Language Facilitator as Reinforcer

As communicators, we continue to interact with individuals who provide positive feedback and reinforcement. Each of us avoids communicating with certain individuals who are nonresponsive, caustic, or overly critical. Children avoid certain potential conversational partners for many of the same reasons. If SLPs want children to communicate with them, then they must be people with whom children want to communicate.

Children respond most readily to adults who convey genuine caring and respect for them. These attitudes are conveyed by meeting the child halfway. Adults who desire to be effective conversational partners must appreciate the world from a child's perspective. Events easily understood by an adult may be quite incomprehensible to a young child. It may help to recall that for children the world is full of wonder and delight, full of things that cannot be explained, and full of magic.

Adults demonstrate concern for children and adolescents when they are willing to attend to children, to listen, and to accept their topics. As much as possible, intervention should be nonintrusive, with facilitators providing supportive, evaluative feedback to the child. By reducing the authority-figure persona, demonstrating an attentiveness and a willingness to adopt the child's topics, and remaining accepting while providing evaluative feedback, the SLP can send a message of acceptance of the child as a partner.

Few child linguistic responses are totally wrong. Even seemingly incorrect utterances demonstrate the child's understanding of the situation and of the underlying relationships. Acceptance of the child includes acceptance of these utterances. Usually, some portion of the utterance can be reinforced.

Child: I need ear-gloves.

SLP: That's right, they are like little gloves for your ears. We call them ear*muffs*. Here, let me help you put on your earmuffs.

The partner has accepted the child's utterance, recognized the child's understanding of the situation, corrected the utterance, and left the child's ego intact.

The intervention setting itself should "create and sustain an atmosphere containing fun, surprise, interest, ease, invitation, laughter, and spontaneity" (Cochrane, 1983, p. 160). In such an atmosphere, children will be eager to participate. One of my best lessons on verbal sequencing used mime, complete with whiteface. The children enacted familiar everyday event sequences, such as making breakfast, while other students tried to guess the name of the sequence. After the correct guess was given, the actor stated each event in the sequence while performing it. Finally, each actor attempted to reconstruct the sequence verbally. The lesson was messy, fun, enjoyable, and thoroughly successful.

Children also respond favorably if the facilitator occasionally plays the clown or buffoon. I may wear a cooking pot on my head in order to evoke a response. On other occasions, I purposely may make incorrect verbalizations or actions. I've even dressed as a chicken. These behaviors add to the magic of the communication situation and encourage children to communicate in an accepting atmosphere.

Close Approximation of Natural Learning

Language intervention strategies should approximate closely the natural process of language acquisition. The strategy should be communicative in nature and should use language as it naturally occurs (Mahoney & Weller, 1980). Teaching language devoid of its communicative function deprives the child of intrinsic motivation and of one essential element of generalization.

Natural language models—parents, teachers, aides, and others—should be the principal resources for implementation of language intervention (Broen & Westman, 1990; Crais, 1991, 1992; Hazel, 1990; Whitehurst et al., 1991). These individuals serve as language models with or without the SLP's input. Their potential as language facilitators can be exploited best, however, when they are guided in content selection and trained in facilitative techniques. When using these language facilitators within the child's everyday situations, the role of the SLP changes to that of collaborator.

Following Developmental Guidelines

The language development of typical children can guide the selection of training targets. As a group, these children develop language in a similar, albeit individualistic, manner. Generally, language form is preceded by function, with easier, less complex structures being learned first. Children use the language they possess to accomplish their language goals. These uses are the framework within which new forms develop. The overall result is a hierarchy that suggests steps for training language.

Of course, no SLP would ever adopt a language intervention hierarchy without adaptations for the child and the contexts in which he or she functions. Slavish adherence to a developmental hierarchy is inappropriate for two reasons. First, the typically developing child's hypothesis testing of language rules occasionally results in nonproductive strategies. For example, young children learn a few irregular past tense verbs early in their language development. On learning the regular past tense *-ed* rule, these children apply it to the previously learned irregular verbs. This tactic results in such delightful forms as *eated* and *sitted*. No SLP would wish to adopt these forms as training targets, even though they appear in the language of children developing typically.

Second, good teaching may suggest alternative hierarchical teaching patterns (Elbert & McReynolds, 1985; Powell, 1991). For example, children developing typically acquire the verb *to be* as both an auxiliary verb and as a main verb or copula. In intervention, therefore, these forms might be targeted separately. Our knowledge of carryover suggests, however, that we train them together, making little distinction between the forms and aiding generalization.

Developmental hierarchies can act as guides for intervention. These hierarchies suggest several subprinciples:

1. Language evolves from nonverbal communication means.
2. Social and cognitive prerequisites are necessary for the child to use language in certain ways.
3. Simple rules are acquired before more difficult ones.
4. Development is not uniform across all aspects of language.
5. At different levels of development, children act differently.

Each subprinciple has several implications for intervention.

Because language has evolved as a sophisticated communication means from a nonverbal communication system, intervention with children who are low functioning should begin with other systems, such as gestures, and progress toward symbol use. In addition, the SLP needs to be mindful of the many ways in which a message may be sent by any communicator and to note development within the nonlinguistic and paralinguistic realms, as well as within the linguistic.

Although social and communicative prerequisites are important prior to the appearance of first words, these prerequisites cannot be overlooked with later development. The SLP should be aware of the prerequisites for successful communicative behaviors at the functioning level of the child. The child learning plurals need not be able to count but must have a notion of one and more than one. Likewise, successful use of *why* questions and answers requires an ability to reconstruct events in reverse. These cognitive skills may need to be taught prior to attempting the linguistic manner for noting this knowledge.

Similarly, the child needs to understand the requirements and demands of different communication situations to communicate effectively within them. For example, the requirements of classroom give-and-take are very different from having a face-to-face conversation or from talking on the telephone.

As with much learning, simple rules are combined and modified or enlarged to form higher-order rules. By carefully analyzing each new training target and monitoring progress, the SLP can ensure that the child possesses the appropriate rules for new learning. It is best not to change too many aspects of the training situation at one time. For example, words used frequently by the child should be selected to train longer utterances. New words and new forms together are too challenging.

Children with LI will not present textbook examples of language development hierarchies. Language development and impairment can be very individualistic and may not follow the dictates of a developmental hierarchy. Aspects of language will develop at rates influenced by perception and cognition, opportunity, needs, and training. Of more importance for intervention is the designation of training targets that help the child function more effectively within the everyday environment.

Finally, the language rules observed by most children at each level of development are valid for those children at that time. For example, young children say such things as "Mommy eat" and "More juice," which demonstrate adherence to simple word sequencing rules based on semantics. "Mommy eat" is not a defective form of some longer adult sentence. Children demonstrate rules appropriate to their level of linguistic competence. Requiring adult rule use negates the uniqueness of children and dismisses the importance of child rules as a step in the acquisition process.

At various levels of intervention, it is appropriate to target child rules rather than the more difficult adult ones that will be trained later. The child with LI who is forming negatives, such as *no + noun + verb,* should make a logical progression to *noun + no + verb,* rather than to the adult rule with full auxiliary verb. To require children with LI to use adult sentence forms seems ridiculous, especially when we do not require such behavior from children developing typically. As adults, we sometimes think that the adult way of doing things is the only way.

Even the expectation that a child will use a new or adultlike language rule or feature following brief periods of intervention may be unrealistic (Fey, 1988). Children developing typically learn and extend or retract their language rules gradually after many encounters and trials. Over time, these rules come to resemble those of adults. Therefore, it is inappropriate to expect near perfect performance from children with LI shortly after a target is introduced. Rule learning is complicated and time-consuming. In addition, children with LI may form rules very different from those intended by SLPs, therefore necessitating additional training.

As the child progresses, the language training should be modified accordingly. In other words, the SLP *ups the ante* (MacDonald, 1985) or requires performance just above the child's current functioning level.

Following the Child's Lead

Often, the expectation that a child will not communicate effectively becomes self-fulfilling. If facilitators expect the child to communicate and plan for it, the child will.

It is important that the facilitator attend to the content and intent of each child utterance and respond appropriately. Thus, "teaching occurs when the child is attending and because the language being taught to the child is a positive consequence" (Warren & Rogers-Warren, 1985, p. 7).

Language facilitators can choose either to direct and maintain the child's attention or attend to what interests the child (Kovarsky & Duchan, 1997). Although the former is a trainer-oriented approach (or adult-centered) that gives the trainer virtual control of the entire interaction, it may not be the most effective approach. For example, children with MR are less likely to follow such trainer attempts to redirect attention (Landry & Chapieski, 1990). In contrast, these children learn object-vocabulary relationships more easily at least when the trainer follows their attentional lead (P. Yoder, Kaiser, & Alpert, 1991; P. Yoder, Kaiser, Alpert, & Fischer, 1993).

A more child-centered approach guarantees joint or shared reference, enhances semantic contingency, and reduces noncompliance by the child (McDade & Varnedoe, 1987). With semantic contingency, the adult comments on the child's topic or previous utterance, thus facilitating processing by the child. Children appear to attend most to and be best able to comprehend speech during joint-attention activities (Tomasello & Farrar, 1986).

Responses to child actions or utterances provide contextual support (Duchan, 1997). Such support aids the processing of children with MR who have memory storage and retrieval problems that complicate encoding and decoding (Mervis, 1990).

The child's verbal behavior should be interpreted by others in terms of its intention, rather than viewed as inappropriate or incorrect. In other words, a request is still a request even though the form may be wrong, the item desired misnamed, and so on.

When the adult has an agenda different from that of the child, the interaction is diminished. Such interactions are at cross-purposes and are faulty (Duchan, 1997).

Children signal those things in which they are most interested by their actions or through verbalizations. This gauge can be used to keep child interest and motivation high in the intervention setting. Often, I will say to a child, "What toy do you want to play with?" Although the topic is open-ended, the technique is very specific—as we see later—permitting a flexible choice of topic.

When the child initiates an interaction and is responded to accordingly, the value for learning is greater than when the child's initiation is ignored or penalized (Duchan, 1984). Ignoring or penalizing the child will result in a decrease in future initiations.

While observing a lesson in a training apartment in preparation for a young man's move to his own apartment, I overheard the following exchange:

SLP: What are you doing?

Client: (Matter-of-factly) Dusting furniture.

SLP: Good. What else are you doing?

Client: You live in apartment?

SLP: You didn't answer my question. What…

The client obviously was interested in living arrangements and would have joined such a conversation willingly if the SLP had followed his lead. The SLP should follow the client's content and manipulate the conversation to encourage the desired language features. Continued use of directive responses by this SLP will diminish the client's initiating behavior.

Active Involvement of the Child

Language acquisition occurs with the active participation of the learner. Language learning is not a passive process. In like fashion, more rapid learning occurs when the child with LI is participating actively in some event. In general, the more actively involved the child, the greater and more stable the generalization. Ideally, intervention should consist of motivating participatory activities with the potential for a variety of language use contexts (Duchan, 1997).

Heavy Influence of Context on Language

Context can be a big determiner of what is said and how it is said. Language is a socially based cultural form whose use reflects an individual's linguistic, interpersonal, and cultural competence within a given contextual situation (Rice, 1986). The individual's knowledge of the event or situation influences the way he or she uses language in that situation.

Language intervention should occur within the contexts of everyday events and within the context of conversational give-and-take or of other communication events. The language facilitator needs to create a rich context in which the child with LI can experience a variety of linguistic and nonlinguistic stimuli and be supported in his or her linguistic attempts. The integration of talking and listening within conversations should be emphasized.

The content for these dialogues is the common experience of the intervention setting. Ideally, this setting reflects or is a part of the child's everyday environment. The child and the facilitator talk about the focus of the activities used in training. The skillful facilitator can manipulate both the linguistic and nonlinguistic context to attain desired targets from the child.

Familiar Events Providing Scripts

A *script* is an internalized set of expectations about routine or repeated events organized in a temporal-causal sequence. As such, scripts contain shared event knowledge based on common experiences that aid and enhance memory and comprehension (Constable, 1986; Furman & Walden, 1989; Lucariello, Kyratzis, & Engel, 1986; K. Nelson, 1986). Scripts provide structure that describes appropriate sequences of events in particular contexts.

Routinized events for which children have scripts provide specific situations in which children can learn appropriate language (Kim & Lombardino, 1991). Familiar activities of high interest, such as making popcorn, pudding, or cake, can be used as the contexts for language intervention. The event sequences contained in scripts can be used to teach language expression and comprehension and recall (Duchan, 1986b; 1997; Kim & Lombardino, 1991; Ross & Berg, 1990).

Scripts have been used to improve both functional communication and group play among preschoolers (Neeley, Tipton, & Neeley, 1994). In addition, verbal routines and expansions have been linked to changes in MLU and generalization of language performance across different partners, contexts, and interactive styles (P. Yoder, Spruytenburg, Edwards, & Davies, 1995).

Naturally, scripts will differ with a child's maturational level and, to some extent, with the individual, although even very young preschoolers remember events in an organized manner similar to adults in general structure and content. As children mature, their scripts become longer, more detailed, and contain more options ("Sometimes…"), alternatives ("You either…or…), and conditions ("If…, then you…") (Fivush & Slackman, 1986; K. Nelson, 1986; Slackman, Hudson, & Fivush, 1986).

Individual differences may be the result of different experiences. In general, specific event experience is more important than age alone (Chi & Ceci, 1987; Ross, 1989; Ross & Berg, 1989). The resultant personal scripts are more important for memory than a vague generic notion (Ross & Berg, 1990). Individual experience becomes especially important when we consider intervention with CLD children.

Designing a Generalization Plan First

Considerations of generalization are essential to treatment program design and should be identified prior to beginning training. Table 9.2 is a suggested generalization plan format. In designing such a plan, the SLP considers the individual needs of the child and environment and the relevant variables that will affect generalization.

TABLE 9.2 Possible generalization plan format

Training targets:

Identify settings, situations, and persons across which training can occur.

Settings:

Persons	Situation:	Situation:	Situation:	Situation:	Situation:	Situation:	Situation:	Situation:
P								
e								
r								
s								
o								
n								
s								

Cues:

Consequences:

Generalization Variables

To ensure generalization to the everyday environment of the child, the SLP must manipulate the generalization variables most likely to result in that outcome. The variables that affect generalization can be grouped as content and context variables (Table 1.2). Content variables include the training targets and training items. Context variables include the method of training, language facilitators, cues, contingencies, and location of training. Each of these variables and considerations for intervention as they relate to a functional model is discussed in this section, expanding on the brief presentation in Chapter 1.

Training Targets

As mentioned previously, teaching the complex process of language use as discrete bits of language actually can retard growth. Language intervention should be relevant to the particular needs of the child within the communication environment and target the language process, rather than language products or units. Therefore, intervention must answer two questions (Warren, 1985):

1. What will be the function of the forms and content we are teaching?
2. Are the forms and content being trained in the context of communication events in which the intended function can actually be accomplished?

In general, more frequently used targets are more relevant to the child's world and, therefore, are more likely to generalize. Communicative utterances observed to occur in the home, albeit incorrectly, can be introduced in therapy as natural outcomes of the context. Once introduced, they can be modified by the facilitator.

Language "is often acquired more rapidly and used more effectively if the skill called 'communicative interaction' is established first" (Rieke & Lewis, 1984, p. 44). Language targets need to be those that increase the effectiveness of the child as a communicative partner. The first goal of intervention should be successful communication by the child at the present level of functioning.

As mentioned, developmental guidelines can aid target selection but should be followed cautiously. Remember that a development "description" of normal acquisition is not a "prescription" for the way language must be taught (deVilliers & deVilliers, 1978).

In forty-three published language-intervention studies, those that used goals approximating a developmental sequence were more successful that those that did not (Bryen & Joyce, 1985). In general, most earlier emerging forms can be learned in fewer trials and prior to later emerging forms. In addition, earlier emerging forms seem to generalize more readily into the child's use system and at a higher level of use (Dyer, Santarcangelo, & Luce, 1987).

A functional model would suggest teaching forms useful in the natural setting while attending to the developmental order of these forms (Dyer et al., 1987). Although the development of typical children can serve as a general guideline, the overriding criterion for target selection should be to aid the child in communicating what is necessary in the contexts in which she or he most frequently communicates. This practical approach is especially important for children who experience pragmatic difficulties, such as with TBI or psychiatric disorders (Audet & Hummel, 1990; Ben-Yishay, 1985; Russell, 1993).

The best way to determine need is through environmental observation. If, for example, the child frequently requests items in the environment but is generally ineffective, then requesting might be chosen as a target. When there is very little opportunity for a possible training target to occur, it might be best to identify other content for training.

Infrequent opportunity for possible training targets to occur may be the result of low environmental expectations or requirements for the child to produce these forms or functions. For example, there may be few opportunities for children to ask questions when there is little expectation that they will do so. In such cases, low expectations can become self-fulfilling. The communication environment may need to be restructured to facilitate use of newly acquired communication skills.

The SLP should identify both targets and everyday situations in which each target is likely to occur and in which its use will be affected by and, in turn, affect the context. For example, questions should be trained in situations in which they make sense and in which they perform their intended function of gaining information. SLP instructions such as "I'm coloring a picture. Ask me what I'm doing" violate the function of questions. Usually, we do not ask questions for which we already have the answer. Similarly, the SLP's attempt to elicit an answer with the instruction "What am I doing?" also violates the function of questions and answers. Although we might wonder about the mental capacity of SLPs who do not know what they are doing, we can modify both the situation and the cue to elicit an answer more appropriately. For example, the SLP might sit behind a screen, give clues, and ask the child, "Can you guess what I'm doing?"

Training Items

The SLP should plan to train enough examples of the feature being targeted to enable the child to generalize to untrained members (Stremel-Campbell & Campbell, 1985). For example, it is neither desirable nor possible to train all noun-verb combinations. The goal should be to train enough examples from the noun class in combination with examples of the verb class so that the child will generalize the rule *noun + verb* to all members of these two classes. Obviously, this process is being simplified in this discussion, and more planning and thought are required.

In addition, a sufficient number of items must be trained so that the child can determine both the relevant and irrelevant aspects of the communication context. For example, words or phrases such as *yesterday, last week,* and *in the past* are relevant to use of the past tense. The child forms a hypothesis that states, "In the presence of *yesterday, last week,* or *in the past,* use the past tense." Other aspects may be irrelevant, such as the specific nouns, pronouns, or verbs used. For example, the pronoun I is irrelevant and can be used with any tense. If the child is trained to use the form *Yesterday, I...*, *Last week, I...*, and *In the past, I...*, the resultant incorrect hypothesis might be "In the presence of I, use the past tense." Knowledge of both the relevant and irrelevant aspects of the context are essential for learning.

Not all word classes require the use of all training targets. For example, nouns do not require the past tense marker *-ed*, and *tomorrow* does not require a past tense verb. The child needs to learn those response classes in which the target is required and those in which it is not.

Initially, training response classes should be similar so as to limit irrelevant dimensions. For example, the child first may learn to use regular past tense with *yesterday*. Such words as *today* do not signal the tense as clearly and should be introduced later. Gradually, more irrelevant dimensions, such as longer sentences, are introduced.

When a particular syntactic form or function is being targeted, it is especially important to select content words or utterances already in the child's repertoire. With the targeting and introduction of new topic words, the SLP selects familiar structural frames. This principle is called "new forms–old content/old forms–new content" (J. MacDonald, 1985).

Processing constraints found in all human beings reflect the limited capacity of the brain to process information. When these boundaries are reached, performance sacrifices or tradeoffs must occur in one area because of demands in another. For example, children omit more grammatical markers in longer, more complex sentences than in shorter, less complex ones (Nakayama, 1987). Children with LI are particularly susceptible to these constraints because the automatization of linguistic processing takes longer. Training items that exceed the information-processing constraints of these children may result in inadequate learning and poor generalization (J. Johnston, 1988a).

Often a language feature fails to generalize because the child has not learned the conditions that govern its use. For example, if the child learns by imitation, he or she internalizes the variables that affect imitation, not the variables found in conversation. In order for a behavior to generalize to another context, such as conversation, the behavior must be related to the variables found in that context.

Because the young the child lacks metalinguistic awareness, rule explanation is not a viable clinical tool. The SLP must structure the environment so that linguistic regularities are obvious.

Contrast training is one method of overcoming generalization problems (Connell, 1982). In contrast training, the child learns those structures and situations that obligate use from those that do not. For example, use of the third-person -*s* marker is required with singular nouns and third-person singular pronouns. The child must recognize also that plural nouns and other pronouns do not require this marker. "By contrasting sentences which obligate a target form with minimally different sentences which do not...the learner can recognize which parts of sentences occur regardless of the presence or absence of the target form" (Connell, 1982, p. 235).

Conversational use requires recognition of the linguistic contexts within which the training target does or does not appear. The identification of other contexts, such as events, facilitators, and settings, also should be accomplished. Using several different contexts ensures that the child does not identify the SLP and the therapy setting as the only contexts in which to use the language being trained.

Ideally, functional training uses multiple examples (Stremel-Campbell & Campbell, 1985), such as the several categories of linguistic response classes or training items, several facilitators, and several settings. This feature is essential for generalization.

Method of Training

In the past, language was taught much as one would teach any other complex behavior, and intervention centered on individual discrete behaviors. The goal was to increase the frequency of targeted language features. Language, however, is a set of rules that allow a person to use these language features in communication contexts to express intentions.

A rule is an abstraction that describes similarities. Language is rule governed. Thus, the goal of intervention should be to learn the abstract rules, rather than the behaviors that reflect these rules. Many methods of teaching language do not reflect this goal (Connell, 1987b). There is a discrepancy between the goals and the methods of teaching.

It is not practical with most children and most intervention targets simply to explain the language rule being trained. Instead, training needs to be limited to observations of the rule being applied within situations that contrast the critical conditions that apply to the rule (Connell, 1987b). For example, can you imagine trying to teach regular past tense to a child as follows:

When a verb is used in the past, an -*ed* is added to it to produce a past tense verb, as in *walk/ walked.*

Instead, we might teach regular past tense in the following manner:

Every day I *walk,* yesterday I *walke **d.***

Every day we *talk,* yesterday we *talke **d.***

The word *yesterday* tells us to add the /t/ sound. Now you try it. I'll start.

Every day I walk, yesterday I _____.

Every day they rake, yesterday they _____.

The SLP's role is to provide organized language data to the child as an illustration of rule use. Thus, the child would be presented with paired minimally different situations that do and do not invoke the rule (Connell, 1987b). For example, these situations could be sentences in which the use of a form, such as pronouns, is alternately appropriate and inappropriate. Pronoun use might be contrasted with noun use.

SLP: We're going to play imagination. I'll tell you about something in my mind and you try to find the picture. I'm thinking about a *ghost.* **He** has a big nose. Wow, you found that really fast. Okay, you think of something else.

Child: It has blue eyes.

SLP: I don't know what you're talking about. What's the name of it?

Child: A doll.

SLP: Um-hm. What about the doll?

Child: It has blue eyes.

SLP: I found the doll with blue eyes. It's easy when I know what you're talking about. Try another. I'm thinking…

Child: Thinking of a dinosaur and he's got sharp teeth.

SLP: Oh, I know which dinosaur has the sharp teeth.

By presenting these contrasting situations and encouraging the child to practice, the SLP helps the child amass the data necessary to identify the critical elements of the rule. Once the child is aware of the critical elements, the SLP has the flexibility to present these elements in any communication situation.

The strength of the rule-teaching approach is in the way it simplifies the learning task by condensing relevant input and highlighting critical conditions (Connell, 1987b). Unfortunately, not every form has a direct link to some function. The passive voice, for example, does not have a clear function and may be used to answer, comment, reply, declare, and so on. Forms that do not have a clear direct function are more difficult to teach. Rules based on abstract grammatical categories are also difficult.

Functional techniques are effective because they incorporate behavioral principles and also use the context of naturally occurring conversations that can be modified systematically by the language facilitator. For example, the following exchange might occur with a child for whom we have targeted future tense.

SLP: That sounds like fun. What about tomorrow?

Child: Zoo?

SLP: What about the zoo?

Child: Go zoo.

SLP: Now?

Child: Go zoo tomorrow?

SLP: You **will?** John **will** too, right. Tomorrow you both…

Child: Will go zoo.

SLP: I love the zoo. I wonder what **will** happen there.

Generalization is more likely than with more structured approaches because the cues used resemble the varied ones found in communication events. In addition, the child's attention is focused on objects and events in the environment while the child is receiving linguistic input about those objects and events (Warren & Kaiser, 1986a).

A functional model provides a dynamic context for teaching language. Language training that works for the child in communication events should generalize to those events. The focus should not be merely the correctness of the child's language, but its communicative potential (Bauer & Sapona, 1988).

In general, functional intervention in combination with more structured remediation facilitates both acquisition and generalization of language targets to usage within natural environment situations. The functional approach involves (a) selecting appropriate language targets for the child and environment, (b) arranging the environment to increase the likelihood that the child will initiate, (c) responding to the child's initiations with requests for elaboration of the target forms, and (d) reinforcing the child's attempts with attention and access to objects in which the child has expressed interest (Warren & Kaiser, 1986b). Interactions between adults and children arise naturally in unstructured situations, such as play, and can be used systematically by the adult to give the child practice in communication.

The child signals a topic by demonstrating interest or requesting assistance. Thus, the child provides the topic and the opportunity for the facilitator to teach the language form (Duchan, 1986b). The child is more likely to talk and be more interested in the content of this talk if the topic has been established by the child.

Within these communication contexts, the SLP models the responses that fulfill the child's communication goals. Because the purpose of language already is established in the natural environment, form and content may be learned more easily. In short, the child is taught a more effective way to communicate within a particular context (Audet & Hummel, 1990). The SLP also models behaviors for the caregivers in order to facilitate training and increase the likelihood that situations will occur in which the child is successful.

When the desired interactions do not occur, the SLP can manipulate the environment to enhance its language-training potential (J. Norris & Hoffman, 1990a). Both linguistic and nonlinguist aspects of the context can be altered to elicit the desired communication.

Activities can be planned around communication contexts that are highly likely to occur for the child. Training outside the normal environment should be as close to that environment in materials, situations, and persons as possible. Activities should include the child's usual reasons for talking and typical topics, rely on previous experiences and introduce new ones, use familiar focuses of communication, and include the child's normal communication partners (Spinelli & Terrell, 1984).

Each child's individual learning or cognitive style also must be considered by the SLP. Children are most comfortable with new experiences and information presented in a manner consistent with that style. In part, learning styles are culturally based, a consequence of accumulated experience (Saville-Troike, 1986; B. Terrell & Hale, 1992). For example, extended families, such as those in many Asian and Hispanic cultures, may foster a less independent style of learning than more nuclear families. Studies also have demonstrated that African American children benefit from incorporation of physical activity and movement into the learning situation (Hale-Benson, 1986, 1990a, 1990b).

The SLP must recognize that events within the child's everyday environments will differ in the amount of structure provided by the event itself (Duchan, 1986a). Some contexts are highly planned and scripted or routinized, such as bathing or eating, whereas others are relatively free and open, such as playing. The communication demands and the expectations on the child vary accordingly. Language intervention must recognize what the child brings to each context and what is demanded in return. New information should be organized to meet the functioning level of the child (J. Norris & Hoffman, 1990a).

Routines may provide the best vehicle for training the child who is noninteractive. The child can ease into participating through repeated exposure to a routine in which the facilitator models actions and communication. Because the event is prescribed and expectations are known, there is some security for the child. Likewise, discussions of familiar events, such as a birthday party, provide a script for communicating.

Routine event knowledge shared with a communication-facilitating adult provides the scaffolding for communication. Routines provide structure and expectations, freeing cognitive-processing abilities for linguistic processing (Lucariello, 1990). Overall, varied linguistic features are more likely to occur in familiar, meaningful contexts (Lucariello et al., 1986). Language treatment based on play and daily life experiences is similar to normal language-learning processes.

By considering why and how children use words and gestures, the SLP increases his or her ability to provide the most natural and optimal situations for eliciting and teaching communication. The combination of appropriate context and specifically targeted language features facilitates maximum carryover and generalization outside the clinical environment (Kunze, Lockhart, Didow, & Caterson, 1983).

Data from a number of studies indicate that functional intervention (a) teaches target skills effectively, (b) aids generalization to nontraining settings, times, and persons, and (c) improves both the formal and functional aspects of language (Warren & Kaiser, 1986b). The technique works well with a variety of age groups and populations with LI and with a variety of specific language responses. Language training generalizes to classroom and home settings and to teachers and parents. In addition, the general effects of the technique are beneficial to the overall language learning and functioning of the child (Rogers-Warren & Warren, 1985).

Language Facilitators

If the goal is language use within the child's everyday context, then the lone SLP working only in a clinical setting is limited as to what he or she can accomplish. The brevity of child-SLP contact necessitates the use of a wider variety of social contexts, including various communication partners. These partners supply a strong social base for intervention, providing a reason for language use (Paul, Looney, & Dahm, 1991). The SLP need not question *whether* these partners should be involved, but rather *how* they should be involved (Olswang & Bain, 1991).

The appropriate partners to be used in training will vary with the age and circumstance of the child. Whereas parents may be appropriate for preschool children, they may have more limited interaction with their school-age children for whom teachers and peers may be more effectual. Classroom approaches are discussed in Chapter 12. Successful use of the language taught in intervention programs depends, in part, on the expectations of these significant others in the child's environment.

Parents have been successful language facilitators with children having a variety of LI types (Broen & Westman, 1990; Fey, Cleave, Long, & Hughes, 1993; Whitehurst et al., 1991). Most success has been reported for children in early stages of language and cognitive development (Girolometto, 1988; Tannock, Girolometto, & Siegel, 1990; Weistuch & Brown, 1987; Whitehurst et al., 1991; P. Yoder et al., 1991).

It is often difficult for toddlers with LI and their parents to establish mutually rewarding interactional patterns. Such children are less likely to succeed in a preschool setting. Their experience level and their success in communicative interaction are often minimal, and they may exhibit poor listening skills. Children who are not successful in communication often become resistant or negative and develop attention-getting behaviors.

The child must have the opportunity to communicate; thus, the facilitator must be attentive and responsive. The facilitator must consistently recognize the child's attempts to communicate and provide appropriate responses (Wilcox, Kouri, & Caswell, 1990). Parents need to be taught more than just modeling, and their progress as trainers must be monitored (Fey, Cleave & Long, 1997).

Communication partners, such as teachers and parents, can be an effective part of an intervention team if they are trained and monitored thoroughly (Jimenez & Iseyama, 1987). The facilitator must be trained in both (a) the *how,* or the best teaching techniques, and (b) the *what,* or the goals and materials for intervention. Training of facilitators can be accomplished in a combination of ways, including direct training and modeling, in-service training, and the use of telephoned and written/illustrated instructions.

Children with severe language impairment accompanying such disorders as ASD and MR usually have serious problems with conversational interactions, primarily due to the complex nature of such interactions. In general, these individuals have difficulty organizing, coordinating, and monitoring all of the various elements that comprise these interactions, such as topic initiation and maintenance, presupposition, turn taking, conversational repair, and the like (Mirenda & Donnellan, 1986).

Caregiver Conversational Style

According to the interactional model, the difficulties experienced by these children reflect their everyday contexts more than their so-called disorder. If this is so, then conversational partners must assume some of the responsibility for the communication of these children. For example, the quality and quantity of spontaneous conversational behavior of children with LI are inversely related to the number of verbal initiations and directives by their adult conversational partners.

Partially in response to these children's language deficits, adults modify their own language. Mothers of children with LI repeat more than do mothers of children developing typically. Most of these maternal repetitions are imperatives (demands) or directives (commands), which also correlate negatively. The frequency of parental self-imitations is negatively correlated with the rate of language growth. In a highly directive interaction style there is no necessary connection between the directive and any utterance of the child.

Adult verbal control of interactions also seems to affect adversely the verbal output of children with LI. For example, although the question-answer style of adult communication may aid children functioning around age 2 to maintain a conversational topic, it can discourage children from commenting outside the topics initiated by the adults (Mirenda & Donnellan, 1986). As children with disabilities and those without move beyond this developmental level, the use of a question-answer strategy is counterproductive to the goal of spontaneous conversational behavior.

An adult directive style includes verbal conversational behaviors that (a) control and initiate conversational topics, (b) lead the conversation, and (c) structure the nature of the child's contribution (Mirenda & Donnellan, 1986). These behaviors ensure a cohesive and fluent conversation at the expense of the child's spontaneous initiations.

In contrast, the use of an adult facilitative style of conversation can increase the use of topic initiations, questions, and topic comments by children with LI (Mirenda & Donnellan, 1986). An adult facilitative style (a) allows the child to control and initiate conversational topics, (b) follows the child's conversational lead, and (c) encourages the child to participate in various ways.

The facilitative adult is less interested in conversational flow than in providing an opportunity for the child to participate and to assume control of the conversation. Specific behaviors that define each style are given in Table 9.3.

Several conversationally based parent-training programs have demonstrated an increase in parent responsiveness and a decrease in directiveness toward their preschool children with LI (Broen & Westman, 1990; Mahoney & Powell, 1986; Weistuch & Lewis, 1986). Other changes include increased willingness to follow their child's lead, more equality in turn balancing, shorter parental MLU, and fewer questions.

Mothers who receive facilitative training are more responsive to and less directive of the children's behavior than are untrained mothers (Girolometto, 1988). These changes in parental behavior are related causally to such child language changes as increased MLU, increased number of utterances, increased lexicon, and improved standardized test scores. Children whose parents receive training initiate more topics, are more responsive, use more verbal turns, and have a more diverse

TABLE 9.3   Characteristics of the directive and facilitative styles

Directive	Facilitative
Initiate at least half of the topics of conversation.	Initiate fewer than half of the topics of conversation.
Use direct questions to initiate most topics.	Use indirect questions or embedded imperatives to initiate most topics.
Use primarily direct questions and occasional imitations or expansions to maintain topics.	Use primarily direct statements, encouragements, imitations, expansions, or expansion questions and occasional direct questions to maintain topics.
Do not ask for clarification directly, relying instead on encouragement, imitation, and expansion strategies.	Use direct clarification questions or statements when necessary and appropriate.
Do not allow lapses in turn taking to occur, but use direct questions to require the child to respond.	Allow lapses between turns to occur and after a short wait, initiate topics as noted above.

vocabulary. These results suggest that the effect of parental conversational strategies may be greater on semantics and pragmatics than on linguistic form.

An increase in the percentage of semantically related or contingent utterances can, in turn, provide greater opportunity for topic maintenance and turn taking. With more opportunity to participate, the child gains more control over both the adult's behavior and the exchange process.

Children's spontaneous verbalizations can be enhanced when adult facilitators provide a high level of verbal feedback coupled with little verbal directing (Broen & Westman, 1990). Examples are given in Table 9.4. Data from several studies suggest that children's conversational abilities can be increased by adult behaviors that are highly responsive to the children's spontaneous communicative behaviors.

Language facilitators plan their role in the communication event and their communication turns to maximize the learning opportunity for the child. Within each turn, the facilitator responds to the child while troubleshooting the child's previous utterance, maintains the conversation by taking a meaningful turn, and provides an opportunity for the child to respond (see Table 9.4) (Craig, 1983).

The use of parents, teachers, and others as language facilitators does not diminish the role of the SLP. It is essential that he or she remain very involved in the intervention and also become a facilitator. Whereas parents sometimes find it difficult to adapt their behavior to a more facilitative style, SLPs can more readily provide this input on a consistent and uniform basis (Fey et al., 1993). Best results seem to occur when other facilitators receive frequent, regular, structured training, including role-playing and critiques.

Family-Centered Intervention

There is a distinct difference between parental involvement and family-centered or family-focused services in which all family members participate (Crais, 1991). Public Law 99-457, regarding education of special needs populations, focuses on the family as integral to intervention, recognizing the characteristics of the family that transcend any single individual. In a family-centered model, families are treated as valued, equal partners and are encouraged to participate at all stages of decision making. Families are recognized as a constant in the child's life, while special services are recog-

TABLE 9.4   Examples of minimally directive verbal feedback to children

Child: I went to the zoo, yesterday.
Partner: Oh, that's one of my favorite spots. I love the monkeys best.

Child: I have a birthday party, tomorrow.
Partner: Oh, that should be fun. What do you want for your birthday?

Child: We went whale watching on vacation.
Partner: I've always wanted to do that. Bet it was exciting. Tell me about it.

Child: My picture is a cowboy.
Partner: A big cowboy on a spotted horse.

Child: I'm gonna be a ghost for Halloween.
Partner: Don't come to my house; I'm afraid of ghosts. I think I'll be a witch and scare your ghost.

In each of these five exchanges, the adult followed the child's lead by commenting on the child's topic and then cueing the child to provide more information or waiting for a reply.

nized as more transient by nature. In such an arrangement, the SLP-family relationship becomes a collaborative one. The aspects of this collaborative model are presented in Table 9.5.

Although each family is individualistic, culture is one of the most important influences on it, affecting such aspects as structure, interaction, function, and life cycle. Family *structure* includes the number of individuals and types of relationships, but more important, the cultural values and beliefs about family structure. Members of Asian American families that a majority-culture SLP might consider to be distant relatives may be very important in decision making involving the child with LI.

Family *interaction* is the way family members relate and the roles they play within the family. The relative importance of certain roles will vary with the culture. For example, a child who is an unmarried adult will be treated very differently, depending on the family background. Interactions are governed by the cohesion of the family, its adaptability or ability to change, and patterns of communication (Summers, Brotherson, & Turnbull, 1988). Japanese American forms of communication may seem extremely formal to a SLP from the majority American culture.

Family *functions* are the responsibilities that families are expected to assume for their members. Again, this aspect of families varies widely across cultures. Some cultures may value overprotection of children more than the SLP's goal of increased independence.

Finally, family *life cycle* describes the changes in families over the course of their development. Nuclear families may have periods of isolation after children have grown or in old age, whereas extended families may not experience this phenomenon.

With infants, toddlers, and preschool children, the SLP is required to design an Individualized Family Service Plan (IFSP) for the child and family. The IFSP is a plan for service, not for treatment alone, and represents a team effort that includes the family (Polmanteer & Turbiville, 2000).

TABLE 9.5   Guidelines for implementing a family-centered collaborative model

Define your role and explain your approach to intervention.

Convey respect by

1. Providing real choices for the family and encouraging them to make decisions
2. Providing requested information and services immediately
3. Ensuring confidentiality
4. Recognizing cultural/ethnic values, traditions, and beliefs
5. Explaining the purposes of procedures and methods
6. Providing a rationale for procedures and methods
7. Ensuring a role for the family in both assessment and intervention
8. Meeting at times and locations convenient for the family
9. Attending to family concerns before professional concerns

Ensure that the family attends all discussions and decision-making meetings. Use language that can be comprehended easily by the family.

Speak to family members forthrightly, completely, honestly, and in an unbiased manner.

Design intervention plans to fit the family's routine.

Be flexible in intervention planning.

Source: Adapted from Crais (1992); B. Johnson, McGonigel, & Kaufmann (1989); McWilliams & Winton (1990).

The origin of family-centered services is in functional theories such as those espoused in this text. The child is seen as an individual within complex relationships that are affected by the child and affect the child in return. The SLP has a perspective from which he or she views the child. Members of the family offer differing perspectives. These diverse points of view can offer insight into the communication of the child and help to explain her or his behavior from the perspectives of those closest to the child. If families are going to be the vehicles for change for children, the SLP must try to understand each family's perceptions, feelings, concerns, and understanding of their child with LI (Polmanteer & Turbiville, 2000). IFSP recommended practices are presented in Table 9.6.

Cultural Considerations

Cultural identity is not a stereotype. Families within the same culture differ. Recognition of cultural contributions by the SLP, however, increase the likelihood of appropriate and effective intervention. Table 9.7 presents guidelines for SLPs to follow when interacting with culturally diverse families.

SLPs should be mindful of the differing expectations and perceptions of various ethnic and racial minorities. The role of parents, the expectations for children, and the attitudes toward disability, medicine, healing, self-help, and professional intervention within a minority population should be understood thoroughly prior to intervention. Children and professional intervention services are viewed quite differently across Asian, Hispanic, and African American cultures. Likewise, the SLP's conversational style may have a great effect on future involvement with members of that community (Matsuda, 1989). Successful SLP-family collaboration should be characterized by mutual respect, trust, and open communication (Wayman et al., 1990). These characteristics only evolve when the SLP is sensitive to the cultural background of the families with whom he or she interacts.

The model of intervention proposed in this text is based on North American psycholinguistic research of white, middle-class families and, therefore, contains an implicit cultural bias (van

TABLE 9.6   Recommended practices for implementing Individualized Family Service Plans (IFSP)

Team members include family members and selected members of the family's informal network of friends, neighbors, and other service providers, plus professionals such as the SLP.
Community and culture must be considered in assessment and intervention.
Family members sign the IFSP.
Family members' assessments of the child's skills are included in reports and in the IFSP.
Family members provide information on the child's communication and communication partners.
Of interest are the language(s) used, stylistic variations, roles, modes of communication, and adult expectations and teaching style.
IFSP outcomes
Are written in the family's language and avoid professional jargon.
Reflect the family's concerns and priorities shared by the team.
Reflect beneficial changes identified by the family
Services are provided by multiple agencies listed on the service plan in settings that are typical for the child's age peers who have no language impairment.

Adapted from Polmanteer & Turbiville (2000); Scheffner Hammer (1998).

TABLE 9.7   Guidelines for interacting with culturally diverse families

Do not make assumptions based on cultural stereotypes.

Cultural rules govern each encounter for both the family/child and the speech-language pathologist. Be aware that responses to stimuli, such as a clinic room, may be very different across cultures.

Learn about the cultures of the families and the children you serve.

Use cultural mediators or interpreters when necessary.

Learn to use words, phrases, and greetings from the culture of the family/child.

Be patient; allow more time for interactions. Use as few written instructions as possible, unless a family member has good English reading comprehension. Allow time for questions.

Recognize that the family may not be prepared for the amount of professional-family collaboration found in functional approaches.

Encourage family input without embarrassing family members. Involve the family to the extent that they wish to be involved.

Ensure that goals and objectives of the professionals and the family match.

Involve the cultural community when possible.

Source: Adapted from Lynch & Hanson (1992); Wayman, Lynch, & Hanson (1990).

Kleeck, 1994). Other cultures may not value either child talking or child conversational initiation or feel especially predisposed to accommodate the needs of young children. In addition, the two-party conversational interactions proposed may not be appropriate for the childrearing practices of other cultures. Indeed, the very foundation of child and parent as equal conversational partners may be anathema to some clients' beliefs and practices.

The parent-as-caregiver model found in white, middle-class, North American homes is less characteristic of African American, Latino, Native American, and Hawaiian communities in which siblings take a greater responsibility. Samoan and Mexican American children also participate in more multiparty and fewer two-party interactions.

Family-centered training must be culturally congruent with each individual family structure and belief system (van Kleeck, 1994). The model proposed in this text will need to be adapted to best serve families with various cultural backgrounds.

Training Cues

If one accepts the premise that pragmatics is the governing aspect of language, then the SLP must be concerned with the context within which training occurs. Certain linguistic and nonlinguistic contexts require or provide an expectation of certain linguistic units.

In part, the problem of lack of success in generalization is due to response *programs* "in which children are taught specific responses to specific, often carefully worded, directions or questions" (Rieke & Lewis, 1984, p. 49). The child's everyday world lacks this careful control. The everyday context contains many irrelevant stimuli that do not and cannot elicit trained communication behaviors.

At the same time, parents and teachers may be presenting cues and prompts in such a diverse manner as to inhibit learning. They can be trained to focus their attention and to manipulate the environment to elicit the behaviors desired (Lucariello, 1990). Within an approach in which conversational partners respond to all communication attempts by the child and prompt additional presponses, an increase in the number of child utterances and vocabulary is associated with increased talking and the use of questions by the adult (Kaiser & Hester, 1994).

Relevant, common stimuli within the everyday communication context can serve, however, to elicit the child's new language targets if these stimuli are included in the training (Stremel-Campbell & Campbell, 1985). Targets can be trained across several behaviors, facilitators, and settings to ensure generalization. For example, the child's toys or everyday items and daily routines become part of the training.

The systematic introduction of increasingly more irrelevant stimuli from the communication environment into the training context has been termed "loose" training (Stremel-Campbell & Campbell, 1985). The overall goals are for the newly trained behavior to be emitted in response to a variety of stimuli and for a single stimuli to result in a variety of responses. These goals can be achieved by using concurrent behaviors, response variations, and linguistic and nonlinguistic cue variations. In concurrent behavior training, relevant and irrelevant stimuli are presented together so that the child learns which ones affect the newly learned behavior.

Response variation teaches the child that several responses can be used to achieve the same communication goal. For example, a drink can be attained by saying, "Want drink," "Drink please," "May I have a drink?" "I'm thirsty," and, "Are you as thirsty as I am?"

Verbal and nonverbal cues can be varied to ensure that the child does not become dependent on one stereotypic stimulus. Too often, the traditional approaches rely on very narrow and somewhat stilted cues unlike those found in conversation. The use of these traditional cues, such as "Tell me the whole thing," may result in training characterized as "apragmatic pseudoconversational drills" (Cochrane, 1983). Pragmatically, the cues do not make sense—for example, asking a question to which the speaker already knows the answer. As a result, the conversations within which training occurs are little more than drill with a conversational veneer.

Use of a functional conversational approach requires the SLP to assess thoroughly the effects of certain cues and to explore the possibilities of eliciting language with a variety of linguistic and nonlinguistic cues (Constable, 1983). Those SLPs who rely on traditional cues are unaware of the rich variety of cues available for creating contexts in which language targets can occur.

Contingencies

Once the language facilitator has elicited language from the child in a conversational manner or the child has initiated language, the facilitator can begin to modify that language if necessary. In short, the child's utterance is the stimulus to which the facilitator responds. These responses or contingencies help form the context for the child's utterance.

Natural maintaining consequences should be identified prior to beginning training. As much as possible, these consequences should be related directly to the response. Such consequences as "Very good" and "Good talking" should be avoided (Stremel-Campbell & Campbell, 1985). When the child message ("I saw monkeys") and the consequence ("Good talking") are unrelated, the child's language fails to retain its communicative value. Instead, communication behaviors can be maintained by conversational responses ("Oh, I think monkeys are funny. What did they do?"). Often, simply attending to the child is sufficient to maintain the child's participation.

As much as possible, conversational consequences should be semantically and pragmatically contingent and should serve to acknowledge the child's utterance. *Semantic contingency,* the relatedness of a parent's or facilitator's response to the content or topic of a child's previous utterance, has a positive effect on the rate of language development. In the above example, "I saw monkeys," the adult response is semantically contingent.

It is possible to increase acquisition and spontaneous production of language-form targets without requiring the child to produce the targeted form at all (Camarata, K. Nelson, & Camarata, 1994; Nelson, Camarata, Welsh, Butkovsky, & Camarata, 1996). Responses in the form of conversational recast-sentence responses that retain the child's meaning but recast the grammar have been demonstrated to be superior to imitation by the child. Yet, many SLPs continue to use imitation as a primary teaching technique. Recasts will be explained more fully in Chapter 10.

Adult speech that is semantically contingent decreases the amount of processing the child has to do to understand and analyze the structure and meaning of the adult's utterances. The sharing of a conversational topic and common vocabulary decreases the child's memory load for processing and increases the ease of immediate language production. The facilitator's utterance provides a prop or scaffolding for the child's own analysis and production. For children with expressive vocabulary delays, the semantic contingency of adult responses has more effect on a child's language than does the structure of the adult response (Girolometto, Weitzman, Wiigs, & Steig Pierce, 1999). In contrast, frequent topic changing or refocusing of the child's attention by the adult impedes the child's language acquisition.

It is not enough, however, just to comment on the child's topic. In the following example, the facilitator's response is semantically contingent but lacks *pragmatic contingency*.

Child: I want cookie, please.

Facilitator: Johnny wants a cookie.

The facilitator's response should make sense within the conversational framework. In this example, more appropriate responses would be, "What kind of cookie do you want?" "Okay, but just one," "Help yourself," and, "No cookies until after lunch." This example shows that such contingencies as "Good talking" violate pragmatic contingency and do not help continue the interchange. The child's language is reinforced more naturally when its purpose and intention are met.

In brief, behaviors that attempt to increase the child's participation in the interaction, that is, a child-centered interactional style, enhance the child's language skills. By relinquishing some control and adopting the child's topics, language facilitators can ensure more child participation and interest. This interactive, child-centered style can be the therapeutic model for children with LI.

Overall, in the clinical setting it is important that facilitators accept a child's utterance as representative of the child's understanding of the world and of the requirements being asked. Answers considered wrong by the adult may, in fact, represent the child's somewhat different perspective. The child's response meaning can be negotiated by the facilitator and the child as the conversation continues. This degree of acceptance translates into indirect acceptance of the child.

Location

As noted in Chapter 1, location of training includes both the physical location in which training occurs and the conversational context formed by the child and the facilitator. In many ways, the conversational context is more important for generalization because it does not depend on physical setting and transcends the clinic, classroom, and home (J. Johnston, 1988a). In the light of the flexibility of these natural communication sequences, training is more a matter of *how* than *where* (Craig, 1983).

Physical Location

When possible, training should occur wherever the child is likely to use the newly trained language skill. Most communication takes place within familiar events that influence the way the participants communicate. For example, storytelling, conversation, and classroom participation have different rules for participation that affect the language used. Therefore, language intervention should take place within these types of discourse events as they occur in the child's everyday physical locations. The everyday environment provides natural and familiar stimuli for intervention and for generalization facilitation (Caro & Snell, 1989). Children with lingering pragmatic deficits, such as those with TBI, are particularly in need of environmentally based intervention (Russell, 1993).

Obviously, parents and teachers will need to be trained for their new roles as language facilitators. Parents may come to the clinic or the school to be trained. If this is not possible, evening group sessions or written guidelines can be used. Even if the parents only modify their expectations for the child, this will help with the generalization of language training.

Conversational Context

Language must be evaluated and trained within some dynamic context in order to make sense. Language and communication are influenced heavily by the context of what precedes and follows (linguistically and nonlinguistically) and by the expectations for participation with that specific context. For example, the expectations for storytelling are different from those for conversation. Ordering at a fast-food restaurant presents different expectations from chatting with a friend on the phone. Each event follows certain scripts.

Sentences trained out of context are, therefore, more difficult for the child to learn. The SLP is not training static forms but a generative, versatile system. The contextual expectations and scripts must be examined prior to beginning intervention within each context.

Conversations provide a dynamic context in which language serves a purpose or function. Although these conversational sequences may mirror natural sequences, the SLP and other language facilitators are mindful of the teaching situation and the facilitator-child model (Craig, 1983). Communication strategies can be provided to the child as needed (Spinelli & Terrell, 1984). Teaching approaches used previously can be adapted to this setting to approximate more closely conversational exchange.

Conclusion

By carefully considering the variables that affect generalization, the SLP can modify training to maximize this effect. Targets and design decisions can be made on the basis of the likely effect on generalization and on ultimate use within the events and situations of the child's everyday environment. Language can be elicited and modified by using techniques that mirror the conversational style used by the child's usual partners within these contexts. Motivation is provided by the child's desire to participate in enjoyable activities with responsive and attentive adults.

Facilitators should adhere to the following guidelines:

1. Expect the child to communicate.
2. Respond to the child's topics and initiations.
3. Respond conversationally and build the child's utterances into longer, more acceptable ones.
4. Facilitate communication within the everyday activities of the child.
5. Cue the child in a conversational manner to elicit the language desired.

All of these principles are discussed in Chapter 10.

10

Manipulating
Context

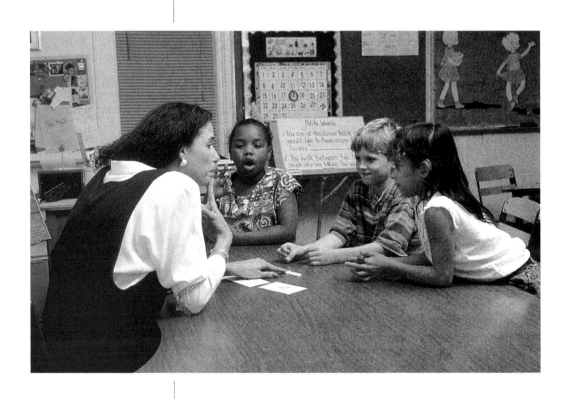

Language is pragmatically based in that the demands of the nonlinguistic and linguistic context give rise to both the form and content of the language expressed. Therefore, a primary goal of language intervention should be for the child to learn the appropriate language skills to function effectively within everyday communication contexts or environments.

Within each activity, the facilitator strives to provide an active experience with language use. It seems appropriate, then, that the SLP and other language facilitators learn to manipulate these contexts to provide the child the maximum learning possible. The facilitator's role is "to accept the child's spontaneously occurring verbal or nonverbal behavior as meaningful communication, interpret it in a manner that is contextually appropriate, and become a collaborator with the child in communicating the message more effectively" (J. Norris & Hoffman, 1990b, p. 78).

When language can be used to achieve goals within everyday communication contexts, the chances of generalization to these contexts increases. Language acquires a purpose or function. The training becomes functional in nature.

In this chapter we explore various strategies that can be used to manipulate the nonlinguistic and linguistic contexts in which language occurs. These strategies can be used within the everyday activities of the child and, thus, can become a part of that natural environment. As much as possible, natural and conversational strategies are recommended. But the reader should be forewarned that there may be even better, more interactional ways to train children than are presented here.

Nonlinguistic Contexts

Speech-language pathology is so oriented toward linguistic forms of communication that it is easy to overlook the nonlinguistic aspects. Yet, the nonlinguistic context—what happens in the environment—offers a rich source for eliciting language. The SLP can manipulate the nonlinguistic contextual cues to elicit desired language and to ensure that the child initiates language. All too often, the training paradigm of the child with LI allows the child little control. Therefore, the child assumes a passive, responsive role to the SLP's linguistic cues.

Certain nonlinguistic contexts naturally elicit more language than do others. For most adults, cocktail parties are more likely to elicit language than are theater engagements. Inherent in the theater experience is the necessity to remain silent during the performance, and we can become irate when this expectation is violated.

Some situations also dictate the type of language used. Most adults do not question and challenge sermons—at least not while the sermon is being delivered. In contrast, learning situations, such as in a classroom, are supposed to encourage questioning. Fast-food establishments are likely to elicit demands or requests.

If targets have been selected to help the child communicate better, then the SLP already has identified the contexts in which the child attempts these targets. In other words, the nonlinguistic contexts that are highly likely to elicit the target are known. Although the child is expected to perform, the SLP believes that the performance will be in error because the target was chosen from aspects of language with which the child has experienced difficulty.

Likewise, the SLP has some control of the topics the child will discuss. The facilitator's role is not to change the topic but to discover through contextual manipulation what topics the child will choose (Hart, 1985).

Ideally, the nonlinguistic context serves to elicit the target language behavior; the SLP then can help the child modify the target into a correct form for that situation. In theory, the child who makes a meaningful response in context will be interested in that response and motivated to change it in the desired manner. This corrected response should generalize more easily to everyday use because it is being trained within the context of everyday events and conversations.

Table 10.1 contains a sample of nonlinguistic contexts and the type of language each may elicit. Small group projects or tasks usually elicit lots of language from children. For younger children, role-play and dress-up are good contexts for language. Routines also can be established within the home or the classroom for asking for desired objects or privileges.

Within these nonlinguistic contexts, language may be elicited through the use of delays, introduction of novel elements, oversight, and sabotage (McLean & Snyder-McLean, 1988b). Delaying or waiting for the child to initiate communication is often a very effective strategy, especially after the child has mastered a desired behavior (Hart, 1985). Too frequently, adults do not expect the child to communicate, and this expectation becomes self-fulfilling when the adult communicates for the child.

The language facilitator waits for the child to initiate the interaction. The facilitator may sit near the child and look questioningly or display some interesting item while looking at the child (Hart, 1985). When the child looks at the adult, the adult does not speak for a specified period of time unless the child does. If the child does not verbalize, the adult models or prompts the desired verbalization. Upon successful completion, the child is given the desired item.

If the item is edible, it should be small and quickly consumed. In a camp situation, I was able to maintain communication initiations of a small child with ASD over eight days with two large sugar cookies crumbled into very small pieces. Nonedible items may be used for specific, limited tasks, such as gluing one piece of colored paper to another and then returning it to the facilitator.

Novel or unexpected events can be introduced into the situation to evoke communication. Most individuals will notice and remark on such events. For example, a kitten, guinea pig, or bright toy might be found in an unexpected spot. Even children functioning at the single-word level will comment on elements in the situation that are novel, different, or changing.

Oversight or forgetting by the facilitator will elicit language from the child eager to become the teacher. I often play dumb, forgetting object locations or children's turns. Needed objects, such as glue or scissors, can be omitted or used in unusual ways.

Finally, sabotage of activities or routines involves taking actions or introducing elements that will not permit the activity to continue or to be completed (Constable, 1983; Lucas, 1980). My favorite example is the classroom teacher and aide who would buckle the children's boots together and turn their coats inside out sometime during the day. One can imagine the chaos at the end of the day and all of the language elicited as children requested assistance.

Linguistic Contexts

The goal of language use within a conversational context necessitates a thorough evaluation of the linguistic cues used with children in the training situation. Cues such as "What do we say?" and "Now, tell me the whole thing" are examples of pseudoconversational cues mentioned previously.

Eliciting language through constant prodding or interrogation can be unpleasant and result in less talking by the child. Such communication is one-sided, with the child assuming the role of receiver or occasional reluctant speaker (McDade & Varnedoe, 1987).

Linguistic contexts can be divided into those that model language with or without a child's response, those that directly and indirectly cue certain responses, and those that do not cue these

TABLE 10.1   Nonlinguistic contexts and language elicitation

Turn taking and requesting objects:

Provide only one plastic knife for children to share as they make a fruit salad.

Provide one highly desirable outfit in the dress-up corner of the class.

Provide only enough art supplies for half of the children and request that children share equipment.

Following directions and directing others:

While working in a group, re-create the teacher's construction-paper collage. The teacher should be careful not to supply precut paper or to help children with the color tints. The goal is to get the children to ask for help and to direct others and themselves.

In groups of two, duplicate a cake decoration previously completed by the teacher.

As a group, plant seeds in cups as the teacher has done previously. A more involved project might involve planting a garden, keeping the different crops straight, and making signs.

Bake while following a written or pictured recipe.

Put together a model by following written or oral directions.

Play dumb. By making lots of mistakes, the teacher can have children direct or correct the behavior.

Have a child explain how to do something known by only that child.

Have children direct each other through activities blindfolded.

Have the child be the teacher.

Requesting information:

Give only partial directions for completing a task.

Put objects that the children need for a task in an unusual location so that they will need to ask for the location.

Introduce visually interesting items but do not name them or explain their function to the children.

Giving information:

Have children explain class projects to children from another class.

Have children explain class projects to parents at a special event or Parents' Night.

Have children tell about events they experienced: for example, summer vacation, a weekend trip, a birthday party. This task and explaining how something is accomplished are excellent vehicles for sequencing.

Have children request information from children who need to improve their ability to give information.

Have children tell make-believe stories.

Reasoning:

Have children try to float or submerge objects in water. Include objects that float and those that do not so that the children must find various combinations.

Build a suspension bridge from straws, string, toothpicks, and tongue depressors.

Design a city with transportation, schools, recreation facilities, and residential, industrial, and business areas.

Play initiative games in which groups of children must solve a common problem.

Make large projects in connection with class projects. For example, children might design the "perfect" world, make montages that demonstrate male and female roles, or design a board game, such as On the Way to Your Birthday, that illustrates stages of fetal development.

Continued

TABLE 10.1   *Continued*

Requesting help:

Pose problems that children cannot solve themselves.

Sabotage activities, such as holes in paper cups, dried markers and paints, glue bottles glued shut, not enough chairs, missing gloves and hats, and so on. The list is endless.

Imagining and projecting:

Set up a drama or dress-up center. Set up a puppet stage with a variety of characters.

Set up simulated shops and stores or a housekeeping center.

Role-play. (Role-play can elicit a variety of intentions.)

Protesting:

Play dumb, as in forgetting to give children peanut butter and jelly with which to make sandwiches.

Miss a child's turn or withhold needed objects.

Violate a routine or an object function by using objects in novel or nonsensical ways.

Give a child too much of something or more than is needed.

Put away objects before the child is finished using them.

Ask a child to do something that is not physically possible (but safe).

Initiations:

Pose problems and wait for children to initiate communication.

Ask children to talk to lonely animals for you.

Source: Author's experience; Constable (1983); Kunze, Lockhart, Didow, & Caterson (1983); Staab (1983).

responses. A particular utterance will cue one type of behavior but not others and, thus, can be used in contrast, training to teach contextual discrimination.

Modeling

In comparative studies, the efficacy of the modeling approach has been demonstrated repeatedly. *Modeling* is a procedure in which the SLP produces a rule-governed utterance at appropriate junctures in conversation or activities but does not ask the child to imitate. The technique compares favorably with more active techniques, such as question-answer, that require responses by the child (Weismer & Murray-Branch, 1989).

Modeling can be used in any of the following ways:

1. As a high-frequency response in very structured situations
2. As general language stimulation containing a number of language targets simultaneously
3. As an element in comprehension training in which the child points to pictures that illustrate the utterance modeled

In general, modeling closely approximates the language-learning environment of children developing typically and is an effective language-learning strategy for the child with LI (Lucas, 1980).

It is expected that the child will acquire some aspect of the language behavior of the facilitator and use it in a similar context later. Unlike direct instruction techniques, interactive modeling considers the child to be an active learner who abstracts the rules used in forming utterances and associates these utterances with events and stimuli in the environment.

It is best to model the training target for the child prior to attempting to elicit the target. Within such *focused stimulation,* the SLP produces a high density of the targets in meaningful contexts without requiring the child to respond (Cleave & Fey, 1997). Two varieties of this stimulation are *self-talk* and *parallel talk.* In self-talk, the SLP talks about what he or she is doing, whereas in parallel talk, discussion centers on the child's actions. Obviously, activities must be chosen carefully to provide sufficient opportunities for the target to occur.

Focused stimulation should be semantically and pragmatically appropriate (Fey et al., 1993). The target feature is presented frequently while little pressure is placed on the child. The following is an example of focused stimulation within a conversational context:

Child: Mommy made hamburgers. Mommy made 'tator salad.

SLP: **She** must be a good cook. What else did **she** make?

Child: A cake.

SLP: **She** did? Yummy. Did **she** cook any hotdogs?

Child: Uh-huh.

SLP: **She** made a very nice picnic for the family. Did **she** get to play any games or did **she** just work?

The language feature being targeted—the pronoun *she*—appears in the initial part of the sentence or in elliptical utterances. Such frequent modeling plus recasts of the child's utterances have been effective in facilitating use of certain language structures (Camarata, Nelson, & Camarata, 1994; Camarata, Nelson, Welsh, Butkowski, Harmer, & Camarata, 1991; Watkins & Pemberton, 1987).

Once a target has been modeled thoroughly, the SLP asks the child to respond in a manner similar to the model. Children who are young, low-functioning, or delayed may need imitation training, with a complete model presented immediately before their response. *Imitation* is a procedure in which the child repeats the language behavior of a facilitator, with the expectation that the child will acquire some aspect of the facilitator's language.

Imitation can be used as a first step in programs to teach specific language targets (Connell, 1987a, 1987b) or as a correction procedure when the child fails to respond or responds incorrectly. The procedure has been used successfully with several types of LI. By monitoring the child's progress, the SLP can provide varied cues, including partial models and/or delayed imitation.

The child may respond also to questions for which the SLP has modeled the answers. Initially, the modeled answer may follow the question, but this format can be altered so that the answer precedes the question, is given partially, or precedes the question by increasingly longer periods of time. The SLP might also model the type of response desired, although not the exact one.

Although the modeling procedure seems stilted in writing, it can be applied very flexibly and works well with groups of children. In small groups, children who have acquired a certain target can serve as models for those who have not. By varying turns, the SLP ensures that sufficient models are provided for different children with different targets. In a reversal of roles, the SLP can serve as a model for the child, while the child cues the SLP.

Modeling may be less effective than other, more structured methods (K. Cole & Dale, 1986; Connell, 1987a). Whereas modeling is effective in changing the behavior of children developing typically, it is less effective than imitation with children with LI (Connell, 1987a). More structured approaches include imitation, elicitation in the form of fill-ins, stimulation, and comprehension training.

Direct Linguistic Cues

Linguistic cues for certain targets can be direct or indirect. Direct elicitation techniques might include the following target questions:

To elicit...	Use...
Verbs	"What is he doing (are you doing)?" Use any tense. A benefit is that the question contains the target tense.
Noun subjects	"Who/what is verbing?" Again, the tense can be altered for the situation.
Noun objects	"What is he/she verbing?" Tense can be altered for the situation. Obviously, verbs that do not take objects should not be used.
Adverbs or adverbial phrases	"When/where/how is he/she verbing?" Tense can be altered. "How" questions can be used also to elicit process answers, as in "How did you make the airplane?"
Adjectives or adjectival phrases	"Which one...?" Tense can be altered. There should be an obvious contrast between choices for the response, such as *big* and *little*. These differences might be noted prior to questioning. Responses of a particular type can be modeled, as in "Which one ate the cookie, the littlest bear, the middle-size bear, or the biggest bear?" To keep the child from responding, "That one," the SLP may want to cover the child's eyes or use some barrier.
Specific words	Completion sentences, as in "She is playing in the _____." Rising intonation after the last spoken word will signal the child to respond. If the SLP plays dumb or acts forgetful, the child's behavior makes more sense conversationally.

Substitution requests also can be used. For example, pronouns can be substituted for old information. The facilitator might make a statement, such as giving one descriptor ("The dog is little"), and then ask the child to make a comment ("What can you tell me about the dog?"). This procedure also can take the form of a guessing game, as in "Is the dog little? Well, if the dog isn't little, what can we say?"

Although these linguistic cues are conversational in nature, they will seem very nonconversational if used in nonlinguistic contexts in which they make no sense pragmatically. Questions should be used when the facilitator really desires the answer and when the child is interested in the topic of discussion.

The SLP can model a response prior to asking the child a question, for example, "I think I want the yellow one. What about you?" This type of cue is more likely to elicit a longer utterance and is more conversational in tone.

One variation of the direct linguistic cue is a *mand model* (Hart, 1985; Rogers-Warren & Warren, 1985; Warren & Kaiser, 1986a, 1986b). This technique has been used effectively with preschoolers and with children with SLI (Olswang & Bain, 1991). This procedure follows a routine that is established prior to beginning any activity. The routine serves as a chain in which one stimulus cues the next. The mand-model approach usually is used for teaching new language features.

Access to desired items is through an adult, who determines the criterion for acceptability. In this way, the adult, not the object, becomes the stimulus for talking. According to this procedure, "it is likely to be not so much what the teachers do—the forms of language they model—as the interactional context in which the adults' models occur that facilitates children's progress in language learning" (Hart, 1985, p. 81).

In the four-step mand-model training sequence, the adult first attracts the child's attention by providing a variety of attractive materials. This inducement may not be necessary if the child already displays an interest. Thus, the adult establishes joint attention with the child. In the second step, after the child has expressed interest, the adult (de)mands, "Tell me about this," or, "Tell me what you want," requesting a behavior trained previously. If there is no response, the adult moves to step three and prompts a response or provides a model to be imitated. In step four, the adult praises the child for an appropriate response and gives the child the desired item.

Preschool peers can be trained to use the mand-model technique effectively (Venn, Wolery, Fleming, DeCesarem, Morris, & Cuffs, 1993). Production may generalize to unprompted productions.

Indirect Linguistic Cues

Indirect linguistic cues are more conversational and situational in nature. For example, when attempting to elicit questions, the SLP might use unfamiliar objects hidden in boxes to set the non-linguistic context. Beginning with "Boy, is this neat," the SLP peeks into the box. An exchange might continue as follows:

Child: What's in there?

Facilitator: This. (Takes the object out. Waits.)

Child: What is it?

Facilitator: A flibbity-jibbit. It does everything.

Child: What it do?

It is easy to see the interplay of nonlinguistic and linguistic cuing.

Another indirect linguistic technique requires the SLP or language facilitator to make purposefully wrong statements. A child's clothing can serve as the focus of this conversation, a technique I have dubbed "the emperor's new clothes."

Facilitator: (Touching child's red sweater) What a nice blue blouse.

Child: This no blue blouse.

In both examples, the child has given a final response that may be something less than what is desired. The SLP now can respond and begin to shape the child's previous utterance into an acceptable form.

These examples are only a very few of many indirect techniques. Others examples are listed in Appendix F.

Contingencies

Conversational consequences can be divided roughly into those that do not require a child's response and those that do. Each type provides some feedback to the child, and each differs with the functioning level and degree of learning exhibited by the child.

Contingencies Requiring No Response

Contingencies that require no response from the child are nonevaluative or accepting in nature and can be used to increase correct production or highlight incorrect production for self-correction. When the child initiates or responds to some cue, the facilitator focuses full attention on the child, creating joint focus on the child's topic. Because the child has established the topic, it now acts as a reinforcer for the child and can be used to modify the child's language. Techniques used to modify the child's response include *fulfilling the intention, use of a continuant, imitation, expansion, extension* and *expiation, breakdowns* and *buildups,* and *recast sentences.*

By *fulfilling the intention* of the child's utterance, such as handing the child a requested item, the facilitator signals the child that the message was acceptable as received. No verbal response is required.

A *continuant* is a signal that a message has been received and acknowledged. These signals usually consist of head nods or verbalizations, such as "uh-huh" and "okay." Continuants fill the speaker's turn by agreeing with the previous utterance.

In *imitation,* the facilitator repeats the child's utterance in whole or in part but makes no evaluative remarks. Rising intonation, signifying a question, is not present. Again, this behavior acknowledges the child's previous utterance. Imitation is especially helpful to the child when correctly produced features of interest are emphasized ("She is riding the bike"). Imitations might be preceded also by phrases such as *That's right* ("That's right, she is riding the bike").

In contrast to imitation, expansion or recast/expansion is a more mature, or more correct, version of the child's utterance that maintains the child's word order, for example:

Child: It got stolen by the crook.

Facilitator: Uh-huh, it *was* stolen by the crook.

The use of expansion as a teaching tool is very limited for children functioning above about 30 months of age. In a variation of expansion, the SLP can prompt the child to imitate the expansion, although such requests disrupt the flow of conversation. A more appropriate variety of expansion for older children is a reformulation in which two or more child utterances are combined into one utterance that includes the concepts of each, as in the following:

Child: The dog bit the man. The man ran away.

Facilitator: Oh, the dog bit the man, who then ran away.

At low levels of child grammatical production, the use of expansion and cloze, or fill-in-the-blank, procedures by adults produces more responses, more interpretations, and more syntactically complex utterances by children than does a question-and-answer procedure (Bradshaw, Hoffman, & Norris, 1998).

For older children, extension is a more appropriate response. *Extension* is a reply to the content of the child's utterance that provides additional information on the topic, as in the following:

Child: It got stolen by the crook.

Facilitator: Oh, I wonder if the crook stole anything else.

Much of our behavior in conversations consists of replies to the content of the other speaker, and these comments can be used effectively regardless of the age or functioning level of the child. Extensions signal the child that the facilitator is attentive and interested.

Breakdowns and buildups consist of dividing the child's utterances into shorter units and then combining them and expanding on the child's original utterance. The purpose is to help the child understand intrasentential relationships. I use this strategy as my hearing-impaired and senile great-great-uncle used to do to aid the processing of information, mulling it over before commenting.

Child: It got stolen by the crook.

Facilitator: (Emotional, disbelieving) It was. (Hmmm) It was stolen. Stolen by the crook. (Disgusted) By the crook. (Finally) It was stolen by the crook.

This strategy works well, especially if the SLP or facilitator plays dumb or uses a silly puppet who just does not seem to get things right. The child may shake his head or say, "Uh-huh," in agreement between the facilitator's utterances.

Finally, *recast sentences* are a changed form of the child's utterance that maintains the same relations as the original and immediately follows the child's utterance. Recasts repeat at least one of the major lexical items while modifying other constituent parts of the utterance.

Child: It got stolen by the crook.

Facilitator: Was it stolen by the crook?
        OR
        It was stolen by the crook?
        OR
        The crook stole it.
        OR
        Did the crook steal it?

These sentences can be recast in whatever form the SLP has targeted, although comments are easier for children than question forms. Although children with SLI can benefit from the use of them, recasts must be produced in much greater quantity than found in typical conversation to be of value (Proctor-Williams, Fey, & Frome Loeb, 2001).

If the child says little, the SLP can recast his or her own utterances. If the child will not stop talking, the SLP can interrupt with "yeah" or "uh-huh" and insert a recast sentence.

Contingencies Requiring a Response

Contingencies that require a response are used when the child is able to produce the target reliably but has failed to do so or has produced the target inaccurately in conversation. A skilled use of both nonlinguistic and linguistic contextual cues should set the stage for production of the target in a situation in which it makes good pragmatic sense. As a fully participating conversational partner, the child has an interest in the conversation and in his or her own utterance. Thus, the child is motivated to modify production in order to maintain the conversation and receive the adult's attention.

Most of these contingencies note the child's error, or require the child to find the error, and request that the child produce the target more correctly. A second contingency type requests repetition or a correct or expanded utterance to strengthen correct production. A hierarchy of both types, ranging from contingencies used in initial training to those used when the target is learned, would be *correction model/request, incomplete correction model/request, reduced error repetition/request, error repetition/request, self-correction request, contingent query, repetition request, expansion request,* and *turnabouts.*

In a *correction model/request,* the facilitator repeats the child's entire utterance, adding or correcting the target that was omitted or produced incorrectly, for example:

Child: I *builded* a big tower out of blocks.

Facilitator: I *built* a big tower out of blocks. Now you say it.

The child is requested gently to repeat the facilitator's model.

Initially, the target may be emphasized to aid the child in locating the corrected unit. Later training might restate the child's utterance as a question, as in, "You *built* a big tower out of blocks?" Obviously, there are some language features such as omitting *am,* that cannot be modeled in a question, such as *you are....*

Because the entire utterance is desired in the child's response, the facilitator should act confused to maintain the conversational nature of the interaction.

Facilitator: You *built* a tower out of big blocks? No, you *built* a big tower out of blocks? Oh, I'm confused, tell me again.

In a correction model/request, the child is provided with a complete or only slightly altered model of the correct utterance.

The facilitator should require the child to produce correctly only those units that are currently targeted for intervention. It is difficult for some facilitators to reinforce utterances even when they contain errors, as in the following example:

Child: I *builted* the most biggest tower out of blocks.

Facilitator: You *built* the biggest tower out of blocks?

Child: Yeah, I *built* the most biggest tower out of blocks.

Facilitator: Uh-huh, how big was it?
           OR
           Yeah? What kind of blocks did you use?
           OR
           Oh! Where is the tower now?

A conversational approach requires the language facilitator to remain focused on the target and on the hierarchy of teaching strategies being used.

In contrast to a correction model/request, an *incomplete correction model/request* provides only the corrected target. The child must provide the rest of the utterance, as follows:

Child: I *builded* a big tower with blocks.

Facilitator: Built.

Child: I *built* a big tower with blocks.

Initially, the child will need a cue to repeat the utterance with the corrected target.

As the child begins to exhibit some success at self-correcting, the facilitator can offer *choice-making:* "Is it *builded* or *built*?" The facilitator must be careful to use this form occasionally when the child's initial utterance is correct as well as when it is incorrect. Otherwise, the child will recognize that the question is only used when he makes an error. In addition, the location of the correct answer should vary so that the child does not develop a strategy of always picking the first or second answer.

Once the child has learned the target reliably within more structured situations, the language facilitator can use other techniques that require the child to supply the missing or correct target. With *reduced error repetition/request,* the facilitator repeats only the incorrect structure with rising intonation, thus forming a question. This contingency informs the child that the language unit in question is incorrect and must be corrected, for example:

Child: I *builded* a big tower with blocks.

Facilitator: Builded?

Child: Built.

The facilitator's question is more conversational than the cue found in correction model/requests and is less disruptive to the flow of conversation. If the child fails to recognize the error, the facilitator can provide a corrected model by using an incomplete correction model/request.

With *error repetition/request,* the facilitator repeats the entire utterance with rising intonation. The child must locate the error or omission and correct it, as in the following:

Child: I *builded* a big tower with blocks.

Facilitator: I *builded* a big tower with blocks?

The emphasis on the error can be increased or decreased as needed. For example, increased emphasis might be used to aid the child in finding the error. If this technique is unsuccessful, the facilitator might provide a reduced error repetition/request.

Once the child's target knowledge is reasonably stable, the facilitator can use the error repetition/request even when the child is correct. This procedure helps children scan their productions spontaneously and to self-correct.

A *self-correction request* does not provide the child with a repetition of the previous utterance. Instead, the facilitator asks the child to consider the correctness of that utterance from memory, for example, "Is/was that right/correct?" and "Did you say that correctly?" If the child is unsure, the facilitator can provide an error repetition/request.

In contrast to the somewhat stilted tone of the self-correction request, the *contingent query* is very conversational. It is concerned more with comprehension of the message being sent than with specific targets. Nonetheless, this technique can be used effectively to signal the child that something may be amiss with the production. The child is left to scan recent memory to determine where communication breakdown occurred.

Use of contingent queries should be limited because they can disrupt communication and frustrate the speaker who is continually asked to repeat. Young school-age children dislike having to repeat more than once or twice.

Contingent queries may be specific or general, depending on the abilities of the child. In response to the sentence "I *builded* a big tower with blocks," the facilitator might respond, "What did you do with blocks?" "What did you do?" or simply, "What?" If the child falsely assumes that his or her production was correct and merely repeats the error or omission, the facilitator might use a self-correction request.

Correct productions of the target can be reinforced by asking the child to repeat. With a *repetition request*, the facilitator simply says, "Tell me that again," or, "Could you say that again?" This technique also can be used conversationally, implying that the listener missed some portion of the transmission, not that the transmission was in error.

If the child produces the target correctly but in a smaller unit than desired, such as a one-word response following a reduced error repetition/request, the facilitator can use an *expansion request*. The typical cue "Tell me the whole thing" is not conversational in tone. It is better for the facilitator to fake confusion and ask for a total restatement, as in the following example:

Facilitator: Built? What was *built?* Who *built* it? I get so confused. You better tell me again.

The advantages of using this routine to elicit language from children were discussed previously.

Turnabouts may be more effective than repetition requests and are more conversational in nature. In a *turnabout,* the facilitator acknowledges the child's utterance or comments and then asks for more, as in "Uh-huh, and then what did you do?" or "Wow, what will you do next?" or "That sounds like fun; what happened then?"

The turnabout technique has been taught to high school peers and parents and has been used effectively in conversation with children with LI (Hunt, Alwell, & Goetz, 1988, 1991). This partner-as-facilitator strategy reportedly can improve conversation skills significantly.

The *wh-* questions used in turnabouts should be of a topic-continuing nature and thus support the child's efforts to maintain the topic (P. Yoder, Davies, Bishop, & Munson, 1994). This style of responding is especially helpful to preschool children and children with LI.

Several relational terms also may be used in open-ended utterances to aid the child in providing more information of a specific nature. For example, the facilitator might repeat the child's utterance with the addition of *but* to elicit contrary or adversative information, or *and* to elicit complementary information.

Child: We played games at the party.

Facilitator: What fun. You played games at the party *and…*

Child: And we had cake and ice cream.

Other types of relationships and terms are as follows (J. Norris & Hoffman, 1990b, pp. 78–79):

Temporal	*and then, first, next, before, after, when, while*
Causal	*because, so, so that, in order to*
Adversative	*but, except, however, except that*
Conditional	*if, unless, or, in case*
Spatial	*in, on, next to, between, etc.*

These contingencies can be arranged in a hierarchy similar to that in Table 10.2. This arrangement will differ with the language unit being targeted. The facilitator who is familiar with this hierarchy can respond to the child's utterances in a manner that enhances language stimulation and facilitates language learning.

TABLE 10.2   Hierarchy of conversational contingencies

For the examples, the child's utterance is "I sawed two puppies." The facilitator should use the contingency farthest down on the list that ensures the child's success with minimal input.

Conversational Contingency	Example
Correction model/Request	I *saw* two puppies. Can you tell me again? (The cue to say it again is optional, unless the child does not repeat spontaneously.)
Incomplete correction model/Request	*Saw.* Can you tell me again? (Again the cue is optional.)
Choice-making	Is it *saw* or *sawed*?
Reduced error repetition/Request	Sawed?
Error repetition/Request	I *sawed* two puppies?
Self-correction/Request	Was that right?
Contingent query	I didn't understand you. Say it again, please. (Other options include *Huh?* and *What?* or, in this example, *What did you do?*)
Expansion request	Tell me the whole thing again.
*Repetition request	Tell me again.
*Turnabout	You did? I love puppies. What did they look like?

Example of hierarchy in use:

Child: I sawed two puppies.
Partner: Was that right? (Self-correction request)
Child: Uh-huh.
Partner: I sawed two puppies? (Error repetition/request)
Child: Yeah.
Partner: Sawed? (Reduced error repetition request)
Child: Saw. I saw two puppies.
Partner: Uh-huh, tell me again. (Repetition request)
Child: I saw two puppies.
Partner: I think I love puppies more than kittens. Where did you see them? (Turnabout)

*Used with complete, correct responses.

Conclusion

Both the nonlinguistic and linguistic contexts can be manipulated by the SLP and other language facilitators to teach language to the child and to encourage use of structures recently acquired. By using the various techniques described in this chapter, facilitators can maximize interactions with the child with LI. Although it would be ideal if facilitators used the full range of techniques, even the adaptation of some would help make learning more conversational in nature.

11

Specific Intervention Techniques

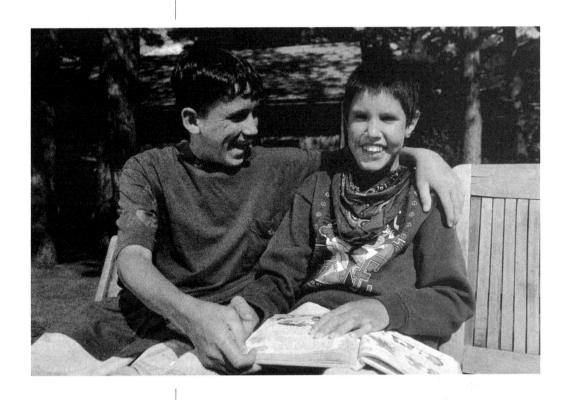

A number of training techniques effectively teach the use of linguistic features to children with LI. The success of intervention varies with the particular linguistic feature trained, the manner and duration of the training, and the characteristics of the individual child (Leonard, 1981).

Often, SLPs must make decisions about candidacy for intervention services. Such decisions are driven by caseload size, scheduling, or budgetary constraints. In addition, school districts may have policies governing candidacy. Although children with both low cognitive and low language performance often are excluded or given low priority, they benefit more or at least as much from intervention as children with higher IQs and low language abilities (Cole, Coggins, & Vanderstoep, 1999; Fey, Long, & Cleave, 1994).

Prior to beginning intervention, the SLP should examine all deficit areas for a given child and apply a "What's the point?" criterion (Lilius, 1993). In short, the SLP is concerned with the importance of individual deficits on the child's overall communication. Each deficit should be evaluated to the extent that it contributes to the child's communicative functioning. Deficits that greatly affect functioning should be targeted first for intervention. Those that do not affect overall communication fail the "What's the point?" test.

It is important that the SLP consider generalization at the beginning of intervention and make crucial training decisions on the basis of generalization to the use environment. Even in a direct teaching approach, at least a portion of each lesson should involve the conversational context. Intervention that focuses solely on linguistic form can result in limited progress and lack of generalization (Goetz & Sailor, 1988; Halle, 1988). Preferable are specific situations in which language form skills are necessary, such as ordering in a fast-food restaurant and using the telephone (Mire & Chisholm, 1990).

In general, in this chapter we discuss a developmental hierarchy of intervention, modified where appropriate by sound teaching principles. It is important to remember that development is a gradual process with much overlap between structures. A child will reach performance levels gradually, and it is unrealistic to expect 90 to 100 percent correct performance for many language features when they are initially targeted. It may be more practical to expect a lower performance level followed by a plateau and then further change. During these plateaus, other features can be targeted.

Development is also not "domain-specific" (Kamhi & Nelson, 1988). Rather, changes in one area of language can affect other areas, just as overall developmental changes can affect language.

When possible, apply the functional approach explained throughout this text. Use it as your overall model. At all levels of instruction, some elements of the functional intervention model can be used.

Intervention should be fun and challenging, using real conversational exchanges between the child and partners wherever possible. Thus, both partners are involved actively in the process.

In this chapter we explore some proven and some promising techniques for language intervention. For clarity, I have divided the chapter into four aspects of language: pragmatics, semantics, syntax, and morphology. We discuss hierarchies for training and techniques that lend themselves well to each area. The final portions of the chapter deal with the special needs of CLD children, early intervention, and the clinical application of computers.

The best intervention presents language holistically so that the child can experience newly acquired language as it is used in communication. Some SLPs accomplish this goal by targeting skills in more than one area of language or by using a stage approach in which a few training targets from a stage of development are targeted simultaneously. The holistic aspect of intervention is discussed at the end of the next section, and suggested activities are presented in Appendix G.

Pragmatics

As children mature, they gain increasingly more complex categorizational or word-associational strategies and increasingly more complex organizational word and structure systems. The most appropriate and effective way of expressing oneself depends on a number of variables that are stylistic, socioemotional, personal, and contextual. In other words, linguistic variation is the result of skills in pragmatics or language use.

Many children do not use language as an effective tool for learning about their environment. They do not ask questions or request materials. Making mistakes and being corrected is easier for them than asking questions. They wait for the environment to act in some way, and then they respond. Often, adults in the child's world lose their expectation that the child will initiate communication.

What passes for effective communication varies with the communication situation and with the age of the child. For example, with young adolescents the SLP may need to target academic and personal-social success. As the youth nears adulthood, academic concerns yield to vocational ones (Larson & McKinley, 1993). The communication skills required for success in these contexts vary considerably. Intervention might begin at the point of communication breakdown (Nippold, 1993). In general, adolescent conflicts with peers are easier to modify than those with adults, and personal difficulties are easier than vocational ones (Selman et al., 1986). Targeting peer interactions is especially important for children with SLI because social acceptance is so dependent on effective and appropriate language (Hadley & Schuele, 1998). Highly verbal and fast-paced peer interactions are real-life situations that should be included in training for maximum generalization to occur.

Traditional language intervention goals, however, are usually product rather than process oriented (Wilkinson & Milosky, 1987). In other words, language forms are targeted, whereas language use is tangential. Although a theoretical shift has occurred toward pragmatic models of language, many treatment programs continue to emphasize syntax and semantics. In general, communicative context is used only to create fun or as an afterthought relative to generalization.

Children can acquire very complex forms without totally comprehending them. It is essential, however, that they understand the functional qualities or use of the form (Snow & Goldfield, 1983). Thus, the effect of communicative need overrides the effect of syntactic complexity. We might do better to identify and train pragmatic behaviors and to teach the appropriate contexts in which to use these behaviors. When targeting pragmatics, form errors should be ignored unless they interfere with the intended purpose of the child's utterance.

When appropriate, however, forms can and should be targeted within a functional context. For example, the SLP might teach requesting as a function of the goal of gaining information, action, or materials. The SLP can help children identify the goal first and then the form that goes with each goal. Subsequently, he or she may teach alternative forms for such requests.

Through role-playing and the use of videotaped interactions, the SLP can teach the child to identify situations in which the desired information, action, or material was requested inadequately, inaccurately, or inappropriately. The SLP also can train either repairs and reattempts or requests for clarification. Likewise, he or she can help the child to identify the requested goal of another speaker and to respond appropriately.

The SLP may target a number of pragmatic skills within a single lesson and should use many everyday events and play activities to teach a single pragmatic skill. For example, telephone conversations teach acknowledgment of the interaction, conversational opening and closing, topic maintenance, and referential communication. The use of situational cards and different voices on the other end of the phone can help the child adapt to differing situations. Pretending that he or she is lost or cannot see, the SLP can teach requesting and giving assistance and information, roles, and following directions.

Construction toys used to copy a model, such as Legos, clay, and Play-Doh, or construction paper can teach requesting assistance, referential communication, giving and following directions, and topic maintenance. More difficult tasks will require more assistance.

Several children's stories can be enacted to help the child learn roles. Recitation of stories or nursery rhymes to different audiences will aid growth of register. The use of different puppets or dolls or different costumes will aid the learning of role taking.

Finally, the SLP can use any number of activities for referential communication. Children can describe objects seen in Viewmasters, on computers, or through periscopes, felt in paper bags, or hidden. Such activities as I Spy and Twenty Questions also aid referential communication growth and foster requesting and giving information.

If we "provide the child with the tools and an opportunity to be a successful communicator…the child has been given a purpose to maintain linguistic communication" (Lucas, 1980, p. 201). These tools might take the form of communicative intentions or conversational abilities.

Intentions

Children select and acquire utterances that are communicatively most useful. This fact explains why request forms and words that mark the initiation of favorite activities are acquired before labels and descriptive terms (K. Nelson, 1981a). In training, however, the SLP is concerned with the breadth of illocutionary functions that the child is able to express.

The following section addresses the training of several intentions illocutionary functions (Bedrosian, 1985, 1988; Constable, 1983). In Chapter 12, some methods to be used in the classroom are discussed. Appendix F also provides several indirect linguistic cues useful for eliciting different functions.

Calling for Attention

Calling for someone's attention requires the presence of a person whose attention the child seeks or who is essential to completion of a task. In general, children seek attention from adults who provide it. Adults or other facilitators might give the child an object within a situation and ask him or her to take it to an adult who, for the purpose of training, initially ignores the child. The child also might be asked to relay a message to someone else.

Facilitators should attend to the child as soon as the child requests attention. If the child continually demands attention or uses inappropriate behavior to get attention, the facilitator will have to set some limits, such as only responding in certain situations and never responding to inappropriate behavior.

The form is usually the child calling the facilitator by name or gaining attention by some other means, such as tapping the listener's shoulder, moving into the visual field of the listener, leaning in the direction of the listener, or using eye contact. The child also may specify how the facilitator should respond.

Requests for Action

Requests for action can be trained at mealtime, within small group projects, or during almost any physically challenging task. Again, the child assumes that the facilitator can provide what is requested.

The facilitator will need to design situations in which children require assistance to complete the task. To encourage requesting, the facilitator can use initiative games in which children must solve problems. Tasks also may be sabotaged (see Table 10.1). As in requests for objects, attention is gained first, and the form of the utterance is interrogative or imperative.

Requests for Information

Children with LI often do not see other persons as sources of information and may produce few such requests. Although the environment can be manipulated to encourage requests for objects and actions, it is not as easy to encourage or increase the child's need and desire to seek information.

Requests for information require that the facilitator omit essential information for some novel or unfamiliar task, such as an art project, a new game, or some challenging academic task. Objects unknown to the child may be introduced without being named or their purpose explained. The child can be prodded gently to ask questions if asking does not occur spontaneously.

The child must recognize both the need for this information and that another person possesses the knowledge. Recognition of need is often the most difficult aspect of this training. Confrontational naming tasks, with objects known and unknown to the child, may encourage initial requesting for information. The form of requests for information is either a *wh-* or *yes/no* interrogative with rising intonation.

The facilitator also might encourage the child to ask questions by questioning him or her about other people's feelings or actions of which the child has little knowledge. The child then can be cued with "Why don't you ask (name)?" This tactic can be used with confrontational naming tasks as well.

The child should be expected to ask questions that reflect the forms the child is capable of producing. The facilitator's verbal responses discussed in Chapter 10 can be used to help the child modify incorrect, inappropriate, or immature responses.

Requests for Objects

The facilitator can easily train requests for objects within art tasks, group projects, snacktime, job training, or daily living skills training, such as dressing and hygiene. It is essential that the child actually desire the object he or she is to request and that the facilitator can provide it.

The facilitator can change the environment to increase both the opportunities for requesting and the caregiver behaviors that direct the child's attention to these opportunities. Many situations, especially those with groups of children, provide an opportunity for overlooking a child's turn, thus encouraging requesting. Of particular importance is a coordinated program designed to teach requesting for the everyday environment by approximating that environment and training those within it to model and elicit requests. Table 11.1 includes general guidelines for caregiver elicitation techniques.

This intention usually begins with eye contact or some attention-getting behavior, such as using a name. The form, usually accompanied by a reaching gesture, is interrogative or imperative and specifies the desired object. Form training can occur within the actual need situation.

Responding to Requests

Responses may take the form of an answer to a question or a reply to a remark. These forms are very different and require different skills.

In responding to questions, children must recognize that they possess the answer and that they are required to reply. Initial training should disregard the correctness of the answer in favor of reinforcing answering in general. At this stage, teaching *wh-* question responses should reflect the *appropriateness-before-accuracy* pattern found in early question development (Parnell et al., 1986). In a situation in which the facilitator asks about objects known to the child, it is fairly certain that the

TABLE 11.1   Guidelines for caregiver elicitation of requests

Make statements throughout the day about objects that the child might prefer. Wait for a response.

Use elicitation behaviors to accompany high-interest activities and play. These behaviors include the following:

Modeling with an imitative prompt. Facilitator provides a model of a request and asks the child to imitate.

Direct questioning. Facilitator asks, "What do you want?" or "What do you need?"

Indirect modeling. Facilitator provides a partial model followed by an indirect elicitation request, such as, "If you want more *X,* let me know (or, "ask me for it") or, "Would you like to *X* or *Y?*"

Obstacle presentation. Facilitator requests that the child accomplish some task but provides an obstacle to accomplishment.

"Please get me the chalk over there." (There is no chalk.)

"Pour everyone some juice." (The container is empty.)

General statement. Facilitator makes a verbal comment about some activity or object that the child might want to request. The facilitator entices the child.

"We could play Candyland if you want to."

"I have some Play-Doh on that high shelf."

Set up specific situations to elicit requesting.

Provide direct and indirect models as often as possible without requiring the child to imitate.

Provide a model at appropriate times when the child appears to need assistance or is looking quizzical.

Have the child attempt difficult tasks in which help is occasionally needed.

Respond *immediately* and *naturally* to any verbal request.

Source: Adapted from Olswang, Kriegsmann, & Mastergeorge (1982).

child will give the appropriate answer, although it might be inaccurate. The information requested can expand gradually to conform to the child's ability to respond.

Replying is more difficult to teach because a response is expected but not required. The child's response may be in the form of nonlinguistic compliance or a linguistic response. Children's comprehension of different requests will vary with age (Ervin-Tripp, 1977). Table 5.5 contains the ages at which different types of requests are understood. The child can be helped to recognize the need to reply by physical signs from the SLP or the passing of an object.

The child's ability to reply may be hindered by an inability to determine the topic or to formulate a response. The facilitator may enhance linguistic processing by having the child repeat the request. Over time, the facilitator can modify this procedure to whispered imitation, mouthing, and silent repetition until the process is internalized. He or she can help children in identifying important information in requests and in formulating responses.

The SLP can elicit denials by giving the child something other than what he or she requested or by giving the child something undesirable. The child can reject either an action or proposal. The speaker uses emphatic stress, and the utterance is in a negative form.

Statements

Show-and-tell, discussions, and current-event activities help children state information. During discussions of high-interest topics, such as dating, holidays, pets, or competitive games, the facilitator can encourage children and adolescents to offer their opinions. The facilitator also can use mock radio and television broadcasts. With a little cutting and some paint, he or she can convert a large appliance box into a console television from within which children can deliver daily newscasts of information.

The facilitator may either know the information the child is sharing or not. In the first instance, the child is recalling a shared event; in the latter, the child is presenting new information and can assume that the facilitator has very limited information. Each situation has different informational needs and requires some presuppositional skill to determine the necessary amount of information to convey.

The form is declarative. Initially, the child must secure the listener's attention and state the discussion topic. Statements can be expanded into narratives whose purpose is also to convey information.

Conversational Abilities

More than other areas of language intervention, the training of conversational abilities requires the use of actual conversational situations. Ritualized communication that interferes with interpersonal communication, such as echolalia, can be modified gradually into acceptable and conventional routines, such as greetings, conversational initiations, and requests for repair (Lord, 1988; Lord & Magill, 1988; Magill, 1986). Social routines can be memorized and practiced in different situations that help the child become more flexible in their use. Variations can be taught through different facilitators and situations. For example, one does not offer to shake hands when the potential partner has her or his arms full (Lord, 1988). If nothing else is accomplished in training, the child learns appropriate entry into conversations (Prizant & Wetherby, 1985).

For adolescents with conversational deficits, it's recommended that intervention occur within structured, conversation-focused, small-group activities (Nippold, 2000). The atmosphere should be positive with plenty of opportunity for success. Within this context, the SLP models, followed by teen practice, then peer analysis and feedback with the use of videotapes and small group discussion (Hess & Fairchild, 1988). Scripted sequences and role-play are very helpful.

Presupposition

The speaker's semantic decisions are based on her or his knowledge of the referents and the situation and on *presuppositions,* or social knowledge of the listener's needs. The speaker needs to provide information that is as unambiguous as possible. In other words, the speaker and the listener need to share the same linguistic context.

Often, children with LI are unaware of their audience's needs (Bliss, 1992). With maturity, children developing typically are increasingly able to perspective-take, the greatest growth occurring in middle childhood. In contrast, children with LI seem to improve little with age. Breakdown could occur in social-cognitive processes and/or linguistic production (Bliss, 1992). Significant improvement can occur, however, from training speakers to be aware of listener needs.

The two aspects of this training are (a) what information to relay and (b) how much. The first can be trained with descriptive or directive tasks in which the child is the speaker. The listener tries to guess or draw the described object or to follow the directions. The facilitator can use barrier games, in which he or she places an opaque barrier between the speaker and the listener, for teaching speakers to be aware of their listeners' needs (Wallach, 1980). Some clinical materials are available commercially (McKinley & Schwartz, 1987). Because the speaker and the listener do not share the same nonlinguistic context, the bulk of the information must be carried by the linguistic element in an unambiguous manner if the listener is to comprehend.

When the child is the listener, the SLP can send ambiguous or incomplete messages or directions to give the child an opportunity to identify the missing semantic elements. Obstacle courses are also a good vehicle through which the child can be directed or direct others.

Training the correct amount of information to transmit may be more difficult. Of course, giving insufficient information in the tasks mentioned in the last paragraph would make the directions difficult to follow. The SLP can train children to give more, as well as more accurate, information. For the child who gives too much information, these tasks may be trained initially one descriptor or one step at a time. These tasks then can be grouped into multidescriptor or command steps so that the child experiences offering more information. The relating of very discrete or limited events, such as combing your hair or washing your face, also can control the amount of information to be relayed.

The SLP can help the child monitor his or her own production to know when redundancy occurs. The SLP can gently remind the child that certain information was relayed previously. In subsequent training, the SLP can quiz the child about the novelty of information presented.

Referential Skills

Referential skills include identifying novel content and describing this content for the listener. Children with LLD have been trained successfully to use referential skills through the use of barrier games (Bunce, 1989). The description of physical attributes is somewhat easier to teach than are relational terms, such as location.

It may be best to pair a child with LLD with another child, rather than with an adult, because the child with LLD may assume that the adult partner intuitively knows the object or is pretending not to know. Thus, the child may provide less information to an adult partner.

Topic

Topic performance is an important intervention target for the following reasons (Bedrosian & Willis, 1987):

1. Its use is one means of coordinating conversations and actions, thereby fostering development of interpersonal relations.
2. It regulates the sequence of a conversation.
3. It involves the initiation of conversation.
4. It requires listening and comprehension to maintain the flow of conversation.
5. It provides a framework for making relevant contributions.

In short, topic offers an encompassing framework for considering other language skills.

Unlike greetings, which vary only slightly across situations, topics and methods of topic introduction and identification are context-dependent (Lord, 1988). Topic identification is a complex process that develops gradually through school age and adolescence. A successful strategy is to engage in whatever everyone else in the conversation is doing.

Topic Initiation.   *Initiation* is the verbal introduction of a topic not currently being discussed. Children often do not understand the purpose of conversations or are reluctant to introduce topics for discussion. Topic initiation, a form of conversational manipulation, implies an active conversational strategy. The child with LI may not be adept at introducing topics clearly or may have very limited topics (Dollaghan & Miller, 1986). Children with ASD or TBI may introduce unusual or inappropriate topics (Rumsey et al., 1985).

Adolescents with moderate-to-severe MR have been taught to initiate a topic through the use of facilitator waiting and through training in the purpose of conversation (Downing, 1987). In the first step of training, the facilitator maintains eye contact for 10 seconds but does not speak. Planned delay can be an effective strategy for prompting clients to initiate conversation.

If the child does not initiate the conversation during this wait, the facilitator can explain the purpose of conversation and the enjoyment that can result (Downing, 1987). He or she also can describe the roles of speaker and listener. Then the facilitator returns to the waiting strategy. If the child still does not respond, the facilitator can suggest that the child find something of interest to discuss by looking through a magazine. The facilitator then returns to the waiting strategy. If the child fails to initiate again, the facilitator can model a topic initiation.

Some children fail to initiate conversations and topics because of a history of failure. It is important that the facilitator focus fully on the child when he or she initiates and follow the child's lead. The facilitator should try not to interrupt the child.

The facilitator might first teach the child to gain the listener's attention. When the child inadequately introduces a topic, the facilitator can request further information to identify the topic. Focused activities, such as describing pictures or a shared event or following directions, will show the child the need to share the referent with the listener.

The facilitator initially can tolerate inappropriate topics to give the child some success. Gradually, the facilitator can discuss the inappropriateness of these topics and gently steer the conversation to more appropriate ground. He or she can suggest topics ("Maybe you'll tell me about…") and leave it for the child to initiate. The facilitator also can train the child to ask other people about their likes and dislikes, favorite foods, sports, TV shows, or exciting trips or vacations in order to include other-oriented topics in the child's repertoire.

Traditional therapy often centers on the immediate context and may inhibit generalization by failing to incorporate displacement or nonimmediate contexts. In part, the discussion of the immediate context is related to the stimulus items used with children. To increase the frequency of memory-related topics, the facilitator can encourage the child to talk about feelings or activities engaged in prior to the conversation (Bedrosian & Willis, 1987). Elicitation can be direct ("What did you do yesterday?") or indirect ("I wonder what you did yesterday"). The facilitator can encourage the child to ask the same information of the language facilitator. In addition, she can engage the child in activities and then ask the child to discuss what was done. The SLP can provide feedback in the form of expansions of the child's utterances. Future-related topic initiations are similar, such as discussing what the child will do next. The use of such conversationally based strategies can increase nonimmediate topic initiations, as well as the general level of syntactic performance (Bedrosian & Willis, 1987).

Topic Maintenance.   The SLP can continue the conversation by commenting on the topic the child initiated and by cuing the child to respond (Downing, 1987). The SLP can use turnabouts—usually a comment followed by a cue for the child to respond, such as a question—to keep the conversation flowing and on-topic. Questions should make pragmatic sense; that is, the facilitator should not know the answer prior to asking. Table 11.2 is a list of various turnabouts.

Off-topic responding may indicate that the child is inattentive or cannot identify the referent or topic presented. Children who are inattentive may be distracted easily and need help determining the focus of their attention. Children with ASD may make off-topic comments because of a lack of

TABLE 11.2   Variety of turnabouts

Type	Example
Tag	*Child:* Baby's panties.
	Mother: It's the baby's diaper, *isn't it?*
Clarification (contingent query)	*Huh?*
	What?
Specific request	*What's that?*
Confirmation	*Horse?*
	Is that a hippopotamus?
	(Hand object to partner and give quizzical glance)
Expansions	
Suggestions	*I want one.*
Corrections	*No, it's a zebra!* (Expectant tone)
Behavior comment	*You can't sit on that.*
Expansive question for sustaining conversation	*What would the police officer do then?*

Source: Drawn from Kaye & Charney (1981).

assumed background information and experience or a lack of realization that such background is available (Lord & Magill, 1988; Rutter, 1985).

The facilitator can help the child who cannot sort through the information to identify the referent or topic through the use of questions and prompts that highlight those semantic cues of importance to the child (T. Williams, 1989). Practice conversations with various partners and topics can provide an opportunity to learn and generalize. The facilitator can keep the child on-topic with such cues as "Anything else you can tell me about (topic)?" and, "Tell me more about (topic)." Later, he or she can use contingent queries to keep the child on-topic.

When the facilitator and the child have shared the same experience, the facilitator can act as a guide to keep the child on-topic. The facilitator also can help the child sequence events through the use of questions ("Then what happened?") or probes ("Are you sure that happened next?").

The facilitator should avoid dead-end conversational bids. Dead-end bids result in a short response that ends the interaction. A common dead-end bid is the overused "What did you do today?" to which every child knows the answer: "Nothing."

Duration of Topic.   The facilitator may help the incessant talker by using very limited topics with definite boundaries, such as "What animals did you see at the zoo?" If the child strays beyond the topic, the facilitator should interrupt. He or she then can remind the child of the topic and gently bring him or her back to it.

The facilitator also should alert the child when he or she has provided enough information or is redundant. Such phrases as "You've already told me about *X*" or "I'll only answer that question one more time" help the child establish boundaries.

Children who provide too little information can be encouraged to provide more with "Tell me more." The SLP also can play dumb with such utterances as "Well, I guess it was pretty boring if that's all that happened." In general, children remain on-topic longer when they are enacting scenarios, describing, or problem solving (Schober-Peterson & Johnson, 1989).

Turn Taking

It is important not to initiate turn-taking training while also attempting to train topic maintenance. Too many new training targets may confuse the child. The facilitator may have to tolerate off-topic comments initially to correct inappropriate turn taking.

Turn taking can begin at a nonverbal, physical level. The facilitator and the child can pass items back and forth as they use them. The item then can become the symbol for talking. Many structured games also require turn taking. The facilitator also can provide a turn-taking model by imitating the child. He or she can use verbal games and motion songs with groups of children. Later, the facilitator can use turnabouts or a question-answer technique to help the child take verbal turns. Nonlinguistic cues, such as eye contact and nodding, can signal the child to take a turn. The facilitator can decrease questioning gradually in favor of these nonlinguistic cues and wait for the child to take a turn. He or she can teach the child attention-getting devices, such as increased speaking volume, to gain a turn. The facilitator can change conversational partners for those with whom the child is more assertive and initiates more frequently. Games in which the child directs other people are highly motivating.

Turn taking is appropriate if it does not interrupt others. The child who is overly assertive and who continually interrupts may need to be reminded not to do so. The SLP might focus instruction on identifying when speakers have completed their turns. He or she also should explain appropriate interruptions, as in emergencies. Structured exchanges through use of an intercom or mock police radio may help children understand the importance of turn allocation. Structured games, such as Twenty Questions, also foster turn-allocation learning.

Conversational Repair

Through monitoring, each conversational partner detects and reacts to conversational breakdowns by other people when she or he is speaking and by one's self when a partner is speaking (Markman, 1981). Children with LI often seem unaware of the distinction between understanding and failure to understand and rarely act when they do not.

The SLP may modify comprehension monitoring through the use of audiotaped language samples in the following training sequence (Dollaghan & Kaston, 1986):

1. Identification, labeling, and demonstration of active listening
2. Detection of and reaction to inadequate signals
3. Detection of and reaction to inadequate content
4. Identification of and reaction to comprehension breakdown

Although this sequence can be trained easily in an audiotaped mode with first graders, generalization to actual conversational use should not be neglected. The introduction of puppets, dolls, or role-playing at each step can facilitate this generalization. Written scripts may be used with older children.

Comprehension monitoring can be facilitated when the child takes an active role in the process. The child is taught first to identify, label, and demonstrate active orientation to listening behaviors, such as sitting, looking at the speaker, and thinking about what the speaker says (Dollaghan & Kaston, 1986). After learning to distinguish successful and unsuccessful performance of the three active listening behaviors, the child labels and demonstrates each. The child also might repeat the previous speaker's utterance or reply to such questions as "What did (name) just say?"

Next, the child is taught to detect and react to *signal inadequacies,* such as insufficient loudness, excessive rate, or competing noise. These concrete obstructions that prevent representation of the message are relatively easy to identify and enable the child to learn the difference between understanding and not understanding (Dollaghan & Kaston, 1986).

Within everyday activities, the facilitator can encourage contingent queries from the child by mumbling or talking too fast. This technique works especially well when giving directions needed to complete some fun task. The facilitator occasionally can ask the child, "What did I say? How can we find out?"

Once able to identify signal inadequacies, the child can be taught a variety of responses for requesting clarification. Requests may include general appeals, such as "Pardon?" (or "What?"), "I can't hear you," and "Wait…Now say it again" (or "Again please"), or more specific requests, such as, "Talk louder please" (or "Louder"), "Could you talk more slowly?" (or "Slow down"), and "Did you say *X*?" It is best to begin with more general requests and then move to more specific ones. The request form should reflect the child's overall syntactic level.

Next, the child can be taught to detect and react to *content inadequacies,* such as inexplicit, ambiguous, and physically impossible commands. For example, because inadequate content may not always be obvious, the SLP can ask the child to repeat the message to himself or herself and/or to the speaker and to attempt the task demanded (Dollaghan & Kaston, 1986). Again, the child is taught various methods for requesting clarification of inadequate content. Requests may include "What do you mean?" "Which one?" "Where?" "I can't do that" (or "I can't"), "Do you mean *X*?" and "That doesn't make sense."

This part of the training can be great fun, with the facilitator making outrageous statements and ridiculous demands of the child. I still remember the expression on the face of a child with Down syndrome whom I had asked to get into his lunch box. He or she can insert intentional content inadequacies into any number of daily activities.

Finally, the facilitator can teach the child to identify and react to messages that exceed his or her comprehension capacity by the presence of unfamiliar lexical items, excessive length, and excessive syntactic complexity. This level of comprehension breakdown may be the most difficult to detect because of the often abstract nature of the breakdown.

The child can practice identification and reaction in the form of clarification requests in real-life situations in which these difficulties are likely to occur. Most novel activities include unusual jargon that the facilitator can use to confuse the message. For example, cooking offers such words as *ladle, simmer,* and *skillet.*

Requests for clarification might include "Say those one at a time" (or "One at a time"), "That was too long for me," "I don't know that word" (or "I don't know"), "Can you tell me a different way?" "What does *X* mean?" (or "What do you mean?"), and "Can you show me?" (or "Show me"). As training progresses, the child should learn to identify the point of actual breakdown for the speaker.

Narration

Language intervention with narratives may focus on the organization of the narrative, cohesion, or comprehension. The length and complexity of narratives is positively related to the amount of exposure to narratives in intervention (Gummersall & Strong, 1999). Modeling and practice are especially important. Specific targets will vary with the maturity of the child.

Narrative Structure

Young children use a script-based knowledge organization system. Although older children and adults retain this system, they also use taxonomic or categoric knowledge for processing (Mistry & Lange, 1985).

Scripts are sequences of events that form unified wholes. When this event sequence is placed in linguistic form, it is called a *text*, the basis of narratives. You'll recall that narratives generally are organized by a story grammar consisting of a setting statement and one or more episodes that include an initiating event, a reaction by the main characters to the event, a plan, an attempt to respond to the event, a consequence or outcome to the event, and a reaction or an ending (J. Johnston, 1982b; Stein & Glenn, 1979).

Knowledge of episode structure forms a framework within which the child can interpret complex events and unfamiliar content. The SLP can facilitate development of internalized narrative schemes or story grammars through the following (Hewitt, 1992; N. Nelson, 1986b):

1. Involve children in organized activities, such as daily routines, to help them organize their own real-life scripts.
2. Use scripted play in which children enact everyday activities that gradually become more variable and less contextualized.
3. Read and tell real-life stories with clear scripts.
4. Help children transfer from activities to linguistic organization by telling them narratives with clearly structured story grammars and then having them dramatize the stories.

These exercises may be performed orally or in writing.

Scripted play is especially useful with preschool and early school-age children and will be discussed in detail in Chapter 12. Initially, it is very important that the scripts describe familiar motivating events, such as going to the market or getting ready for school. The script should be introduced and discussed prior to play, with expectations stated.

> Today, we're going to play "shopping at the market." How many of you have gone shopping with someone? Good. Whom did you go with, Tiera? Okay, and whom did you go with, Andre? Good. What do we buy at the market? Uh-huh. Yes. Good. I have some things right here. What's this, Jewell? Good. What's this, T. J.? Right. Do we buy this at the market? That's right, we don't buy this at the market. What's this, Rochelle? Good. Do we buy this at the market? Good, that's right, we do. What is the first thing that happens when you get to the market? (And so on.)

The script is played and discussed afterward.

With each replaying, the children change roles, modify the events, and use less concrete objects. As children become more adept at recounting the script, the SLP encourages telling of the narrative without an enactment. Again, familiar roles and situations are used. These procedures work especially well with groups of children and will be discussed in more detail in the following chapter on classroom intervention.

The SLP can facilitate production of event descriptions by having children describe familiar events as they occur or as recalled from slides, pictures, or videotapes (Duchan, 1986b; Lewis, Duchan, & Lubinski, 1985). Children can role-play and describe familiar events as they occur. One of my favorite language lessons, mentioned previously, included mime and the acting out of familiar situations. Later, these events were described without role-playing.

Pictures of familiar events as the child draws them can be used for sequencing. The facilitator can help the child identify the setting and characters by asking him or her to describe the picture; for example:

Facilitator: Well, what do we have here?

Child: This is me in the kitchen, and I'm making breakfast.

Facilitator: So, we might say, "This morning, I was in the kitchen making breakfast." What did you do first? (Or Then what happened? or What's this next picture?)

After completing a step-by-step description, the child can be encouraged to tell the entire narrative.

Episodic knowledge can be taught through the use of children's books. Book selection should be based on the following criteria (Naremore, 2001):

- Familiar event scripts
- Pictures that support the episodes
- Clearly sequenced episodes
- Appropriate length and language level
- Stories "pretested" for retelling by the SLP

The actual story is not of prime interest. The SLP should select stories that contain all episodic elements. Intervention can begin with a mediated approach by discussing with the student the importance of stories for communication.

After reading the book together, the SLP helps the child analyze the story following a "problem-solution-result" format. Learning structure is the goal. Terminology is not. The SLP helps the child break the story into pieces, identify the parts, and recombine them again into a cohesive narrative. For children who can't relate to books, the SLP can construct one-episode narratives of experiences familiar to the child. Pictures and real objects may aid the child's participation.

Narratives can be retold repeatedly, although retelling is not the overall goal. Ideally, the child will use internalized knowledge to compose and comprehend conversational and book-based narratives (Naremore, 2001).

Narrative telling can be extended in both speech and in writing. If the child is able to retell a story with two or three complete episodes, she or he is probably ready to begin composing original narratives (Naremore, 2001). This can be accomplished within a story context with the SLP supplying the supporting structure initially. The SLP begins a story and the child furnished the final story grammar element. Gradually, the SLP supplies fewer episode portions. In each narrative, the child completes the story by supplying the final elements until he or she can compose an entire narrative. The teaching of longer written narratives will be discussed in Chapter 13.

Children then can progress to fairy tales or their own stories. The facilitator can use questions to move children to more sophisticated ways of organizing and expressing concepts and relationships. Chapter 12 includes a discussion of replica play and narratives in the classroom.

Narrative discourse is the next logical step. Children should have the opportunity to practice forms of narration within a variety of role-playing situations (Heath, 1986b). Narratives can be cued by statements such as, "Tell me what you did at…" or "Tell me how you did…".

It is unclear whether cohesion can be taught directly. Increased organization may reflect maturation of children's cognitive-social-linguistic knowledge system (K. Nelson, 1985). Contextualized training can provide the structure needed to foster the development of cohesion in children's communication.

Cohesion

It is best to teach story grammar structure prior to cohesion (Liles, 1990). Although the two are related, it is possible for a narrative to have a good story grammar and poor cohesion. Cohesion requires some metalinguistic skill because the narrator must pay attention to the text apart from the sequence of events being presented.

Cohesion is of five types: conjunctive, referential, substitutive, elliptical, and lexical. (Lexical cohesion, using terms such as *yesterday, in the future, prior to,* and *ate/will eat,* is difficult to measure reliably and is very individualized. It will not be discussed here.) *Conjunctive* reference is the easiest form of cohesion to teach. Children's oral narratives can be collected and transcribed into a "book." Use of conjunctions and the relationships expressed can be analyzed. Simple stories containing various clausal relationships also can be read to children. In a retelling, a child usually will not express relationships and conjunctions that he or she does not use.

Once the child's narrative relationships and conjunctions have been analyzed, the SLP can begin to introduce other conjunctions. A developmental order of introduction may be helpful, although the first priority should be conjunctions omitted or used incorrectly in the relationships expressed. For example, in "…stoled all his money. He robbed a bank. He was starving…," cause and effect are suggested but without the use of *because.*

The SLP can introduce narrative relationships with or without a conjunction and then, using a question-answer technique, prompt the child to produce the desired conjunction. If the child responds incorrectly, the SLP can reread or retell the relevant portion of the narrative, model a response including the conjunction, discuss the meaning, and prompt the child to respond again. The important aspect of the training is an understanding of the relationship expressed, not a regurgitation of the correct conjunction. The final stages of training would include original narratives produced by the child.

Referential cohesion uses nouns, pronouns, and articles to designate old and new information in the narrative. Again, questions and answers can be used to direct the child as a narrative is told. Retellings by the SLP might use a *cloze* technique, in which the child fills in the appropriate word. Gradually, less narrative-structured and more expository materials can be introduced. It is more difficult to comprehend and produce cohesion without the narrative frame.

Comprehension

Narrative comprehension can be improved by beginning with predictable narratives concerning everyday events or routines familiar to the child. The child's internalized event script aids both comprehension and recall. As in scripted play, variations in the narrative are introduced gradually, and the text moves to more unfamiliar and fictionalized events and stories. Comprehension and recall can be facilitated by having children draw or write event sequences.

Before beginning a narrative, review it with the child. Help the child bring his or her knowledge to the task. This prenarration task is discussed in detail in Chapter 12.

Data suggest that the use of subjectivity or the character's thoughts and feelings can enhance comprehension of fictional narratives (Hewitt, 1992). Children can be taught to focus on a character's thoughts and feelings as a way of making sense of the events in the narrative. Thus, the child focuses more on the reasons for and outcomes or results of events within the narrative. There are no right or wrong answers; rather, the child's responses explain events in a manner comprehendible to the child.

Semantics

Semantic intervention consists of several different but related levels of intervention. Word meanings form relationships with other words that help categorize and organize not only the language system but also cognitive processes, particularly for older children. For this reason, semantic intervention involves a variety of interrelated intervention strategies much more complex than simply training vocabulary words.

At its core, word meaning consists of concepts or knowledge of the world. Words do not name things, but rather refer to these concepts. These conceptual complexes are formed from many experiences with the actual referents.

The process of forming and organizing concepts may reflect general cognitive organization and, in turn, influence that organization (N. Nelson, 1986b). Semantic training must recognize the importance of these underlying concepts and include cognitive aspects of concept formation. Several commercial resources are available for training cognitive skills essential for conceptualization (Cimorell, 1983).

Inadequate Vocabulary

Reference, or *meaning,* is the relationship of a sign or word to the underlying concept. Different strategies are used by different children and by the same child at different developmental times to construct meanings.

Children with LI often use one strategy exclusively or predominantly. For example, the meanings expressed by some children with ASD seem to be unanalyzed, situationally related "chunks." Children with MR are often deficient in their ability to form complex concepts. Other children may have conventional concepts but experience difficulty relating these underlying concepts to linguistic symbols or words.

The SLP may assist with the building and extending of individual reference systems by providing situations in which children encounter the physical and social world. Dynamic events seem to encourage early concept development better than do static ones (N. Nelson, 1986b). Therefore, feature learning can be enhanced by focus on movement, contrast, and change. The most successful strategy is to (a) build on an experiential or prior knowledge base and establish links to new words, (b) teach in meaningful contexts, and (c) provide multiple exposures (Nagy & Herman, 1987). The experiential base is important, especially for the child below age 7. The child should have the opportunity to have meaningful, real experiences.

World knowledge, or what the child knows about her or his world, is very important for vocabulary growth. Early word meanings are acquired within event-related experiences, especially predictable, everyday routines and their accompanying scripts (N. Nelson, 1986b). Gradually, meanings generalize and decontextualize. Between ages 5 and 9, the child developing typically reorganizes her or his vocabulary from event-based processing to more linguistic, semantic-based processing.

Groups of children on a field trip can experience the world by touching, smelling, and even tasting an old log and describing the sensation. Language facilitators can encode features of events and entities to which children attend (N. Nelson, 1986b). Older elementary school children can learn from the experiences of others, much as adults do.

Vocabulary is acquired in a two-phase process. First, words are *fast-mapped*—a small portion of the meaning is acquired on the first exposure. The child's world and word knowledge affect which features of the definition she or he acquires. The second phase is a later, more gradual one in which repeated exposure results in a more complete map of the word's meaning.

Children and adolescents with LI need to learn how to use the context to establish word meaning (McKeown & Curtis, 1987; Nippold, 1991; R. Sternberg, 1987). Contexts provide a number of cues that can be classified as temporal (time), spatial (location), value (relative worth), stative descriptive (physical description), functional descriptive (use), causal (cause and effect), class membership (type), and equivalence (similarity/difference). Class membership and functional descriptive are the easiest for children, whereas stative descriptive seems to be the most difficult (R. Sternberg, 1987). Context should be established for the child prior to introducing the word numerous times. The child will need help in determining what he or she knows from the context and repeated exposures. Novel word learning is enhanced when words receive emphatic stress while being presented within stimulus sentences (Ellis Weismer & Hesketh, 1998). Stress is important given the difficulty children with SLI have in using syntax to acquire lexical items (Rice, Cleave, & Oetting, 2000). In this format, meaning, use, and word class (i.e., noun and agent) membership coalesce. Narratives also may provide a context for introducing a novel word (Crais, 1987).

No one likes to give verbatim definitions. Learning benefits if the child and the facilitator can use the word to discuss a relevant topic in context. It is important to remember that the child may not need a full adult definition when the word is first introduced. A less full definition may suffice (Kameenui, Dixon, & Carnine, 1987).

The facilitator should not expect dictionary definitions from children below age 12. By that age, however, the child developing typically should be able to define words, draw conclusions, and make inferences.

Child and adult definitions, especially categorical ones, seem to be organized around a prototype or best exemplar. Examples given to the child should be of the prototype, or best exemplar, variety, as these will enhance learning of salient features. In addition, the SLP should expose children to multiple examples of events and things in familiar contexts in order to perceive these features of events and entities. Language facilitators can act as mediators, framing, focusing, and providing salient features of experiences for the child (N. Nelson, 1986b).

Within activities, children can be encouraged to describe features. Descriptors then can be used to determine similarities and differences and to label the world. Instead of naming unfamiliar entities such as types of leaves, children can be encouraged to stretch their existing language and give descriptive names, such as *five-pointed leaf tree*.

Facilitators also can target words used frequently at home and school in everyday activities and events. In general, it is easier to learn words for known concepts than to learn both words and concepts (Crais, 1990). The choice of which words to teach should be based on the likely frequency of use, typical development, need within the classroom and use in textbooks, and likelihood of the child learning the word from context alone (Graves, 1987). Even slang expressions might be taught to aid socialization, especially among adolescents (D. Cooper & Anderson-Inman, 1988).

Training should include words along with others that mean the same (synonyms), sound the same (homonyms), or are opposites (antonyms). This training will help the child organize language for easy storage and retrieval of information. Prefixes and suffixes are also important, as is syllabication. The child's existing meanings can be consolidated by building on the child's current vocabulary while correcting errors and misconceptions of meaning (Elshout-Mohr & van Daalen-Kapteijns, 1987).

Understanding and training should progress from these general meanings to more specific ones. It is important for the child with LI to expand meanings beyond the often obvious best exemplars. Training also should proceed from more contextual meanings, as in "hit the ball," to less contextual, more figurative meanings, such as "hit the roof," and multiple meanings, such as "a hit musical." Abstract terms, such as *except, instead,* and *until,* should be targeted last.

The semantic features of words can be analyzed to expand the characteristics associated with words and to aid categorization (Crais, 1990). Words can be classified according to their semantic features, as in Figure 11.1. Sorting tasks perform a similar function, and children can be encouraged to make their own associations.

Multiple meanings should be related to specific academic subject areas or contexts. The facilitator should help the child understand that meaning varies with context (Graves, 1987).

A root-word strategy can be used with school-age children to help them discover meanings and their modifications (Crais, 1990). Suffixes are easier to learn than prefixes and should be introduced first (see morphology section of this chapter). Prefix training should begin with concrete, easy-to-define prefixes, such as *un-,* and proceed to more abstract ones. The most frequently used prefixes in American English are *un-, in-, dis-,* and *non-.*

Materials should provide for adequate semantic development. Pictures are too abstract for some children; single examples too limited. "Materials that isolate word meanings from the total concept are too abstract" (Lucas, 1980, p. 21). Referents should be presented in a variety of ways to build a total concept. Varying contexts provide for maximum usage and exposure. Storytelling in which a novel word must be used is also a good strategy and uses context to facilitate use.

	Transportation	Four-wheel	Two-wheel	Engine-powered	Pedal-powered	Runs on rails
Motorcycle	X		X	X		
Bicycle	X		X		X	
Car	X	X		X		
Bus	X	X		X		
Train	X			X		X

	Animals	Bird	On farm	Wild or zoo animal	Gives milk	Four-legged
Chicken	X	X	X			
Duck	X	X	X			
Cow	X		X		X	X
Elephant	X			X	X	X
Goat	X		X		X	X

FIGURE 11.1   Analyzing semantic feature similarities.

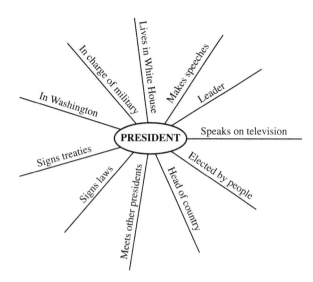

FIGURE 11.2   Spidergram of word meanings and associations.

Many commercially available games can be used as is or modified for vocabulary training, including Boggle, Pictionary, and Scrabble (Beck, McKeown, & Omanson, 1987; Graves, 1987). Semantic organizers, such as spidergrams, can be used to build associations. Children can use semantic organizers to "brainstorm" or to tell all they know about a word (C. Nelson, 1991). Figure 11.2 is a typical spidergram.

Children also enjoy creating words that do not exist in the dictionary or giving existing words new definitions. Such original words can be used along with real words to try to encourage children to make educated guesses about the meaning (Atkinson & Longman, 1985; Hall, 1984). Table 11.3 contains several original words.

Semantic Categories and Relational Words

Meaning extends beyond the word level. As children develop beyond the single-word level, they are able to encode meaning in the form of the utterances produced. Words with the same referent can

TABLE 11.3   Examples of sniglets

Sniglet	Definition
Bathquake	n. The violent quake that rattles the entire house when the water faucet is turned to a certain point.
Lotshock	n. The act of parking your car, walking away, and then watching it roll past you.
Maggit	n. Any of the hundreds of subscription cards that fall from the pages of a magazine.
Petrool	n. The slow, seemingly endless strand of motor oil at the end of the can.
Shoefly	n. The aeronautical terminology for a football player who misses the punt and launches his shoe instead.

Source: Adapted from Hall (1984).

fulfill different semantic roles or cases that specify the relationships among those referents. Table 7.7 presents the most common cases or semantic classes. Thus, the child forming a sentence must keep in mind both the referent and the semantic role.

Words and phrases also modify the meaning of basic syntactic elements by indicating qualities, such as perceptual attributes, manner, and temporal aspects, and relationships between larger sentential units, such as additive (*and*) or causal (*because*). As a listener, the child can only comprehend other people to the extent that she or he understands the various relationships underlying their utterances.

Semantic Classes

The SLP can teach words to children and place the words in different semantic classes. A portion of word definition is the semantic class into which a word can be placed. The SLP also can teach other word types that relate to that class. Children with LI may find it difficult to identify and use semantic classes of words.

The agent function usually found in the subject position of a sentence offers a unique example for semantic category training (Connell, 1986b). English is a subject-prominent language in which a large number of morphosyntactic and transformational elements are associated with the subject of the sentence. These elements include subject-verb agreement, as with the verb *to be* and the third-person singular, present tense marker; pronouns; and auxiliary verb inversions in questions. These elements are not critical to the content of a sentence, and they can be omitted without greatly affecting the understanding of the sentence.

The SLP may facilitate teaching these elements by teaching the concept of *subjecthood* (Connell, 1986b). The SLP can accomplish this by using a functional approach in which he or she teaches the child the purpose of a subject.

The function of a sentence's subject, represented by a noun or a noun phrase, is to designate the perspective used in the sentence. In contrast, the topic designates the focus of discourse. If the sentence contains action, the agent designates the actor. In the sentence "John ate the salami" (Connell, 1986b, p. 482), all three elements are the same. In "*John* was arrested by the police" (ibid.), *John* is the topic and the subject, but *police* is the agent.

Subjects can be identified by the pronouns used with them. Subjects take nominative case pronouns, whereas topics and agents may take different types. Subjects also agree with predicates, whereas topics and agents need not.

The SLP can train children to identify the topic and the subject by using the following forms (Connell, 1986b):

1. Objective   nominative   verb/
   case   +   case   + *be* +   adjective/
   pronoun   pronoun   adverb/noun
   (*Him,*   *he*   *is*   *running*)
2. Nominative case pronoun + *be* + verb/adjective/adverb/noun
   (*He*   *is*   *running*)

The first is taught in response to a "Which one is…?" type of question, and the second in response to a "What is the man doing?" or "Who is…?" type of question. Children can induce the function of the subject and its separateness from the topic by the varying sentential contexts in which they are used.

Children can learn each sentence form by imitation and then in response to questions within ongoing activities. Training should begin with the second sentence type because it is included within the first. Once children have learned the formats, the questions can be alternated. Later, the habitual or simple present form of the verb, such as *eat* or *drink,* can be introduced to teach children subject-verb agreement within the same subject-highlighted format.

Other semantic classes may be taught in a similar manner. Table 11.4 presents suggestions for training.

Relational Words

Relational words fulfill many functions in language. Relationships may be based on quantity or quality and may be general or specific. Other relational words are used to mark location and time. Conjunctions are relational words that relate one clause to another. Each type of relational word requires specific considerations.

In general, relational terms can be acquired through descriptive tasks, in which the child must differentiate between one entity and another, or through narrative tasks, in which the child must aid the listener to differentiate characters. The SLP can help the child initially by keeping the task context-bound and by controlling the number of items or characters. By playing dumb or acting confused, the facilitator can help the child provide additional or essential information. Narratives are

TABLE 11.4   Suggestions for training semantic classes

Instrument
Initially, this class can be trained in the final position of the sentence, preceded by the word *by,* as in "The wood was split *by his axe*." Position and the preposition *by* act as signals for this class. This class can also be signaled by the verb use, as in "John *used the rake* to gather the leaves." This sentence type can be prompted by questions such as "How did...?" and "What did John use to...?"

Patient/Object
This class may be taught initially by using the final position in the sentence as a direct object to transitive verbs. Question prompts such as "What did Carol throw?" may be used to elicit this class.
   It is somewhat more difficult to teach this class in the subject position because that position is usually occupied by an agent. If agents are taught in response to a *who* type of question, patients might use *what,* as in "What grew in the park?"

Dative
The dative class is most frequently and obviously used as an indirect object. This function can be clearly signaled initially by use of the prepositions *to* and *for.* Question prompts can include these cues and the word *whom,* as in "For whom did Mary buy the flowers?"

Temporal, Locative, and Manner
These classes are relatively easy to teach because each has specific questions that prompt usage. Prepositions, such as *in, on,* and *at,* are used with these functions, as are *to, with,* and *by,* which are used to mark other semantic class use.

Accompaniment
The final position in the sentence and the preposition *with* should be used in training to signal this class. A *with whom* question prompt can be used to elicit response.

also effective vehicles for acquiring conjunctions, especially when the facilitator synthesizes larger, more conceptually complex sentences based on those of the child.

Quantitative Terms. A child does not need to be able to count to learn quantitative terms. Initial training can begin with the concepts of *one* and *more than one*. The second concept can be marked variously by *many, much, some,* and *more*. Such terms as *these* and *those* should be introduced with some caution because of deixis, or interpretation from the perspective of the speaker. Deixis is mentioned in the pragmatics portion of this chapter and is covered briefly in the following section.

The distinction between *many* and *much* is complex and should be ignored with children functioning at a preschool level. In general, *many* is used with regular and irregular plural nouns, such as *cats, shoes,* and *women*. In contrast, *much* is used with mass nouns—nouns that refer to homogeneous, nonindividual substances, such as *water, sand,* and *sugar.* It is not surprising that children have difficulty with the two terms *much* and *many.*

Before going beyond the quantity words mentioned, the child must learn to count and have a concept of the relative values of different numbers. In other words, the child must know that 4 is greater than 2, not that 4 merely follows in a sequence.

Later quantifiers can include words such as *few* and *couple*. These can be followed by other quantifiers, such as *nearly, almost as much as,* and *half*. Table 11.5 presents common quantitative words. The ordering of these words in the noun phrase is very important and is discussed in the syntax section of this chapter.

Qualitative Terms. Qualitative terms include such words as *bigger* and *tallest,* which use the *-er* and *-est* morphological markers, and such phrases as *as big as, not as wet as, smaller than,* and the like. Table 11.5 also presents common qualitative terms. In general, children learn to use the comparative *-er* before the superlative *-est,* and training should follow that pattern. It is best to begin with the regular use of these two markers before introducing exceptions, such as *better* and *best*. Words can be expanded into phrases, for example, *bigger* to *bigger than.*

TABLE 11.5   Common quantitative and qualitative terms

Quantitative	Qualitative
One, two, three, four...	Big, little, long, short
Many, much, lots of	Large, small, fat, thin
Some, few, couple	Soft, hard, heavy, light
More, another	Same, different, alike
Nearly, almost all	Old, young, pretty, ugly
As much/little as	Blue, green, red, ...
Plenty	Hot, cold, warm, chilly
Half, one-fourth, two-fifths	Wide, narrow
10%, 75%	Sweet, sour
Units of measure: Inch, foot, mile, cup, pint, quart, gallon, centimeter, meter, kilometer, liter, ounce, pound, gram, kilogram, acre	Nice, mean, funny, sad
	Fast, slow
	Smooth, rough
Clean, dirty	Angry, afraid
Empty, full	Comparative and superlative relationships: *-er, -est,* as *x* as, *x-er* than

Children seem to acquire concepts one semantic feature at a time. A corollary to this hypothesis is that broad, nonspecific concepts (e.g., *big*) are learned before more specific concepts (e.g., *long*). In this example, *big* refers to overall size, whereas *long* refers to size only in the horizontal plane.

The SLP should introduce terms and relationships in the order in which comparative terms develop. Table 11.6 includes common pairs of comparative terms and the approximate age at which most children can use them correctly.

In general, conceptual word pairs are acquired asymmetrically, one prior to the other, on the basis of their polarity. Children ages 3 to 7 appear to learn the positive-pole member of conceptual pairs, the one that represents more of the dimension characterized by the conceptual pair, prior to learning the negative member (Bracken, 1988). For example, *big* and *little* are opposite poles of the dimension *size. Big* represents more size and is, therefore, the positive member. These data suggest that positive members should be taught first to children with LI. In addition, positive-type comparisons should be taught before negative ones. In other words, *bigger than* should be introduced before *smaller than* and *not as big as.* Positive comparisons seem to be easier for children to process.

Spatial and Temporal Terms. Several words are used to mark both space or location and time and, thus, are potentially confusing. Among the most commonly used words in English are prepositions, such as *in, on, at,* and *by.* Each of these small, seemingly insignificant words has several definitions. In the syntax section of this chapter I discuss prepositional training. In addition, other words, such as *first* and *last,* also note place and time.

Spatial concepts are best taught first in relation to the child; then with "featured" or fronted objects, such as a television, chair, or person; and finally with nonfeatured objects, such as a wastebasket or a ball (Edmonston & Thane, 1990). The latter is more difficult to learn because it involves deixis.

TABLE 11.6 Common comparative word-pairs

Positive-Negative (age)	Positive-Negative (age)	Positive-Negative (age)
same-different (36–60 months)	inside-outside	high-low (42–60 months)
in front of-behind (48–54 months)	over-under (42–48 months)	forward-backward
into-out of	front-back (48–52 months)	happy-sad
top-bottom (48–54 months)	above-below (66–72 months)	old-young
rising-falling	right-wrong	large-small (78–84 months)
healthy-sick	heavy-light (30–48 months)	long-short (horizontal) (54–60
big-little (30–48 months)	tall-short (30–84 months)	months)
deep-shallow	loud-quiet	hot-cold
thick-thin	sharp-dull	dark-light
hard-soft (30–42 months)	solid-liquid	tight-loose
smooth-rough	full-empty (36–48 months)	a lot-little
more-less (42–72 months)	with-without (48–54 months)	fast-slow
all-none	arriving-leaving	early-late
old-new	first-last (60–66 months)	always-never
before-after (66–72 months)	on-off (24–36 months)	
open-close	up-down (36–60 months)	

(The overall order does not reflect the order for teaching conceptual pairs.)

Source: Bracken (1988); Edmonston & Thane (1990); Wiig & Semel (1984).

In general, vertical dimensions are learned before horizontal. Horizontal front and back terms, such as *in front of* and *behind,* are learned before horizontal side-to-side terms, such as *beside* and *next to.*

The order of temporal term learning reflects the underlying concepts of order, simultaneity, and duration (Edmonston & Thane, 1990). Terms that denote order, such as *before, after, first,* and *last,* usually are learned before terms for simultaneity, such as *at the same time, during* and *when.* Duration terms, such as *a long time,* generally are acquired last.

Children with psychological disorders have difficulty with the concept of time and with event boundaries. Thus, changing activities is often difficult. Intervention needs to begin with awareness (Audet & Hummel, 1990). The use of timers or other reminders can help these children monitor and regulate their behavior. Concrete event boundaries, such as the completion of a project, can aid transitions. Schedules and/or pictures of sequential events also may increase awareness.

In general, it is better to begin with concrete definitions and progress to more abstract ones. For example, with *first, last, before,* and *after,* training can begin with objects in a line. The facilitator can have the child touch individual objects, then a short sequence of objects, and finally a reverse sequence. Objects should be used before terms for events and the concept of time sequencing.

One context is not enough for teaching concepts of space and time. The greater the number of contexts, the more learning and generalization that will occur. Language can be used to help the child organize the environment by marking experiences of space and time. Table 11.7 includes common spatial and temporal terms.

The SLP can use direction following and activities to train children about space and time. It might be best to begin with routines that the child knows, such as those that occur at home or in the classroom, and then move into less familiar activities, such as using a pay telephone or changing a tire, in which the child must rely more on linguistic input.

Later, the SLP can use sequenced pictures or storytelling in the training. Pictures may seem very abstract to some children, especially school-age children with MR and preschoolers, and should be used with caution.

Deixis and the use of deictic terms are very difficult concepts to teach. The facilitator who takes the role of speaker and prompter for the child violates the roles in a conversation. The simple example of *here* and *there* is illustrative.

The request "Put the ball *here*" is said from the speaker's perspective. To the listener, the speaker's *here* is most likely *there.* If the speaker then shifts to the listener's (the child's) perspective and says, "Yes, put it *there,*" it may confuse the child further.

TABLE 11.7   Common spatial and temporal terms

Spatial			Temporal		
next to	under	in front of	next	today	days
before	over	behind	before	tomorrow	weeks
after	below	beside	after	calendar dates	hours
on, on top	corner	right	in, to	months	minutes
in, into	bottom	left	soon	seasons	through
in between	inside	through	later	numerals for years	away from
between	outside	high, tall	now	morning	toward
middle	side	upside down	above	afternoon	sometimes
above	end	together	yesterday	evening	

When training the child about deictic terms, it is best to sit next to the child so that you can share a perspective. From this shared perspective, some deictic terms, at least those for location, would be similar. Another facilitator, puppet, or prerecorded tape may act as the other conversational partner. The teaching of deixis is discussed also under the topic of pronouns in the syntax section of this chapter.

Conjunctions.   The SLP should teach conjunctions in the order in which they develop by noting for the child the relationships expressed in each (Klecan-Aker, 1985). For example, *because* represents cause and effect and may not be fully acquired until about age 12 by children both with LLD and without. Table 11.8 presents the general order of conjunction acquisition. The conjunction *and* can first be taught to combine entities, as in "cats *and* dogs." In a cooking activity, the facilitator might say, "Which two types of cookies do you like best?" or, "Tell me your two favorite types of cookies." In similar fashion, *but* can be used for like/dislike distinctions ("I like cookies, *but not beets*").

A *main clause* + *conjunction* + *subordinate clause* format can be employed initially to help the child acquire the underlying relationship. For example, sentences might be presented as follows:

We wear a coat *because* it is cold.
We wear a coat *if* it is cold.
We wear a coat *when* it is cold.

Once the child understands these relationships, the order of the clauses can be reversed, as in "Because it is cold, we wear a coat."

Next, the SLP can present new clauses for the child to complete. He or she also may use a break down and build up technique, as described in Chapter 10, in which the child identifies clauses and conjunctions and then reconstructs the sentence (Klecan-Aker, 1985).

Word Retrieval and Categorization

Word-finding difficulties can result from two possible sources (Kail & Leonard, 1986). The first is lack of elaboration or lack of a well-established, thorough representation of the word within the child's lexicon. Word knowledge is related to storage ability in that growth in word knowledge results in a larger storage capacity. An increased lexicon requires greater semantic networks in which to group words. In general, children who exhibit difficulties often have less extensive vocabularies and poor word knowledge (Kail & Leonard, 1986).

The second source of problems is in retrieval. In general, children with this problem are less efficient in retrieving words from storage. Whereas elaboration difficulties may occur alone, retrieval

TABLE 11.8   Acquisition order for English conjunctions

and	because	although, while, as
and then	so, if, when	unless
but, or	until, before-after	therefore, however

Data from studies are very variable, and this list is only a rough guide.

Source: Based on Bloom, Lahey, Hood, Lifter, & Fiess (1980); L. Lee (1974); Wiig & Semel (1984).

problems usually do not and may be an additional difficulty found in some children with elaborative problems (Kail & Leonard, 1986).

A number of activities have been suggested that facilitate word-finding skills (McGregor & Leonard, 1989; Wing, 1990). Children appear to benefit from both elaboration and retrieval activities (McGregor & Leonard, 1989). Word-finding activities can be incorporated easily into a number of everyday activities and conversations about these activities.

Prior to beginning intervention, it is important to determine the source of the problem (German, 1992). The SLP should derive naming data from a variety of activities to be certain of the cause of the problem. In general, children name real objects and colored pictures with a higher accuracy than black-and-white (Barrow, Holbert, & Rastatter, 2000). Naming words in a meaningful context is also performance enhancing. In short, children with poorly established word meanings have a semantic storage problem. In contrast, those with word-retrieval problems on words that they understand have poor retrieval skills. Finally, some children have problems in both areas. These last children should receive intervention services that combine the goals of the other two.

Children with storage problems have difficulty understanding and retrieving words that are not stable in their memory. Inadequate storage is the result of shallow meanings, reference-shifting problems, and poor analytical and synthesizing skills (German, 1992). The goal of intervention is to improve word knowledge and storage.

Those with retrieval-only problems have difficulty with search and recovery. Somewhere in the process of discriminating the desired word from among competing words and constructing the phonological specifications for production, the process breaks down (Bjork & Bjork, 1992). The goal of intervention is to improve access.

Memory storage seems to be affected by the depth or level of processing. In general, recall is best for words processed at the deepest levels, which are elaborative by nature (Lockhart & Craik, 1990). Theoretically, acoustic processing, such as rhyming, is surface processing; categorical is midlevel; and semantic/syntactic is deep.

Words are remembered in relation to other words and form meaning networks. Such relationships might be morphological (Nagy et al., 1989). When one member of the family is accessed, it activates others. These relationships are based on meaning, not just linear sound or letter strings. In other words, *ride* might elicit *drive* or *pedal* but not elicit *stride,* *cad* might elicit *villain* but not **cadet***.*

Semantic similarity and, to a lesser degree, phonetic similarity do affect judgments of relatedness. Networks of semantic-related morphemes are part of each individual's memory system. Thus, *stain, stained glass,* and *stainless steel* are perceived to be related.

Elaboration training focuses on organization of the child's lexicon and generalization of word meanings to everyday use (Kail, 1984; Kail & Leonard, 1986). In children developing typically, increased word knowledge results in increased storage strength. In short, a larger vocabulary means a more extensive database.

In elaboration training, the SLP can use semantic focus strategies, such as nonidentical exemplars and word comparison tasks. The SLP presents nonidentical exemplars, or examples of the word in several linguistic contexts, to enrich the child's definition and word associations. Nonidentical exemplars for house might include *dollhouse, housefly,* and *greenhouse.* In comparative tasks, the SLP expects the child to identify similarities and differences between two words with related meanings, such as *house* and *hotel.*

A mnemonic or "key word" strategy (Parente & Herrmann, 1996) also might be used to aid elaboration and recall of new vocabulary. New words are linked with acoustically or visually similar words with which the child is familiar. For example, *dogged* might be linked with *dog*. This initial linkage is modified by the child through use to a semantic one with deeper processing.

Pictures and written descriptions may be used to link two words. A known word is used to aid learning and storage of an unknown one. In the above example, a *dog* would be portrayed being stubborn or determined (dogged). Under the picture, it might read *The **dog** was **dogged** and would not give up.* Other examples are given in Figure 11.3. The key word now becomes the retrieval cue.

Children using this approach reportedly are able to recall 50 percent more definitions than those taught vocabulary by a more traditional method. In addition, the combined picture and sentence format appears to be more effective than either used separately (Condus, Marshall, & Miller, 1986).

Children seem naturally to enjoy word games and word play, and these teaching strategies can be incorporated into many types of activities. As a communication partner, I like to get very "confused" and use words in silly ways. Children laugh and freely correct their somewhat slow-witted communication partner. Retrieval training may include categorization tasks, such as naming members of a category or identifying the category when given the members. Categories include animals, clothing, grocery items, and the like. Categories also may be formed by the initial sounds of words and by rhyming.

As a group, children with LI are less likely than children developing typically to discover semantic organization strategies on their own and usually require more examples to determine a basis for organization and for generalization of organizational skill. Word-retrieval errors should demonstrate the predominant organizational framework of the child and alert the SLP to the patterns that need strengthening.

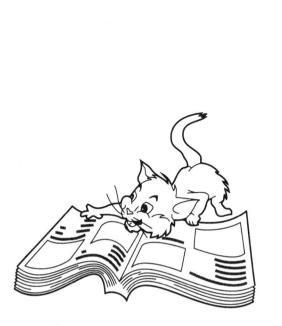

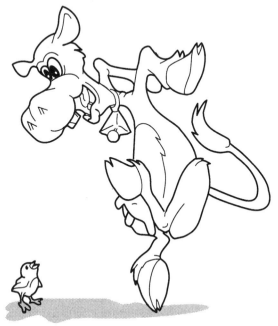

The **cat** is ordering from the **catalog**.   The **cow** is a frightened **coward**.

FIGURE 11.3   Examples of mnemonic strategies.

Categorization tasks, especially such familiar ones as Saturday morning cartoon shows, in which the child names members of the category, facilitate recall by building associational and categorical linkages between words. We usually recall a word by first accessing the category to which it belongs. Of course, the possibility still exists that the child will access the right category but retrieve the wrong member.

Categorization tasks can be elaborative in nature when members of more than one category are presented together. For example, the items *chair, bed,* and *table* can be classified as furniture; *chair, swing,* and *bicycle* are things on which you sit; and *bicycle, car,* and *bus* are vehicles. The facilitator could present these items together and ask the child to classify them in as many ways as possible.

Training might begin with actual objects and children making piles of objects that go together (Parente & Herrmann, 1996). As a child, I sorted my comic books by main character and my baseball cards by team. Similar tasks are found in several everyday activities. Children can make collages in school of things that go together. After objects and pictures, then words can be used. Entities might be classified by description (e.g., cold) or by function (e.g., things that you ride on). The facilitator should encourage the child to use as many different sensory descriptions as possible to describe objects.

Objects, then pictures, and finally words can be sorted and then used to facilitate cognitive organization (Parente & Hermann, 1996). After sorting, the child can be asked to recall the categories. Once the child has recalled categories, he or she can be asked to recall members. Categories might include semantic/hierarchical groupings, perceptual similarities, and rhyming, spatial, and locational groups. Everyday tasks such as preparing grocery lists, organizing chores, or planning items to take on vacation have more relevance than arbitrary groupings.

Verbal training should begin with common words for everyday concrete objects (Nippold, 1992). Familiar everyday objects and events should be used. This notion is sometimes difficult for adults to understand, especially if they are attempting to bring interest and variety into the training. I am reminded of a teacher who tried to teach zoo and farm animal categories but found the children very unresponsive. Both categories were outside their realm of experience. When one child suggested the category of animals seen "squashed" on the highway, every child became a participant. Although the example is somewhat gruesome, the lesson for SLPs is very practical. Everyday natural environments provide specific cues that aid memory (Nippold, 1992).

Word-retrieval difficulties can be helped by (a) naming/descriptive tasks ("It's a bicycle; you ride on it by peddling"), (b) associational activities ("Red, white, and ____"), and (c) sentential elaboration tasks based on syntactic characteristics of two words drawn at random ("The *trailer* was parked near the *restaurant* while the driver ate") and open-ended fill-ins and completions ("We eat with a ____") that involve deeper levels of processing (Casby, 1992). Word-sorting tasks can aid in the development of categorization and recall skills. Taxonomy charts, especially for newly introduced classroom content, also can help children develop categorization strategies.

Although semantic strategies appear to work well, they are not the only ones. With some children, a combination of phonological and perceptual strategies may also be effective (Wing, 1990), although semantic elaboration and retrieval activities produce better results than phonological strategies alone (McGregor & Leonard, 1989). In phonological training, the child participates in segmentation exercises such as rhyming, initial sound matching, and counting syllables and phonemes. The rationale for this method is that, in part, breakdown is the result of poor phonological representation of the word. Phonologically based treatment that focuses on words that begin with the same phoneme and words that sound alike can reduce semantic substitutions (McGregor, 1994). The child is trained to think about the first sound in the word when retrieving.

Perceptual training involves imagery activities, such as simultaneous picture and auditory exposure, visualization with eyes closed, and silent name repetition. This procedure progresses to matching pictures to a "memorized" sample of names.

The facilitator can help a child note perceptual and functional features and attributes that determine how members are categorized. The child with LLD will have particular difficulty abstracting salient features and, therefore, will have difficulty forming categories based on these features. One mediational strategy might be to teach the child to ask a set of questions to establish an association between a new item and something familiar. Questions might include the following (Parente & Hermann, 1996, p. 50):

What does it look (sound, smell, taste) like?
What does it mean the same thing as?
What groups does it belong to?
Who is it commonly associated with?

It is important that children note a similar attribute on more than one object. Otherwise, children may begin to associate certain attributes with specific items. For example, several very different objects may be described as *wet*. This kind of task naturally leads to categorization. Attributes should appear also in many different linguistic forms.

Categorical identification by the facilitator seems to be the best cue for recall. By naming the category, the facilitator can help the child locate the desired word. Partial word cues also may help the child and are less confusing than synonyms. Sentence completion and nonverbal, gestural cues are also aids. Even the most effective strategies have limitations, suggesting that some children have severe deficiencies in the size, elaboration, or organization of their lexicons (McGregor & Windsor, 1996).

Speed and accuracy of retrieval are important. In general, retrieval speed and accuracy are correlated (German, 1986/89, 1990; Guilford & Nawojczyk, 1988; Wiegel-Crump & Dennis, 1986). In children developing typically, speed and accuracy improve with maturity. Retrieval using picture cues is easier than naming to a descriptive cue. Naming to a rhyme is the most difficult (Wiegel-Crump & Dennis, 1986). Several retrieval strategies are listed in Table 11.9. In intervention, retrieval units should move from single words to discourse.

As mentioned previously, it is important to keep in mind the "What's the point?" criterion. The relationship of responses to naming exercises and word finding in conversation is unknown. Overall, responses to pictures may be of relatively little value. At a minimum, it is essential that training include a strong conversational element to ensure generalization of word-finding skills (Dennis, 1992).

It may be helpful to teach the child strategies for circumventing blocks (German, 1992). Synonyms, category names, and multiword descriptions may enable the child to continue the conversation and to work through the word-retrieval difficulty. Compensatory programming, such as modifying classroom tasks, also may aid the child with word-retrieval difficulties (Table 11.10). It is essential that those in the child's home and classroom modify expectations and cue the child in the most advantageous manner.

Comprehension

Very young children, lacking good word definitions, use their knowledge of familiar event sequences to structure their responses (Paul, 1990). Familiar events provide scripts that aid comprehension.

TABLE 11.9   **Word-retrieval strategies**

Retrieval strategies		Descriptions
Attribute cuing	Phonemic cuing	The initial sound, vowel nucleus, digraph, or syllable is used to cue the target word.
	Semantic cuing	The category name or function is used to cue the target word.
	Graphemic cuing	The graphic schema is used to cue the target word.
	Imagery cuing	A revisualization of the referent is used to cue the target word.
	Gesture cuing	The motor schema of the target word action is used to cue the target word.
Associate cuing (story for book)		An intermediate word is used to cue the target word.
Semantic alternates	Synonym/category substitutions	Semantic components (synonym or category words) are substituted for the target word.
	Multiword substitutions	Semantic components (functions or descriptions) are substituted for the target word.
Reflective pausing		Constructive use of pausing is used to reduce inaccurate competitive responses.

Remedial strategies		Descriptions
Stabilization of phonological specifications	Rehearsal	Students practice saying or writing the target words five times alone and then in five different sentences.
	Rhythm + rehearsal	Each syllable is marked with a tap during the above rehearsal of the target word.
	Segmenting + rehearsal	A line is drawn between each syllable during the above rehearsal of the target word.
Rapid naming		Students rapidly say names of and phrases with target words until their response time is reduced.

Source: German, D. J. (1992). Word-finding intervention for children and adolescents. *Topics in Language Disorders, 13*(1), 33–50. Reprinted with permission.

Even later, when children and adults rely on lexical and syntactic cues, it is still easier to comprehend information in familiar events and contexts.

In early preschool, the child matures from reliance on the immediate context to reliance on stored experience for interpretation. This stored experience is called *world knowledge.* The child uses world knowledge to structure a "probable event" strategy of interpretation. Only gradually does the child gain the ability to rely on word order.

By late preschool, ages 3½ to 5, word order is used more consistently for interpretation (Tager-Flusberg, 1989). Linguistic knowledge becomes the preferred comprehension strategy, although no clearly dominant strategy is evident. Preschoolers still rely more readily on contextual knowledge.

TABLE 11.10   Classroom oral questioning modifications for word-retrieval problems

Word-Finding Profile	Content Areas	Classroom Activity	Recommended Modifications for Teacher	New Materials
Difficulty retrieving specific words: inaccurate namer	All	Oral questioning	1. Use multiple-choice frames 2. Accept volunteer participation only 3. Provide target word cues (e.g., initial sound, syllable) 4. Use questions that require yes/no or true /false response	Advance organizer
Difficulty retrieving specific words: slow namer	All	Oral questioning	1. Prime student for questioning 2. Give student additional time to answer 3. Use multiple-choice frames 4. Use questions that require yes/no or true /false response	List of possible questions

Source: German, D. J. (1992). Word-finding intervention for children and adolescents. *Topics in Language Disorders, 13*(1), 33–50. Reprinted with permission.

It is not until ages 5 or 6 that children use syntactic and lexical interpretation more consistently (Keller-Cohen, 1987). They still make errors, of course, usually by ignoring clausal boundaries and interruptions in the flow (Wallach & Miller, 1988). By ages 7 to 9, children are more sensitive to boundaries, embedding, and temporal connectives.

Humor in the form of jokes, a school-age development, requires extensive use of linguistic interpretation. The linguistic incongruity in the punch line must be understood in order for the joke to be funny.

Children with a range of LIs perform similarly on language comprehension tasks (Bishop, 1982). They exhibit poorer comprehension than their peers developing typically (D. Bernstein, 1986; Nippold, 1985; Spector, 1990). In general, there is a greater tendency among school-age children with LI to rely solely on word-order strategy and to retain this strategy longer than do children developing typically (F. Roth & Spekman, 1989a).

Preschool children with LI overuse word-order strategies earlier and use of world knowledge less than their peers (Lord, 1985; Paul, Fisher, & Cohen, 1988; Tager-Flusberg, 1985). As a result, the comprehension strategy is less flexible and there are fewer alternative strategies than in children developing typically (Paul, 1989a, 1989b). It is not surprising that higher interpretative skills, such as those used to comprehend humor, are often not observed in children with severe LI.

Even mature language users rely on world knowledge to some extent (Milosky, 1990). *Comprehension* consists of both decoding the syntactic and semantic information and interpreting that information based on the linguistic and nonlinguistic context and world knowledge. While comprehension intervention is a worthy goal in and of itself, I should caution that training word recognition alone does not ensure production of newly learned words (Kiernan & Gray, 1998).

The goal of intervention is to teach the child to retrieve relevant word and world knowledge as a comprehension aid and to help the child decide how and what to remember from what he or she hears or reads (Trabasso & Van Den Broek, 1985). Comprehension and memory are aided by familiar, meaningful contexts; thus, intervention should occur within familiar routines and locations (Milosky, 1990). The degree and type of experience the child has with events strongly shapes his or her expectations and, thus, comprehension. Meaningful activities are more comprehensible; they make more sense.

The level of involvement also affects memory and comprehension (Lehnert & Vine, 1987; Miall, 1989). The more involved the child, the more he or she comprehends and recalls. Songs, nursery rhymes, and finger play can be used to help the child make active associations between words and the nonlinguistic context (Paul, 1990). The repetitive nature and limited focus of such activities help shape expectations and aid comprehension and memory. In "Where Is Thumbkin?" the structure is *where…here* with the phrases repeated several times. Similarly, "Farmer-in-the-Dell" uses an *agent + action + object* format in each verse (*The farmer picks a wife…*) (Paul, 1990).

Finally, comprehension intervention should be pleasurable. Fun activities keep children engaged, a necessity for comprehension and comprehension training. Involvement is fostered by facilitator feedback. A pleasing manner encourages responding and making use of the feedback (Paul, 1990).

Initial comprehension training may need to be very concrete and highly contextual. Preschool children benefit more from direct labeling instruction than from less direct use of narratives (Kouri, 1994). The use of gestures and a slower rate of talking by the language facilitator also enhances comprehension by young children (Weismer & Hesketh, 1993). As children approach school age, training should become more decontextualized, similar to many of the literate activities found in school.

Comprehension training might begin with recall from pictures or objects and progress to literal recall of one or more details from verbal sources. Gradually, the SLP can require the child to recall more details. Later, the child can detail these in sequence, possibly using sequential pictures, photographs of past events, or comic books as aids. Daily events can provide a script to aid comprehension. Next, the SLP can require the child to relate cause and effect from familiar or recently read narratives. Once able to reconstruct these relationships, the child can begin to make inferences, to draw conclusions, and to predict outcomes from stories, riddles, and jokes. Finally, the child can learn to synthesize information and create subjective summaries of the meanings of narratives, TV shows, or movies.

To assist comprehension, the SLP can shape question-response strategies by manipulating the semantic content, complexity, context, and function (Parnell & Amerman, 1983). The therapy process moves from simple, context-embedded questions to the use of questions in more abstract contexts, while controlling the length of the questions to highlight semantic content (Moeller et al., 1986). In the first stage, the facilitator attempts to build awareness and enhance emerging skills by using topics of high interest as the question contexts. The facilitator concentrates on establishing repeatable responses to yes/no questions by using a second adult as a model, multiple-choice alternatives ("Did the ball roll under the sofa? Yes or no?"), visual cues to signal that a response is desired, and the child's natural, everyday contexts.

In stage two, early-developing *wh-* question forms become the targets, and yes/no questions are used to highlight the semantic content desired. Take, for example, the question, "What is the girl wearing on her head?" A nonresponse, an inappropriate response, or an inaccurate response might be followed by "Is she wearing a shoe on her head?" If the child responds negatively, the prompt would be "That's right, what is she wearing on her head?" Print, pictures, or signs can be used to highlight the *wh-* words and, thus, emphasize the information desired. These prompts can be faded gradually. In the third stage, new *wh-* forms are added systematically. In the final stage, stimulus content is shifted gradually from concrete, predictable, factually based academic topics to more abstract, less predictable conversational ones.

School-age children might manipulate objects or pictures and match them with the sentences heard (Wallach & Miller, 1988). For example, the child might be told to place a small red ball on top of a large yellow box. Similarly, the child might select a picture described by the facilitator from among a set of pictures. Written cues also could be used.

The child also might match sentences with similar meaning. Synonyms can be introduced. Metalinguistic skills can be enhanced by tasks in which the child judges similarity and difference among sentences (van Kleeck, 1984).

Figurative Language

Figurative language consists of idioms, metaphors, similes, and proverbs. Idioms are a form of figurative language that is particularly troublesome to comprehend for school-age children with LI and for CLD children (Lutzer, 1988; Seidenberg & Bernstein, 1986). The most common error is literal interpretation. Although idioms are a concise, colorful, and intriguing way to express complex meanings, they are very diverse and, thus, difficult to learn as a group. Idioms vary along several continuums, including single-words-to-clauses, colloquial-to-formal, and concrete-to-abstract.

Difficulty with idioms can affect classroom comprehension because of their frequent occurrence (Nippold, 1991). Approximately 11.5 percent of teacher utterances contain at least one idiom, with a range from 4.7 percent in kindergarten to 20.3 percent in eighth grade (Lazar et al., 1989). Similarly, 6.7 percent of the sentences in textbooks contain idioms, with a range from 6 percent in third grade to 9.7 percent in eighth (Nippold, 1990).

The meanings of idioms are inferred gradually from repeated exposure in context. In addition, idiom learning requires metalinguistic skills and is closely associated with familiarity with the idiom and skills in reading and listening comprehension (Nippold, Moran, & Schwarz, 2001). Children with LI may lack a strategy for determining meaning. Some common idioms are listed in Table 11.11.

Intervention should begin with comprehension of transparent or easily decipherable idioms. Narratives may be the best teaching milieu because of the contextual support (Nippold, 1991). The child can be instructed prior to the narrative that it will contain a certain idiom and that he or she will be able to figure out the meaning from the story. Questions can be used throughout the narrative to help the child attend to important information. Answers can be redirected to ensure that the child is attending to salient points. After repeated exposure and the child's correct interpretation, he or she can be encouraged to invent his or her own narratives that illustrate use of the idiom. Finally, conversationally appropriate use can be discussed and role-played.

Proverbs depend on their context to be good advice. Sometimes *he who hesitates is lost,* but at other times, it's best to *look before you leap.* The context in which the idiom is used also facilitates

TABLE 11.11   Common American English idioms

Topics

Animals
    A bull in a china shop
    As stubborn as a mule
    Going to the dogs
    Playing possum

    A fly in the ointment
    Clinging like a leech
    Grinning like a Cheshire cat

Body Parts
    On the tip of my tongue
    Raise eyebrows
    Turn the other cheek

    Put your best foot forward
    Turn heads

Clothing
    Dressed to kill
    Hot under the collar
    Wear the pants in the family

    Fit like a glove
    Strait laced

Colors
    Grey area
    Once in a blue moon
    Tickled pink

    Has a yellow streak
    Red letter day
    True blue

Foods
    Eat crow
    Humble pie
    That takes the cake

    A finger in every pie
    In a jam

Games and Sports
    Ace up my sleeve
    Cards are stacked against me
    Got lost in the shuffle
    Keep your head above water
    Paddle your own canoe

    Ballpark figure
    Get to first base
    Keep the ball rolling
    On the rebound

Plants
    Heard it through the grapevine
    Resting on his laurels
    Shrinking violet

    No bed of roses
    Shaking like a leaf
    Withered on the vine

Vehicles
    Fix your wagon
    Like ships passing in the night
    On the wagon

    Don't rock the boat
    Missed the boat
    Take a back seat

Tools and Work
    Bury the hatchet
    Has an axe to grind
    Hit the nail on the head
    Jockey for position
    Throw a monkey wrench into it

    Doctor the books
    Has a screw loose
    Hit the roof
    Nursing his wounds
    Sober as a judge

Weather
    Calm before the storm
    Haven't the foggiest
    Steal her thunder

    Come rain or shine
    Right as rain
    Throw caution to the wind

Source: Compiled from Clark (1990); Gibbs (1987); Gulland & Hinds-Howell (1986).

understanding. The ability to explain proverbs lags behind the ability to select an appropriate interpretation from a list of possible meanings (Nippold, 2000).

The ability to interpret and use proverbs develops during late elementary school and continues into adulthood and is related to reading and metalinguistic abilities. With this in mind, the SLP is advised to teach proverb interpretation within the context of reading (Nippold, 2000). Working in small groups, adolescents can discuss interpretations. The SLP uses structured modeling and practice strategies, such as the use of contextual cues, questions, and analysis, to help teens become independent learners. Through both asking and answering factual and inferential questions, adolescents learn to interpret the context. Analysis of the main characters' motivations, goals, actions, and feelings further aid interpretation. Finally, adolescents need help determining the relationship between the proverb and their own lives.

Training for proverbs can follow a similar form. In general, concrete proverbs are easier to interpret than abstract, and familiar easier than unfamiliar (Nippold & Haq, 1996).

Microcomputers can be used to teach figurative language comprehension. Computers have special advantages, including inherent motivation, active involvement, nonjudgmental feedback, and an independent, self-paced mode of operation (Fitch, 1986; Sanders, 1986).

Unfortunately, commercially available software does not reflect current developmental knowledge, does not offer a clear rationale for instructional methods, and does not offer comprehensive instruction (Nippold, Schwarz, & Lewis, 1992). In addition, these programs provide for little or no customizing and offer only minimal use of animation, graphics, synthesized speech, or sound effects that might aid children with reading problems. At best, current computer software can complement intervention by the SLP (Nippold, Schwarz, & Lewis, 1992). Each SLP should analyze software carefully to determine the best way to use it. In addition to concerns for content and instructional methodology, the SLP should consider the compatibility of computer-based intervention and his or her teaching style.

Verbal Working Memory

Although the depth and breadth of this topic is beyond the scope of this text and the topic fits only loosely—if at all—under semantics and comprehension, I would be remiss were I not to mention verbal working memory given the deficits mentioned in Chapter 2, especially for children with SLI. Verbal working memory can be strengthened in several ways. For example, the SLP can help children focus on a task by explaining its purpose, importance, and what it will accomplish (Ylvisaker & DeBonis, 2000).

The SLP will need to slow the rate of presentation and decrease the size of processing units. These can both be increased gradually as training progresses. The SLP can use verbal repetition tasks in which the number of syllables and words are gradually increased. Unrelated words are theoretically more difficult than words in a sentence, the more typical conversational processing task. For the child who is not attending or is distracted, however, syntactic cues may be missed or go unused.

In any listening task, including conversational and classroom use, the child will need to bring past knowledge to bear. The SLP can help the child build a knowledge base by using tasks that are familiar to the child and/or revolve around a theme. The child and SLP can discuss key words and relationships prior to beginning.

Through explanation of the importance of syntactic cues and the use of cloze procedures, the SLP can help the child attend to these features. In the cloze procedure, the child must process the sentence in real time to be able to complete it. Verbal absurdities can also be used and the child asked to explain them. The SLP must be careful not to exceed the processing capabilities or the language abilities of the child.

The use of linguistic cues of many types—such as phonemic, syntactic, semantic, and pragmatic—can be integrated and explained. Through the use of successively longer sentences, the SLP can manipulate cues to aid in the interpretation of cloze sentences. For example, the SLP might present a short sentence such as "We eat _____." Children working in small groups brainstorm possible words to finish the sentence. In like fashion, the SLP presents alternative choices, and the children discuss why these are acceptable or not based on the information given. Obviously, in this example, several words are acceptable.

After completing the discussion, the SLP presents the same sentence or a very similar one with more information, such as "We eat at _____," and the exercise continues. The importance of verbal working memory is very evident, especially as the sentences become longer.

Processing within actual use contexts is the goal of intervention. Each session should provide real conversational activities within which the SLP can monitor each child's behavior and aid participation.

Syntax and Morphology

Although language use improves syntax, the reverse is not true. It is important, therefore, that syntactic training be as conversational as possible.

When language forms or constructions are taught outside a communication context, the forms may be mastered without the knowledge of how to express ideas within and across these forms (J. Norris & Bruning, 1988). In addition, utterances produced in context strengthen cohesion and relationships across linguistic units.

The linguistic techniques discussed in Chapter 10 are particularly applicable to syntactic and morphologic training. Methods requiring an imitative or spontaneous response by the child are reported to be superior to those presenting only a model, although focused stimulation can be very effective (Connell & Stone, 1992). Feedback is also very important.

During training, it is important that the facilitator control for vocabulary and/or sentence length, especially when teaching new structures. If the facilitator changes too many variables at one time, it may confuse the child or make the task too complex for successful completion.

The facilitator should be careful not to require metalinguistic skills beyond the child's abilities. Although recognition and comprehension usually precede production, judgments of correct usage do not. Judging a sentence to be grammatically correct is a metalinguistic skill that develops in the middle elementary school years. Asking children to form sentences with selected words also requires metalinguistic skill. In short, any task that requires the child to manipulate language abstractly takes some degree of metalinguistic skill.

The development of syntactic and morphologic forms is well documented and provides a guide for intervention. In the following section, hierarchies for intervention with several different forms are discussed. The purpose is to offer general guidelines for the ordering of structures to be taught.

Just as development is a gradual process, especially for older children and adolescents, so too is intervention. It may be unrealistic to expect error-free production following teaching (Nippold, 1993). Some low-frequency forms are difficult even for adults.

Morphology

Inflectional suffixes develop early and lend themselves well to teaching within a conversational milieu. Other morphemes may best be taught in a more explicit manner first, beginning with derivational suffixes, followed by prefixes (Rubin, 1988). Explicit training is not recommended for preschool children. The unique learning style of children with SLI also may make explicit rule learning less effective (Swisher, Restrepo, Plante, & Lowell, 1995). Common bound morphemes are listed in Appendix E. Because derivational relationships are complex and irregular, memorization is of little value as a learning tool (Adams, 1990). It is essential that the child understand the changes in meaning that are occurring.

Although data for school-age morphological development are scarce, some suggestions for the method of teaching do exist. These are presented in Table 11.12. Training should begin with the most transparent and most common morphemes and proceed toward those that are more complex and cause phonological and orthographic or spelling changes.

The school-age child should be taught to analyze from derived words to word stems and to synthesize from word stems to derived words (Moats & Smith, 1992). Meaning relationships should be emphasized. The metalinguistic skill of awareness of word structure is essential to the analysis of complex structures. These skills should be taught and used at all levels from word imitation to conversational use.

Young school-age children who read and have some metalinguistic skills can be taught to differentiate word structures (Rubin, 1988; Rubin et al., 1991). Words can be contrasted on the basis of structure and rhyming, as in *money-funny, wise-pies,* and *pinned-wind,* or on small structural changes that affect meaning, as in winner-winter.

Middle-school children can be taught complex derivational morphology (Moats & Smith, 1992). Training can occur in both the oral and written modes. Training for middle-school children also should include Latin and Greek roots because of the frequency of these in science, math, and social studies (Henry, 1990).

Verb Tensing

Although the typical 2-year-old has a notion of action words, the child does not understand the many forms these verbs can take; nor does the child comprehend other verbs that express notions such as state.

TABLE 11.12   Suggested order for teaching morphemes

1. Establish awareness of syllables and sounds. Practice counting both.
2. Identify roots and affixes. Practice pronouncing and defining roots and affixes in contrasting words that are similar in sound or appearance, such as *happy-sunny,* and *include-conclude.*
3. Generate a formal definition in the form "A/An *X* is a (superordinate category) that (restrictive attributes)."
4. Discuss relationships with other words.
5. Use words in meaningful contexts and in analogies and cloze activities.
6. Use words in reading activities if appropriate.
7. Introduce spelling and spelling rules if appropriate.

Source: Adapted from Moats & Smith (1992).

Verb learning takes several years, with the rules being mastered slowly. Verbs are very difficult for children with LI, partly because of the many ways they are treated syntactically and morphologically.

The teaching of verb tensing can be adapted easily to everyday activities in which children discuss what they are doing at present, did previously, or will do in the future. Art projects and building toys are especially useful. Appendix G offers a number of activities for targeting verb tensing.

Training should begin with protoverbs, such as *up, in, off, down, no, there, bye-bye,* and *night-night.* These verblike words usually are used in relation to some familiar action sequence. General purpose verbs, such as *do,* might be targeted next.

More specific action verbs should be introduced in their uninflected or unmarked form. The facilitator can cue by asking what a child is doing or by directing the child, "Tell X to (verb)." To facilitate learning, action word meanings might be taught with specific actions or objects. Children first describe their own actions, not those of others. While playing, the facilitator can hide his or her eyes or turn away from the child and ask, "What are you doing?" Although the cue requires an *-ing* ending on the verb in the response ("Eating"), this form is not required of the child at this level of training. I usually simplify my question to "What do?" The response is "Eat" or "Eat cookie."

Familiar event sequences, such as play or routines, facilitate action verb usage because of the mental representations of these sequences that children possess (K. Chapman & Terrell, 1988). These event sequences enable the child to focus on the communication, rather than on the extralinguistic elements of the event (Constable, 1986).

Once the child is able to form simple two- and three-word utterances with an action word, as in "Doggie eat meat," the present progressive verb form can be introduced without the auxiliary verb. The SLP can model this form through self-talk and parallel talk. The SLP can cue the child to use this form with "What's doggie doing?" or "What's he doing?" Pronouns, such as *he,* must be used with caution at this level because many children with LI use very few.

At this level of training, the child only needs to deal with the immediate context. A sense of time beyond the present, however, is essential for further verb training.

The SLP can use a few high-usage irregular past tense verbs, such as *ate, drank, ran, fell, sat, came,* and *went,* to introduce the past rather quickly and to forestall overgeneralization of the regular past *-ed,* the next target form. With both past tense forms, storytelling, show-and-tell, and recounting past events are good vehicles for training and use. Initially, the facilitator can ask the child a question like "What did you eat (or other action verb)?" to teach the child the form. When the child responds with "Cookie" or another entity, the facilitator can reply, "What did you do with cookie?" Later, the sequence can begin with the question, "What did you do?" The child responds, "Ate cookie," or, "I ate a cookie." It is important that question cues not violate pragmatic contingency, which requires that questions make sense. Facilitators should not ask questions to which they know the answers. This strategy is achieved easily by asking about unobserved actions or having a puppet ask questions.

Before training additional verb forms, the SLP should introduce singular and plural nouns and subjective pronouns because the child will need these for the third-person singular present tense *-s* marker and for present tense forms of the verb *to be.*

The SLP can introduce the third-person marker with singular and plural nouns. Subjective pronouns can be introduced gradually. He or she can elicit the third person marker with such cues as "What does he do every day (all of the time)?" or such fill-ins as "Every day, the girls (verb)," or "All of the time, he (verbs)."

The SLP should not target the phonological variations of the *-ed* marker (/d/, /t/, and /ɪd/) and those of the third-person *-s* (/s/, /z/, and /ɪz/) in initial training. When the marker is first being emphasized in training, the SLP should use one form exclusively, such as the /d/ or the /s/. As the emphasis on the marker becomes more natural or lessens, its cognate can be introduced without any fanfare. Be careful: it's not the "d" or "s" sound, but /d/ and /s/.

Facilitators should not expect the child to understand the phonological rules relative to ending sounds and added markers. Usually de-emphasis of the marker's sound will allow the child to produce naturally either two voiced or two unvoiced sounds at the end of each word. The /Id/ and /Iz/ markers should be avoided until much later. Children developing typically usually employ the cognates by late preschool. It takes them a few more years to acquire the /Id/ and /Iz/ forms.

Use of pronouns enables the child to begin training on the verb *to be* both as an auxiliary verb and as the copula or main verb. Because the form is *noun (or pronoun) + be + X,* in which the X can be a noun, adjective, adverb, or verb with *-ing,* these two forms can be trained together, thus facilitating carryover. The distinction between auxiliaries and main verbs is too complex to try to explain here. As a rule, the uncontractible form is taught first, the uncontracted contractible next, and the contracted contractible form last.

The verb *to be* is a "regularist's" nightmare, with different forms for various persons and tenses. Therefore, different forms should be introduced slowly. Children developing typically generally learn the *is* form first.

Other auxiliary verbs, such as *do,* also can be introduced to facilitate the development of more mature negatives and interrogatives. The negative form of *do* can be elicited with "Tell X (some person) not to *verb.*" *Do, can,* and *will/would* appear first in the negative form in the language development of children developing typically. In other words, *can't, don't,* and *won't* appear before *can, do,* and *will/would.*

Using the present progressive form *be + going,* the child can begin to form early future tense forms. Facilitators should be willing to accept this form because it marks the concept (Bliss, 1987).

Training should begin with *going to noun,* as in "going to the zoo," before *going to verb,* as in "going to eat." The former is more concrete and does not require use of an infinitive phrase, such as *to eat.* The more mature *will* form of the future tense can be introduced later.

Guidelines for training *can, do,* and *will/would* include the following (Bliss, 1987):

1. Allow some delay between mastery of one form and introduction of another in order to avoid confusion.
2. Use self-reference in the form of either first-person pronouns or the child's name initially because this is the first referent associated with these forms.
3. Link these forms with actions because this is the first association of children developing normally.
4. Initially, use short utterances with the word at the end in order to increase saliency ("Can you jump?" "Yes, I *can.*") Use the popular Bob the Builder refrain "Can we do it?" "Yes, we *can.*"
5. Provide meaningful situations in which the concepts and forms serve some purpose.

An explanation of guideline 4 is in order. Children with SLI have particular difficulty with verbs, verb endings, tenses, and verb phrases (Hadley, 1998a). These children are more likely to use an auxiliary verb if it is included in the preceding sentence, but both the form and location must be considered (Leonard, Miller, Deevy, Rauf, Gerber, & Charest, 2002). Although the exact form of the verb does not need to be in the preceding sentence, some forms do facilitate others. For example, use of *are* facilitates *is.* The sentence-final position (Yes, we *can*) also facilitates learning, but the sentence-initial position as in questions (*Can* we do it?) does not (Fey & Frome Loeb, 2002).

With the addition of the future tense, the child now can discuss the past, present (progressive), and future. Language activities can now include planning, execution, and review.

After teaching other auxiliary verbs, the SLP can introduce *modal auxiliaries*. These are helping verbs that express mood or feeling, such as *could, would, should, might,* and *may.* The shades of meaning across the various modal auxiliaries are often very subtle, and the facilitator should not expect mature usage for some time. Most adults have difficulty with the distinction between *may* and *might.*

Finally, the SLP may wish to target verb particles, multiword units, such as *pick up* and *come over,* that function as verbs. Although verb particles emerge in early preschool years, they are not fully acquired and differentiated from prepositions until age 5 (Goodluck, 1986; Tomasello, 1987; Wagner & Rice, 1988).

The particle—*up, down, in, on, off*—may either precede or follow a noun phrase, as in *kick **over** the pumpkin* or *kick the pumpkin **over***, or follow pronominal noun phrases, as in *kick it **over***. Prepositions, in contrast, always precede noun phrases, even those with pronouns, as in *over the box* or *over it*. The acquisition of verb particles is especially difficult for children with LI, possibly because they are unstressed units and may appear in either position vis-à-vis the noun phrase (Watkins & Rice, 1991).

Particles should be introduced with a limited set of verbs used regularly by the child. It might be helpful to use position cues to teach the distinction between particles and prepositions. Particles could be taught following the noun phrase and prepositions preceding. Particles preceding the noun phrase could be introduced later.

Procedures for teaching verb tensing should make sense both semantically and pragmatically (Bliss, 1987). Examples are "I bet you can/can't. Mother, may I?," asking the child to perform various tasks ("Will you please…?"), problem solving ("What will happen if…?" "What might happen if…?"), and role-playing ("What should we do if…?"). Many children's books—discussed in the next chapter—lend themselves to predicting tasks.

Pronouns

Pronouns are extremely difficult to learn because the user must have syntactic, semantic, and pragmatic knowledge. In general, the SLP should teach the underlying concept first and should model appropriate use for the child. Use of pronouns requires an understanding of the semantic distinctions of number, person, and case. The noun in the sentence generally determines use, but the conversational context is also a determinant.

Several parent and teacher practices that make language easier for the child to process may, however, confuse pronoun learning and use. Overuse of nouns or of the royal *we* (e.g., "*We* are tired" to mean that the speaker is tired) model inappropriate use.

Children often avoid making an overt pronominal error by overusing nouns. This mistake can be avoided somewhat in training by limiting the number of referents. For example, if the SLP uses too many characters in a story format, the child may overuse nouns in an attempt to remember who is being discussed. Using nouns can help children use their memory, which is somewhat more limited than that of adults.

In general, the first person *I* should be trained before the second person *you,* followed by the third-person *he/she.* This developmental order reflects increasing complexity with shifting reference and the number of possible referents.

Deictic terms, such as *I* and *you,* are difficult to teach, as noted in the semantics portion of this chapter. A second SLP, facilitator, or child can serve as a model to avoid confusing the child's frame of reference.

Development by children developing typically would suggest that facilitators target subjective pronouns (*I, you, he, she, it, we, you, they*) before objective pronouns (*me, you, him, her, it, us, you, them*). Possessive pronouns would follow (*my, your, his, her, its, our, your, their*), and, finally, reflexive pronouns (*myself, yourself, himself, herself, itself, ourselves, yourselves, themselves*). Although there are exceptions to this hierarchy, it approximates typical development (Haas & Owens, 1985). Subjective and objective case can be taught by location in the sentence.

This hierarchy and the error patterns of young children suggest that reflexives might be trained initially as possessives (*my self*). The exceptions (*himself* and *themselves*) can be introduced later.

One exception to the suggested hierarchy might be third-person singular pronouns. It appears easier for children to learn *her-hers-herself* than *him-his-himself,* probably because of the consistency in the feminine gender (Haas & Owens, 1985). The three feminine pronouns might be trained as a unit before the masculine.

Conversational training with so many varied forms can be very confusing. Initially, the facilitator must target carefully the desired pronouns and practice cues to elicit these forms.

Plurals

To learn plurals, the child must have the concepts of *one* and *more than one.* Numbers or words such as *many* and *more* may serve as initial aids. Begin with comparisions of one item versus many. Cue with "Show me (Touch) more," then respond, "Yes, more block*s*!"

As with the past-tense *-ed* and third-person *-s* markers, the facilitator should not expect mastery of the phonological rules until later. Again, training should begin with either the /s/ or the /z/, gradually introduce the other, and wait some time before introducing /Iz/.

The SLP may wish to introduce a few common irregular plurals to forestall overgeneralization. As mentioned in the semantics section of this chapter, words such as *water* and *sand* are not irregular plurals and present a special case, especially with the modifiers *any* and *much.*

Articles

Articles are extremely difficult for children to learn because of the two different operations they perform. Articles may mark definite (*the*) and indefinite (*a*) reference and also new (*a*) and old (*the*) information. When in doubt, preschool and early elementary school children tend to overuse *the.*

The SLP can use objects and pictures and instruct the child to describe what is seen ("A puppy"). Next, the SLP and the child can describe each object or picture, as in the following exchange:

Facilitator: Tell me what you see.

Child: A duck.

Facilitator: A duck? Let's see. I can tell you that *the duck is yellow. What* can you tell me?

Child: The duck is swimming.

The *an* should not be introduced until the child is functioning at the early elementary school level.

Once pronouns have been introduced, the facilitator can switch back and forth between pronouns and articles, as in the following:

Facilitator: Here's *a* puppy. What can you tell me about *him?*

Child: He has a cold nose.

Facilitator: Who does?

Child: The puppy.

The possibilities are endless within a conversational paradigm. Remember that many Asian languages don't have articles so this feature may be especially difficult for some children with LEP.

Prepositions

Although nine prepositions (*at, by, for, from, in, of, on, to,* and *with*) account for 90 percent of preposition use, these nine have a combined total of approximately 250 meanings. No wonder some children with LI have difficulty with this class of words. Children with LEP will find prepositions especially difficult. Prepositions are discussed briefly in the semantics section under relational terms.
    Development of prepositions suggests the following hierarchy of training:

in, on, inside, out of
under, next to
between, around, beside, in front of
in back of, behind

Such terms as *in front of* and *behind* should be trained initially by using fronted objects, for example, a television. Nonfronted objects can be introduced later.
    In general, children will learn more easily when real objects are used in training. Actual manipulation of these objects, however, may interfere with learning. Such experience may be better at the level of conceptual rather than linguistic training. Spatial and directional aspects should be trained with a number of objects and/or examples so that the child understands the concept separately from any specific referent. Variety may preclude the child's focusing on the objects and referents in favor of the relationship. Large muscle activities also can be used as children go *in* and *out* of boxes or closets, *on* and *off* tables and chairs, and the like. Thus, the child's body becomes a referent (Messick, 1988). Spatial terms may be taught in a naturalistic context of play with puppets, dolls, action figures, or the child's body. In one lesson, I played the tiger who pursued a preschool child *in* the cage, *out* of the cage, and so on.

Word Order and Sentence Types

Word order and different sentence types are best trained within conversational give-and-take, although school-age children and adolescents also may benefit from both oral and written training (Nippold, 1993). Miniature linguistic systems have been used to teach word combinations (Bunce, Ruder, & Ruder, 1985). In these systems, a matrix is developed with one class of words on the ordinate and another on the abscissa. The child need not learn all possible combinations to acquire the rule. Good generalization to untrained combinations has been reported. Figure 11.4 presents some sample matrices and the teaching models that have been effective.

Noun phrases initially can be expanded in isolation. A question-answer paradigm will enable the SLP to target specific aspects of the noun phrase (How many…, Where…, Can you describe…?). Once placed within a sentence, the noun phrase can be expanded in the object position, followed by the subject position. The order of noun modifiers is discussed in Chapter 7 under analysis of the noun phrase (Table 7.17).

Adjectives can be taught in contrastive situations in which the child must distinguish between two objects that differ along one parameter, as in *big ball* and *little ball* (Kamhi & Nelson, 1988). Incorrect or inadequate adjective use in conversation would result in misunderstanding and the misinterpretation of the child's message. In a similar fashion, post-noun modifiers can be used with objects in different locations, as in *the ball in the box* and *the ball on the table.*

Verb phrases and accompanying clause types should be chosen carefully. Specific verbs that clearly illustrate transitive and intransitive clauses might be chosen. Equitive verb phrases and the use of *be* can be trained in elliptical answers to questions, as in *He is* and *We are* responses to questions such as "Who is at the zoo?" The uncontractable form of the verb is very salient in this format, as in *he is* or *they are.* A similar method of teaching transitive and intransitive verbs can be used to teach auxiliary verbs, as in "Who is eating?" and "Who can jump?" (Kamhi & Nelson, 1988).

Using both oral and written techniques, the SLP can aid later-school-age children and adolescents to form longer sentences and more concise sentences and to use more low-frequency structures

	Cookie	Cake	Pudding	Pie	Bread
Eat	X	X	X	X	X
Bake	X				
Mix	X				
Want	X				
Give	X				

	Pet	Dog	Cat	Horse	Ferret
Feed	X	X			
Bathe		X	X		
Groom			X	X	
Walk				X	X
Brush	X				X

Verbs on one axis are combined with nouns on the other to form short phrases. Each combination taught is marked with an *X.* Rule learning will generalize to the untrained combinations.

FIGURE 11.4   Miniature linguistic systems.

and intersentential cohesion (Nippold, 1993). Compound and complex sentences can be formed from the youth's own simpler sentences. Subordinate clauses, such as *who is driving the red car,* can be transformed later into more concise phrases, such as *The girl **driving the red car** is from Iowa.* Low-frequency structures, such as apposition (*Mary **my sister**...or John **the psychologist** will...*), complex noun phrases (*the large red dog with the bushy tail* or *teachers such as Ms. Meeker or Ms. Lilius*), perfect aspect (*has been verbing*), and passive voice (*The cat was chased by the dog*). Finally, intersentential cohesion can be attempted by using adverbial conjuncts such as *therefore* and *however.* Acquisition is often very gradual. Less common types, such as *conversely* and *moreover,* should be introduced to mature language users.

Several strategies discussed in Chapter 10 can be used very effectively to strengthen word order. For example, expansion can provide a more mature model than the child's utterance, and build-up/ break-down strategies help the child analyze relationships.

Table 7.16 presents some guidelines on the acquisitional order of certain sentence types. By the time most children developing typically begin school, they are using adultlike declaratives, imperatives, and *wh-* and yes/no interrogatives in both the positive and negative forms. Later developing forms include clausal and multiple embedding and conjoining, passive voice, and tag questions.

Summary

Although the SLP cannot always use all elements of the functional model simultaneously, he or she usually can use several elements within any given teaching situation. The target selection certainly should reflect the child's overall communication needs. Facilitators within the environment, everyday activities, and conversational give-and-take usually can be adapted to the individual child and language target(s). Some training, such as phonological intervention, may necessitate the initial use of structured approaches. Generalization to conversational use, however, will require incorporating these settings into the training. The SLP can select several targets for a single child or can work on different individual targets with several children within the same activity.

CLD Children

Schools are among the most multicultural institutions in U.S. society. Children newly immigrant are increasingly poor and older than in the recent past. These children are less successful in school than their monolingual classmates speaking English and are more likely to become dropouts. In general, these children are overrepresented in programs for those with special educational needs and underrepresented in programs for the gifted.

Although it is preached that having limited English proficiency is not a disorder, practice is quite different. Children who may lack a foundation in L_1—a deficit that affects learning of English (L_2)— are placed in English-only classes as soon as possible. Instead, these children should remain in L_1 programs until they have a sufficient base.

In addition, most children remain in bilingual programs for only two or three years before being thrust into regular English-only classrooms. Although they may have gained some conversational proficiency with English, most do not possess sufficient English for classroom learning. It is estimated that it takes approximately five to seven years to attain such proficiency. These children often are referred for special education services on the basis of their classroom performance.

In short, the cognitive/academic language proficiency (CALP) acquired in L_1 can be transferred to CALP in L_2. A unitary system of language provides a foundation for both languages. Enhancing either language enhances the entire system, although its effect on a specific language will vary. The child able to manipulate L_1 in decontextualized situations has resultant facilitated learning in L_2.

Our present well-intentioned educational model is based on the belief that immersion in English is the best way to learn English. Children with a deficient base in L_1 nearly always are placed in English-only programs despite the wishes of the child, family, or community. Quantity of input alone, however, is not the answer. Quality time spent conversing with an adult in English could be much more beneficial at initial stages of language learning.

Language in the typical English-only classroom is treated as one of many academic subjects. The bottom-up approach that begins with grammar and builds toward communication requires good metalinguistic skills that may be lacking in the child with an inadequate base in either language.

The solution to this problem can be found, in part, in the model of intervention that we have discussed throughout this book. The child should remain in an L_1 program until she or he has a sufficient language base. Later English-only training should be functional, reflect its ultimate use, and contain a top-down or communication-through-conversation focus.

An individual must develop to a proficient level in one language to benefit fully from instruction in a second one. Children with LEP and children who are bilingual, taught linguistic concepts such as prepositions and pronouns in L_1, and then instructed in L_2 learn these concepts twice as fast as those taught only in L_2 (Perozzi & Chavez Sanchez, 1992). Instruction in L_1 facilitates acquisition in L_2 (Kiernan & Swisher, 1990; Perozzi, 1985). In short, L_1 provides input for comprehending L_2.

It is not true, however, that instruction in either language improves the other. Teaching vocabulary in L_2 has little effect on L_1 when the words are unknown in both (Perozzi, 1985).

In an English-only classroom, the environment should stimulate use and facilitate production and comprehension of English. The teacher should act as facilitator and encourage group work that fosters language use.

Language is meaningful and used for real communication. New vocabulary is introduced in context, bound to experiences, and associated to other words in the child's lexicon. Language is integrated into other subject areas.

Teachers facilitate language acquisition by surrounding children with visual examples of English. The whole language approach discussed in the next chapter lends itself particularly well to an environment of language.

The teacher's speech is modified for vocabulary complexity and use of idioms. He or she speaks more slowly, uses simple sentences, and emphasizes and repeats key words to enhance comprehension. Although the teacher expects children to communicate and raises these expectations as they progress, he or she attempts to keep anxiety low and the motivation for language use high by employing the conversational feedback techniques discussed in Chapter 10.

In the first stage, the teacher will want to focus on preproduction or comprehension in which the child develops the ability to extract meaning from utterances directed to him. In this stage, the child listens and follows simple instructions, responding with gestures, body movements, names, and one-word answers. One type of extended listening experience is called *total physical response* (TPR), in which the child participates in active singing, rhythming, and movement activities that include language. Language is paired with nonlinguistic elements of learning that happen to be a lot of fun. Suggested TPR materials are listed in Table 11.13. In the next chapter, we shall explore the use of children's literature and music.

TABLE 11.13   Suggested total physical response materials

Before the Bell Rings, Prentice-Hall/Alemany
Brown Bear, Brown Bear, What Do You See? Holt, Rinehart & Winston
Chicken Soup with Rice, Harper Trophy
The Children's Response, Prentice-Hall/Alemany
Here Comes the Cat, Scholastic
Jazz Chants for Children, Oxford
Look Who's Talking, Prentice-Hall/Alemany
The Magic of Music, Movement, and Make-Believe, DLM
Mary Wore Her Red Dress, Clarion
More Songs for Language Learning, Communication Skill Builders
Movement Plus Music, DLM
Oxford Picture Dictionary, Oxford
Purple Cows and Potato Chips, Prentice-Hall/Alemany
Songs for Language Learning, Communication Skill Builders
Where Is Thumbkin? Gryphon House

In the second stage, after six months or more of comprehension training with only minimal English production, focus is shifted to simple production with a strong receptive element (Heberle, 1992). The goal is limited English production with continued vocabulary growth. The facilitator uses *yes/no* and *either...or* questions with content that the child has used repeatedly in comprehension training. All production attempts are encouraged, and the child is not penalized for mispronunciation or errors of form. Production is usually at the one-word or phrase level. This stage of English training may last for approximately one year.

In the third stage, the child is required to use a more extensive production vocabulary and to begin to use grammar more correctly. Again, communication, not syntactic learning, is the goal. The facilitator uses repetition and expansion, respectively, to reinforce and correct the child's productions.

Finally, the child progresses to the final stage, conversational fluency. The facilitator still will have to modify the linguistic context to aid the child's production and comprehension.

Children with minority dialects offer a similar challenge. Minority dialects are neither crude approximations of the standard nor haphazard, unpatterned forms. Nor do they reflect disordered language or disorganized thinking on the user's part. These dialects are valid forms of the standard language within themselves, and this validity should be reflected in the intervention planning of public schools. Notions of dialectal superiority reflect prejudicial thinking and have led to educational approaches aimed at eradicating minority dialects. The American Speech-Language-Hearing Association (1983) has labeled this approach "inappropriate."

Bidialectal education should be fostered instead. This approach recognizes the validity of dialects and also the educational and employment needs of the individual. Smitherman (1985) found that only those speakers of African American English (AAE) who master code switching, the successful use of both AAE and a second dialect closer to the standard, achieve educational success. Unfortunately, any discussion of bilingual or bidialectal education has become embroiled in political debate over what some educators call "Ebonics" and the acceptance of English as the only language for governmental use.

As discussed previously, the SLP must not regard dialectal differences as language disorders. Language is impaired when the child demonstrates inappropriate, incorrect, or immature use within his or her dialectal community. This position suggests, therefore, that intervention should teach both minority and standard equivalents for disordered structures (Adler, 1988, 1990). For example, if the child with LI speaks African American English, use of the verb *to be* should be taught in both AAE and the standard. Only this approach truly serves the child, who must function within both a dialectal community and the larger society.

In effect, the linguistic standard (SAE) is taught as a second dialect, or D_2 (L. Campbell, 1993). D_2, the dialect of education, is taught while maintaining the dialect spoken at home and/or in the community. The goal is not eradication of D_1, but proficiency in an alternate dialect (O. Taylor, 1990). Using the child's knowledge of D_1, the SLP can teach the contrasting features of D_2. Role-play can be used effectively to increase the child's knowledge of both dialects and their use environments (Gee, 1989; O. Taylor, 1986b).

Use of Microcomputers

Microcomputers can enhance language instruction when well integrated into an overall language program in a cohesive manner (O'Connor & Schery, 1989; Steiner & Larson, 1991). Primarily a drill and practice tool at present, the computer can complement—but should never replace—face-to-face learning situations.

Children enjoy using computers. Preschoolers prefer computer-based training to traditional therapy drills and desktop activities (Shriberg, Kwiatkowski, & Snyder, 1989). Most training programs are user friendly, lowering the threat to children with LI.

The goals of intervention and the methodology should be established prior to determining the role of the microcomputer and integrating it into the overall plan. It is all too easy to fall into the trap of allowing the computer program to determine intervention goals. This *train-for-the-program* approach is not individualized for each child.

Children with LI are best served by microcomputers when both the child and the SLP actively participate, when computer use is individualized, and when software specific to the intervention goal is used. The most effective integration of the microcomputer occurs when the SLP or other facilitator and the child interact around the program being used, commenting and discussing choices offered and the child's selections. In this way, computer programs can be tuned more to the needs of each child. Similarly, software designed to address specific language problems (Ertmer, 1986; Meyers & Fogel, 1985) is better than generic, mass-market software.

Computer programs should be used with caution. Prior to using any program, the SLP should ask fundamental questions about its theoretical underpinings, the design of studies reporting success, and the clients who will seem to benefit most from program use (Gillam, 1999). Of special concern for functional communication are the naturalness of the approach, its effect on overall communication, and generalization to real-life situations.

Microcomputers seem especially useful for writing training. A four-step approach of prewriting, writing, revision, and publication can be used effectively to teach both writing and organizational skills (Cochran & Bull, 1991). Writing software includes Kidwriter, Explore-A-Story, and Explore-A-Classic for younger school-age children, and Logowriter. Speech synthesizers that can "read" the story heighten the child's awareness of the audience and can have a positive effect on writing (Borgh & Dickson, 1986; Espin & Sindelar, 1988; Kurth, 1988; MacArthur, 1988; Meyer & Rose, 1987; Rosegrant & Cooper, 1987). Possible intervention activates are presented in Table 11.14.

TABLE 11.14   Integrating computer activities into language therapy

Sample language objectives	Word processing activity	Pre-/postcomputer activity	Extended project
Giving directions Taking another's point of view Sequencing events	Copy a recipe Explain special terms or translate for younger children to use	Make the recipe Tell others how it was done Take photograph of finished dish book and display	Collect recipes into a notebook "Publish" the recipe book and display with photographs
Summarizing information Taking another's point of view Using verb tenses	Write daily entry in "speech journal" (5 minutes at end of each session)	Discuss the therapy session Plan what to write	Make a success report for mom, dad, teacher
Initiating topic Using correct question syntax Maintaining topic Changing topic Closing conversation	Write interview plan Write a "dialog" of the interview (focus on content, not punctuation) Based on the dialog, write a biography or story	Watch videotape of interview on TV Interview someone familiar (cook, bus driver, music teacher) Role-play being the interviewer or interviewee	Make "This is Your Life" display Start a school newsletter
Carryover any new syntactic or phonologic skill Sequencing events Explaining what will happen Explaining what did happen	Write a project plan Write a letter asking for permission to have contest Make signs and invitations Write a letter inviting a newspaper or yearbook photographer to the contest After the contest, write an announcement of the winners to be read over the school PA system	Plan a contest Discuss what will be needed Discuss what contestants must do Discuss what makes "news"	Hold a contest (bubble blowing, poster making, ball throwing, Twister)

Source: Cochran, P. S., & Bull, G. L. (1991). Integrating word processing into language instruction. *Topics in Language Disorders, 11*(2), 31–49. Reprinted with permission.

Early Intervention with Presymbolic and Minimally Symbolic Children

Intervention with children who are presymbolic and minimally symbolic can follow many of the principles emphasized throughout this book by being naturalistic, functional, and developmentally appropriate. The child's intervention plan should be based on and should address the needs of all three major areas assessed—child-related variables, environmental variables, and interactional variables—within an overall integrated functional approach. Goals for the child and family should be to move through presymbolic communication to symbolic and for the child to move to more intentional communication. The beneficial effects of treatment for toddlers with language delay can be seen even in areas not targeted for intervention (Robertson & Ellis Weismer, 1999).

It is essential that caregivers be involved in the training. "The child affects and is affected by the entire family system" (Bristol, 1985, p. 49). Therefore, the SLP must work at the level of the dyad, rather than the individual child. Communication is a cooperative venture. A child cannot be taught to communicate by him- or herself. Parents can be taught to enhance their natural role as language teachers, to speak more slowly, and to use less complex, more focused language. As a result, children are more likely to produce more target words, multiword combinations, and early morphemes (Girolometto, Pearce, & Weitzman, 1996).

Ideally, the SLP sees the child daily for individual or group therapy within a classroom or unit setting with the caregiver. If this arrangement is not possible, the caregiver should attend at least once a week or be kept informed about the training through detailed reports and instructions and be trained periodically in group sessions.

The SLP can observe the teachers and aides in the natural classroom environment and make suggestions for improving the quality of the child-caregiver interaction. With instructional staff, training can occur at in-service sessions or in direct instruction following brief observation and data review sessions in the classroom environment.

Training may focus on either expanding the breadth of communication behaviors, such as increasing the number of illocutionary functions or the number of means of expressing current functions, or increasing developmental complexity, such as moving from nonintentional to intentional communication or from presymbolic to symbolic. Idiosyncratic means of communication can be replaced gradually by more conventional means (Carr & Durand, 1985; Donnellan et al., 1984; Schuler & Prizant, 1987; M. Smith, 1985).

Methods of Training

Activities within each child's various interactional environments form the bases for communication and training. Communication and language training occur at natural junctures within these ongoing activities (Rowland & Schweigert, 1989a, 1989b). Three intervention techniques are beneficial: incidental teaching, stimulation, and formal training (Owens, 1982d).

Incidental Teaching

Incidental teaching is a strategy that arises naturally within the child's and caregiver's daily activities or in unstructured situations. In this child-directed strategy, the child controls the focus of the interaction by signaling interest. While enhancing these naturally occurring communication interactions, the caregiver trains or strengthens presymbolic or early symbolic behaviors. In other words, the behavior is trained within the child's daily activities in which it would naturally appear. For example, the child learning about object permanence could encounter natural teaching situations while bathing with nonfloating soap or while searching for misplaced toys. *Incidental teaching is not formal training disguised as fun.* Hidden training, such as preschool action songs, may be just as irrelevant to the context and to the child as formal training, although action songs in another context can aid in valuable concept development.

The caregiver's tasks are to be aware of the learning potential within each situation and to structure events to enhance learning. Caregiver input to the child should match or lead slightly the complexity of the child's language (Owens, 1982d; Prizant & Schuler, 1987). In unstructured activities, such as free play, the child's expressed interest is the key. Caregivers can learn to follow the child's lead and to incorporate training into these interests. Table 11.15 presents examples of incidental teaching.

Unfortunately, this incidental aspect of training is most difficult for caregivers to comprehend. Although it is relatively easy to train caregivers to engage in formal training with children, and it is relatively easy for these caregivers to adapt the training to other environments, it is not as easy for

TABLE 11.15   Examples of incidental teaching

Type of Training	Example
Establishing eye contact	During feeding, the child looks at the facilitator in order to receive a spoonful of food.
Object permanence	While bathing, the facilitator "loses" nonfloating soap in the bath water and states, "Oh, I lost the soap; can you find it?"
Imitation with objects	During daily living skills training, the child imitates the facilitator's use of a comb.
Requesting gesture	At snacktime, the child requests a special snack from those on the table.
Symbol recognition	The child picks out clothes named during dressing.

them to adapt the training to less structured, informal, everyday activities unless directly taught these behaviors.

The SLP can assist caregivers in using incidental techniques by following these suggestions:

1. Keep the training procedures simple.
2. Role-play potential situations with the caregiver.
3. Target a few frequently occurring everyday situations, rather than try to cover every possible situation.
4. Do not require record keeping of incidental teaching.
5. Demonstrate in the actual environment or within real situations.

Caregivers are overwhelmed easily by the plethora of training advice to be used in numerous different potential teaching situations.

Incidental teaching is "ecologically sound." It is more likely than other methods to meet the needs of the family or classroom because it incorporates their daily routines where skills are taught and used. The environment can be arranged so that adults follow the child's lead, such as when they comment on or play with a child-selected toy and engage in turn-taking routines (Yoder, Warren et al., 1994). Children who do not have choice-making behaviors can be prompted by the adult ceasing pleasurable activities and asking "What do you want?" or "Do you want this?"

Stimulation
Stimulation, the way caregivers interact with the child, should be just slightly more complex than the child's functioning to serve as a model. The child will learn best when the model is far enough above his or her competency level to maintain interest but not so far as to frustrate. Table 11.16 presents some suggested stimulation techniques.

Because research has not identified which behaviors are the most effective, caregivers should use as many as are practical. It is best for caregivers to change their own behavior slowly, possibly incorporating one or two techniques and waiting until these feel comfortable before using more. It will not be necessary to use all of the stimulation techniques with every child. Small changes in the current method of interacting, such as increasing the number of verbalizations addressed to the child, may have dramatic effects (Owens et al., 1987). AAC symbols, such as signs, can be learned singly by caregivers, possibly in a "signs of the week" program (Spragle & Micucci, 1990).

Formal Training
Formal training, a third strategy, occurs a few brief times daily. The SLP monitors this training closely for content, procedures, and the child's progress. He or she analyzes each skill to be taught

TABLE 11.16   Suggested stimulation techniques for children who are presymbolic and minimally symbolic

Presymbolic Children
  Speak in short sentences of three to five words containing one or two syllables each.
  Speak about entities in the immediate context.
  Speak slowly with pauses and emphasize content words.
  Use self-talk and parallel talk to describe your own and the child's actions, respectively.
  Gesture or use simple signs when it may aid comprehension.
  Allow time for the child to respond even though she or he may not.
  Establish a communication position vis-à-vis the child's face that is comfortable for the child and that demonstrates a genuine interest in the child's communication efforts.
  Maintain the child's attention by varying the intensity and pitch of your verbalizations.

Minimally Symbolic Children
In addition to the techniques above:
  Attend to all symbolic initiations.
  Gently correct with feedback.
  Expand the child's communication into a more mature form.
  Reply to the child's communication with a relevant and appropriate comment.
  Do not ask too many adultlike questions. They are difficult to process.

Source: Adapted from Owens (1982d).

for antecedent and consequent events and constructs a hierarchy that includes the steps needed for successful completion. With children who are presymbolic, especially those above preschool age, it is essential that training hierarchies consist of small increments of change. This necessitates a task analysis approach that reflects the child's individual style and sequence of learning, the individual cues necessary, reinforcers, success criteria, and content.

Generalization will be affected by the content selected and by the manner and sequence of formal training. Content or training items and the location of training should come from the child's natural environment. The SLP must analyze the child's communication environment to determine whether there are natural opportunities for the behavior to occur.

The reinforcement should reflect the child's environment in order to aid generalization. Parents should be trained to respond as naturally as possible. Conversational replies are usually be best. Conversational responding, such as "Um-hm, that is a horsie, big horsie," is appropriate and aids generalization to conversation because of its inherent conversational nature.

Child development studies have demonstrated the reinforcing power and teaching potential of *expansion, extension,* and *imitation,* discussed in Chapter 10. All three provide feedback on acceptability of the child's utterance within a conversational context. Similar responses can be used with the child's presymbolic behaviors, such as imitating a child's action or expanding it into a more complex action.

Course of Training

Training should focus on both the child's communication system and presymbolic or early symbolic skills. The communication system is expanded and moved ever closer to symbolic communication while the child is learning presymbolic cognitive, social, and communicative skills.

Establishing and Expanding the Communication System

Facilitators should be careful to note the signal value to the child of excess behaviors before beginning intervention. In addition to possibly using self-injurious and self-stimulatory behavior in initial communication, the SLP can rely on additional techniques, such as behavior chain interruption.

Self-Injurious and Self-Stimulatory Behaviors. Self-injurious, tantruming, and aggressive behavior may signal either frustration and a desire to escape or a call for attention (Carr & Durand, 1985). Although excess behavior cannot be allowed to continue to the child's detriment, punishment should be paired with reinforcement of less destructive, more socially acceptable communication behaviors. To the degree that such behavior signals escape, attention getting, or demand, the frequency should decrease with the learning of more socially acceptable methods of signaling this information (Carr & Durand, 1985; Donnellan et al., 1984; Durand & Kishi, 1986; L. Meyer & Evans, 1986; Reichle, 1990; Robinson & Owens, 1995).

Self-stimulatory behaviors can be treated differently and used as reinforcers for behaviors that are less likely to occur. Please note that I did *not* say reinforce self-stimulation. The child is allowed to engage in self-stimulatory behavior when the SLP elicits a social or communication behavior.

The child's limited repertoire of behaviors may be expanded through gradual modification or the introduction of more appropriate alternative behaviors to signal intentions. The SLP must decide whether to maintain the child's present method of signaling intentions, modify it, or train new signals. In general, such signals may be maintained if they are not part of a perseverative pattern, if their intention is easily discernible, and if they do not call undue attention to the child (Reichle et al., 1988). It is important that the signal be clearly differentiated from others and be socially appropriate (Theadore et al., 1990). The SLP must find ways to prompt or cue the acceptable communicative behavior prior to the inception of excess behavior in order to decrease and control the excess behavior. It must be stressed that not all excess behavior is socially motivated and, therefore, amenable to reduction with the introduction of functional communication.

Behavior Chain Interruption. Interruption strategies have been used effectively with individuals with severe MR and multiple disabilities (Romer & Schoenberg, 1991). Establishment of a communication system might begin with behavior chain interruption strategies, such as *resonance training*. In resonance training, the facilitator cradles the child and rocks slowly while speaking about the action. This training should not be attempted without consultation with the physical therapist to ensure that handling and positioning are optimal. A large mirror in front of the pair provides feedback on the child's reaction.

Initially, the facilitator is interested primarily in child responses that signal the child's realization that someone has intruded on his or her space. The child may try to help the facilitator rock by pushing in the direction of the rocking. Although such behavior signals compliance and acceptance, this movement should not serve as a signal when the rocking stops, because it is part of the movement itself. The pushing is, however, an indication that the child is motivated to signal, and the facilitator physically prompts a signal, such as tapping the floor. The prompted signal is followed by continuation of the rocking. The prompt is faded gradually.

After several sessions in which the child has signaled for the activity to continue, the facilitator changes the criterion and will not begin rocking initially until the child signals. The facilitator and the child assume the rocking posture but do nothing until the child signals. At first, this signal probably will need to be prompted. More important than the signal is the lesson that through communication the child can affect the environment. Development of other related behaviors may occur.

As the facilitator moves from a cradling position to a side-by-side or facing one, he or she is in a better position later to attempt such training as physical imitation, an important presymbolic skill. This phase of training is called *coactive movement.* With fewer and fewer prompts, the child learns to follow an increasingly diverse set of facilitator behaviors.

The facilitator can attempt similar behavior-chain-interruption training with any behavior pleasurable to the child, such as listening to music. The behavior is interrupted and a signal prompted for it to resume (Goetz, Gee, & Sailor, 1985; P. Hunt, Goetz, Alwell, & Sailor, 1986). Once the signal is used consistently, training moves to initiation. Interruption strategies can be used within a number of pleasurable routines and expanded to include passively blocking a child from the next action, delaying presentation of an item needed for task completion, placing needed items out of reach, and removing needed items (P. Hunt & Goetz, 1988).

Close physical proximity, touching, and a gentle, pleasant manner and voice may help establish an initial communication system. If the child does not respond well to touching or to close proximity, initial assessment and training may have to focus on toleration and desensitization, which usually are accomplished by pairing touching with a pleasurable or reinforcing stimulus.

The SLP can expand the communication system to include environmental *tangible symbols* (Rowland & Schweigert, 1989a), signals, and gestures, such as having the child reach for, touch, or look at common objects prior to beginning everyday activities in which they will be used. For example, the SLP might require the child to look at or touch a toothbrush before brushing. The toothbrush becomes a tangible symbol for brushing and later can signal that activity. Initially, to avoid confusion, the toothbrush used to signal may be the one actually used for brushing, but later brushes should be separate to preserve the signal quality of the nonused one. At the next level of training, the child uses the tangible symbol to initiate the event. The child is using a primitive augmentative communication system.

The SLP must be careful at this point in training to ensure that the child engages in communication interaction using the tangible symbols, not just in associational tasks. The objects should be used also to request, protest, and signal notice (Rowland & Schweigert, 1989b).

Nonverbal Communication

Nonverbal communication systems, whether gestural, vocal, AAC, or a combination, are especially important. Within this communication framework, the child learns valuable lessons on turn taking, initiation of communication, responding, and a variety of communication intentions.

The rate of intentional nonverbal communication, including gestures, is a good predictor of spontaneous word production later (Calandrella & Wilcox, 2000). Intentional communication is communication with the purpose of achieving some outcome, communication with a predetermined goal. To be effective, intentional nonverbal behaviors must be coordinated with the behaviors of caregivers. It does little good to request a cookie if no one is there to provide it or if adults in the child's environment ignore the child. This simple example demonstrates the importance of including caregivers in the training as language facilitators.

Within intervention to establish and maintain the child's intentional nonverbal communication, the SLP targets a variety of communication intentions of illocutionary functions. It is within these intentions, such as requesting, signaling notice, and giving, that first words or other symbols appear.

Intentions can be established by responding to unintentional child behaviors believed by the family and SLP to signal some information. Unintentional behaviors are performed without considering the audience and in an inconsistent manner. For example, the child may reach consistently for a desired object but not signal an adult for help. The reach can be interpreted as a request for that object. Intentional communication behaviors already present in the child can be shaped into more appropriate, typical, or recognizable signals. For example, tantruming to obtain a cookie can be gradually modified into something more acceptable.

Presymbolic Training

Obviously, not every behavior of the child developing typically is an appropriate training target. Nor should the SLP assume that infant development scales identify the skills that children with LI need. These scales often include a variety of activities, many unrelated to symbol use. The SLP should select presymbolic targets judiciously, choosing those that affect communication and symbol use. A long list of prerequisites actually may prevent children who are presymbolic from learning to communicate.

The SLP can determine presymbolic targets by beginning with skills important for the language development of children developing typically, such as means-ends, turn taking, and gestures, and modifying these targets on the basis of his or her training rationale (Table 11.17) (McLean & Snyder-McLean, 1988b). Each possible presymbolic target should be evaluated on the basis of how it will facilitate the development of symbol use for a specific child.

All training is considered in relation to the three strategies of incidental teaching, stimulation, and formal training. Training procedures and sequences mentioned below are equally applicable, whether the child's ultimate form of communication is speech, an augmentative system, or a combination. Recognition and receptive training with augmentative systems can begin at a relatively low level of presymbolic functioning. Presymbolic training is not ignored, however, because productive use of augmentative symbol systems require a level of cognitive functioning at least as high as that for verbal symbols.

Symbolic Training

Symbolic training is superimposed on a gestural, gestural-vocal, or AAC base trained previously. At the symbolic level, the dual nature of training in communication and prerequisite skills becomes one as the child's communication system becomes more symbolic in nature.

TABLE 11.17   Determining presymbolic training targets

Presymbolic Cognitive and Social Skills +	Client Communication Needs =	Training Targets
Object permanence	Semantic knowledge of objects	Functional use of objects. Appearance, disappearance, and reappearance of objects.
Means-ends	Semantic knowledge of objects	Repeat action with pleasurable outcome. Object manipulation. Indirect means, such as pulling string or winding toy. Tool use.
Gestures	Influence others	Generic (basic, constant) behaviors used to signal. Hierarchy from contact to distal signals. Range of signals.
Turn taking	Interact with others	Joint action routines—Ritualized pattern with a specific theme, following a logical sequence in which each participant plays a specific role, with specific response expectations essential to successful completion.

Source: Adapted from McLean & Snyder-McLean (1988b).

Symbols should be taught for referents that are established clearly in the client's meaning system. Attempts to teach referential concepts and symbols simultaneously may confuse the child (Romski & Sevcik, 1989). He or she may associate the symbol with the teaching context, rather than with the referent.

It is important that symbolic training remain functional and fulfill a broad range of communication intentions, whether the means of transmission is verbal or AAC. All too often, training deteriorates to the child's responding to such cues as "What's this?" in the hope that the response will be used spontaneously on some future occasion.

Initially, each lexical item should correspond to a specific pragmatic function. General symbols, such as *want, more,* and *no,* might be used. Specific symbols, such as *juice* or *hot,* also may be trained, but they, too, should be function-specific. Children who are minimally symbolic have difficulty generalizing the use of a symbol across several illocutionary functions (Calculator & Delaney, 1986; LaMarre & Holland, 1985).

Careful selection of individual symbols requires a study of the child's environment that is sensitive to the child's needs. Whether the child is using AAC or a verbal communication mode, the SLP should select vocabulary that is "individualized, functional, and dynamic" (Yorkston, Honsinger, Dowden, & Marriner, 1989, p. 102). Vocabulary should enhance the child's functioning in multiple environments frequently throughout the day, be age appropriate, and be valued by both the child and the caregivers (L. Brown et al., 1988). Vocabulary is dynamic and should be updated continually as the child and the child's environment, knowledge, and needs change (Beukelman, McGinnis, & Morrow, 1991). The lexicon should be "open-ended," capable of modification.

Standardized vocabulary lists do not provide a sufficiently thorough lexicon for the individual child. Such lists, if adopted, are inefficient because they contain many words that are rarely used (Yorkston, Smith, & Beukelman, 1990).

Even lists of the most frequently used words of peers who are developing typically may be of little value in vocabulary selection because they include such words as *to, a, it, am,* and *and* (Beukelman, Jones, & Rowan, 1989), which are abstract and difficult to teach, especially at the single-symbol level of communication. Lexicons based on frequency of occurrence by the individual child within different natural communication contexts may yield a short but highly useful list of symbols.

The child should be involved in vocabulary selection to the best of his or her abilities. The SLP can observe daily activities and "script" them for possible vocabulary needed. Caregivers, too, can suggest vocabulary. The SLP should be careful to select symbols that reflect the child's needs. If symbols chosen relate only to basic needs, however, the system's use will be very restricted (Morrow et al., 1993). Table 11.18 is a list of the words most commonly selected by caregivers.

Too often, training concentrates on limited use of nouns, ignoring the rich presymbolic functional communication of children developing typically. It is assumed by trainers that nouns are easier to learn and more functional than other types of words (Beukelman et al., 1991). Social-regulative terms, such as *please, thank you, excuse me, I'm sorry, I'm finished, be quiet, stop, help, more, good, yes, no, I want, hello,* and *good-bye,* also can be learned easily and can increase normalization of communication (Adamson, Romski, Deffenbach, & Sevcik, 1992; Buzolich, King, & Baroody, 1991). Symbols learned but not used by the child are of little value; thus, the need for such words must be established first.

The SLP can use a combination of the gestural intentions already present and verbal and nonverbal cues to vary the child's behavior. For example, symbols are first trained in imitation to cues, such as "Say ____" ("Sign ____," "Point to ____," etc.), when the child demonstrates an interest in

TABLE 11.18　Most common caregiver-selected words for training

afraid	close	goodbye	library	popcorn	take
alone	coat	grandfather	lie (down)	potatoes	talk
alphabet	coke	grandma	little	pretty	teacher
am	cold	grandmother	living room	pull	telephone
apple	comb	grandpa	love	purple	thank you
applesauce	come	grapes	mad	push	thirsty
are	computer	green	magazine	puzzle	tired
arm	cookie	grits	make	radio	toast
bad	crazy	ham	McDonald's	read	toilet
ball	cry	hamburger	meat	record player	toothbrush
banana	dad	hand	medicine	red	toothpaste
bathroom	dance	happy	milk	restaurant	towel
bedroom	dining room	has	mom	ride	truck
behind	dirty	hat	mouth	roast beef	t-shirt
beside	doctor	head	need	root beer	turn
between	down	hear	no	run	tv
bicycle	draw	hello	nose	sad	ugly
big	drink	help	numbers	school	under
black	ears	home	oatmeal	see	underwear
blanket	eat	hospital	on	shirt	up
blocks	eggs	hot	open	shoes	upset
blue	elbow	hotdog	orange	shorts	walk
boat	empty	how	outside	sick	want
book	eyes	hungry	over	sing	was
break	fall	hurry	pancakes	sit	water
broken	fat	hurt	pants	sleep	were
brown	feel	I	paper	smell	wet
bus	fight	ice cream	park	soap	what
buy	fish	in	pear	socks	when
cake	fix	is	peas	soft drink	where
candy	foot	jeans	pencil	soup	who
car	french fries	juice	pie	spaghetti	why
carrots	funny	kiss	pizza	stand	work
carry	game	kitchen	plane	stomach	write
cereal	give	knee	play	stop	yellow
chest	gloves	know	playground	store	yes
chicken	go	laugh	please	supermarket	yuck
church	good	leg	poor	sweater	zoo

Source: Morrow, D. R., Mirenda, P., Beukelman, D. R., & Yorkston, K. M. (1993). Vocabulary selection for augmentative communication systems: A comparison of three techniques. *American Journal of Speech-Language Pathology, 2*(2), 19–30. Reprinted with permission.

or desire for an entity. This verbal cue is accompanied by a nod that signals the child to respond. The trainer also may prompt by beginning the response for the child.

Verbal imitative cues should be minimized and decreased as soon as possible to decrease possible dependence. This reduction is especially true for children with ASD who may develop echolalia. Child-initiated communication may not occur unless it is planned.

The verbal cue "Say" ("Sign," "Point to") can be faded gradually and the response shifted to the visual nodding cue. The child now will respond with the name after the trainer names the object and nods. Gradually, the verbal model is faded. Because the child will name in response to a nod, he or she can be cued in other ways to get a range of illocutionary and semantic functions. It is possible to train a variety of functions for each symbol, thus increasing the child's repertoire.

Words, signs, and visual symbols are learned faster for requesting than for labeling (J. Goodman & Remington, 1993). General symbols for *want* or *more* have broad application and will occur frequently, thus enhancing generalization to the transfer environment (Reichle, 1990). General symbols can be paired with object and event names to form longer utterances, such as "Want juice" or "More book."

Initially, the SLP should require both gestures and verbalizations of the child because there is often a lack of correspondence between the two with young learners (Guevremont, Osnes, & Stokes, 1986a, 1986b). Unless the child chains the verbal and nonverbal behaviors, correspondence between the two may not occur. Through training that uses two items, one desirable and one not, the child can learn to make specific requests for the desirable one (Piche-Cragoe, Reichle, & Sigafoos, 1986). The trainer modifies intonation and gestures that accompany a single symbol to model a variety of functions.

The SLP should target also a variety of semantic functions, such as agent, object, and action. Initially, children use action-related symbols called *protoverbs*. These verblike symbols, which accompany specific actions children perform, include *up, down, no, on-here, inside, there, get-down, bye-bye, night-night,* and *out*. Gradually, each symbol acquires broader meaning and becomes decontextualized.

Multisymbol combinations should be trained gradually. It is vital that the child not be introduced to too many new training targets simultaneously. Lexical items should be learned prior to being taught in symbol combinations (Mineo & Goldstein, 1990). At this point, receptive comprehension and expressive production seem to be mutually beneficial, and it might be best that the child has many exposures to the semantic pattern targeted, such as *agent + action,* prior to requiring comprehension or production (Goldstein, 1985).

The training of any specific semantic construction, such as *action + object,* requires precise cues that target that construction. Table 11.19 presents conversational cues and training prompts that have resulted in children's generative use of the *action + object* construction and subsequent generalization across settings, partners, and interactive styles (Warren, Gazdag, Bambara, & Jones, 1994).

Modified Milieu Approach.   Within the classroom, a modified version of the milieu or mand-model approach described in Chapter 9 can be used with children who are presymbolic to teach them requesting, commenting or declaring, and two-word combinations (Warren et al., 1994; Warren, Yoder, Gazdag, Kim, & Jones, 1993). The techniques generalize across different materials, settings, teachers, and interactive styles.

Requesting and commenting have been targeted because these are the earliest developing intentions and the most frequent illocutionary functions in the presymbolic period (Bates, O'Connell, & Shore, 1987; Wetherby et al., 1988). In addition, these are the building blocks for later symbolic communication (Snow, 1989).

The milieu approach uses naturally occurring situations and prompts child responses to those situations. The environment is arranged so that the child can select a toy for play. The adult follows the child's lead with the toy and initiates familiar turn-taking games. Within this activity, the trainer uses the techniques described in Table 11.20.

Augmentative Communication.   The ease in learning augmentative communication systems depends on the child's overall developmental and communication level, the system chosen, and the

TABLE 11.19 Cues and prompts for generative use of action + object

Behavior	Definition	Example
	Degree of support Events that immediately (3 seconds or less) preceded a child's utterance	
Conversational cues		
Verbal stimulus	A nonobligatory verbalization (i.e., does not require a response) that may have stimulated child speech. This category included "systematic comments" by the adult that included the target training form but did not require its use in response.	*T:* "You're washing all the cups." *C:* "Wash cup." *T:* "I have a toy dog." *C:* "Want dog."
Question	Verbalization expressing inquiry and requiring a verbal response	*T:* "What are you (he/she) doing?" *T:* "What do you want me to do?"
Target question	A question requiring a target response (e.g., action-object). Target questions do not correct and cannot be preceded by a training prompt for the same target response.	*T:* "What do you want to do?" *T:* "What is this/that?"
Training prompts		
Elaborative question	A corrective question that indicates through content or tone that the preceding child verbalization was incorrect or inappropriate and requires the child to make another attempt at stating the target response. By default, a target question that follows a training prompt for the same response is coded as an elaborative question.	*C:* "That." *T:* "What toy do you want?" (elaborative question) *C:* "Big block." (target) *T:* "What do you want me to do?" (target question) *C:* "Open." *T:* "Open what?" (elaborative question) *C:* "Open jar." (target)
Mand	An instruction requiring a verbal response from a child.	*T:* "Tell me what to do." *T:* "Use words."
Model	A demonstration of a verbal response with direct emphasis on a word or phrase that requires child imitation.	*T:* "Say, 'blow bubbles.'"

Source: Warren, S. F., Gazdag, G. E., Bambara, L. M., & Jones, H. A. (1994). Changes in the generativity and use of semantic relationships concurrent with milieu language intervention. *Journal of Speech and Hearing Research, 37*, 924–934. Reprinted with permission.

training method (Mirenda & Locke, 1989; Mizuko, 1987). Although the exact level of development necessary for a truly functional communication system is unknown, this factor should not be ignored even for low-level gestural systems. Several factors related to AAC systems also determine ease of learning and use.

Symbol transparency or "guessability" is important in system selection and training. In general, the more a representation or symbol resembles the real object, the more transparent it is (Ecklund & Reichle, 1987; Mirenda & Locke, 1989; Mizuko, 1987; Sevcik & Romski, 1986; Vanderheiden & Lloyd, 1986). Thus, pictures or manual signs that resemble their referents are more transparent and eas-

TABLE 11.20   Techniques in a modified milieu approach

Requesting

Prompt-Free Approach: Hold up a highly desirable item, obtain eye contact, and wait, gazing at the child with raised eyebrows and quizzical look.

    If child produces request correctly, respond to illocutionary function of the utterance with a comment, possibly a semantically related two-word utterance, and give the item to the child.

    If no response or incorrect response, provide assistance to complete.

        If no eye contact previously, say, "Look at me." Recue.

        If no response or incorrect response, provide a verbal/sign/graphic (picture on communication board) model.

            If no response again, provide physical assistance to sign or point.

Prompted Approach: Either stop activity and ask, "What do you want? or hold item needed to resume an activity and ask, "Do you want this?"

    Wait.

    If child produces, request correctly, respond to elocutionary function of the utterance with a comment, possibly a semantically related two-word utterance, and obtain the item for the child.

    If no response, incorrect response, or incomplete response, provide assistance to complete.

        If no eye contact previously, say, "Look at me." Recue.

        If no response or incorrect response, provide a verbal/sign/graphic model and a physical pointing model toward the object.

            If no response again, provide physical assistance to sign, point to symbol, or point to the object.

        If incomplete response, say "What?"

Commenting

Frequently model commenting. Focus on what the child is attending to (joint attending) and verbalize ("Wow" or "Good" or "Yuk"). Cue child to imitate, with "Say _____" or "You say it."

    If child imitates, respond conversationally.

Fade model as spontaneous use increases.

Physically back away and attend elsewhere as novel items are introduced. Respond to child's vocalizations as if they attract your attention.

Labeling

Establish joint attending with the child and verbalize the name of the item of focus.

    If child imitates label, respond to the illocutionary function of the utterance and expand into semantically related two-word utterance.

    If label incorrect, give corrective feedback ("No, that's a horse"). Cue the child to imitate.

Respond to spontaneous utterances by expanding or extending the utterance.

Source: Adapted from Kozleski (1991); Warren, Yoder, Gazdag, Kim, & Jones (1993); Wilcox, Kouri, & Caswell (1991).

ier to learn. The Amer-Ind, or American Indian, Sign System is extremely transparent. Nearly 50 percent of the one-handed signs can be guessed by unfamiliar viewers (C. Campbell & Jackson, 1995).

    It is also important to remember that whereas whole systems may be more or less transparent, individual signs or symbols vary greatly (Bloomberg, Karlan, & Lloyd, 1990). In addition, judgments of transparency by children developing typically and by adults do not necessarily reflect the perceptions of children with LI (Bloomberg et al., 1990; Dunham, 1989). Nor does the level of transparency correlate with the task of learning to use a symbol system or with specific skills needed for learning such as visual perception (Sevcik, Romski, & Wilkinson, 1991).

Other determiners of the ease of manual sign learning are symmetry, inclusion of a portion of the body, and concreteness. In general, signs are easier to learn if both hands move symmetrically and the body is touched in some way, and if the signs are concrete rather than abstract (Kohl, 1981). Bilateral arm movements may be difficult for someone with motoric involvement (J. Keogh & Sugden, 1985).

Intervention.   Often, the concept that symbols have a function is the most difficult aspect of training for children who are presymbolic (Romski, Sevcik, & Pate, 1988). Initial contact between an aided symbol and the client might occur "by chance" (Murray-Branch et al., 1991). When the child accidentally touches the shape, he or she is given the referent. Gradually, the child makes the association, and behavior becomes more purposeful. The size of the shape is reduced as the child becomes better able to discriminate. Next, requesting is trained by using a physical prompting technique.

Children must learn that they can effect change through symbol use. Initially, the child is trained to select the one representation or symbol presented. Foils, such as an uninteresting item or a blank picture, then are introduced. Two-item choices are trained next. The facilitator might use a modified vending machine device, using light, sound, and symbol cues to train children to choose (Romski et al., 1988). In similar fashion, a child might use eye contact to signal a request.

Children with more severe or multiple disabilities may have difficulty moving from gestural communication to abstract symbols. For children using aided systems, the transition to symbols might begin with the easier task of match-to-sample (Saunders & Spradlin, 1989). In match-to-sample, the child picks from an available group of objects, pictures, or symbols the one that matches the "sample" held by the trainer. Obviously, matching an object, such as a ball, to another sample object would be easier than matching a picture or symbol to an object. Before moving to this more symbolic task, the SLP should ensure that the child can match both objects to objects and pictures or symbols to their like members.

Mentioned previously, tangible symbols, or representations in the form of objects or pictures with a clear perceptual relationship to the referent, can form a link between gestural and symbolic systems of communication. Actual objects or identifiable packaging might be used. Between the actual object and color photo representations, the following three levels of representation might exist (Rowland & Schweigert, 1989a):

1. Associated objects, such as a shoelace to represent a shoe
2. Shared feature objects, such as a cookie refrigerator magnet to represent a real cookie
3. Artificial associations in which an object appears on the communication board and also is attached to the referent, such as a wooden apple on the cafeteria door to represent meals

The learning of symbolic systems, such as Blissymbolics, can be enhanced by the addition of pictographs that emphasize the meaning (Raghavendra & Fristoe, 1995). Examples are presented in Figure 11.5. Pictographs can be faded gradually as the child learns the symbol.

A *cue-pause-point* method (McMorrow, Foxx, Faw, & Bittle, 1987) has been effective in teaching responsive use of signs (Foxx, Kyle, Faw, & Bittle, 1988). In this method, the child is taught a signed answer and then must await the appropriate question. Pauses are used at critical points to en-

Term	Standard Blissymbol	Enhanced Blissymbol

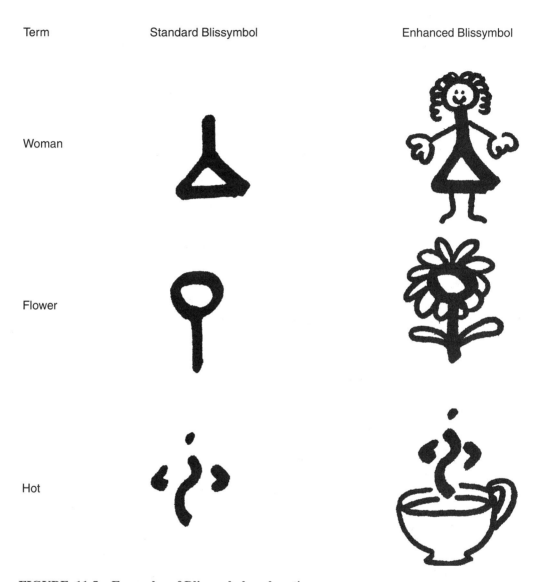

Woman

Flower

Hot

FIGURE 11.5   Examples of Blissymbol explanations.

Source: Adapted from Raghavendra & Fristoe (1995).

courage responding. Table 11.21. presents the training steps in sequence. As the prompts are removed systematically, the signs are maintained and generalized to novel questions.

Once the child has learned the response, the first cue can be omitted and the SLP can use the pause to wait for the child to initiate an utterance. For example, if frosting holiday cookies, the SLP can organize all the materials on the table, then await a request from the child. If no request is forthcoming, the SLP use an open-ended prompt, such as "If you want to help, just let me know" or "Tell

TABLE 11.21   *Cue-pause-point* **method for teaching responsive use of signs**

Step I	Ask a question, such as "What's that?" or "Where's _____?" or "What do we eat with?" Present signed answer. Pause prompt: Hold finger up to prevent signing until cued again.
Step II	Ask a question, such as "Where's _____?" or "What do we eat with?" Point prompt: Point to object that answers question.
Step III	If incorrect response to Step II, train object or item name by sign imitation.
Step IV	If correct in Step II, cover the object and repeat Step II.
Provide feedback at each step.	

Source: Adapted from Foxx, Kyle, Faw, & Bittle (1988); McMorrow, Foxx, Faw, & Bittle (1987).

me what you want." If there is still no response, the SLP can wonder aloud "How can we frost cookies?" "What do we need to frost cookies?" or "What should we do first?" Assuming that the child wants to frost cookies, the SLP might next try choice making, such as "Do you want to mix frosting or read a book?" Should the child still not respond, the SLP can use a partial physical prompt followed by a full physical prompt. Physical prompts are hand-over-hand assists that shape the child's hand into a sign or activate the device. Notice that the SLP has attempted initially to be as conversational as possible and to increase both child participation and initiation.

To forestall the child's learning of responsive communication behaviors only, the SLP can train requesting, mentioned previously, and commenting. Commenting allows the user to convey an attitude or opinion and includes expressions such as *wow, yuk, fun, I don't like this,* and *great.* These can be learned first through modeling, then by direct cuing ("You could say _____"), and finally by indirect cuing ("What would you say?") (Buzolich et al., 1991). Finally, eye contact, a nod, and/or an expectant delay can be used to cue as mentioned previously.

There are a number of organizations and websites that can support the SLP training AAC. Internet resources are presented in Table 11.22.

Generalization.   A lack of generalization of augmentative system use may result from (a) facilitator-centered or facilitator-controlled training, (b) unintelligibility of the child's system as used, (c) the precedence within training of the system over the communication process, (d) nonuse of natural settings, and (e) nonusers' lack of response in the natural environment (Calculator, 1988b). One survey of children with severe/profound MR who were learning signing found that augmentative training (a) frequently ignored receptive comprehension, (b) was taught primarily through imitation while rarely encouraging spontaneous use, (c) was rarely taught in meaningful situations outside the therapy setting, and (d) often chose vocabulary that was irrelevant to ongoing activities and interests of the child (Bryen, Goldman, & Quinlisk-Gill, 1988).

Intervention should focus on encouraging flexible use of various modes of communication (Downing & Siegel-Causey, 1988). Instead, the means of transmission and/or the code may be taught separately from the communication function of the symbols. The goal of training becomes learning the system, rather than optimizing communication. This inflexibility is obvious when a child who is nonspeaking is required to rely on an augmentative response, such as signing "no" when a head shake would suffice. Flexibility can be maintained by continual training to upgrade the child's symbol system and device.

TABLE 11.22   Augmentative/alternative communication (AAC) and assistive technologies (AT) resources

sarahblack@aol.com	Alternatively Speaking (newsletter)
ussaac@northshore.net	United States Society for AAC
www.aacproducts.org	Communication Aid Manufactures Association
www.abledate.com	Search engine for assistive technology
www.asha.org	American Speech-Language-Hearing Association
www.ATAcess.org	Alliance for Technology Access
www.atk.lsi.ukans.edu	University of Kansas AT info
www.augcomm.com	Links to AAC
www.closingthegap.com	Closing the Gap (newspaper)
www.creative-comm.com	Creative Communication
www.csun.edu	Center on Disabilities, California State University
www.dinf.org/csun97	Maryland AAC curriculum
www.dynavoxsys.com	DynaVox System, Inc.
www.frame-tech.com	Frame Technologies
www.ilp-online.com	Independent Living Center AT info
www.isaac-online.org	International Society for AAC
www.mic.ucla.edu	UCLA Microcomputer Team
www.msu.edu/~artlang	Artificial Language Laboratory, Michigan State University
www.news-4-you.com	Weekly newspaper for AAC users
www.orin.com	Origins Instruments
www.pecs.com	Picture Exchange System
www.pluk.org	Family guide to AT
www.resna.com	Rehabilitation Engineering and Assistive Technology Society of North America
www.trace.wisc.edu	Trace Research and Development Center, University of Wisconsin

Targets should be functional, such as requesting aid or objects from other people, rejecting or protesting, and commenting (Calculator & Jorgensen, 1991; Reichle, 1990). Thus, the child learns to control acquisition and refusal of specific entities within the environment. In general, requesting is easier to train than are the other functions (Reichle et al., 1988). The child might touch desired items to signal a request. Both preferred and nonpreferred items should be offered so that the child must make an active choice. Once a choice is made, the facilitator can probe the child's choice by offering two items: the requested one and another. The SLP can expand requesting behaviors with the use of a generalized request signal, such as *want* or *more*. He or she can place the printed symbol for *want* or *more* before the child as he or she reaches for desired items. The child touches the signal in the process of reaching for the item.

The child might signal protest or rejection by pushing away unwanted objects. An instructional prompt to touch a rejection or protest signal can be delivered prior to offering items that are predictably refused (Reichle, 1990). The child might be taught also to use a general rejection signal (*no*) in different situations (Keogh & Reichle, 1985). The comment function can be taught by using object names or labels (Keogh & Reichle, 1985). Initially, commenting serves a notice function that directs the attention of others and may be signaled by a generalized "look" or "notice me" signal. For ease of learning, separate lexical items should be used for different functions.

Vocabulary size can be increased by the flexible use of multimodality responding (Mirenda & Schuler, 1988; Morrow et al., 1993). If the child can shake his or her head "no," there is no reason at the onset of AAC use for the child to be forced to use a symbol or sign to replace it. Children developing typically use many modes of communicating. Multimodality communication assumes that any devices to be used be present in the communication environment and functioning. To violate this axiom is to risk device abandonment by the child.

Multimodality communication may be more difficult for some children because of the different memory tasks involved (Iacono, Mirenda, & Beukelman, 1993). Pictures and visual symbols require recognitory memory; signs and speech require recall memory.

Symbols used for many illocutionary functions can give the child a very flexible system (Owens, 1982d). Too often, augmentative communication users exhibit a limited range of illocutionary functions (J. Light, 1988).

Training should stress both receptive comprehension and expressive production rather than focusing on only one mode. In general, expressive learning of signs is best for symbols previously known receptively in speech (Clarke, 1987; P. Light, Remington, Clarke, & Watson, 1989). Children tend to overselect the visual model in expressive training and to ignore the verbal name for the symbol being taught. This problem can be overcome by training receptive use first or by using differential sign training in which the cue alternates between verbal-visual and verbal-only (Remington & Clarke, 1993a, 1993b).

Because generalization from simulated environments to the transfer or natural environment is difficult for many presymbolic clients, AAC systems should be trained within a wide variety of functional activities as these naturally occur in the transfer environment (Calculator, 1985, 1988b; Calculator & Jorgensen, 1991; Falvey, 1986; Falvey, Bishop, Grenot-Scheyer, & Coots, 1988; Guess & Helmstetter, 1986; Kangas & Lloyd, 1988; Orelove & Sobsey, 1987, Siegel-Causey & Downing, 1987). When trained within everyday activities, communication becomes relevant to the child's world. AAC use should be integrated into other services, such as occupational therapy or adaptive physical education. Each may require a specialized vocabulary that, if using a device, should be available while in those activities. Unfortunately, training, even with AAC, too often consists of unnatural, out-of-context, mass-trial formats (Helmstetter & Guess, 1987).

The spontaneous use of AAC can be a problem for both the user and the communication partner or nonuser. Compared with speakers, AAC users have fewer conversational partners and engage in shorter exchanges (Kraat, 1985). Caregivers may know few signs and use them only infrequently outside training (Bryen et al., 1988; Bryen & McGinley, 1991).

Although AAC can improve the quality of the communication, at present most users still have considerable delay as they produce their responses. Production time can be decreased for aided systems by the placement of items on a communication board, by the vocabulary selected, by careful analysis of the child-device interface, and by multimodality responding.

For more advanced children, especially those with motoric difficulties, who are able to type their messages, communication can be painfully slow. Studies of speed increase have focused on lessening the necessary keystrokes in any given message (Higginbotham, 1992), completing a child's electronically generated message on the basis of the most frequent words used (Newell et al., 1992) and prestoring prefixes, suffixes, and lexicons (Creech, 1989; Schwejda, 1986; Swiffin, Arnott, Pickering, & Newell, 1987; Vanderheiden & Kelso, 1987; Woltosz, 1988).

In general, the nonuser partner assumes a disproportionate responsibility for the conversation (Buzolich & Wiemann, 1988; Farrier, Yorkston, Marriner, & Beukelman, 1985). With little expectation that the user will participate, nonusers may talk around the user, fall into a yes-no probing strategy, answer their own questions or comment before the user can answer, use less mature language, and anticipate a response and preempt (Goosens & Kraat, 1985). These modifications cause the user to lose control of the conversation. In turn, the child may underfunction or behave as if he or she is much more limited (Calculator, 1985; Houghton et al., 1987). This is the result of insufficient motivation to communicate. The child adopts a pattern of passivity and learned helplessness (Basil, 1992; Kraat, 1985; J. Light, 1988).

Nonuser partners can change their behavior, but doing so requires that the SLP instruct them in the use of the AAC too. Instruction is especially important if the expectations and demands of the environment are dissimilar from those used in teaching the user. While AAC is used to initiate and maintain conversations both at home and in school, the school environment is more directive (Sevcik, Romski, Watkins, & Deffebach, 1995).

The SLP should encourage use of the child's AAC system whenever possible throughout the day by using incidental and stimulation techniques. In general, the more the child and the caregivers use the system, the more it will generalize. The key to successful learning and use is a system that is easy to use, an ability by the child to be understood, and a motivation to imitate and use the system in response to natural cues in everyday contexts (Halle, 1987; G. McGregor et al., 1992; Rotholz, Berkowitz, & Burberry, 1989).

Communication Environment Manipulation

The SLP can modify the child's communication environment in several ways to enhance communication and training. After a thorough analysis of the communication demands placed on the child, he or she identifies high- and low-communication contexts by location, activities, and communication partners.

High-communication contexts are encouraged and increased. These high-communication contexts often offer ideal opportunities for incidental teaching.

The SLP modifies or eliminates low-communication contexts. For example, the child's communication behavior may elicit no response from the school bus aide. The facilitator might instruct this person in a few simple methods of conversational responding to increase the communication learning potential of this situation. If the child spends long periods each day in solitary play, these times might be eliminated or changed to parallel group play.

Interactional Changes

Caregivers will need guidance to help them redefine their perceptions of their child's abilities (Sameroff & Feise, 1990). This change of attitude may require helping caregivers reassess communication breakdowns and identify subtle ways in which their child may be communicating. Caregivers should be encouraged to alter nonfacilitative strategies. Initial caregiver training might begin with the following three principles (MacDonald, 1985):

1. Everyone engages in some form of communication.
2. Every communication occurrence has the potential for reciprocity.
3. Expectation of one partner affects motivation of the other to initiate communication.

Children learn to the extent to which they communicate in contexts that support these endeavors and are reciprocal and balanced (MacDonald & Carroll, 1992b).

Possible targets for caregiver interactional training might include learning to abandon his or her own agenda and to follow the child's lead, to establish joint attention and action, to give the child the freedom to make meaningful choices, to balance turn taking with no one partner dominating, to be less directive, to respond in a semantically and pragmatically contingent manner, and to use a variety of illocutionary functions and a child lexicon (Dobe, 1989; Holton, 1987; MacDonald, 1989; Mac-Donald & Carroll, 1992b; Manolson, 1985; Theadore et al., 1990; J. Young, 1988). Essentially, the adult is learning to fine-tune her or his communication for the abilities of the child. Possible changes in caregiver behaviors are listed in Table 11.23.

TABLE 11.23   Possible changes in caregiver behavior as a result of training

Balancing conversational partnership with child
Physically prompt child to take a turn.
Wait expectantly.
Allow enough time for child's turn.
Follow the child's lead.
Respond in meaningful ways to keep the conversation going.

Matching the child's linguistic abilities
Respond to movements and sounds with similar ones.
Expand one-word utterances to two words or short phrases.
Add something to the child's turn that is slightly more mature.
Act like the child in interactions.

Responding contingently
Respond to even the slightest behaviors.
Pay attention to appropriate behavior while ignoring immature or disruptive behavior.
Respond immediately to imitated behaviors.
Be fun to be with; be a reinforcer.

Being nondirective
Limit questions and directives to authentic ones.
Wait and expect.
Match child's language and cognitive level.
Engage child in conversations of more than one turn.
Follow child's lead but expect that he or she will follow yours on occasion.

Becoming emotionally attached
Balance your turns for length.
Match the child's interest and communication.
Respond sensitively.
Share the lead; be nondirective.
Enjoy your time together.
Reduce stress by focusing on play, not achievement.
Avoid negative judgments.
Concentrate on keeping the interaction going, rather than on correcting the child.

Source: Adapted from MacDonald & Carroll (1992b).

Even minimum instruction in training techniques is beneficial and enables some caregivers to adopt suitable teaching strategies spontaneously. Feedback from the SLP regarding the application of newly acquired teaching skills, however, is the critical element.

The caregiver can elicit trained responses within the home or classroom through environmental manipulation (McNaughton & Light, 1989). After the child is taught to respond to *need to communicate* situations, the caregiver restructures needs-meeting situations within daily routines so that the child's needs are not anticipated but are dependent on communicative behavior. The behavior becomes situationally dependent and makes sense in context, rather than dependent on a verbal prompt from the facilitator (Halle, 1987).

The caregivers can structure elicitation situations, such as turn-taking games, choice making, enticement with desirable items, and assistance requesting (McNaughton & Light, 1989). Once a skill is learned, the child is required to use that skill to obtain desired entities or privileges for which it was not formerly required. Previously accepted behaviors are no longer sufficient.

A strategy of *waiting,* or time delay, has been used effectively to enhance spontaneous use of trained communication behaviors (Charlop, Schreibman, & Thebodeau, 1985; Gobbi, Cipani, Hudson, & Lapenta-Neudeck, 1986). This procedure is most effective when the child desires some item or has to communicate to complete a task.

Interactive routines in which the child has some expectation from past events offer an opportunity to create a need to communicate (McLean et al., 1991). The facilitator can wait as the child anticipates and, hopefully, signals. Other effective strategies for child initiation are *introduction of novel elements, oversight,* and *sabotage* (McLean & Snyder-McLean, 1988b).

Finally, the stimulation behaviors discussed previously can be a helpful guide for caregiver interactional behaviors. The following are additional conversational suggestions (MacDonald & Gillette, 1986):

Structure the activity for give-and-take.

Follow the child's lead.

Imitate the child.

Wait for the child to take a turn.

Signal the child to take a turn.

Chain responses by using turnabouts, in which a turn includes both a response to the child's turn and a cue for the child to take another turn.

Summary

Children who are presymbolic and minimally symbolic have special needs that often relate to the very purposes for communication. If these children are going to communicate more effectively, there must be a reason for doing so. In addition, the environment must provide models and respond to the child appropriately. Initial communication training cannot be an isolated affair; by its nature, communication is central to all human interactions. Communication will not generalize to the everyday use environment unless that environment becomes a facilitative one for such behavior. Only an integrated, functional intervention that targets both the child and the environment can hope to change effectively the child's current behavior. Throughout the day within each child's natural communication environment, caregivers use the three intervention techniques of incidental teaching, stimulation, and formal training.

Conclusion

Even though you may feel overwhelmed by all the recommendations in this chapter, we have discussed only a small percentage of the available intervention techniques. Limited space necessitates a rather cursory examination of these procedures. SLPs should seek further information in source materials or in published clinical materials. In addition, they will conceive their own creative and innovative methods for intervening with children with LIs. It is hoped that these methods will be adapted to fit the conversational model presented in Chapters 9 and 10.

Not all specific language problems are treated easily with a functional approach, but the entire model does not have to be discarded. Caregivers, for example, are a valuable resource and can be used in various ways, whatever the specific language problem being targeted. Likewise, training can occur in meaningful contexts within everyday events.

12

Classroom Functional Intervention

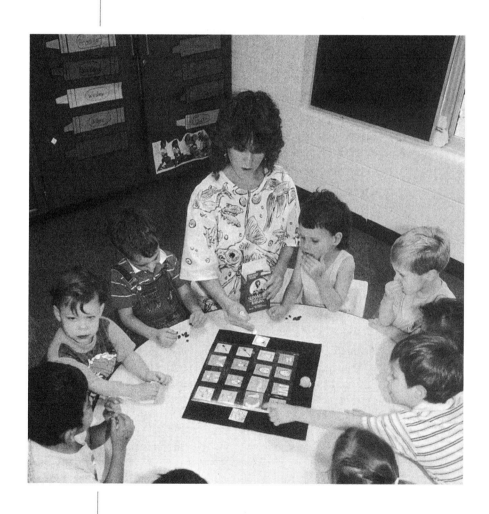

In school, children encounter the language of instruction, which presents discourse experiences that are very different from the child's previous conversational interactions (N. Nelson, 1985; Ripich & Spinelli, 1985). Language is treated in the abstract as children learn to talk about it and to manipulate it to learn about other things. Metalinguistic skills are very important (Gottschalk, Prelock, Weiler, & Sandman, 1997). The child with inadequate language skills or inadequate strategies for making sense of different situations is apt to become lost (N. Nelson, 1989).

More than for communicating with other people, "in school, language must also be used to regulate thinking, to plan, reflect, evaluate, and to acquire knowledge about things that are not directly experienced" (J. Norris, 1989, p. 206). On an oral-to-literate continuum (Westby, 1985), school tasks are at the extreme literate end, requiring the child to understand and express information displaced from her or his own experiential base. Language itself creates the context in which information is conveyed to other people so that they can comprehend it and understand an event without having shared in the experience.

The SLP supports the child's communication efforts in the following ways (Duchan, 1997):

Socially, by modifying his or her role and modeling appropriate roles for the child and by creating contexts in which the child can take varying roles.

Emotionally, by preventing ostracism and by aiding the child to resolve conflict and to be tuned to the needs of others.

Functionally, by redesigning contexts when needed by the child and by helping all children achieve their communication goals.

Physically, by arranging the environment for maximum participation.

Communicatively, by providing scripts for participation.

The goal is for each child to be successful with diminishing adult support. Language is an "interactional phenomenon" and, as such, is a tool for achieving social aims and for making sense of the world and of others (Kovarsky & Maxwell, 1997).

Language intervention should reflect more closely what we know about language development and use (N. Nelson, 1986a, 1988a; Wallach & Miller, 1988). Functional intervention treats language as it occurs throughout the child's many experiences. Assessment and intervention that flow from this model stress language processing within a variety of relevant contexts, such as the classroom (L. Miller, 1989).

A functional approach to intervention shifts the focus from the child as the source and solution of the language problem to a holistic view that includes the child and the child's language uses and learning strategies, the contextual demands, the expectations and beliefs of other people within that context, the child's interaction, the context, and the child's communication partners (L. Miller, 1989). Thus, the focuses of intervention become the contexts that surround the child with LI and the manipulation of these contexts.

The classroom's cognitive activities are an excellent context for stimulating language growth (Moses & Maffei, 1989). Within the classroom's constructive activities, children create, change, relate, and compare entities; set goals; encounter and try to overcome problems; make errors; reflect on success or failure; and note problem-solving procedures.

The functional model discussed throughout this text can be adapted to these differing classroom needs. In fact, some of the recent changes in education, such as inclusion and collaborative teaching, espouse some of the same principles we have been discussing. In this chapter, we will examine these trends and propose some models of classroom intervention. Following that, we will describe the new role of the public school SLP and elements of a classroom intervention model, including specific intervention targets for preschool and school-age children. Finally, we will discuss implementation of classroom intervention.

Background and Rationale: Recent Educational Changes

Language training within the school classroom offers a special challenge for the SLP and the classroom teacher. School systems throughout the United States and Canada are adopting and modifying many models of intervention to provide more appropriate and effective intervention. These new models reflect recent educational changes in inclusion and collaborative teaching.

Inclusion

Educational legislation in the United States has resulted in increased educational benefits for children with disabling conditions. One outcome of this legislation, intended or not, was two parallel educational systems: one for children developing typically and another for children with disabilities. Special education included separate placement, separate teachers, and a separate curriculum. Special services such as speech-language pathology usually were accomplished by removing the child from the classroom.

As a result, the *pull-out,* or *isolated therapy model,* of intervention prevailed in public education (Marvin, 1987). The pull-out model tends to fragment the child's intervention, especially if the child needs more than one pull-out service. Such patchwork schedules are extremely difficult for children with few strategies for making sense of the world. Increased need results in increased fragmentation until there is little continuity, and the child's progress suffers as a result (Bashir, 1987). Usually, there is little generalization with the pull-out model, and the content of such intervention may be irrelevant to the child's classroom needs (Anderson & Nelson, 1988).

Larger criticisms—just or otherwise—of the overall separate special-education model include the inherent segregation, the focus on labeling and categorization of children, the "slow it down, water it down" educational approach, and a general frustration with a "once in, never out" treadmill. Beginning in the 1980s and continuing today, a movement has developed to raise education standards for all children and to share decision making through more local control and more teacher-parent shared involvement.

These changes have led to inclusive schooling and to the Regular Education Initiative (REI). **Inclusive schooling** is an educational philosophy that proposes one integrated educational system based on each classroom becoming a supportive environment for all of its members—children and teachers (S. Stainback & Stainback, 1992; W. Stainback & Stainback, 1990). The notion does not envision an end to special education. These services still will be essential.

Instead of separate systems of education, inclusive schooling proposes a unitary system of education adaptive enough to meet individual children's needs in a flexible manner. The result is (a) a shift in focus from the deficits to the abilities of children with special needs, (b) collaborative learning, (c) curriculum-based intervention, and (d) placement of all children in regular-education classrooms, with special services as needed (Silliman, 1993).

REI is the movement toward an educational continuum that extends from regular-education class-rooms for most children through regular-education classrooms with special services to adaptive environments for a small majority of the children most severely involved (Hoffman, 1993). At the latter end of the continuum, children will require services from trained professionals and curriculum-based intervention services to enhance their classroom participation. For example, in reading readiness training, children with LLD need explicit, systematic, and intense instruction in areas such as phonological awareness and letter-sound relationships (Silliman, Bahr, Beasman, & Wilkinson, 2000).

Ideally, children developing typically will serve as models for children with LI, although integration alone may be insufficient. In such classrooms, preschool children with LI will spend a considerable amount of time talking with adults (Weiss & Nakamura, 1992). Model children developing typically are chosen carefully and trained in simple techniques that will facilitate communication for children with LI (Weiss & Nakamura, 1992). Children in self-contained special education classrooms often do not form friendships with children developing typically and thus often do not have typical peer models (Roller, Rodriguez, Warner, & Lindahl, 1992).

The result is not an end to special education, but rather a change in emphasis and a new way of educating children. The intent of inclusive teaching is increased educational opportunity for all children.

Change is not without its problems. More than a quarter of SLPs surveyed feel that inclusion is not appropriate for all children with LI even though it results in better carryover and provides good language models for these children (Bell, 1995). The most frequent complaints are that there are too many students to serve and not enough time for individual attention.

Collaborative Teaching

The negative effects of pulling children out of class to receive speech and language services are not found when these services occur in the classroom. Ongoing classroom activities can serve as the basis for intervention, with content coming from the child's assignments and projects and the interactions of the classroom (Wallach & Miller, 1988). Thus, intervention is relevant for the environment in which it is being used. In addition, the child can benefit from the social dynamics of the classroom (N. Nelson, 1988b).

The variety of formats for classroom intervention includes the following (Blank & Marquis, 1987; Catts & Kamhi, 1987; DeSpain & Simon, 1987; Dudley-Marling, 1987; L. Miller, 1989; Simon, 1985):

1. The SLP team-teaches with the regular classroom teacher and other specialists, usually the resource room teacher (J. Norris, 1989; Roller et al., 1992). This teaching may include both specialists teaching small groups simultaneously, or one specialist, such as the teacher, working with the larger class, while the other, such as the SLP, works with a smaller group. Goals and objectives, individualized educational plans (IEPs), and the monitoring and reviewing of individual programs are the team's joint responsibilities.

2. The SLP provides one-on-one classroom-based intervention with selected students in the classroom by using course materials (N. Nelson, 1989). The intervention usually centers on language strategies for classroom use.

3. The SLP acts as a consultant for the classroom teacher and other specialists. As such, he or she advises (not supervises) personnel, assisting primary caregivers with intervention strategies. Consultative models of intervention usually involve joint goals and objectives that the classroom teacher implements. The SLP assists the classroom teacher in modifying curriculum, instruc-

tion, and assessment to facilitate the success of children with LI. Within a therapeutic partnership, the SLP helps the teacher set objectives, reinforce and modify behavior, and assess progress (Ehren, 2000). This collaborative consultation model is the one most frequently suggested in the professional literature (Marvin, 1987). This model is very flexible and may include elements of several other formats. Because this model has obvious advantages for generalization (Damico, 1987), it is the basis for discussion in this chapter.

4. The SLP provides staff training and curriculum development to the school or district.

The model for discussion incorporates some elements of each of these formats, although primary emphasis is on the collaborative format.

Collaborative teaching is a combination of consultation, team teaching, direct individual intervention where needed, and side-by-side teaching in which the teacher and the SLP share the same goals for individual children (Montgomery, 1992a). In partnership, the SLP and the classroom teacher combine their efforts to serve children with LI. Parents are also members of the intervention team. The collaborative-consultative model stresses interaction and integration of the knowledge and expertise of the individuals involved (Confal, 1993). The approach is a problem-solving one in which all participants share the responsibilities of decision making, planning, and implementation. All aspects of speech and language services are built around the skills a specific child needs to function better in the classroom environment. The many evolving models of collaboration vary with the SLP's therapeutic perspective, the degree of child- and family-centeredness, the amount of guided inquiry and cooperative group work, discourse scaffolding, and prevention (Prelock, 2000).

Collaborative teaching also involves active choices by children. Within limits, children can select the focus of learning just as they can select the topic of conversation. In this way, children have a stake in what is being learned. They are actively involved.

This model includes, but is not limited to, the following elements:

1. The SLP provides in-service training for staff and parents.
2. The classroom teacher helps identify potential children with LI through observation of classroom behavior. The SLP evaluates the speech and language skills of these children and others who fail speech and language screenings. Such evaluations are an ongoing and integral part of the intervention process.
3. The SLP, classroom teacher, and aide provide individual and small and large group intervention services within the classroom and the curriculum. In addition, the SLP continues to provide individual or small group therapy outside the classroom to children in need.
4. The classroom teacher, aide, and parents interact daily with the children in ways that facilitate the development of language skills.

The SLP is not a paraprofessional aide for the classroom teacher. To use the context of the natural environment, the SLP should be in that environment and use communication situations occurring in that context. Thus, the SLP increasingly provides individual and group intervention within the classroom and conducts small group activities in which newly acquired language skills are used.

Classroom training has been shown to be effective in increasing both elicited and spontaneous language production (Dyer et al., 1991; Haring et al., 1988; Koegel, Dyer, & Bell, 1987; Koegel & Johnson, 1989; Scott, 1995). With very young children, a classroom intervention model for teaching an initial lexicon is superior to individual intervention methods in generalization of learned words

(Wilcox et al., 1991). When the SLP and classroom teacher plan collectively but work independently in the class, even children not enrolled in language intervention benefit. This model can be used also to train phonology within everyday classroom activities (Masterson, 1993a). In short, the collaborative classroom model is both effective and cost-efficient (Langenfield & Coltrane, 1991).

These results reflect the more numerous natural opportunities for communication available in typical situations and contexts of the classroom and with the many potential language facilitators in the classroom (L. Miller, 1989). Ideally, the classroom provides an interactive model in which a high density of language features are modeled and used in a conversational format embedded in familiar, ongoing activities (K. Cole & Dale, 1986; N. Nelson, 1989; Snyder-McLean & McLean, 1987). For collaboration to be successful, "each member of the team must be comfortable with his or her teaching style and must be willing to take risks" (Roller et al., 1992, p. 366).

Real conversations and meaningful activities provide motivation and experiences that are usually not available in isolated individual intervention targeting discrete bits of language (Bricker, 1986). Activities are meaningful and experience based. Communication is child initiated and controlled. The SLP, teacher, and other children respond to the child's naturally occurring communication (Bricker, 1986; Fey, 1986). In this way, naturalistic classroom intervention is consistent with the principles of whole language.

Summary

Educational trends, including inclusive schooling and collaborative teaching, have combined to change the teaching and remediation of language. In many schools, the SLP is working with children and their language impairments within a naturalistic language curriculum in regular education classrooms.

"Speech-language pathology…is moving away from the behaviorism of the past sixty years and its fragmented view of language…moving toward a more dynamic and integrated construct of language proficiency" (J. Norris & Damico, 1990, p. 219). The principles we have been discussing in this book are a near perfect match to the demands of this intervention situation.

Role of the Speech-Language Pathologist

Any classroom intervention model raises questions about the SLP's role and about others' expectations of the intervention team. These questions include the following:

What is my new role? Who am I?

Are there special language needs within the routines of the classroom situation?

How do I address individual needs within a classroom?

How do I justify my new role to an administration that gauges my work in individual contact hours?

What is the relationship of language arts and language remediation?

How do I educate teachers?

The classroom model is still evolving, and there are no quick answers. Our discussion of the elements of the classroom model addresses some of these questions.

The SLP is a problem solver who, with the guidance of a few principles, applies and adapts a variety of methods in seeking solutions. In the final analysis, the model of intervention that evolves is a blend of the child's needs and the desires of the school, the individual teacher, and the SLP. The SLP will assume the roles of co-teacher, consultant, and direct service provider and will be integrated fully into the classroom (Farber, Denenberg, Klyman, & Lachman, 1992).

The SLP is the school's language expert. As such, he or she advises administrators, teachers, and special needs committees about children and language impairment. The SLP is also responsible for speech and language assessment, for the planning and implementation of all speech and language programming, for record keeping, and for training personnel who will work with the children with LI.

Relating to Others

Functional intervention such as that in the classroom necessitates coordination of intervention goals and schedules. This coordination requires that the SLP interact daily with a variety of individuals.

Classroom Teachers

The SLP is uniquely qualified to assist the classroom teacher in assessing each child's level of functioning, analyzing the language requirements of various activities and materials, and developing intervention strategies in conjunction with the classroom teacher. He or she helps the teacher identify children with LI and suggests techniques to facilitate development. This is an ongoing process, accomplished through in-service training and individual consultation and training, as well as with co-teaching within the classroom. Both teachers and SLPs rank team teaching and one teach/one drift as the most appropriate model for collaborative teaching (Beck & Dennis, 1997). Team teaching is supplemental teaching in which one team member adapts the material for children with LI. In one teach/one drift one member teaches and the other assists students as needed.

The SLP and the classroom teacher have unique skills that they can use to help each other and the child with LI. The SLP understands language development and the remediation of speech and LI. The classroom teacher knows each child and understands the use of large and small group interactions for teaching.

Difficulties usually arise over turf or territory. The classroom teacher may feel threatened by the presence of another "teacher" in the classroom and may resent being shown how to talk to students to maximize each child's language learning. The SLP may feel like a classroom aide, undervalued for his or her expertise. These differences and potential problems should be discussed openly prior to beginning intervention. Each professional's role should be delineated and clearly understood. The SLP and the classroom teacher should exchange clear and valuable information. This ongoing exchange is especially important at the beginning of intervention.

It is imperative that the SLP avoid the "tutor trap" in which she or he becomes a glorified classroom aide (J. Norris, 1997). The SLP needs to focus on each child's clinical goals while being mindful of the classroom requirements for each child. Classroom requirements should not dictate clinical content. In addition, the SLP should work to enhance the classroom environment as well as to change the child's language.

Some SLPs voice concerns about becoming a classroom aide or "watering down" therapy for the entire class that they should be providing to individual children. It is important to retain a therapeutic focus. This requires the interrelated steps of planning and implementation (Ehren, 2000). Planning requires intervention services for children that target skills underlying the curriculum. In implementing intervention, the SLP should focus on the goals for children on the caseload and not on general educational activities. Examples of classroom *dos and don'ts* are presented in Table 12.1. The role of the SLP is not to provide specific curriculum teaching or tutoring nor to relieve the teacher of the responsibility to teach all students in the class.

The SLP and the classroom teacher are part of the intervention team and should contribute in that fashion. Each has special expertise to impart. Neither one is there to spy on the other, and their personal opinions of each other have no place in the classroom.

Parents

Not all parents can or wish to participate in their children's speech-language intervention. Parents tend to fall into three identifiable groups, the largest being those who desire participation. Next are those who desire no participation, and the smallest group is composed of parents who only want more information (Andrews, Andrews, & Shearer, 1989). The first group of parents can be involved in planning and implementation of intervention, and parents who want information can be served through parent meetings and in-service training.

School Administrators

The SLP's new role may require some education of the administration. Traditional patterns of instruction change slowly, and administrators may not understand generalization and the need to provide language remediation within the classroom. Caseload dictates and contact hour requirements may have to be modified to accommodate the classroom model. Both teachers and SLPs agree that finding enough consultative time is a big problem (Beck & Dennis, 1997).

Administrators will need to be impressed with the increased efficiency gained through the co-teaching of the SLP and the classroom teacher. Discussion should center on how best to serve the children and how to use professional time commitments most efficiently.

Finally, the SLP's new role should be viewed within the perspective of a comprehensive school or districtwide program that includes early childhood intervention, bilingual and bidialectal services, and the training of English as a second language (Koenig & Biel, 1989). Public law is dictating an extension of speech-language and educational services to these children.

TABLE 12.1   Examples of *dos and don'ts* of classroom speech and language services

Do...	Don't...
Help child to identify the important information on a math worksheet and decide on a way to perform the operation.	Help the child complete the math problems.
Teach relevant vocabulary by focusing on the words and figurative language of the science text that may be difficult for the child with LI, and encourage the teacher to establish a language learning center.	Preteach the science vocabulary next chapter.
Co-teach a social studies lesson by guiding the students with LI to practice the language strategies learned in therapy. Simple note cards containing reminders can be given to each child.	Co-teach a social studies lesson for all students without addressing the IEP goals of the children with LI.

Source: Adapted from Ehren, (2000).

Language Intervention and Language Arts

Classroom teachers and administrators are sometimes confused about the difference between language arts and language remediation. Unless this distinction is clear, the SLP's role also may be misunderstood, especially as it relates to classroom intervention. *Language arts* accomplishes several things:

1. Provides children with labels for the language units they have been using in their speech
2. Requires children to stretch their language abilities into new areas, such as fictional and expository writing
3. Enables children to have language growth experiences, such as performances
4. Helps children reason and problem solve by using linguistic units

All of these valuable accomplishments presuppose that each child has a well-formed language system. Children with LI are at risk of failure.

In *language remediation,* the child is taught language units or behaviors that are not present or are in error in the primary mode of communication—that is, in language transmitted via speech. Secondary modes, such as reading and writing, are a concern when problems with oral language affect them. Through training, teachers and administrators become aware of this distinction and of the valuable contribution of each to the child's education.

Elements of a Classroom Model

The model consists of identification (assessment), intervention, and facilitation. In each phase, the classroom teacher and the SLP, although a team, have individual inputs that affect the delivery of quality services for the child.

Identification of Children at Risk

Teachers play a vital role in identifying children with LI. Most teachers are not trained in language development or impairment, and the SLP must alert them to the behaviors that signal a possible impairment.

Teacher training can be accomplished in in-service sessions. Teachers also can be given aids to use in identifying a potential language problem. Table 12.2 presents a list of some signs for recognizing children having difficulties in the classroom. Appendix H contains an analysis format for classroom interactions that can guide teachers in determining the locus of breakdown in communication interactions in the classroom (Vetter, 1982). Table 12.3 or its adaptation might be used by teachers for referral to the SLP.

Teachers should be trained to observe and describe classroom behaviors as precisely as possible. The SLP's complaint that teachers refer children who have rather nonspecific vocabulary problems or are inattentive reflects poorly on the SLP's training of teachers in LI and its manifestations. Teachers are a valuable source of raw data on classroom performance when they know what to observe and measure.

In addition, the SLP and the classroom teacher can identify the individual classroom's or grade level's special communication requirements as a gauge against which each child can be measured to

TABLE 12.2   Recognizing children with language impairment in the classroom

The child may have some or all of the following:
  Seems to fail to understand and follow instructions.
  Is unable to use language to meet daily living needs.
  Violates rules of social interaction, including politeness.
  Lacks ability to read signs or other symbols and to perform written tasks.
  Has problems using speech to communicate effectively.
  Demonstrates a lack of appropriate organization and sequence in verbal and written efforts.
  Does not remember significant information presented orally and/or in written form.
  May not recognize humor or indirect comments.
  Seems unable to interpret the emotions or predict the intentions of others.
  Responds inappropriately for the situation.

Source: Adapted from N. W. Nelson (1992).

assess achievement. Called *curriculum-based assessment,* this method uses the child's progress within the school curriculum as a measure of her or his educational success (Tucker, 1985). Children are assessed against the curriculum within which they are expected to perform. Thus, intervention focuses on changes in the child's behavior that are relevant to the educational setting.

From preschool through high school, the curriculum not only becomes more difficult but also changes in the types of demands made on the student. These changes are as follows (Wiig & Semel, 1984):

Preschool: Learning focuses on sensorimotor, language, and socioemotional growth with materials that are manipulative, three-dimensional, and concrete.

Early grades (K–2): Learning focuses on perceptual-cognitive strategies with materials that are one dimensional, abstract, and symbolic.

Middle grades (3–4): Learning places higher demands on linguistic and symbolic skills with less direct instruction. The child is expected to make inferences, analyze data, and synthesize information.

Upper grades (5–6): Learning focuses on content areas, with the child expected to recall past learning and display fluency with basic academic skills.

Middle and high school: Learning emphasizes lectures in content areas, with students expected to reorganize material as they listen and to gain the main or important points. From 75 percent to 90 percent of the day may be spent receiving information.

By identifying the overall requirements for the class, the teacher has provided a list of potential skills with which the child with LI may experience difficulty. Some school districts have identified skills that children need to succeed in each grade. Table 12.4 presents some of the skills needed in the first three grades.

In addition to the school's official curriculum, which is an outline of the material to be learned in each grade, children encounter several other curricula (N. Nelson, 1989). These include the *de facto curriculum* that is actually taught and the cultural and school curricula needed to succeed within each context. The expectations of the latter are often very confusing for the child with language-processing problems. The implicit expectations of individual teachers and other children form a fourth curriculum.

TABLE 12.3   Teacher referral of children with possible language impairment

The following behaviors may indicate that a child in your classroom has a language impairment that is in need of clinical intervention. Please check the appropriate items.

_____   Child mispronounces sounds and words.

_____   Child omits word endings, such as plural -*s* and past-tense -*ed.*

_____   Child omits small unemphasized words, such as auxiliary verbs or prepositions.

_____   Child uses an immature vocabulary, overuses empty words, such as *one* and *thing,* or seems to have difficulty recalling or finding the right word.

_____   Child has difficulty comprehending new words and concepts.

_____   Child's sentence structure seems immature or overreliant on forms, such as subject-verb-object. It's unoriginal, dull.

_____   Child's question and/or negative sentence style is immature.

_____   Child has difficulty with one of the following:

_____ Verb tensing	_____ Articles	_____ Auxiliary verbs
_____ Pronouns	_____ Irregular verbs	_____ Prepositions
_____ Word order	_____ Irregular plurals	_____ Conjunctions

_____   Child has difficulty relating sequential events.

_____   Child has difficulty following directions.

_____   Child's questions often inaccurate or vague.

_____   Child's questions often poorly formed.

_____   Child has difficulty answering questions.

_____   Child's comments often off-topic or inappropriate for the conversation.

_____   There are long pauses between a remark and the child's reply or between successive remarks by the child. It's as if the child is searching for a response or is confused.

_____   Child appears to be attending to communication but remembers little of what is said.

_____   Child has difficulty using language socially for the following purposes:

_____ Request needs	_____ Pretend/imagine	_____ Protest
_____ Greet	_____ Request information	_____ Gain attention
_____ Respond/reply	_____ Share ideas, feelings	_____ Clarify
_____ Relate events	_____ Entertain	_____ Reason

_____   Child has difficulty interpreting the following:

_____ Figurative language	_____ Humor	_____ Gestures
_____ Emotions	_____ Body language	

_____   Child does not alter production for different audiences and locations.

_____   Child does not seem to consider the effect of language on the listener.

_____   Child often has verbal misunderstandings with others.

_____   Child has difficulty with reading and writing.

_____   Child's language skills seem to be much lower than other areas, such as mechanical, artistic, or social skills.

TABLE 12.4 Some possible language skills needed in the first three grades

First Grade. The child will be able to:
Recognize correct word order auditorily.
Identify singular and plural common nouns and proper nouns.
Identify regular and irregular past and present verbs.
Identify descriptive and comparative adjectives.
Use nouns and pronouns, adjectives, and verbs correctly in sentences, including verb-noun agreement.
Give and write full sentences.
Categorize words by opposites, by sequence, by category, and as real/nonreal.
Retell a story.
Identify the main idea in a paragraph.
Classify narrative and descriptive writing.
Rhyme words and identify words that begin with the same sound.
Identify declarative and interrogative sentences and use correct ending punctuation for each.
Capitalize the first word in a sentence, days, months, people's names, and the pronoun *I*.
Alphabetize.
Give directions and explanations and follow two-step directions.
Read aloud.
Listen attentively and courteously to others.

Second Grade. In addition to the skills needed for first grade, the child will be able to:
Use correct word order.
Identify incomplete sentences.
Recognize singular and compound subjects of a sentence.
Identify possessive and plural nouns, contracted verbs, and superlative adjectives and use correctly.
Capitalize holidays, titles of people, books, stories, and places.
Identify correct comma use.
Use an apostrophe in contractions.
Identify the topic sentence and sentences that do not relate in a paragraph.
Write an explanation or set of directions.
Address an envelope.
Write rhyming words to complete a poem.
Identify figurative language and synonyms.
Recognize characters, plot, setting, and the major divisions in a story or play, and the difference
    between fiction and nonfiction.
Tell and write a clear, original story.
Use the title page and table of contents in a book.
Use the dictionary for spelling and meaning.
Read critically for sequence, main idea, and supporting details.
Use tables and graphs as sources of information.
Recognize types of poetry.
Listen discriminately for rhyming, sequences, and details.

Third Grade. In addition to the skills needed for first and second grade, the child will be able to:
Identify imperative and exclamatory sentences, simple and compound sentences, and run-on sentences.
Recognize compound predicates in a sentence.
Recognize articles and conjunctions in sentences.
Use an exclamation point.
Use an apostrophe in possessive nouns.
Define a paragraph and identify the main idea and supporting sentences.
Write a paragraph, a book report, and a letter with correct capitalization and punctuation.
Write a clear, original story with title, beginning, middle, and end.
Recognize the difference between biography and autobiography.
Use a dictionary for pronunciation.
Use an encyclopedia, telephone book, newspapers, and magazines as references.
Identify compound words, homophones, and homographs.
Use prefixes and suffixes.
Read critically for sequence, main idea, and supporting details.
Organize information by category and sequence.
Recognize real and make-believe, relevant and irrelevant, and factual and opinionated statements.
Identify characteristics of different types of narratives.

The SLP first must become familiar with the curricula that affect the individual child with LI. He or she can assess the child through a combination of interview and observation of the child's ability to meet the language demands of the curricula. The interview phase can provide information on the curricular expectations, and observation can focus on the specific linguistic demands made of the child.

An analysis of the linguistic demands must consider all aspects of language and the many reception and production modes. Such an analysis should note metalinguistic skills demanded in these various aspects and modes (N. Nelson, 1989).

An educational language assessment should focus on the child's oral and written abilities and capacity to learn, rather than on his or her deficits (Silliman, 1993). Data are gathered by direct testing and real-life observation within the classroom. The level of support necessary for learning is determined, including evaluation of the effectiveness of various instructional and intervention strategies. Most standardized tests are too global, and more specific measures should be used to measure the child. The parents and the teacher, as well as the child and the SLP, should participate.

The SLP follows up these reports and collects her or his own data within the classroom setting. These data can be corroborated by further testing and sampling.

Teachers should be informed about the results of such testing and sampling and advised on the best methods of intervention. Classroom teachers can be apprised periodically of the child's progress and involved intimately in the intervention process.

Assessment with Preschool Children

The SLP is interested in pragmatic abilities at both the utterance, cross-utterance and cross-partner, and event levels; semantics, especially the child's lexicon, and language structure; and narrative form and story grammar rudiments. Additional areas of importance for literacy education include role-play and representational play, decontextualization, literacy, and adaptations for non-oral responding (Culatta, 1992; Culatta, Horn, Theodore, & Sutherland, 1993; Westby, 1988).

Play is particularly important for preschool children, especially as a context within which to experiment with language (Westby, 1988). Of particular importance are the level of decontextualization, thematic content, organization, and self/other relations (Culatta, 1992; Culatta et al., 1993; Westby, 1988). Play can be very context-bound, using only real objects, or relatively decontextualized, using imaginary or symbolic objects. The familiar versus unfamiliar themes of play are also important for later intervention. The organization of play can demonstrate cohesion, logical connections with the theme, and planning. Finally, the roles the child takes and assigns may be important for later training and may tell the SLP something about the child's ability to take the perspective of others and to style and code switch.

Decontextualization of the child's language is important for later reading and is demonstrated by reference to nonpresent entities and to past and future tense. Reading is very decontextualized because all meaning comes from print and little from the physical context.

Even though the child cannot read, literacy skills are important for further development. The SLP is interested in the child's comprehension of text, knowledge and awareness of print, and sound-symbol associations and decoding abilities.

Finally, non-oral methods of communicating are important. These include gestures, facial expression, and body posture, but also drawing and "writing."

Assessment with School-Age Children and Adolescents

In addition to considering the language features mentioned in Chapters 5 through 8, the SLP is interested in the child's language as it relates to the specific requirements of the classroom. An authentic, or real, assessment should be a *train-test-train* procedure, with both the SLP and the classroom teacher acting as "participant observers," determining the best instructional strategies for individual children (Silliman, 1993). Such an evaluation consists of systematic observation of real teaching and learning in the classroom that yields meaningful information on student progress on an ongoing basis.

Systematic observation might include rating scales and checklists, narrative records, and descriptive tools by the teacher, SLP, and student (Silliman, Wilkinson, & Hoffman, 1993). Possible rating scales for use with school-age children and adolescents are listed in Table 12.5. Teacher logs, notes, journal entries, and student assignments and self-evaluations should be gathered to ascertain the child's oral and written language skills. Of interest is the amount of scaffolding or structure and assistance needed by the child for success.

Interviews with the student are also helpful (N. Nelson, 1992). Students can be asked to describe their most difficult and easiest subjects and their strengths and weaknesses, to relate recent classroom events that made them feel bad and to prioritize changes they would like to make in themselves and in the classroom and manner of instruction.

The SLP may gain additional information by informally sampling the child's performance. For example, the SLP might compare a secondary school child's notes with those of a higher-performing student in the same class (Larson & McKinley, 1987). Audiotapes of classroom instructions can be analyzed to determine the level of complexity that each child must be able to process. The SLP might collect samples of the child's oral reading or help the child complete assignments, noting the child's language-related work skills.

TABLE 12.5   Tools for assessment of classroom skills

Observation/Interviews

Clinical Discourse Analysis (Damico, 1985a)

Environmental Communication Profile (Calvert & Murray, 1985)

An Interview for Assessing Students' Perceptions of Classroom Reading Tasks (Wixson, Bosky, Yochum, & Alvermann, 1984)

Pragmatic Protocol (Prutting & Kirchner, 1983, 1987)

Self-Attribution of Students (SAS) (Marsh, Cairns, Relich, Barnes, & Debus, 1984)

Social Interactive Coding System (SICS) (Rice, Snell, & Hadley, 1990)

Spanish Language Assessment Procedures: A Communication Skills Inventory (Mattes & Omark, 1984)

Spotting Language Problems (Damico & Oller, 1985)

Systematic Observation of Communication Interaction (SOCI) (Damico, 1985b)

Testing

Classroom Communication Screening Procedure for Early Adolescence (CCSPF-A) (Simon, 1987)

Curriculum Analysis Form (Larson & McKinley, 1987)

Interactive Reading Assessment (Calfee & Calfee, 1981)

Lindamood Auditory Conceptualization Test (Lindamood & Lindamood, 1979)

Pre-Literacy Skills Screening (Crumrine & Lonegan, 1998)

Test of Awareness of Language Segments (Sawyer, 1987)

Within the language curriculum, the SLP would want to investigate several specific language features. Within the classroom, children use language for self-monitoring, directing, reporting, reasoning, predicting, imagining, and projecting thoughts and feelings. Of interest is the breadth of functions demonstrated in conversation and narration.

School semantic features include abstract terms, refinement and decontextualization of word meanings, the ability to define words, multiple word meanings and figurative language, organization of a semantic network, and use of metalinguistic and metacognitive terms (N. Nelson, 1985; Pease, Gleason, & Pan, 1989). Semantic networking, or relating ideas to a theme, is an important skill for children to acquire (Heimlich & Pittelman, 1986). Those with better-formed, more-extensive networks are better able to comprehend and follow a topic or theme (Westby, 1990). Networks can be evaluated by having the child name everything he or she can related to a given topic or category or place pictures and words into categories. Matching and categorization tasks can be used. Picture tasks can be made more challenging by the use of pictures with differing perspectives.

Success in the classroom requires that the child be able to explain decision making, to discuss mental processes, and to reflect on mental processes of others and him- or herself (Wellman, 1985). Metalinguistic and metacognitive terms are listed in Table 12.6. Some terms are acquired prior to school age, but many are not mastered until adolescence.

Syntax and morphology gradually change throughout the school years. Initially, structure is more complex in oral language rather than in written, but this reverses. Therefore, the SLP is interested in the structure of both. (See Chapters 6–8.) Analysis would include clause and T-unit length and elements of the noun phrase and verb phrase. Cohesive elements such as pronouns and conjunctions are especially important (French & Nelson, 1985; Nippold, 1988a).

Poor readers and writers often have poor cohesive skills and are unable to go beyond a single sentence or bit of information (Irwin, 1988). Linguistic cohesion relies on a set of semantic and syntactic relationships or ties, such as reference, substitution, ellipsis, conjunction, and lexical. Reading and writing are discussed in detail in Chapter 13.

Narrative and expository writing and speaking also should be analyzed. Difficulty at these levels may signal underlying problems. Narrative analysis is discussed in Chapter 8.

Pictures can be used in an assessment to elicit both oral and written samples. Of interest are the clarity of cohesion and the types employed (Irwin & Moe, 1986). Questions based on the student's reading can be used to evaluate comprehension of text cohesion.

For children with word-finding difficulties, the SLP can analyze reading and writing errors to determine the strategies used by the child. Even though a word is incorrect, it may be semantically

TABLE 12.6   Common metacognitive and metalinguistic terms

afraid	assert	assume	believe	concede	conclude
confirm	disgusted	doubt	embarrass	feel	forget
guess	happy	hypothesize	imply	infer	interpret
know	mad	predict	propose	proud	remember
sad	surprised	talk	think	understand	

or syntactically acceptable. For example, in the following sentences incorrect words may or may not make semantic or syntactic sense.

Target:	He went into the *house.*	
	He went into the *home.*	Semantically and syntactically acceptable
	He went into the *hotel.*	Syntactically acceptable but semantically unacceptable
	He went into the *heavy.*	Semantically and syntactically unacceptable

The types of substitutions made may highlight the type of processing—auditory or visual—being used by the child. Categorization strategies may also be revealed.

Word substitutions may signal word-retrieval problems. A curriculum-based assessment should attempt to identify the discrepancy between the child's knowledge of classroom content and his or her ability to retrieve it (German, 1992). The SLP should note the presence of word-finding strategies discussed in Chapters 3 and 7.

Auditory discrimination and articulation skills are important for spelling and should be assessed. Similarly, phonemic awareness is important for writing and reading.

As language becomes more complex in school-age and adolescent years, the assessment and intervention tasks also become more challenging. Add to this deficits found in reading and writing and the task becomes even more formidable. Reading and writing assessment and intervention will be discussed in Chapter 13.

Elementary and High School Curriculum-Based Intervention

Children with LI may need assistance transitioning from preschool to kindergarten and elementary school (Prendeville & Ross-Allen, 2002). Not only is the child-to-adult ratio increased but children are also expected to work increasingly in small groups and to negotiate using language. In addition, there is also increased expectation for the child to work independently while receiving less individualized support. The curriculum is different and language based, as is the manner of instruction (Rosenkoetter, 1995). Children need instruction and activities that help them "bridge" to the curriculum (Masterson & Perrey, 1999). Planning for each child's transition should be systematic, individualized, timely, and collaborative involving both the family, classroom teacher, and SLP. Through collaborative intervention, the SLP can model interactive teaching styles and help the teacher to combine listening, speaking, reading, and writing activities into each lesson but structured in such a way as to ensure success for children with LI (Farber & Klein, 1999).

Within the classroom, the SLP can work with individuals or small groups of children and adolescents while the teacher works with the rest of the class. Group projects can provide the context for intervention by using the techniques discussed in Chapter 10. Other children can serve as models. If the teacher and SLP are working on similar projects, the teacher can observe the SLP and use some of his or her techniques. Small group instruction is efficient and effective and increases generalization and interaction (Shelton, Gast, Wolery, & Winterling, 1991).

An axiom of the classroom is "Busy little hands are productive ones" (Pearson, 1988). Group activities may center on art or construction projects using modeling clay or Play-Doh, pegboards, beads, puzzles, construction paper and glue, and the like.

Children's individual needs can be addressed if the SLP or teacher carefully interacts with each child in ways that foster the targeted aspects of language. Signs posted conspicuously will remind the teacher or aide how to interact with each child. With planning, this training can be accomplished individually even in groups of children.

The goals of classroom intervention are for the child to learn new ways of communicating and to have ample opportunity to practice newly acquired skills (McCormick, 1986). The environment should be responsive so that the child learns that language can have some effect on that environment. "Communication intervention should focus on increasing the frequency of communicative behaviors, shaping production of increasingly more sophisticated language functions, and encouraging expression of familiar functions with more advanced language forms" (McCormick, 1986, p. 125). The language of effective classroom communicators is characterized by fluency of word-finding skill, coherence or content organization, and effectiveness and control (National Council of Teachers of English, 1976).

The child's learning within the classroom is a function of individual learning style and the environment. Both must be considered when assessing or attempting to intervene with learning. The language of the child's classroom and materials can provide the context and content for intervention. A number of sources provide intervention materials for use within the classroom curriculum (Cosaro, 1989; Hoskins, 1987; Larson & McKinley, 1987; N. Nelson, 1988a; Pidek, 1987; Simon, 1985; Wallach & Miller, 1988).

With advancing grades, the emphasis shifts increasingly to independent work and to listening and note-taking abilities. Rules become implicit and children are expected to work independently (Westby, 1997). Each of these tasks is extremely complex. Intervention helps students learn strategies for analyzing various tasks and for determining the steps to take to accomplish them. The SLP might teach language-impaired students time management skills, study skills, critical thinking, and language use (Buttrill, Niizawa, Biemer, Takahashi, & Hearn, 1989). He or she might develop a book of listening activities for teacher use within the classroom (Cosaro, 1989). Other innovations that might help children with LI organize their day and make sense of the classroom include encouraging use of a daily planner, helping teachers add graphic input to lectures, defining concepts and vocabulary, cuing to guide reading comprehension, developing guided questions to help children make inferences, discussing how to answer questions, and helping children to identify main ideas for note taking (Norris, 1997).

Study skills training might include text analysis, study strategies, note taking, test-taking strategies, and reference skills. Through text analysis, the child can be helped to understand the organization of texts and their more efficient use.

Study strategies might include active processes for reading, such as identifying the main ideas and reviewing periodically to organize the material. Children also can learn associative and other memory strategies.

Critical thinking is the collection, manipulation, and application of information to problem solving. Language is an integral part of this process. Therefore, the child with LI may experience difficulties with organizing information and with decision making. Likewise, sophisticated metalinguistic judgments also would be difficult. Critical thinking training might target the three components of general thinking, problem solving, and higher level thinking (Buttrill et al., 1989).

General thinking includes observation and description, development of concepts, comparisons and contrasts, hypotheses, generalization, prediction of outcomes, explanations, and alternatives. *Problem-solving skills* include analyzing the problem into smaller parts, developing options, predicting outcomes, and critiquing the decision. *Higher level thinking* includes deductive and inductive reasoning, solving analogies, and understanding relationships. These tasks are increasingly more abstract and require greater reliance on linguistic input.

Analogies are particularly difficult for children with LLD. Analogical reasoning can be taught through a two-phase model in which steps for solving analogies are taught in Phase I and bridging activities to specific academic areas are taught in Phase II (Masterson & Perrey, 1994). Phase one targets the following skills:

Encoding	Translating each term into an internal representation of its attributes.
Inferring	Establishing the relationship of the first pair.
Mapping	Using the first relationship to identify a similar one in the second pair.
Applying	Picking the answer that has the same relationship as the first pair.

Activities and instruction are presented in Table 12.7.

With increased emphasis on lectures at the secondary level, listening skills become even more important. In general, good listening skills are highly correlated with good overall language performance. Students can be taught to tune in to what they hear and to listen actively. Subsequent training can focus on recognition and understanding of lecture material. The child's semantic, syntactic, and morphological repertoire can be expanded as a base for comparison with new information from lectures. Such training might include word meanings, relationships and categories, sentence transformations, active and passive voice, embedding and conjoining, and segmentation (Buttrill et al., 1989). Through critical listening training, the child learns to supply missing information, complete stories, find important information, and recognize absurdities in spoken information.

In oral language production, the child can express the language repertoire trained receptively. In addition, the child can sharpen word-retrieval and figurative language skills. The SLP can teach children to verbalize important critical reasoning skills, such as questioning, comparing, and analyzing, and to discuss a task or topic and to give examples. Elementary school children and adolescents can also be taught metapragmatic awareness in order to judge inconsistencies, inadequacies, and communication failures. The SLP can help students with LI understand response requirements for relevancy and thoroughness (Gottschalk et al., 1997; Kaufman, Prelock, Weiler, Creaghead, & Donnelly, 1994).

The SLP can enhance written-language training by using computers and topics of interest to the child. Computer intervention can have a positive effect on language, especially vocabulary, and even can improve social-interactive skills (Schery & O'Connor, 1992). Organizational skills gained in critical thinking training can be used in expressive writing training.

Finally, the SLP can enhance conversational skills by role-playing and practice. The child with LI can be helped to identify different communication contexts and their requirements.

Written information can be used to train oral language skills. Within a conversational or small group framework, this written information can be used for practice in communicating between speaker and listener (J. Norris, 1989). Written material can be controlled systematically to ensure that it is well organized and cohesive and that it offers a variety of topics, roles, and situations.

Prewritten textual information allows the SLP to teach language holistically, using all aspects of language, rather than fragments (Laughton & Hasenstab, 1986). The use of social interactions enables the child to learn language as an integrated social-cognitive-linguistic experience.

Adolescents can offer a special challenge if they are not treated with respect or included in intervention decisions. Pull-out services are not practical because the student will miss required classes. In addition, exiting and entering a class calls attention to the teen in a manner perceived as negative (Holzhauser-Peters & Andrin-Husemann, 1990).

TABLE 12.7   Training analogical reasoning skills

Phase I: Mediated Instruction

Session 1
- The four component processes are presented and defined.
- Applications of the processes are demonstrated by the instructor.
- Students apply the processes in the solution of a horse: a picture of a foal: a picture of a cow: (a picture of a calf) and perceptual analogies (⊞ : □ :: ⊗ : ○)
- Students participate in group practice problems and in independent practice in the form of worksheets.

Session 2
- Component processes are applied to verbal analogies.
- Review the previous day's lecture, move to group practice, and end with individual practice.

Session 3
- Component processes are used during reading activities.
- Students begin with analogies in sentence form (e.g., "At night we seen the moon, but in the day we see the ?").
- Analogies at the paragraph level are presented (e.g., "Astronauts are much like the pioneers of the Old West...").
- The importance of identifying key phrases such as *it is like, similar to,* and *for example* that potentially signal analogies in spoken and written communication is discussed.

Session 4
- A story is read to the students and they must describe other situations that would be analogous to the story, offering both explanations and justification for their decisions.

Session 5
- Focus is on encoding skills.
- The students are given a topic, such as dinosaur eggs.
- They brainstorm as much general information as possible about eggs, such as how eggs look, how they are used, etc.
- They then choose a list of attributes that are specific to the topic (i.e., dinosaur eggs) and rate the attributes by importance.

Session 6
- Focus is on *inferring* skills.
- Before reading a story, students look at the pictures that are included.
- They offer hypotheses about which elements seen in the pictures will be relevant to the outcome of the story.

Session 7
- Focus is on mapping skills.
- Students list the characters in a story, along with their attributes such as personality and physical characteristics and/or jobs or other roles in the story.
- They then compare and contrast the characters on the basis of these attributes.

Session 8
- Focus is on application skills.
- Students answer comprehension questions at the end of a story.
- They discuss potential sources of information (e.g., generated by the reader or found in the text) that can be used to solve questions.
- Using this information for discussion, the students then work through the questions to find the most appropriate response.

Continued

TABLE 12.7 *Continued*

Phase II: Bridging

Session 9, Science
- Measurement skills are addressed.
- Session begins with a discussion of different forms of measurement and when each is appropriate.
- Students then discuss situations in which one measurement must be converted into another. The use of maps may be chosen as the example.
- Students will then draw the classroom to scale on the chalkboard.
- Session ends with students generating other situations in which one form of measurement must be converted to another.

Session 10, Language Arts
- Students read the story *The Giving Tree* by Silverstein.
- Students generate a list of attributes for the boy and the tree and then use these attributes to compare and contrast the characters.
- Students then describe other relationships that are analogous to the boy and the tree.

Session 11, Interaction with Peers
- Various social situations dealing with peer interactions are presented to the class, such as teasing, peer pressure to use alcohol/drugs, vandalism, and shoplifting.
- Students discuss and/or role-play possible ways to handle each situation and talk about the advantages and disadvantages of each solution.
- Emphasis is placed on using experience gained from past interactions to determine appropriate solutions for present scenarios.

Session 12, Life Skills
- The instructor helps the students work through a situation in which a recipe that feeds four people must be increased to feed all the people in the class.
- The students then generate other situations in which determination of the solution would be analogous to increasing a recipe.

Session 13, Social Studies
- Current events such as pollution, gun control, or television ratings are discussed.
- The instructor leads the students in discussion of past events that are analogous to current events (e.g., child labor laws, prohibition).
- Students then generate a list of possible future events that would also be analogous.
- The use of principles or laws that have proven to be either helpful or harmful in the past will be discussed in relation to current or future events.

Session 14, Recreation
- Activities focus on money.
- Students are given an "allowance" for which they must formulate a budget containing specific items.
- The instructor helps the students generate analogous "budgets," such as time management or nutritional/diet-control systems.

Session 15, Vocational Day
- Activities deal with interactions with adults.
- This session follows the format of Session 11, but focuses on relationships with adults such as parents, coaches, and teachers. Topics may include following rules, dress codes, and punctuality.
- Students talk about analogous relationships they may encounter in the future, such as employer, spouse, or government institutions such as the IRS.

Session 16, Math
- The instructor helps the student determine the best buy when presented with two sale ads (e.g., 1 cassette for $3.94; 3 cassettes for $9.99. Which is the best buy?)
- Students discuss other analogous situations in which such comparative information would be important.

Source: Masterson, J. J., & Perrey, C. D. (1994). A program for training analogical reasoning skills in children with language disorders. *Language, Speech, and Hearing Services in Schools, 25,* 268–270. Printed with permission.

It is the very structure of the adolescent's day that highlights the need for some stability in the teen's language input. Many adolescents plateau at grade levels well below assigned grade (Schumaker & Deshler, 1988). These students need more time than short classes allow. In addition, each teacher's contact with individual students is limited to class periods. No one is responsible for the teen's overall language functioning and success (Larson, McKinley, & Boley, 1993). Some school districts have designed program prototypes that attempt to meet some of the needs of adolescents (Larson & McKinley, 1987; Larson et al., 1993; Work, Cline, Ehren, Keiser, & Wujek, 1993).

Essential to any successful adolescent program is destigmatization and the awarding of credit. Rooms selected for language group classes should be mixed with other classes. Classes should have names similar to other classes, such as "oral communication skills," rather than "speech therapy." The giving of credit aids motivation and gives the SLP clout and credibility (Larson et al., 1993).

A program such as Contextualized Adolescent Language Learning (CALL) Curriculum (Ehren & Mullins, 1988) may serve as a model. It consists of two strands, academic and functional. The academic portion targets items in the regular curriculum, while the functional emphasizes immediate daily living demands. Academic targets can be emphasized by the SLP during classroom teaching.

The overall intervention model might incorporate elements of two instructional approaches called strategy-based and systems models. The **strategy-based intervention model** assumes that learning problem-solving strategies is more powerful than learning factual content and will generalize more readily (McKinley & Lord-Larson, 1985). Teaching includes strategies for verbal mediation and for the organization and retrieval of linguistic information (Buttrill et al., 1989; J. Norris, 1989; Tattershall, 1987; Wallach & Miller, 1988; Wiig & Semel, 1984). This model is highly appealing because of its potential for generalization outside the intervention setting.

In contrast, a **systems model** assumes that the source of the language impairment lies in the interactions of the child, the primary caregivers, and the content to be learned. Thus, learning is a function of this complex system (N. Nelson, 1986a). Intervention strategies should reflect the child's varying learning needs across several learning contexts (N. Nelson, 1989; Wallach & Miller, 1988).

Although classroom group intervention may suffice for some children with mild language problems, others will need individual services. This service can be accomplished in the classroom, through the more traditional pull-out model, or both. The functional conversational model is still very appropriate, as noted in Chapter 9. Children also may work individually within the classroom, using computer-aided instruction (Schetz, 1989).

The SLP can demonstrate individualized targets and techniques for the teacher with the child or discuss them in meetings with the child's teachers, aides, and parents. Parents who cannot receive instruction in individualized training techniques are better used as general facilitators, rather than as direct trainers.

Language facilitator education can be accomplished in in-service workshops and at parent meetings. The SLPs should not try to impart all of his or her knowledge to teachers, aides, and parents at these meetings. A general outline of language development and an introduction to principles of instruction will suffice.

Linguistic Awareness Intervention within the Classroom

In addition to providing individual or group services within the classroom setting, the SLP can increase linguistic awareness itself for all children. Within such activities, the SLP can be especially mindful of the needs of those children with LI. Each child should be encouraged to participate at her or his ability level.

Preschool

Whole class, preschool, preliterate activities may include replica and role-play, narrative development, and the use of children's books. Each contributes to the general notion of narration and narrative form.

Replica and Role-Play.   Play and narrative development are very similar (Westby, 1988). For children developing normally, the language of social make-believe play and the language of literacy have similar functions (Pellegrini & Galda, 1990). Language must be modified for the audience or participants, meaning must be conveyed, language is elaborated, and there are cohesive ties and integrated themes.

The imaginative function of the language of play is acquired during preschool. Typically not performed during solitary play, imaginative language is more characteristic of social interactional play. The language is also very explicit in order to convey meaning crucial to directing such play ("You be the baby now"). Language is used to refer to objects within the situation ("*This* is my horse") and to negotiate and compromise ("Okay, you can talk like that if you're the baby"). Integrated themes are evident in the beginnings and ends of play episodes, in the temporal organization, and in the enactment of everyday events or previously heard or seen narratives (Pellegrini, 1985).

Imaginative language is heavily influenced by context. Both boys and girls prefer replica toys, such as dolls, a simulated store, dress-up, and boys also prefer blocks. Toys generally are used as props for their intended purposes. Older preschoolers and kindergartners are more willing to use ambiguous props and to assign meaning (Pellegrini & Perlmutter, 1989).

Preschoolers use language forms in their play that later are used in school literacy events. Linguistic verbs used in play are a good predictor of reading ability later. School success is also dependent, in part, on a child's ability to comprehend and use these linguistic verbs. Finally, reading is often in the temporal sequential mode similar to the narratives found in play.

Play has been used effectively to increase language skills of preschool children developing typically. Children can make significant gains in play-related conversation, vocabulary, and sentence lengthening. Other cognitive and social benefits also occur.

Unfortunately, many children with disabling conditions do not play like children developing typically (Westby, 1988). Sometimes, they do not have the experiential base for replica and role-play. Thus, their event representations may be dissimilar. All children are more likely to engage in interactive communication when they share a social script. In addition, children with LI often are isolated in the regular preschool class, engaging in solitary play. Given the importance of play for later narrative development, it is essential that these children have normalizing play interactions.

As mentioned previously, play would be assessed within the framework of an overall communication assessment. In addition to concern for language features and narrative skill for story retelling and generation, the SLP is interested in play analysis relative to decontextualization of props and language, thematic content of the scripts presented, organization, and the roles assigned by the child to him- or herself and others (Culatta et al., 1993; Westby, 1988). Also of interest are emerging literacy skills (Culatta et al. 1993; Edmaiston, 1988). These skills include recognition of situationally dependent print, such as a stop sign; independent interactions with a book; book handling skills; book knowledge, such as retelling, asking questions, and pointing to a page and its parts; and letter and sound recognition.

Prior to beginning play training, the SLP must plan the event carefully (Culatta et al., 1993; Sonnenmeier, 1992). First, he or she must create a play script. Theme selection should be based on the child's familiarity with the theme or script and the child's level of play. It is best to begin with everyday events. Table 12.8 presents events based on familiarity. For a child unfamiliar with replica play, the SLP might select getting ready for school or going to the market. By providing a supportive context, familiar routines are natural events within which language occurs. Our goal throughout this text has been for the child to have language that works in everyday situations.

Some events emphasize roles; others emphasize sequences. For example, riding on the school bus is more role-dependent, while making a cake is sequential. Different types of events should be chosen over time to aid generalization.

A note of caution is in order. Event representations vary with cultures. A child in a preschool classroom from a different culture may not readily adapt to the event chosen. Even within the "American culture" experience, children respond differently on the basis of race and ethnicity, family income and education levels, and geographic location.

Next, the SLP determines each child's involvement in planning and develops the script. Children unfamiliar with play should be very involved in planning so that the play can be explained and have some contextual reference. The script should begin with one sequence and progress to multischeme events. More detail should be added gradually, along with more story grammar components.

Once children have progressed through this type of replica play, they can reenact selected texts from children's books. Appendix I includes a list of children's books for reading and enactment. The use of literature is discussed in following sections.

Decisions will need to be made about roles, props, repetitive elements in the narrative, and elaboration. In general, children with disabling conditions should be assigned initially to familiar roles. Props should be real objects. Gradually, roles can be modified and reassigned, and prop use can become more decontextualized and symbolic.

Table 12.9 presents a possible format for the training of play. The script is presented first in such a way as to provide a context for play. General play and the specific theme of this particular play are discussed. Then the adult models the appropriate roles. Children then re-create the event. This step is replayed many times with varying roles and elaboration of the basic theme.

TABLE 12.8   Themes for training replica play

Every Day	Once in a While	Very Seldom	Fantasy*
Getting ready for school	Baking a cake	Going to the zoo	Being the teacher (police, grocer, mommy, etc.)
Getting dressed	Having a birthday party	Going to the circus	
Eating lunch	Going to a birthday party	Seeing a parade	
Riding on the school bus	Getting a haircut	Going on a boat ride	Being a dinosaur
Going in the car	Going to the doctor	Going on an airplane	Going to Mars
Getting a bath	Going to the market	Visiting _____	Piloting a plane
	Celebrating (holiday)	Going to an amusement park	Being a caveman hunting animals
	Going to church or temple	Going to a show/concert	Painting a picture
	Eating at McDonald's		Flying with wings

*To preschool children

TABLE 12.9   Sequence of sociodramatic script training

Step 1: Present script.

Step 2: Model roles including spoken parts.

Step 3: Have children re-present event and script. If needed, teacher prompts children for turn changes and for what to say and do. Prompting decreases over time.
  Prompts for motor-gestural response.
    Tell child what to do and give full physical prompt.
      Gradually decrease the prompt to a partial one and then to a physical assist.
    Tell child what to do and gesture or point.
    Tell child what to do.
    Point or gesture.
    Ask child, "What do you do next?"
  Prompts for verbal response.
    Ask child to imitate and present child with model ("You say, 'I want a hamburger'").
    Ask child to imitate and present a partial model ("You say, 'I want...'").
    Tell child it's his/her turn and gesture or point.
    Point or gesture.
    Repeat prior child's behavior and ask, "What do you say?"
    Ask, "What do you say to X (other child's role)?"

Step 4: When children are familiar with roles, reassign.
  Offer fewer prompts.

Step 5: Modify roles and script.

Source: Adapted from Culatta, Horn, Theadore, & Sutherland (1993); Goldstein, Wickstrom, Hoyson, Jamieson, & Odom (1988); Sonnenmeier (1992).

At each juncture, children are encouraged to describe and discuss the event enacted. The language of group discussion and decision making is important for school success and helps more firmly stabilize learning.

Narrative Development.   Training for narrative development and production is similar in many ways to that for play and may occur at the same time or following more advanced forms of replica play. Children enact familiar event sequences with increasing elaboration. Gradually, the events become more decontextualized through the use of puppets or cutouts and imaginary or substituted objects. Children can take turns narrating the story as it continues.

After decontextualized enactment, the narrative is related to the group and retold. With retelling, sequences can become even more elaborated so that a familiar event such as getting ready for school is modified with late arising, no clean socks, burnt toast, no toothpaste, a flat tire, and so on. Preschoolers must be cautioned to stay within the story frame. You do not get attacked by giants at the market nor rescued by the Power Puff girls on the school bus.

Gradually, the SLP can introduce stories with familiar event sequences that have not been enacted by the children. These, too, can be retold and modified by the children. Finally, children's literature can be used and these narratives retold by the children.

Children's Literature.   Despite similarities in socioeconomic status, age, access to materials, and parental expectations, significant differences exist in the activities and interactions with print for children with LI and those developing typically (Marvin & Wright, 1997). These differences are reflected in the poorer letter knowledge, interactive reading skills, story-listening abilities, and discussion of reading skills of children with LI. The normalizing benefits of interactive reading with these children are very important.

Sharing children's literature with preschoolers is not just reading to them. Prereading, reading, and postreading activities can enhance the experience and make it more meaningful, while bonding the class together (Montgomery, 1992a; Owens & Robinson, 1997). Appendix I presents a list of children's books with suggested uses within a preschool classroom.

Children's literature must be presented to children within a framework that makes sense for each child. Books should be introduced by their title and related to world knowledge that children already possess. The following is an introduction to *Brown Bear, Brown Bear, What Do You See?:*

> I'm going to read a book today called *Brown Bear, Brown Bear, What Do You See?* This is the cover. First, what is a bear? It's like a… That's right, Angel. Angel said a bear is like a big dog. Where does he live? Does he live in your house? No, he *doesn't* live in your house. Does he live in your neighborhood? Good, Antonio shook his head "No." He doesn't live in your neighborhood. I wonder if he lives in the woods. Yes, he lives in the woods. And in the zoo, good, Shawna.
>
> Now, this bear is brown; he has brown hair. Who has brown hair? John, point to someone with brown hair. That's your hair, John. Point to…yes, Billie Sue has brown hair. Put up your hand if you have brown hair. Good, Maria…and Katie…and Michel. And my hair is… That's right, Angel, black hair just like you.
>
> Well, our bear has brown hair. Here's a tough one: Do bears have any other color hair?…

As is obvious, the children can bring a lot of information to the task. When the story is read, each child can use her or his personal knowledge to interpret the story.

Notice in my example that some children were allowed to respond by pointing. The SLP can ensure that every child has an opportunity to participate and facilitates their success by structuring their participation.

Often, children with LI do not understand books, temporal and causal sequences, story grammars, or logical consequences. The SLP can guide them.

Within the classroom, books might be used for chanting, rhyming, or predicting activities or for specific language targets. Art activities, sequential memory, and consequential language (if…then) can follow reading. These activities and several resource books are listed in Appendix I. Books can be discussed with children at several levels of discourse and semantic complexity. These levels are presented in Table 12.10.

School-Age and Adolescent

Schools require extensive language skills from their students. Reading and writing are an essential part of the educational system. SLPs can encourage language use and aid development for those experiencing difficulties by actively engaging in classroom intervention. Skills targeted in therapy sessions can be enhanced in classroom application. Classroom linguistic awareness activities might include structuring classroom activities for success and metapragmatics.

Structuring Classroom Activities.   As mentioned, some children find school too frustrating, success too elusive. They give up. Different learning contexts within the classroom can reduce feelings

TABLE 12.10   Levels of discourse and semantic complexity

Discourse levels of book discussion	
Collection:	Relatively unorganized list
Descriptive list:	Utterances coordinated through a central topic
Ordered sequence	Organized by temporal order
Reactive sequence:	Organized causally
Abbreviated structure:	Includes psychological intent and planning
Semantic complexity of book discussion	
Indication:	Nonlinguistic signals, such as pointing
Label:	Naming concrete, observable objects and agents
Description:	Characteristics and relationships
Interpretation:	Observable characteristics used to refer to internal states, motivations, and underlying qualities
Inference:	Own background used to go beyond observable characteristics in a situation
Evaluation:	Likes/dislikes, justifications, summarizations
Metalanguage:	Language applied to reflect on the way language is organized and used

of failure. For example, a noncompetitive environment can keep students task-involved, rather than ego-involved. Motivation is the key. Motivated students are more persistent and more likely to expend the energy necessary to access, monitor, and evaluate their language activities (Butkowsky & Willows, 1980).

The SLP can make all students aware of the metacognitive and metalinguistic aspects of learning and employ strategies that enhance their application. He or she can explicitly teach learning strategies and provide guided practice and feedback. Each student can be guided and encouraged to participate at his or her functioning level.

Students can be aided in recognizing the features that influence comprehension and recall and the processing and retrieval demands of a task. General comprehension strategies to be taught include self-monitoring, drawing inferences, and resolving ambiguities. Study strategies that might be targeted include paraphrasing, summarizing, and note taking (Seidenberg, 1988). In general, metacognitive strategies have been effective in enhancing memory, comprehension, and spelling (Gerber, 1986; Palincsar & Brown, 1986; Wong, 1986).

Metapragmatics.   Children with LI are often unpopular and may seem odd or out of place in the day-to-day communication so common in the classroom. Among teenagers, perspective taking, comprehension of vocal tonal changes signaling emotion, and nonverbal communication are considered important communication skills (Henry, Reed, & McAlister, 1995). Everyday communication is important for classroom success and can be improved by intervention focusing on metapragmatics.

Metapragmatic awareness is a conscious awareness of the ways to use language effectively and appropriately. More precisely, it is the knowledge of common ways of communicating, the ability to detect and judge inconsistencies, inadequacies, and failures, and the flexibility to change communication behaviors in order to increase efficiency (Gottschalk et al., 1997). The SLP can improve metapragmatic awareness by presenting examples of good and poor communication, discussing the differences with students, and role-playing appropriate communication. Videotaped examples of communication may also be employed. Gentle critiques and self-evaluation are essential. Within this model, children have learned to ask questions and to respond effectively (Kaufman, Prelock, Weiler, Creaghead, & Donnelly, 1994).

With the entire class, the SLP can explore strategy-based language intervention (Wiig, 1995). Strategy-based language is used by mature speakers and is characterized by goal identification and fluent, flexible, and efficient communication to reach that goal. The mature speaker is able to take and express another person's perspective and simultaneously formulate and test several communication hypotheses for effective language use. Within intervention, students can be taught to recognize patterns of social communication, to develop options and evaluate their effectiveness, and to organize communication behaviors to integrate communication goals, strategies, and perspectives.

Using scripted social drama as the vehicle for holistic training, the SLP can guide students through the following four steps of training (Wiig, 1995):

1. Awareness of pragmatic features and underlying plans, scripts, and schemes. For example, topic initiations can be signaled by phrases such as *That reminds me…, Speaking of…, You know…, Well…,* and *By the way.*
2. Extending pragmatic awareness to real-life situations.
3. Generalization training across different media, contexts, and partners.
4. Self-directed training to foster independence.

At each level and following each scripted drama, the SLP and the students discuss feelings and reactions, identify alternative strategies, and apply the lessons learned to communication situations within their own lives. The SLP acts as coach while providing scaffolding and support.

Conversational narratives may be taught in a similar manner by first identifying the purpose of a narrative and then constructing the appropriate form to fulfill that function. Sequencing and cohesion can be addressed as the narrative unfolds. Children can be helped to identify the cohesive ties, such as sequencing, word substitutions, conjunctions, and topic-comment relationships.

CLD children with LI might benefit from style-switching activities and an awareness of appropriate use (Fleming & Forester, 1997). Role-playing can provide valuable lessons.

Syntactic structures also can be taught within discourse (Scott, 1995). Awareness activities might begin with modeling. The SLP can "think out loud" and discuss his or her options in a given conversation. Embedded within highly interesting conversations, other activities might include sentence combining and detection and correction of errors.

Summary

The SLP can provide classroom language instruction that addresses the needs of the entire class while enabling every child to participate. The SLP can provide the linguistic scaffolding that teachers often fail to provide, helping children become meaning makers and be successful. In addition, he or she can provide preteaching for the child with LI, helping that child be successful.

Language Facilitation

Language facilitation includes (a) identifying the needs of certain contexts and giving children the opportunity to experience this context successfully and (b) talking to children in ways that facilitate growth and highlight production. The classroom is a special context with its own demands. Facilitative techniques can be used there and in conversational interactions between children and their teachers, parents, and peers.

Classroom Language Requirements

Much of the classroom training should focus on the interactional patterns of the caregiver/facilitator and the child with LI. Most teacher-child classroom interactions consist of providing the right information. The child is taught to provide the correct answer and then be quiet. This behavior does not encourage an interactive conversational pattern (Rieke & Lewis, 1984).

Whereas conversations are relatively egalitarian and observe the rules of turn taking, classroom interactions usually are controlled by the teacher, who allocates turns. In contrast, conversational partners evaluate the acceptability of each utterance, but they are not expected to guess the correct utterance the other desires, as children must do in classroom responding. Finally, conversational turns may be expected but only rarely required. In the classroom, the teacher asks questions that require responses. The abstraction level of certain question forms is difficult for some children. Some question forms demand statement of fact, whereas others expect the child to reason and explain processes that may require inductive or deductive reasoning. Table 12.11 presents ten rules for classroom participation (Sturm & Nelson, 1997).

Often, the type of language used in the classroom is very different from what the child experiences at home. For example, the teacher's language consists of many indirect requests and statements. Questions or statements such as "Can you show us where the answer is written?" and "I can't hear Lori because others are being impolite" contain requests or demands.

There is still plenty of room for conversational give-and-take in nondidactic (non–question-answer) exchanges, however, and these contexts also must be considered. The children have classroom time to participate in social conversation. Classroom programs and materials can be manipulated to maximize the opportunity for interaction. Language functions found in a typical classroom are enhanced through such manipulation.

Often work in the classroom occurs in small groups concerned with some common project. Children working alone have little opportunity to interact with others. Groups should reflect the classroom's composition, with opportunities for children who are high- and low-functioning to interact.

TABLE 12.11   Ten rules for classroom participation

Teachers mostly talk and students mostly listen, except when teachers grant permission to talk.
Teachers give cues about when to listen closely.
Teachers convey content about things and procedures about how to do things.
Teachers' talk becomes more complex in the upper grades.
Teachers ask questions and expect specific responses.
Teachers give hints about what is correct and what is important to them.
Student talk is brief and to the point.
Students ask few questions and keep them short.
Students talk to teachers, not to other students.
Students make few unsolicited comments and only about the process or content of the lesson.

Source: Adapted from Sturm & Nelson (1997).

The skill of knowing how to get things done in the classroom is not usually taught to children, but rather is taken for granted by teachers (Wilkinson & Milosky, 1987). The lack of such knowledge can be problematic for the child with LI asked to work with others to accomplish some task. The usual instructions are to help each other.

The child must be able to request and give information, action, and materials and to make judgments on the correct language and communication behaviors in and out of context. Each child is expected to be able to identify the information needed by all involved to complete a task and also to judge the appropriateness of information that is given.

Classroom language functions include (a) relating socially to others while stating personal needs, (b) directing others and self, (c) requesting and giving information, (d) reasoning, judging, and predicting, and (e) imagining and projecting into nonclassroom situations. Relating socially to others while stating one's own needs contains a number of behavior categories, such as referring to psychological or physical needs ("I want to leave now" or "I'm hungry"), protecting one's self and self-interest ("That's mine"), agreeing or disagreeing ("You're wrong"), and expressing an opinion ("I hated that dessert") (Staab, 1983). This function can be elicited through activities organized around a highly desirable object that is not available to all participants, such as one beanbag for a toss game involving three children.

The "directing self and others" function includes the categories of directing one's own actions, directing the actions of others, collaborating in the actions of others ("You be the mommy, and I'll be the daddy"), and requesting direction ("How do you do this?"). This function can be elicited by requiring children to accomplish some task they cannot do without help. There will also be a need to direct others and to follow others' directions.

The "giving information" function includes labeling ("That's a piñata"), referring to events ("Yesterday, we got a kitty"), referring to detail ("That kitty is black and white"), sequencing ("We went to the party, and then we went to the movies"), making comparisons ("Yours is bigger"), and extracting the general point ("We're making Hanukkah presents"). To elicit this function, the child shares an experience with someone who did not originally share it, as in show-and-tell (Staab, 1983).

Often, classroom discussions involve activities in which the entire class has participated, and children do not feel the need for their information to be as precise or detailed. They presuppose that their classmates share much of the information. This presumption cannot be made when classmates do not share the information.

Requests for information vary with the type of information sought. For example, adults and children tend to use more direct requests when there are few, if any, obstacles to receiving the answer, as in checking short answers to problems (Francik & Clark, 1985). In this situation, the request is very direct: "What's the answer to number 4?"

As children mature, they learn to identify the type of information needed to help a requester. In general, children become more aware of the importance of information specificity. Children are also more likely with maturity to provide information on the process of solving a certain problem, rather than just the answer requested. In responding to the previous question about problem number 4, the child might try to presuppose the difficulties of the requester and respond, "5/8; I converted to 8ths after solving the problem in 16ths." School-age children who provide specific information and process explanations are more likely to be high achievers (Peterson & Swing, 1985).

The "reasoning, judging, and predicting" function includes explaining a process ("When you get lost, you should find a police officer"), recognizing causal relationships ("The bridge fell because it was weak"), recognizing problems and solutions ("This box is too small; get another one"), drawing conclusions ("We couldn't finish the project because there wasn't enough glue"), and anticipating results ("If we pull this cord, the bell should ring"). In general, problem-solving tasks, such as designing or building an object, will elicit this function. Problem solving includes predicting, testing hypotheses, and drawing conclusions.

Finally, the "imagining and projecting" function includes projecting feeling onto others ("I think Carlos is afraid of the ghost") and imagining events in real life or fantasy ("I'm captain of the spaceship *Izits*. All aboard"). This function can be elicited by fantasy play.

Many activities can be projected into imaginings by asking children to imagine that they are some character in a story or what they would do in a particular situation. With older children, different situations can be role-played.

To be successful, children must be able to use all of these language functions with some facility. As noted, activities can be designed to aid this growth.

Talking with Children

Language input is important for later output, and adult interactions with children must facilitate language growth and learning. In a nonthreatening way, whenever possible, the SLP should observe and comment on the use of language by teachers and parents. Teachers are often unaware of the effect their language has on the processing of children with LI. For example, teachers' oral directions may contain a large proportion of figurative expressions and indirect requests (Lazar et al., 1989).

Teachers' responsiveness to the initiations of children with LI is below an optimal level (Pecyna-Rhyner, Lehr, & Pudlas, 1990). In general, teachers respond infrequently and, often, in a manner that terminates the interaction. The teacher's frequent use of directives also may limit child-teacher interactions.

The SLP can efficiently introduce teachers, aides, and parents to facilitative conversational techniques at in-service training sessions or parent meetings. The SLP should help teachers, aides, and parents understand the importance of adult modeling and responding to communicative behaviors. He or she should attempt to decrease the directive style of some parents and teachers in favor of a more conversational approach.

The SLP can provide teachers, aides, and parents with examples of good interactive styles. A handout, such as that in Table 12.12, is often helpful. The SLP should stress the importance of different facilitator behaviors and the need to tailor techniques to the child's individual style and language level.

Whenever possible, the SLP should review these techniques and use them in demonstration with the individual child. Teachers, aides, and parents then can attempt certain facilitative behaviors while the SLP observes.

Peers as Facilitators.   Classmates developing typically can serve well as models and can be taught strategies that promote interaction (Goldstein & Strain, 1988; Handekman, Harris, Kristoff, Fuentes, & Alessandri, 1991; Odom, Hoyson, Jamieson, & Strain, 1985; Wilkinson & Romski, 1995). For example, play interaction between children with LI and peers developing typically increases the play scripts of the children with LI (Robertson & Weismer, 1997).

Sociodramatic or replica play can provide a basis for interaction for preschoolers. With school-age children, many alternative activities can foster interaction and carryover (Hazel, 1990).

Training young children with LI to play with toys has little effect on social interaction. Targeting social skills, such as inviting others to play, is more effective (Kohler & Fowler, 1985). Pairing is very important. Male children with MR seem more likely to respond to male peers than female, although individual children will differ (Wilkinson & Romski, 1995).

TABLE 12.12   Guide for parents' and teachers' interactive style

1. Talk about things that the child is interested in.

2. Follow the child's lead. Reply to the child's initiations and comments. Share his or her excitement.

3. Don't ask too many questions. If you must, use questions such as *how did/do...*, *why did/do...*, and *what happened...* that result in longer explanatory answers.

4. Encourage the child to ask questions. Respond openly and honestly. If you don't want to answer a question, say so and explain why. (*I don't think I want to answer that question; it's very personal.*)

5. Use a pleasant tone of voice. You need not be a comedian, but you can be light and humorous. Children love it when adults are a little silly.

6. Don't be judgmental or make fun of a child's language. If you are overly critical of the child's language or try to "shotgun" all errors, the child will stop talking to you.

7. Allow enough time for the child to respond.

8. Treat the child with courtesy by not interrupting when he or she is talking.

9. Include the child in family and classroom discussions. Encourage participation and listen to his or her ideas.

10. Be accepting of the child and of the child's language. Hugs and acceptance can go a long way.

11. Provide opportunities for the child to use language and to have that language work for him or her to accomplish goals.

Classmates developing typically can be taught to increase communication interaction using a few simple steps. Questions seem to facilitate naturally occurring communication more than directive prompts, although males with MR respond more to comments by peers (Wilkinson & Romski, 1995). Specific techniques for cuing and prompting can be taught but are relatively ineffective and time-consuming to teach (Goldstein & Wickstrom, 1986). The fewer strategies taught, the better (Goldstein & Ferrell, 1987).

One effective method, presented in Table 12.13, is to teach interactive strategies rather than teaching techniques to the peer developing typically and then to prompt and reinforce these strategies

TABLE 12.13   Training peers as facilitators in preschool classrooms

Step 1: Teach peer to interact.
   Introduction
      Explain purpose: To help friend "talk" better.
      Model with another adult.
   Direct instruction.
      Children rehearse and adults critique.
         Adults take role of child with disabilities.
      Posters provide reminders.

Step 2: Prompt and reinforce use of strategies taught. Gradual change with less adult input and fewer peer facilitators and more children with disabilities.
      Teacher prompts ("Remember to have your friend look at you first," "Remember to point").
      Adults should try not to interrupt too much—inhibits children.
      Whisper or point to posters.

Source: Adapted from Goldstein & Strain (1988).

(Goldstein & Strain, 1988). This approach can increase interactions and on-topic responses by children with LI (Goldstein & Ferrell, 1987; Goldstein & Wickstrom, 1986). Peer strategies reportedly continue when teacher prompts decline. Peers can also serve as effective tutors in narrative learning (McGregor, 2000).

One small set of facilitative principles to use with preschool peers can be stated as *stay, play, talk* (Goldstein, English, Shafer & Kaczmarck, 1997):

> Stay close to your buddy
> *Play* together, use the other child's name, and attend to the same objects
> *Talk* while you stay and play

This phrase plus adult modeling, guided practice, and independent practice with feedback and discussion of what it means to be a buddy and of the unconventional communication of some children can provide a model for effective peer training.

School-age peers can be encouraged to interact through cooperative learning, homework monitoring, and language contracts (Hazel, 1990). Cooperative learning fosters interdependence and individual accountability while encouraging face-to-face interactions and interpersonal skills. Students with different language abilities are paired for classroom language projects and rewarded for group achievement (Danserean, 1987).

Homework monitoring is another paired activity. A child who has the skills needed to accomplish the assignment helps a child with LI. The SLP works with both to help them complete their homework, uses role-play to teach the tutor and tutored roles to the tutoring peers, and critiques role-played interactions between the tutors. In addition, the SLP monitors the peers when actual tutoring begins.

Finally, language contracts can be used to decrease inappropriate language behavior (Hazel, 1990). Both the child with LI and the classroom peers must be able to identify the behavior and understand the need to decrease its occurrence. The contract with the class defines the behavior and specifies the cues to reduce the behavior and to elicit a more desirable behavior. It is helpful in eliciting peer cooperation that the class be solicited for suggestions for decreasing the behavior. The contract is reviewed periodically and peers reinforced for success.

Instituting a Classroom Model

The most difficult aspect of the classroom model is its initial institution. The transition from pull-out service to classroom-based, or "push in," service takes careful planning. Central to success is the resolution of the following issues:

> Training of the SLP
>
> Training of other professionals
>
> Establishment of a clear source of authority and responsibility for intervention
>
> Administrative support in the form of adequate space, scheduled time slots, and financial commitment (L. Miller, 1989)
>
> Identification criteria for students to receive services based not on standardized test scores but on classroom language processing and use (L. Miller, 1989)
>
> Responsibility for IEPs (L. Miller, 1989)

The task of changing an entire model of intervention seems overwhelming. It may take three to five years to fully implement a collaborative classroom intervention model. The process is one of evolution, not a solitary event (Ferguson, 1992b). It is essential, therefore, to begin slowly and to prepare parents and other professionals for the change.

The final model will vary with student needs and teacher/SLP flexibility (Brandel, 1992). The teacher and the SLP will need to consult for general language activities and for specific language support of individual children.

First, the individual SLP must train him- or herself. This training includes education in the use of a functional conversational approach and in the school curriculum (Montgomery, 1992b). This text provides one step in that education. Workshops, convention presentations, observation, and further professional reading are also essential. In addition, the SLP should role-play the use of various techniques because they differ considerably from the more traditional behavioral patterns. The SLP might begin by using core curricular materials in intervention (Moore-Brown, 1991).

Classroom teachers can help the SLP become familiar with small and large group instruction. Possibly, the SLP could spend an hour per week in some group activity within a classroom.

Second, the SLP will need to market collaborative teaching in order to recruit teachers and enlist administrative support (Prelock, Miller, & Reed, 1995). A quarterly newsletter and increased visibility at curriculum meetings will educate faculty about the role of the SLP. The SLP can discuss support for language goals in the classroom and inclusion of curricular goals in intervention. Informational meetings, breakfasts, and parent meetings can also be used with demonstrations and videotaped presentations. Administrators can be approached individually. The SLP can present a rationale for collaborative teaching, share scheduling, send brief memos of very successful interventions, invite administrators to attend sessions, and request time at parent events.

Third, the SLP must train other people. The initial purpose of this training is to educate teachers and administrators about the need for classroom intervention. This is best accomplished with in-service training stressing (a) the importance of the environment for nonimpaired language learning, (b) questions of generalization, (c) the verbal nature of the classroom, (d) the practicality and efficiency of classroom intervention strategies, and (e) the need for and desirability of team approaches. A possible in-service training model is presented in Table 12.14 (Prelock et al., 1995).

Administrators may be reluctant to change current one-on-one pull-out services. A more functional classroom model can be presented emphasizing both inclusion and efficacy (Moore-Brown, 1991). It is also important to remember that some children still will require pull-out services for special-skills training. Collaborative teaching is better suited to training of general communication skills (Borsch & Oaks, 1992). Goals and objectives, probably modest at first, should be established prior to implementation (Dyer et al., 1991). At each step in implementation, administrators need to be kept informed of progress.

Several alternative models for collaboration are available (Russell & Kaderavek, 1993). Peer coaching and co-teaching seem especially promising. In peer coaching, the SLP and the classroom teacher work as a team, coaching each other through observation and feedback, commenting on effective teaching strategies (Schmidt & Rodgers-Rhyme, 1988). In co-teaching, each professional focuses on his or her component of instruction on the basis of the curriculum goals of the class. The teacher and the SLP jointly determine student needs, develop goals and objectives and activities to meet them, implement these plans, and evaluate progress (Holzhauser-Peters & Andrin-Husemann, 1990).

Once convinced of the need for such a model of intervention, teachers can begin to learn specific intervention techniques. These techniques may be introduced in in-service training, with individual

TABLE 12.14   In-service training model for collaborating teachers and speech-language pathologists

Session I: Language in the Classroom: Getting Perspective on Collaborating, Sharing Roles, and Teaming
Objectives:
1. To share the perspectives of participants involved in collaborative service delivery on meeting the needs of at-risk students and students with communication disorders in the regular classroom.
2. To recognize those roles shared by teachers and speech-language pathologists as they assess and intervene with students.
3. To understand a transdisciplinary philosophy for teaming, including role exchange, role release, and role support.
Activity: Videotape Viewing of Collaborative Planning Meetings, Classroom Activities, and Follow-Up

Session II: Normal Communication Development and Communication Disorders in the Classroom
Objectives:
1. To understand normal communication and language development in school-age children.
2. To recognize communication disorders common to the classroom.
3. To understand the pervasive nature of language deficits in children with handicaps.
Activity: Role-Playing an Initial Collaborative Meeting

Session III: Identifying and Managing Classroom Language Demands: What Are the Scripts?
Objectives:
1. To gain a broader understanding of the impact whole language and traditional classroom methodology have on the student with communications disorders.
2. To identify scripts in the classroom.
3. To explain a process-based approach for managing classroom language demands.
Activity: Developing and Implementing a Communication Skills "Script" in the Classroom

Session IV: Assessing Communication Problems in the Classroom: A Collaborative Approach
Objectives:
1. To understand curriculum-based language assessment.
2. To provide a framework for collaborative assessment using language-based curriculum analysis, checklists, and observation logs.
3. To suggest ways of establishing collaborative data collection practices during classroom activities.
Activity: Practicing Team Assessment

Session V: Strategies for Managing the Language of Math
Objectives:
1. To recognize the language complexity in the math curriculum and in text materials.
2. To gain skills in adapting curriculum materials for elementary students with communication disorders.
3. To learn strategies for collaborating with students to enhance their performance in math application, computation, and problem solving.
Activity: Explaining Math Problems in Third Grade

Session VI: Using Literature in the Classroom
Objectives:
1. To examine the development of oral and written language.
2. To learn strategies for implementing literature use in elementary classrooms.
3. To recognize and manage the reading difficulties of at-risk students and students with communication disorders.
Activity: Sharing a "Rainbow of Writing"

Session VII: Issues in Collaborative Service Delivery: Scheduling, IEP Development, and Conflict Resolution
Objectives:
1. To explain a process for determining the type(s) of service delivery a student with communication disorders should receive.
2. To recognize the role of regular and special education teachers, parents, and students in developing IEPs for students with communication disorders.
3. To discuss barriers to effective communication when working with a team.
Activity: Conflict Resolution through Role-Play

Source: Adapted from Prelock, P. A., Miller, B. L., & Reed, N. L. (1995). Collaborative partnerships in a language in the classroom program. *Language, Speech, and Hearing Services in Schools, 26,* 286–292.

instruction to follow. Videotaped lessons including children with LI are excellent training vehicles to demonstrate the use of various techniques. Professionals conducting the training should be credible, knowledgeable, and practical. Appropriate materials and hands-on experience are essential to teacher training.

Fourth, clear lines of authority for language intervention must be established. It is vital to the success of this model that roles and responsibilities, as well as authority, be clearly established. This step requires administrative support and a definite statement of policy. New roles and responsibilities should be written into the curriculum, budget, and job descriptions. This step is not a power struggle. No one is in charge of the collaborative intervention. Rather, responsibility is shared and roles shift within the classroom (Prelock et al., 1995).

Fifth, administrative support in the form of space, scheduled time, and necessary financial outlays must be established. It is all too easy for administrators to declare a change in procedures without giving adequate support to ensure success.

The biggest single impediment to implementation is the lack of time (Montgomery, 1992a). The SLP and the classroom teacher must allow time each week to discuss each child's success and to review targets and techniques. Unfortunately, administrators often are unwilling to grant time for these conferences. My experience is that these meetings often occur over lunch or during breaks in the schedule. Although this arrangement is less than optimum, it does allow these essential interactions to occur. A scheduled meeting time of at least a half hour per week is preferred.

Administrators also have difficulty seeing the need to lessen dependence on standardized measures of language. Language test scores offer a quantifiable measure of behavior that can be used for determinations of student needs and progress. Yet, similar measurement can be made against the curriculum and from conversational samples. The implementation of this step requires the joint educational effort of the SLP and the classroom teacher.

Finally, IEPs will need to be written or modified to reflect the change in service delivery. Other members of the intervention team, including parents, will need to be educated on the rationale for such changes. Parents usually accept the classroom model when shown the increased service that their child will receive if the classroom teacher is also a language trainer. Many parents are also happy with the decreased amount of pull-out time.

The implementation phase should progress slowly and carefully because it is new to both the SLP and the classroom teacher. At first, one child in one classroom can be targeted. This can gradually be expanded to include several children in this classroom or one child in each of several classrooms.

The selection of the first classroom is critical. The SLP might begin with a best friend on the faculty, someone willing to learn, grow, and make mistakes (Moore-Brown, 1991). Teacher training should include SLP critiques of teacher use of training techniques. A checklist can ensure objectivity. It might be best for teachers to begin by attempting to integrate a child's newly acquired skills into the daily routine, rather than trying to teach new language skills (Dyer et al., 1991).

The first class taught by the SLP should, likewise, begin cautiously. One goal per lesson is recommended (Ferguson, 1992a). Later, individual IEP goals can be introduced through focused lessons with the whole class.

Undoubtedly, there will be problems in initiating classroom intervention. The SLP is advised to choose the initial child and classroom carefully to ensure some measure of success and to minimize friction with the classroom teacher. Once the SLP and the teacher begin to experience success, other teachers will be more willing to adopt the model.

There will always be administrators, classroom teachers, and/or parents who refuse to accept or cooperate with the implementation of the classroom model. Rather than become discouraged, the SLP should work with those individuals who accept the model and continue to try to educate those who do not. Usually, success with a few children is all that is needed to convince the foot-draggers. The key to success is "establishing a good rapport among the people involved" (Borsch & Oaks, 1992, p. 368).

Conclusion

Functional environmental approaches, as represented by the classroom model, are among the most progressive trends evidenced today (McCormick, 1986). In many school districts throughout Canada and the United States, this model is becoming a reality. Some districts are mandating the change from above, whereas others are experiencing a quiet revolution from below. No change as radical as this one can be accomplished without some difficulties.

The role of the SLP is changing. In many cases, SLPs are being asked to implement intervention models for which they have minimal training. Although such requests are expected in a professional field that is changing and growing as rapidly as speech-language pathology, it does highlight the need for continuing professional education.

Still, the SLP is the language expert responsible for identifying children with LI and for implementing intervention. In this new role of consultant, the SLP enhances this intervention process through others.

By itself, going into the classroom is only the most minimal of changes. In fact, data indicate that many SLPs engaged in a collaborative model are now modifying their intervention style to a more functional one (Roberts, Prizant, & McWilliams, 1995). Although location, such as a classroom, was one of the variables of generalization addressed in the first chapter, it was not the only one. Functional intervention is conversational intervention. A truly functional approach uses language scaffolding techniques within real conversational contexts to accomplish communication goals.

13

Literacy Impairments: Language in a Visual Mode

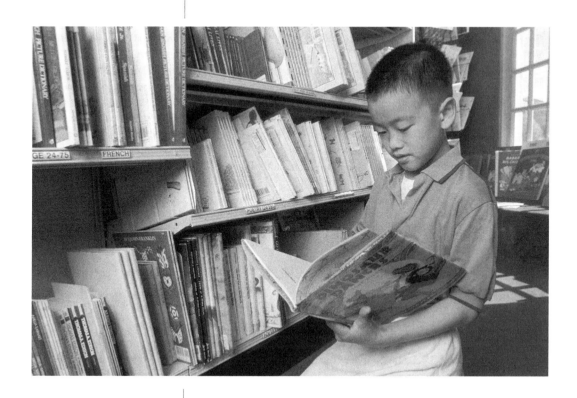

A cross-modal literacy-language connection exists. Each mode influences the other. Changes in one mode ripple into each of the others. Thus, SLPs should be interested in all modes of communication for children with LI.

Only recently have SLPs become concerned with reading and writing. The primary responsibility for teaching reading still rests with the teacher and the reading specialist. The SLP is interested in children's language deficits that influence the acquisition of these modes of communication.

Children with LI are at a high risk for literacy disabilities (Lewis, O'Donnell, Freebairn, & Taylor, 1998). In one study, as high as 60 percent of children designated as having primarily language impairment experienced reading difficulties (Wiig, Zureich, & Chan, 2000). As preschoolers and kindergartners, children with LI are less able to recognize and copy letters and less likely to pretend to read or write, to engage in daily preliteracy activities, or to engage adults in question-answer activities during reading and writing than their typically developing peers (Marvin & Wright, 1997).

SLPs should be involved at the preschool and early elementary school level in preventative intervention for literacy. With older children and adults, SLPs are concerned with improving reading and writing skills.

Recognizing a need, the American Speech-Language-Hearing Association (ASHA) (2001) recommended that SLPs play a role in the promotion of literacy. In short, children with LI are unprepared for literacy instruction because of a lack of preliteracy skills. Key indicators of this lack of skills can be found in their oral language and narrative ability, phonological awareness, alphabet knowledge, phoneme-grapheme (sound-letter) knowledge, spelling and orthographic knowledge, and word awareness (Justice, Invernizzi, & Meier, 2002). All these areas, plus literacy motivation and home literacy, should be assessed prior to formal reading instruction.

Within a preschool or kindergarten setting, the SLP should (1) alert parents to the oral language-literacy relationship, (2) identify children at risk and notify parents, (3) refer parents to good literacy programs, and (4) recommend assessment and treatment in preliteracy skills, such as phonological awareness, letter knowledge, and literacy activities, when needed (Snow, Scarborough, & Burns, 1999). Within the school-age population, the SLP (1) continues to help the child or adolescent develop a strong language base; (2) addresses difficulties in phonological awareness, memory, and retrieval; and (3) addresses difficulties the child is encountering with both narrative and expository or curricular texts.

As we progress through this chapter, I shall address all the topics mentioned so far. For clarity, I have divided the chapter into two major sections, reading and writing. Within each, I have organized the information into sections on development, problems for children with LI, assessment, and intervention. I have tried to be judicious and not include regular reading and writing instruction, subjects more appropriately taught by classroom teachers and reading specialists.

Reading

For the skilled reader, printed words are represented only briefly, both orthographically and phonologically, for processing. Automatic and below the level of consciousness most of the time, each word is represented for less than one-fourth of a second while the brain retrieves all information about that word. The process only becomes conscious when the reader tries to interpret an unfamiliar word based on the context.

Reading ability is highly correlated with spelling ability (Bosman & van Orden, 1997; Greenberg, Ehri, & Perin, 1997; Griffith, 1991). Poor readers tend to be poor spellers (Treiman, 1997). Instruction and advances in one area help the other (Ehri & Wilce, 1987; Uhry & Shepherd, 1993). Reading affects the memory for spelling, which in turn aids reading decoding.

At another level of processing, language and world knowledge are used to derive an understanding of the text, much as one comprehends a spoken message. This comprehension process and the message being decoded are monitored automatically to ensure that the synthesized information makes sense (Snow et al., 1999).

When something goes wrong in the reading process, it becomes less automatic and less fluent. Word decoding or understanding of language relationships expressed in the text may be impaired. Poor vocabulary may hinder understanding. Reading becomes labored and slow. The entire process may not make sense to some children, who may become frustrated and helpless.

Reading Development

Just as in development of language through speech, the development of the basics of reading occurs within social interactions between the child and caregiver(s). At around age 1, parents or others may begin to share books with children. The context is usually positive and conversational in tone with the book serving as the focus of communication.

By age 3, most children in our culture are familiar with books, can recognize their favorite books, and have the rudiments of **print awareness,** such as knowing the direction in which reading proceeds across a page and through a book, being interested in print, and recognizing some letters (Snow et al., 1999). Print awareness includes these skills plus later-developing ones, such as knowing that words are discrete units, being able to identify letters, and using literacy terminology, such as *letter, word,* and *sentence.*

At this age, words may be stored by their visual features, but they lack the phoneme-grapheme (sound-letter) correspondence. Thus, connections in the child's memory for printed words are unsystematic.

Within a year, children are beginning to attend to the internal structure of words such as phonological similarities and syllable structure. This is called **phonological awareness.** Four-year-olds also appreciate both sounds and rhymes. In addition, their vocabularies continue to grow, reflecting the amount of language to which they are exposed on a regular basis (Hart & Risley, 1995).

If the kindergarten curriculum is "literacy rich," children begin to decode the alphabetic system (Snow et al., 1999). Some children develop sight words, words that they can recognize on sight by processing the word shape in context. Some children will begin to "read" based on the first and last letters of a word. Five kindergarten variables seem to predict reading success by second grade: letter identification, sentence imitation, phonological awareness, rapid automatized naming (RAN), and maternal education level. RAN is the ability to label rapidly a series of items and is dependent on the ability to retrieve a phonological pattern from memory.

Although many kindergartners know letter names, their knowledge is incomplete for vowel sounds and many consonant sounds (Ehri, 2000). In attempting to read, they use memorized word shapes, letter names, or guessing. They are unable to decode unfamiliar words.

In first grade, children are introduced to reading instruction and to the sound-letter correspondence called **phonics.** Words read by the child are linked with stored meaning for interpretation. Much of the child's cognitive capacity is used in decoding, leaving little for higher language functions.

As other language skills improve and can be brought to bear on reading, a child's reading begins to become more automatic, especially for familiar words. At this stage, practice is extremely important.

The child with full knowledge of the alphabetic system can read using graphophonemic connections to memory, decode unfamiliar words, and begin to read by analogy or relating unfamiliar words to familiar ones based on spelling. In short, knowledge of the alphabetic system correlates with better reading progress (Morris & Perney, 1984).

Finally, by third grade, the child is expected to do silent independent reading and to use reading texts in different content areas. There is a shift from *learning to read* to *reading to learn* (Snow et al., 1999). The child's oral language skills are essential to comprehension.

Phonological Awareness

Phonological awareness is knowledge of the sounds and the sound structure of words and as such is part of metalinguistics. Among both children developing typically and those with LI, better phonological awareness and better reading skills are related (Cupples & Iacono, 2000). Phonological awareness skills also are the best predictor of spelling ability in elementary school (Nation & Hulme, 1997).

Although important for reading, phonological awareness is an area of development understood better by SLPs than teachers because of SLP training in the sound structure of language. Not a unitary entity, phonological awareness consists of many skills, including syllabication and phoneme knowledge, alliteration, and rhyming. Not all of these skills are required for reading, and their development, while parallel, seems to be independent.

Being able to create a word when a phoneme is deleted and to compare initial phonemes for likeness and difference are two areas of phonological awareness that are particularly important for the development of reading (Stanovich, Cunningham, & Cramer, 1984; Yopp, 1988). In new word creation following phoneme deletion, the child is asked a question similar to the following:

If we take the /s/ sound out of sat, *what word do we have left?*

As this example illustrates, there is clearly a correlation between phonological awareness and verbal working memory (Webster, Plante, & Couvillion, 1997).

Rhyming, on the other hand, seems to be predictive of later reading skill for preschoolers but not for kindergartners. In fact, rhyming is of very little value for reading by first grade.

Within a language, phonemes are organized into syllables, which are salient features for children even in early development. In short, syllables are the organizing units for sounds. For example, vowel sounds in English are to a great extent determined by syllable shape. English, possibly because of the history of the language, has a large, flexible syllable system of both shapes and sizes.

Each syllable can be divided into its initial phonemes, called the **onset,** and the remaining part of the word, or **rime,** which in turn consists of a nucleus or vowel and a **coda.** The onset and the coda in English can consist of up to three consonants. For example, in the one-syllable word *treats,* the onset is /tr/ and the rime is *eats,* which can be further divided into the nucleus /i/ and the coda /ts/. These syllable units will be important for assessment and intervention.

Most teachers have no training in the linguistic structure of English. SLPs can offer phonological awareness instruction to teachers through workshops and in-service training. In addition to training the English phoneme and syllable systems, the SLP should stress the importance of phonological awareness and its integration into the reading curriculum (Hambly & Riddle, 2002).

Reading Problems

Good readers guide and control their behavior. It's purposeful and flexible (R. Anderson, Hiebert, Scott, & Wilkenson, 1985; Baker & Brown, 1984; A. Brown & Palinscar, 1982). In contrast, poor readers lack such strategies, reflecting their misconceptions of the task and their acceptance of failure (P. Johnston & Winograd, 1985; Torgeson, 1980). When children experience repeated reading failure, they become frustrated. They internalize their lack of success. Many children who read poorly become passive, lacking persistence and accepting low self-esteem, and display apathy and resignation (Butkowsky & Willows, 1980). Others will become aggressive or display acting-out behaviors. These affective problems interfere with subsequent learning and development (Winograd & Niquette, 1988).

Children with LI who have average or above-average intelligence may read initially by memorizing word shapes. However, without word attack or decoding skills, by second grade these children begin to fail.

Children with LI are at risk for reading impairment for several reasons (Hambly & Riddle, 2002; Miller et al., 2001; Stanovich, 1986):

- They begin with less language ability and have difficulty catching up.
- They have poor comprehension skills.
- Metalinguistic skills are not developing because of poor overall language skills.
- They have slower linguistic and overall information processing.

Most reading problems are related to deficient phonological processing (Catts & Kamhi, 1999). Even the errors of children with dyslexia are not aberrations and reflect the conventional English phonological system, as do the errors of younger children (Treiman, 1997). Consonant clusters are especially difficult for children with reading impairment and beginning readers.

Children with SLI exhibit more graphophonemic (letter-sound), syntactic, semantic, and pragmatic miscues when reading than other children their age. Comprehension difficulties are revealed in less complete and more confused retellings of what they've read (Gillam & Carlile, 1997).

Deficits in Phonological Awareness

Phonological awareness is fundamental to reading readiness (Bradley & Bryant, 1985; Liberman & Shankweiler, 1985; Snyder & Downey, 1997; Wagner & Torgeson, 1987). Many children with phonological problems also have difficulty reading (Liberman, 1983; Swank, 1994; Torgeson, 1985). Difficulties seem to be related to failure to analyze words into syllables and these, in turn, into smaller phonological units (Bird, Bishop, & Freeman, 1995).

Assessment of Reading

Language deficits associated with reading are often present during the preschool years. Prereading and reading assessment should be a portion of any thorough language evaluation.

Data Collection

Just as all children do not require an oral language assessment, neither do they all require a reading assessment. As mentioned in Chapter 3, language assessments begin with an initial data-gathering step that may include use of questionnaires, interviews, referrals, and screening testing. Table 13.1 presents a checklist designed to identify kindergarten and first-grade school children at risk for language-based reading difficulties (Catts, 1997). No one item alone will indicate a possible problem.

Early literacy can be screened using SLP-designed tasks such as those presented in Table 13.2 (Justice, Invernizzi, & Meier, 2002). For a wider view, data from these tasks can be combined with parental information on home literacy materials and activities.

TABLE 13.1   Early identification of language-based reading disabilities: A checklist

Child's Name: _____   Birthday: _____

Date Completed: _____   Age: _____

This checklist is designed to identify children who are at risk for language-based reading disabilities. It is intended for use with children at the end of kindergarten or beginning of first grade. Each of the descriptors listed below should be carefully considered and those that characterize the child's behavior/history should be checked. A child receiving a large number of checks should be referred for a more in-depth evaluation.

Speech Sound Awareness
❏ doesn't understand and enjoy rhymes
❏ doesn't easily recognize that words may begin with the same sound
❏ has difficulty counting the syllables in spoken words
❏ has problem clapping hands or tapping feet in rhythm with songs and/or rhymes
❏ demonstrates problems learning sound-letter correspondences

Word Retrieval
❏ has difficulty retrieving a specific word (e.g., calls a sheep a "goat" or says "you know, a woolly animal")
❏ shows poor memory for classmates' names
❏ speech is hesitant, filled with pauses or vocalizations (e.g., "um," "you know")
❏ frequently uses words lacking specificity (e.g., "stuff," "thing," "what you call it")
❏ has a problem remembering/retrieving verbal sequences (e.g., days of the week, alphabet)

Verbal Memory
❏ has difficulty remembering instructions or directions
❏ shows problems learning names of people or places
❏ has difficulty remembering the words to songs or poems
❏ has problems learning a second language

Speech Production/Perception
❏ has problems saying common words with difficult sound patterns (e.g., animal, cinnamon, specific)
❏ mishears and subsequently mispronounces words or names
❏ confuses a similar-sounding word with another word (e.g., "The Entire State Building is in New York")
❏ combines sound patterns of similar words (e.g., saying "escavator" for escalator)
❏ shows frequent slips of the tongue (e.g., saying "brue blush" for blue brush)
❏ has difficulty with tongue twisters (e.g., she sells seashells)

Comprehension
❏ only responds to part of a multiple-element request or instruction
❏ requests multiple repetitions of instruction/directions with little improvement in comprehension
❏ relies too much on context to understand what is said
❏ has difficulty understanding questions
❏ fails to understand age-appropriate stories
❏ has difficulty making inferences, predicting outcomes, drawing conclusions
❏ lacks understanding of spatial terms such as left/right, front/back

Expressive Language
❏ talks in short sentences
❏ makes errors in grammar (e.g., "he goed to the store" or "me want that")
❏ lacks variety in vocabulary (e.g., uses "good" to mean happy, kind, polite)
❏ has difficulty giving directions or explanations (e.g., may show multiple revisions or dead ends)

Expressive Language *(continued)*
❑ relates stories or events in a disorganized or incomplete manner
❑ may have much to say, but provides little specific detail
❑ has difficulty with the rules of conversation, such as turn taking, staying on topic, indicating when he/she does not understand

Other Important Factors
❑ has a prior history of problems in language comprehension and/or production
❑ has a family history of spoken or written language problems
❑ has limited exposure to literacy in the home
❑ lacks interest in books and shared reading activities
❑ does not engage readily in pretend play

Comments

Source: Catts, H. W. (1997). The early identification of language-based reading disabilities. *Language, Speech, and Hearing Services in Schools, 28,* 86–89. Reprinted with permission.

TABLE 13.2   Clinician-designed tasks of early literacy screening

Areas	Tasks
Print Awareness	During shared book experience, differentiates written-language units, such as letter, word, and sentence, and identifies direction of print flow, location of cover, functions of books, etc. (Clay, 1979; Justice & Ezell, 2000; Lomax & McGee, 1987) Reads common environmental words (Gillam & Johnston, 1985)
Phonological Awareness	Finds one in three words that differs on the basis of an onset or rime or tells how two words differ on the same basis (Maclean, Bryant, & Bradley, 1987) Produces words that begin with a certain sound or rhyme (Chaney, 1992) Produces a "new" word after one sound has been deleted, as in "Say *cat* without the /k/ sound." (Lonigan, Burgess, Anthony, & Barker, 1998) Takes a word apart, then puts it together again (Yopp, 1988) Identifies the number of phonemes in a word
Letter Name Knowledge	Says the names of upper- and lowercase letters or points to letters named in two modes, at own pace or as fast as possible (RAN) (Blachman, 1984; Justice & Ezell, 2000)
Grapheme-phoneme Correspondence	Produces sound that goes with letter or names the letter that goes with a sound (Juel, 1988). Could also be accomplished with pointing to letter when sound is heard
Literacy motivation	Engages in a variety of literacy events and level of involvement is rated along a continuum from no engagement to high engagement (Kaderavek & Sulzby, 1998)
Home literacy	Parents complete checklist or questionnaire on home literacy activities and materials to determine child's access and participation (Allen & Mason, 1989; Dickinson & DeTemple, 1998)

Adapted from Justice, Invernizzi, & Meier (2002). Readers are advised to read this article for a fuller explanation of the tasks mentioned.

Children who read poorly may exhibit learned helplessness or have negative attitudes toward the reading process. This information can be gathered from interviews with teachers, parents, and the child and by observation within the classroom. Interview questions should include the child's perceptions of the importance of reading and different types of reading and difficulties, along with self-perceptions (Wixson et al., 1984). Scaled responses, such as a 0–5 disagree-agree scale, can be used with statements such as "Reading is difficult for me" or "My teacher helps me learn to read better."

Observation can confirm the child, teacher, and parent responses. Behavioral changes related to learned helplessness, such as nervousness, withdrawal, and aggression, can be noted. Lack of task persistence can be recorded as the amount of time or the number of attempts made in decoding a word or longer unit (P. Johnston & Winograd, 1985). A very high or very low number of requests for assistance also can be a good indicator. In addition, self-verbalizations blaming himself or herself ("I'm so dumb") or others ("This story is stupid" or "Why didn't you tell me I was next?") rather than stating alternative strategies for success ("Oh, this word is spelled like _____, so it's pronounced '_____'") also may signal helplessness.

During more formal testing, either the SLP or the reading specialist might use one of the following standardized testing to determine if the child is functioning within normal limits:

- Test of Early Reading Ability (Reid, Hresko, & Hammill, 2001)
- Gray Oral Reading Test (Wiederholt & Bryant, 2001)
- Woodcock Reading Mastery Test—Revised (Woodcock, 1998)

The Test of Early Reading is designed for children ages 3 to 8 and assesses alphabet knowledge, phonological awareness, and ability to derive meaning from parts. A timed instrument, the Gray Oral Reading Test, is useful with slow readers. Finally, the Woodcock Reading Mastery Test assesses sight vocabulary, nonsense-word decoding, and comprehension.

In a more functional task, the child might also be asked to read curricular materials in an attempt to assess her or his ability to function within the classroom (N. Nelson & Van Meter, 2002). The material should be new to the child to ensure that it has not been previously taught. Reading aloud gives the SLP information on decoding and can be audiotaped for later analysis. If curricular materials seem to be too difficult, the SLP or reading specialist could use graded passages, such as those found in the Qualitative Reading Inventory—III (Leslie & Caldwell, 2000). Regardless of the method of collection, some portion should be read aloud and audiotaped.

Comprehension can be assessed by using questions. Alternative forms include retelling or paraphrasing. Most standardized tests include a comprehension subtest.

Data Analysis

Passages should be photocopied and used by the SLP to record discrepancies noted on the audiotaped reading samples. All attempts at word decoding, repetitions, corrections, omitted words and morphemes, extended pauses, and dialectal usages should be noted by the SLP and analyzed for possible strategies used by the child. There is little danger that children with SLI or LLD will inflate their performance by guessing words correctly, because a part of their reading difficulty is an inability to integrate syntactic, semantic, and textual information (N. Nelson & Van Meter, 2002).

The percentage of words correct on the first attempt should be calculated. Usually, children who experience less than 90 percent correct on their first attempt demonstrate frustration (Leslie & Caldwell, 2000).

Miscues can be analyzed by type at the word level (Nelson, 1994). These include reversals, in which word order is changed; semantic substitutions, in which an acceptable but different word is substituted; syntactic substitutions, in which a syntactically appropriate but semantically nonsensical word is substituted; insertions, in which a word is added; and deletions. The percentage of incorrect but linguistically acceptable words should be calculated as these indicate the use of linguistic cues to predict the correct word.

Graphophonemic miscues should be divided into onsets and rimes. The SLP should note the way in which the child sounds out the words (N. Nelson & Van Meter, 2002). Good readers use several strategies. Common strategies include the following:

- Sound by sound
- By consonant clusters including digraphs ("sh," "th," "on," "ch," "ay")
- Common rimes ("-ack," "-ent," "-ite," "-at")
- Morphemes ("un-," "dis-," "-ly")

Assessment of Phonological Awareness

Phonological awareness is multifaceted and assessment should mirror this fact. In addition, an assessment for phonological awareness should be accomplished within an overall assessment of reading that includes measurement of reading, spelling, phonological awareness, verbal working memory, and rapid automatized naming (RAN).

A thorough assessment of phonological awareness includes rhyming, sound isolation, segmentation, blending, deletion, and substitution. The rhyming portion is only predictive of reading with preschool and kindergarten children.

Formal testing can be accomplished using the Comprehensive Test of Phonological Processing (CTOPP) (Wagner, Torgesen, & Rashotte, 1999) or the Phonological Awareness Test (PAT) (Robertson & Salter, 1997). Designed for ages 5 through 21, the CTOPP includes subtests on deletion of sounds, sound and word blending, segmentation, and phoneme reversal, a difficult memory task. In addition, tasks on the CTOPP also assess verbal working memory and RAN. The PAT, designed for children ages 5 through 9, includes testing of rhyming, segmentation, phoneme isolation, deletion, substitution, blending, sound-symbol association, and word decoding.

Intervention for Reading Impairment

Print awareness can be increased among preschool children with print-focused reading activities (Justice & Ezell, 2002). In contrast to picture-focus strategies that stress characters and actions found in the pictures accompanying the story, print-focus strategies emphasize word concepts and alphabetic knowledge. Print- and picture-focus prompts are presented in Table 13.3. In general, preschool children respond more to print-focused prompts than to print-focused comments by adults (Justice, Weber, Ezell, & Bakeman, 2002).

Parents can be taught to use print-based reading strategies that enhance their children's print-referenced behaviors (Justice & Ezell, 2000). Print-focused prompts are easy to teach, and parents have been successful with only minimal training.

Reading intervention might begin with a two-stage intervention model (van Kleeck, 1995). In stage one, meaning foundation, the reader scaffolds the reading for the child by placing the text in context and asking questions to guide comprehension, much as the SLP books shares with preschool

TABLE 13.3   **Print-focus and picture-focus prompts**

Prompt	Example
Print-Focus Strategies	
Print conventions	*Show me how to hold the book so I can read.* *Do I read this way or this way?*
Word concepts	*Where is the last word on the page?* *How many words do you see?*
Alphabet knowledge	*Find the letter C. Whose name starts with C?*
Picture-Focus Strategies	
Character focus	*Who's this?* *I see a turtle. Can you find it?*
Perceptual focus	*What's that in the tree?* *Show me something that's blue.*
Action focus	*Now what's he doing?* *What happens next?*

Source: Adapted from Justice, L. M., & Ezell, H. K. (2002). Use of storybook reading to increase print awareness in at-risk children. *American Journal of Speech-Language Pathology, 11,* 17–29.

children as explained in Chapter 12. The child learns that print contains the meaning and gains phonological awareness and letter knowledge. In stage two, form foundation, phonological awareness and alphabetic knowledge are emphasized. Phonological training would include syllables and subsyllabic units, such as initial phonemes, or *onsets,* and *rimes,* or the remaining part of the word. Rhyming and alliteration activities also would be used. Training in alphabetic knowledge would include learning upper-case letters, followed by lower-case, copying shapes and letters, sound-letter correspondence, and knowledge of meaning found in books read to the child by others. Four levels of abstraction of meaning are presented in Table 13.4. The first two require concrete skills, such as naming and describing, while the latter two require children to make inferences and to reason.

Later reading intervention might target both linguistic and metalinguistic skills including recognition of key words, use of all parts of the text such as the glossary and the index, and application of general learning strategies, such as graphic organizers (Wallach & Butler, 1995).

Identifying the Main Idea

Children with LI often cannot find the main idea or organizing frame even in simple texts. This task is fundamental to success in comprehension and academic success. The overall organizational abilities of some children may account for reading and writing problems. Incoming information needs to be organized for comprehension.

Structure of narrative and expository texts differs greatly and affects comprehension and memory. Readers or listeners go through a process of deleting, generalizing, and integrating the propositions of a text until they reach a macrostructure that summarizes the propositions presented. This process is dependent on underlying cognitive classification skills and world knowledge. Text often is evaluated for its "goodness-of-fit" to the reader's expectations. World or prior knowledge also provides organizational strategies for writing. Children vary in their ability to make use of prior knowledge (Pehrsson & Denner, 1985).

TABLE 13.4   The four levels of abstraction and the strategies at each level

Level I: Matching Perception	Level II: Selective Analysis/Integration of Perception	Level III: Reorder/Infer about Perception	Level IV: Reasoning about Perception
Comments or questions that:	*Comments or questions that:*	*Comments or questions that:*	*Comments or questions that:*
Label: name an object or person	Describe characteristics: focus on properties or parts of objects or personal quality of characters	Summarize (information in book): describe two or more actions or events in book	Predict (what will happen next or outcome of story)
Locate: locate an object or character	Describe scene: describe actions Skill practice: numbers, colors (letters go under print conventions)	Define (word meaning): Distinguish between fantasy and reality	Problem solve: consider causes of events, formulate solutions, explain obstacles to characters' thinking or actions
Notice: direct attention to a pictured object but do not name	Recall information: focus on prior information presented in book during current reading Cloze: pause to allow child to complete sentence of text	Provide point of view (for a character in the text) Recall information: from previous reading of book Identify similarities and differences (between pictured objects or between story and child's life) Make judgments (about characters, ideas, or objects) Unify pictures: summarize or synthesize information from a series of pictures in book	Explain (story concepts or actions)

Not tied to a level of abstraction:			
Print and book conventions	Talk about how books work (title, author, which way print goes, etc.)		
Interaction	Manage behavior, provide feedback, ask for clarification, imitate child		

Source: van Kleeck, A. (1995). Emphasizing form and meaning separately in prereading and early reading instruction. *Topics in Language Disorders, 16*(1), 27–49. Reprinted with permission.

Informational understanding develops as the readers progressively revise their expectations until they approximate the meaning of the author. Organizational clues supplied by the author enable the reader to interpret the passage and determine the main ideas.

Several textual features signal important information, including graphic features, such as italics, boldface, and type size; syntactic features, such as word order; semantic features, such as summaries and introductions; and schematic features, such as text structure. Of course, it is easiest to determine the overall organization if the topic is stated explicitly in the first sentence.

Good readers are sensitive to the text organization. They "discover" the organizing structure. In general, poor readers are less sensitive to important information. Many children with LI have difficulty comprehending and producing narratives because they fail to realize the internal organization of the text (Yoshinaga-Itano & Snyder, 1985). In general, these children fail to integrate new information with prior knowledge or fail to use the author's clues (Pehrsson & Denner, 1988). Poor readers use a fragmented organization or impose an unrelated structure. Even though third and fourth graders are able to recall important information, they have difficulty deciding what information is important in a text.

Intervention might include comprehension strategies, such as predicting, questioning, clarifying, and summarizing; semantic networking; generative tasks in which the child generates a summary sentence; and familiarization with different text structures (Armbuster, Anderson, & Ostertag, 1987; Richgels, Mcgee, Lomax, & Sheard, 1987; J. Williams, 1988).

In general, by second grade, children are aware of strategies for summarizing text. Strategies used by older children include deletion of unimportant information, deletion of redundant information, substitution of category names for various category members, and selection or creation of a topic sentence. Direct instruction in these strategies results in the best performance (Rinehart, Stahl, & Erickson, 1986; J. Williams, 1986).

Semantic networking or organizing is a method of teaching organization (Heimlich & Pittelman, 1986; Pehrsson & Denner, 1988; Pehrsson & Robinson, 1985; J. Williams, 1988). Helping children organize and reorganize structure during and after reading improves reading comprehension, writing cohesion, retention, and recall (Denner & Pehrsson, 1987; Reutzel, 1985; Schultz, 1986).

Ideas are displayed in semantic networks as clusters resembling spiders. Major ideas are circles or other shapes. Lines form related ideas or connect major ideas. Semantic clusters can be taught with a guided study approach that helps the child develop generalizable strategies. Slowly, students adapt and internalize the methods for reading comprehension and for writing.

Organizational patterns are of two types: cluster and episodic. Cluster patterns are for superordination and subordination. In Figure 13.1, the topic, or superordinate aspect, is in the center. Related ideas radiate outward. Episodic organizers representing change move from event to event as in narration. These also can be used for problem-solution and cause-effect diagrams.

Children can begin to use semantic organizers in kindergarten or first grade, drawing pictures for the sequence of events in a narrative. Older children can write events in each cluster, either to aid recall or to structure narratives for telling or retelling. Variations, such as the story map, can help children develop story grammars (Figure 13.1). Similar diagrams, such as the mind map, can be adapted to various purposes, such as a book report, newspaper article, or argument (Montgomery, 1992a). Likewise, classroom brainstorming can help children realize their prior knowledge by examining all they know about a given topic (Dodge & Mallard, 1992).

As SLPs, we are interested in language and in helping children make sense of the language they receive and produce. Semantic networking is just one method of doing this.

Intervention for Phonological Awareness

Luckily, phonological awareness can be taught to preschool, kindergarten, and elementary school children, so both prevention and remediation can be targeted (van Kleeck, Gillam, & McFadden, 1998). The goals of phonological awareness intervention are (Hambly & Riddle, 2002):

- To help the child learn the English language sound code as a basis for phonics
- To improve the child's reading and writing

With the accomplishment of these goals, not only does reading improve, but so do acting-out behaviors and feelings of helplessness.

Whenever possible, phonological awareness should be taught within meaningful text experiences (McFadden, 1998). In this way, the emergent nature of both literacy and phonological aware-

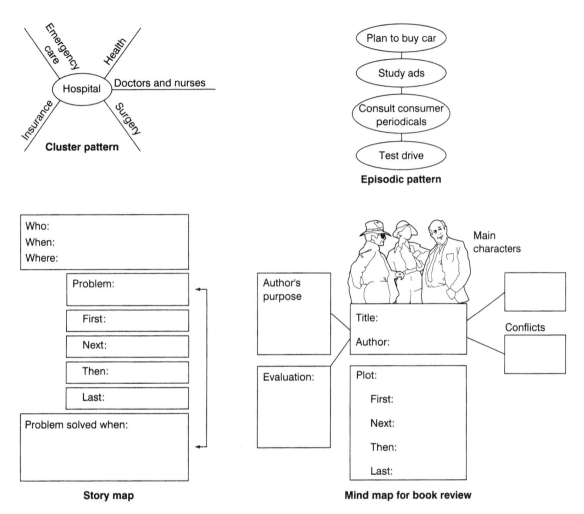

FIGURE 13.1　Examples of semantic networking.

Source: Adapted from Montgomery (1992a); Pehrsson & Denner (1988).

ness can be used. Environmental signs, such as *stop, women,* and *Main Street,* should be used to enhance training.

Within intervention, the SLP addresses segmentation and blending, working at the phoneme and syllable levels. In general, programs focusing on one or two phonological awareness skills yield better results than those that try to teach with a broader focus (National Reading Panel, 2000). At the phoneme level, it seems best to work on sounds within single syllables since cross-syllable training has less effect on overall phonological awareness.

As stressed throughout this text, the SLP should teach skills that will directly impact the child's functional performance. Syllable structure is important for phonemic training. The *Wilson Word List* (Wilson, 1996) is a good resource and is organized by syllables, sounds, and blends.

Intervention can begin with sound recognition and identification, first in the initial position in words. Training should be both receptive and expressive. Next, the SLP and child can move to onset-rime segmentation and blending and finally, to phoneme segmentation and blending. Training can begin—remember the *treats* example—at the onset-rime level (*/tr-its/*), then move to nucleus-coda (*/i-ts/*), and finally to onset-nucleus-coda (*/tr-i-ts/*).

Phoneme segmentation is easier than blending, and intervention should begin with segmentation first. Begin with only two sounds and gradually increase to five or six. Real words are better than nonsense ones and will decrease the memory load for children, although the latter can be added as training progresses. The training should progress from CVC to CCVC to CVCC. Final blends are the most difficult. It's advisable to concentrate on one type of final blend at a time rather than mixing all possible ones together. Memory can also be aided with the use of real objects or pictures. Working at the word level results in more gains than using longer units, such as sentences.

Printed letters can be used to support phoneme learning, especially if letters are used in the classroom. Again, a functional approach tries to incorporate use contexts, such as the classroom, as much as possible. Letters give additional input, are a potential memory aid, and are functional for generalization to reading. For children with deficits in working memory, letters can offer a compensatory visual aid. It is important for the SLP to remember that intervention is for phonological awareness not reading per se. It is very tempting to try to teach reading, but that is not the job of an SLP.

Multisensory approaches are also helpful and can make the training interesting. For example, during auditory training children can respond by dropping objects into cans, stacking toys, playing hopscotch, or taking turns in any number of child games.

Vowels offer a particular problem because of the number and inconsistent spelling in English. Vowels sounds are related to syllable structure, and this relationship will be presented in intervention. The SLP can begin with short vowels because they are the nucleus of the longest syllables, called closed syllables. Closed syllables have rimes that end in at least one consonant and may have a maximum of six phonemes in the word, as in *scrimp*. The rime is VC+ in form. Children can be taught common rimes such as *-ent, -ide, -old,* and *-ick.*

Long vowels can be introduced later, first in the VCe form, in which the "e" is silent, as in *home;* followed by the open syllable with no consonant in the coda, as in *tray* or *she.* Appearing in short syllables or syllables with unusual spellings, long vowels can be taught as intervention assumes more of a reading focus. The inconsistent spelling of long vowels can be seen in *day, weigh,* and *raise.*

Training of the phoneme-grapheme relationship should be approached cautiously following the outline above. Some sound-letter relationships, presented in Table 13.5, are particularly difficult.

The goal of phonological awareness intervention at the syllable level is to help children segment and blend syllables in order to read and spell multisyllabic words (Hambly & Riddle, 2002). Syllables can be introduced as naturally occurring "beats" in a word. Clapping hands or drumbeats can be used to help children recognize and identify syllables. Jaw movements in a mirror can also be helpful, especially if low, open-mouth vowels and elongated diphthongs are part of the syllables used.

Writing

As with all language modes, writing is a social act. Just like a speaker, the writer must consider the audience. Because the audience is not present when the writing occurs, writing demands more cognitive resources for planning and execution than does speaking (Golder & Coirier, 1994; Graham & Harris, 1996, 1997; Scott, 1999).

TABLE 13.5   Difficult phoneme-grapheme relationships

Phoneme	Example	Explanation
/r/-controlled vowels	Thr*ough*, tr*ue*, cr*ew*	Inconsistent spelling
diphthongs	Fl*y*, h*eight*, r*ight*	Inconsistent spelling
/ə/	Sof*a*, tel*e*phone	Stress and spelling interact
/ʌ/	F*u*n, w*o*n, *o*ne	Multiple spellings

Grapheme	Example	Explanation
-nk	Tha*nks*, ri*nk*	Two phonemes /ŋk/
x	Ta*x*i, ma*x*imum	Two sounds /ks/
u	t*u*ne, f*u*n	Two pronunciations /U/ and /ʌ/
Plural -s	Dog*s*, cat*s*, kiss*es*	Multiple pronunciations
Past -ed	Walk*ed*, jog*ged*, collid*ed*	Multiple pronunciations
-pt	Ke*pt*, sle*pt*	Final blend has short stop

Source: Adapted from Hambly & Riddle (2002).

Writing and reading are not simply reverse processes. Rather than creating meaning from the written text and integrating it with background knowledge, the writer uses knowledge and new ideas to create text (Kintsch, 1998). Writing is a complex process that includes the generation of ideas, organization and planning, action based on the plan, revision, monitoring, and self-feedback (Scott, 1999). Writing is more abstract and decontextualized than conversation and requires internal knowledge of the writing form. Forms can be divided into narrative and expository writing.

Expository texts have several forms. The easiest type, especially with familiar content, is sequential or procedurally organized, while others are descriptive with little overall structure. A typical sequential text explains how something is accomplished. Problem-solving, cause-and-effect, and compare-and-contrast genres are the most difficult.

The writing system consists of several processes: text construction, handwriting, spelling, executive function, and memory (Berninger, 2000). Text construction is the process of going from ideas to written texts. This is not the same as actual handwriting and spelling, although all three are correlated. Texts consist of words and sentences supporting the ideas of the writer.

Executive function is the self-regulatory aspect of writing. It's the ability to select and sustain attention, organize perception, and flexibly shift perceptual and cognitive setup, as well as control social and affective behavior (Ylvisaker & DeBonis, 2000). Further, executive function includes realistic self-appraisal of strengths and weaknesses and the difficulty of tasks; the ability to set reasonable goals; planning and organizing to achieve each goal; initiating, monitoring, and evaluating your performance in relation to each goal; and revising plans and strategies based on feedback. Intelligence and executive function are not the same thing, although language use and executive function are interdependent (Stuss & Benson, 1986; Wehmeyer & Kelcher, 1995).

Memory serves the writer in many ways. Working memory stores ideas as they are worked and reworked by the writer. Short-term memory is used for word recognition while writing. Long-term memory provides content and word knowledge as well as overall format. Automaticity of retrieving letters and words from memory and producing them contributes to the quality of text generation.

Writing Development

Obviously, writing and speaking are not the same process. Their development is interdependent and parallel. Many aspects of language overlap both modes, while others are characteristic of primarily one or the other.

Writing development is really the development of many interdependent processes. The mechanics of forming letters and learning to spell develops first, with text generation and executive function developing much later (Berninger & Swanson, 1994).

In the initial phase of writing development, children treat writing and speaking as two separate systems. Children as young as 3 or 4 years of age will "write" in their own fashion. They don't yet realize that writing represents sounds. Most likely, for them writing represents meaning. Even so, writing and drawing are different for young children, and 3-year-olds can differentiate the two. The writing of preschoolers differs from their drawing in distinct ways. Their writing is often arranged in linear strings of units separated by spaces. By age 4, some real letters of the parent language may be included (Tolchinsky-Landsmann, & Levin, 1985). By 5, children can differentiate the writing system of their native language from other languages with different systems, such as Cyrillic or Hangul.

As children learn to write, either at home or through more formal instruction, they expend a great deal of cognitive energy on the mechanics of letter forming and spelling. Letter forming becomes more accurate and finally *automatized,* extractable from memory with only minimal memory resources.

Gradually, the spoken and written systems converge and children write in the same manner as they speak, although speech is more complex. Around age 9 or 10, writing and speaking become differentiated and children become increasingly literate. Gradually, written sentences become longer and more complex than speaking. Within their writing, children begin to display an increasing awareness of the audience's perspective through the use of syntax, vocabulary, textual themes, and attitude (Kroll, 1981). Cohesive devices are used to signal relationships for the reader, and time, location, and perspective are more specific. The syntax selected reflects the purpose of the writing.

In a final phase of writing development, not achieved by all writers, speaking and writing are consciously understood to be separate linguistic codes. The syntactic characteristics of writing are fully understood and the writer has greater flexibility in writing style.

Text Generation

Once children begin to produce true spelling, even if it is unconventional, they begin to generate text. In first grade, text may consist of only a single sentence, as in *My dog is called Spot* or *Today is Chinese New Year.*

Early text formats are usually of the topic-comment type, as in the following:

I like my grandpa. He buy me presents and makes me laugh.

Early compositions usually lack cohesion and use structures repeatedly, as in the following:

I like going to camp. I like to swim. I like to canoe. I like the overnight camp-outs.

Older writers use more variety for dramatic effect. In a similar development, the facts and events characteristic of the variety of young writers evolve into older writers' use of judgments and opinions, parenthetical expressions, qualifications, contrasts, and generalizations (Berninger, 2000).

Overall organization progresses from a linear form to a hierarchical structure. Initially, compositions lack coherence and ideas may be joined in a "free association" pattern. Later ideas may relate to a central idea in a form similar to the centering narratives of young children. Very simple narratives, consisting of a list of sequential events, and expository texts emerge next. At this stage, expository structures include a unifying sentence to provide coherence.

Finally, advanced narratives and expository text develop. Narratives contain temporal events unified by a topic sentence and the narrative elements of story grammar, character development, plot, and dialogue. Expository essays include a unifying topic sentence, comments referenced to the topic, and elaborations on the comments.

Executive Function

It is not until early adulthood that most writers develop the cognitive processes and executive functions needed for mature writing (Berninger, 2000; Ylvisaker & DeBonis, 2000). The reason for the protracted period is the slow anatomical and physiological development of the frontal lobe.

Until adolescence, young writers need adult "scaffolding," or guidance in planning and revising their writing. By junior high school, guidance for young adolescents may take the form of encouragement to preplan.

In late elementary school, children can be guided to revise, but revision is usually limited to one aspect of their writing. Improved short-term memory in primary grades results in improved writing and revision of these aspects of text. By junior high school, teens are capable of revising all aspects of writing. Improved long-term memory results in improved overall compositional quality (Berninger, Cartwright, Yates, Swanson, & Abbott, 1994).

Spelling

Spelling and reading share the same underlying phonological processes but are not simply reverse processes (Perfetti, 1997). Pronouncing spellings, called reading, is easier than writing spellings, which requires a larger amount of information to be extracted from memory (Ehri, 2000). To a large extent, reading requires blending skills while spelling requires segmentation.

Writing and spelling are separate but correlated processes. The two must be coordinated for optimal functioning. Spelling knowledge is working knowledge, not just the applying of memorized rules. Sometimes a speller relies on memory, at others on invention based on spelling and reading experience, and at still others on analogy to familiar words already in memory.

Because spelling is related to other forms of visual communication, it competes with them for cognitive capacity. Excessive energy expended at the visual processing level comes at a cost to higher language functions. Poor spellers generally produce poorer, shorter texts.

Children use knowledge of the sound-letter correspondence and a few rote visual memorizations to spell. Later, they are able to call on multiple learning strategies and different types of knowledge (Rittle-Johnson & Siegler, 1999; Treiman & Cassar, 1997; Varnhagen, McCallum, & Burstow, 1997). This doesn't happen all at once. Spelling development is a long, slow process.

Initial attempts at spelling, called *preliterate,* usually consist of scribbles and drawing (Henderson, 1990). The occasional letter may be strewn within. Because young children are sensitive to syllables, letters represent syllables initially (Treiman, 1994). Later children use some phoneme-grapheme knowledge along with letter names. Gradually, they become aware of conventional spelling and are able to analyze a word into sounds and letters, although vowels will be difficult for some time.

As knowledge of the alphabetic system emerges, the primacy of syllables as a perceptual unit gives way slowly to letters and to a system called "invented spelling." In this *letter-name stage,* the names of letters may be used in spelling, as in *SKP* for *escape* and *LFT* for *elephant* (Henderson, 1990).

By the late letter-name stage, spelling symbolizes the structure of spoken words, but not the rules or memorized sequences that represent the adult spelling system (Treiman & Bourassa, 2000). For example, *sky* may be written as *SGIE.* Say "sky" slowly. It sounds like *SGIE* to me. Other phonetic representations may include cluster reduction or using one letter for each sound grouping. In the latter, a word such as *stripe* might be written as *SIP* in which *S = str, i = I* and *P = pe.* The child lacks full knowledge of the phoneme-grapheme system and has difficulty separating words into phonemes (Treiman, 1993).

Invented spelling is related to an emerging phonological awareness (Lombardino, Bedford, Fortier, Carter, & Brandi, 1997). It is easy to see how each might be included by the SLP in an assessment of the other.

As spelling becomes more sophisticated in the *within-word pattern stage,* children learn about spacing, sequencing, various ways to represent phonemes, and the morpheme-grapheme relationship (Henderson, 1990). The parallel development of reading aids this process. Even kindergarten children begin to notice letter patterns in environmental signs, family names, and favorite reading books (Treiman, 1993).

The child with full knowledge of the alphabetic system can segment words into phonemes and knows the conventional phoneme-grapheme correspondences. The system is also used to facilitate reading.

As the child begins to recognize more regularities and consolidate the alphabetic system, he or she becomes a more efficient speller and the memory load decreases (Ehri, 2000). For example, just 37 rimes generate 500 primary-grade English words (Stahl, Osborn, & Lehr, 1990). Other patterns are morphological, such as *-ing, -ion,* and *-ly,* or sound related, such as "ck" for /k/ in *track, trick,* and *truck,* and silent letters, such as final "e" and the "l" in *walk* and *should.*

Many vowel representations, phonological variations, such as *later/latter,* and morphophonemic variations, such as *sign/signal,* will take several years to acquire (Treiman, 1993). Within the *syllable juncture stage,* the child learns about consonant doubling and stressed and unstressed syllables. Finally, in the *derivational constancy stage,* spellers become familiar with root words and derivations (Henderson, 1990).

Spellings are stored in memory for repeated use. Most likely, word storage is organized into units of letters, such as *st-ack,* rather than by individual letters, as in *s-t-a-c-k* (Ehri, 1992).

Memory helps with familiar words and also for analogy, a common strategy of older children (Bowey & Hansen, 1994; Snowling, 1994). Using analogy, the speller tries to spell an unfamiliar word using prior knowledge of words that sound the same. In trying to spell *pillage,* the speller accesses *village.* This strategy works sometimes but can lead to horrendous misspellings because of the irregularities of English, as in spelling *though* as *thow* because of *row.* Most spellers shift from a purely phonological strategy to a mixed one containing analogy between second and fifth grade (Goswami, 1988; Lennox & Siegel, 1996). As words and strategies are stored in long-term memory and access becomes automatized, the load on cognitive capacity is lessened and can be focused on other writing tasks.

It is estimated the nearly 4,000 words are explicitly taught in elementary school. Spelling words are taken from several sources including published lists, basal spellers, and texts or are specified by the curriculum.

Most spelling is self-taught using a trial-and-error approach (Braten, 1994). Good spellers use a variety of strategies and actively search words for patterns and consistency (Hughes & Searle, 1997).

Writing Problems

Children with oral language impairments will most likely have writing impairments too. For many children with LI, writing difficulties do not decrease with age and the gap widens between their writing abilities and those of children developing typically. The content and organization of their writing suffer as more of their cognitive capacity is used for the lower-level mechanics of writing, such as spelling.

Children with LLD have difficulties with all aspects of the writing process (Graham, Harris, MacArthur, & Schwartz, 1991; McFadden & Gillam, 1996; Roth, Spekman, & Fye, 1991; Troia, Graham, & Harris, 1999; Vallecorsa & Garriss, 1990; Wong, 2000). First, they have little knowledge of the writing process, thus children with LLD fail to plan and make few substantive revisions. Second, because of the time it takes and the difficulties encountered, children with LLD write very little on a given task. Third, clarity and organization are forsaken for spelling, handwriting, and punctuation, although children continue to have difficulties in all three areas. In other words, cognitive capacity is expended on low-order mechanics. Despite this, children with LLD make more grammatical and punctuation errors and produce fewer complex sentences than age-matched peers. They have difficulty with cohesive ties and unambiguous reference. Fourth, spelling often follows a maladaptive pattern in which words that can be spelled are substituted for those that cannot. In the process, meaning suffers.

In narrative writing as in storytelling, children with LI lack mature internalized story schemes (Graves et al., 1994, Montague, Graves, & Leavell, 1991; Roth, et al., 1991; Vallecorsa & Garriss, 1990). As noted in Chapter 8, the oral narratives of children with LI are often shorter with fewer episodes, contain fewer details, and often fail to consider the needs of the listener. Listeners are only rarely given cause and effect or character motivation. The oral and written narratives of children with LI have similar characteristics.

Deficits in Executive Function

When executive function is impaired, communication abilities are diminished, especially in socially demanding or complex linguistic tasks, such as writing. Executive function is especially important for the pragmatic aspects of communication, memory and retrieval, strategic thinking, perspective taking, and generalization. In addition to anatomical and physiological aspects of development, executive function is also vulnerable to academic and social failure. Both may slow development as children begin to realistically assess their abilities.

Executive function impairment is most evident in children with TBI (Sohlberg, Mateer, & Stuss, 1993; Ylvisaker & Feeney, 1995). The high frequency of frontal lobe injury makes executive function particularly vulnerable for these children.

Children with ADHD have been described as inattentive and impulsive, disorganized, unable to inhibit behavior, and ineffective learners, characteristics of those with impaired executive function. In nonexecutive function tasks, such as visuospatial processing, children with ADHD experience no difficulties.

Children with LD minimize self-regulatory processes found in executive functions (Englert, Raphael, Fear, & Anderson, 1988). When they write, they follow a "retrieve-write" strategy in which they write whatever comes to mind, each sentence stimulating the next, with little thought to planning. The result is that they produce and elaborate very little. Revisions are ineffective and can be characterized by seeming indifference to the audience, inept detection of errors, and difficulty executing intended changes (Graham & Harris, 1999).

Deficits in Spelling

As mentioned, writing and spelling are separate but correlated processes. Children with written-language deficits due to LLD, SLI, or other causes may have problems in either or both. In general, children have more difficulty with spelling if handwriting is also a problem (Berninger et al., 1998a).

Poor spellers view spelling as arbitrary and random. To them, spelling is difficult and ultimately unlearnable (Hughes & Searle, 1997). Adults with LD often cite spelling as their primary area of concern (Blalock & Johnson, 1987).

Beyond the obvious difficulties for poor spellers are the parallel deficits seen in reading. Poor spellers have poor word attack or decoding skills and overrely on compensatory strategies, such as use of context for reading words (Bruck & Waters, 1990; Newman, Fields, & Wright, 1993).

The misspellings of the poorest older spellers suggest the following patterns of spelling deficits (Moats, 1995):

- Omission of liquids and nasals in rime or noninitial positions, as in *SEF* for *self* and *RET* for *rent*
- Omission in consonant clusters, especially in the syllable- and word-final positions, as in *FAT* for *fast*
- Omission of unstressed vowel, as in *TELFON* for *telephone*
- Vowel substitutions, as in *TRI* for *try*
- Consonant substitutions that share some articulatory features, as in "t" for "d" or "m" for "n"
- Omission of plural inflections
- Omission or substitution of past tense inflections
- Misspelling of difficult common words, such as *their/there* and *to/too/two*

Overall, these spellers demonstrate primitive phonologically based errors even when they have high levels of orthographic knowledge (Treiman, 1997).

Although most spellers shift to greater use of analogy between second and fifth grade, poor spellers continue to rely on visual matching skills and phoneme position rules because of limited knowledge of sound-letter correspondences (Kamhi & Hinton, 2000). In other words, they continue to use the visual approach to learning that characterizes much younger spellers. In fact, spellers with dysgraphia seem incapable of changing their spelling of certain types of words (Treiman, 1997).

Spelling deficits are only rarely caused by poor visual memory. Usually, deficits in spelling represent poor phonological processing and poor knowledge and use of phoneme-grapheme information.

Assessment of Writing

It is best to employ an evaluative tool that uses data from actual writing in varying contexts. One method of assessing writing in the classroom is through the use of portfolios of children's writing (Paratore, 1995). Portfolios are a collection of meaningful writing selected by the child, SLP, and teacher that contains samples of the child's writing over time, enabling the child to demonstrate progress. The wide variety helps to increase the validity of the sample. Allowing children to contribute fosters self-growth and monitoring. In addition, selection of teacher and SLP choices fosters collaboration. The writing contained within can also be used to demonstrate progress toward IEP goals. Guidelines for portfolio use in an initial evaluation are as follows (Manning Kratcoski, 1998):

- Careful determination of the items to be included for variety over time
- Analysis appropriate for the different types of writing and the goals of the assessment
- Appropriate persons contributing items

Items to be included in a portfolio may include SLP observation notes, work samples, and first drafts of writing samples, such as journal or learning log entries, and projects/papers, final drafts of the same, and peer and teacher evaluations.

As mentioned, the SLP and teacher should collaborate to decide on the type of writing desired (N. Nelson & Van Meter, 2002). Narratives are best for young elementary school children (N. Nelson, 1998). Open-ended tasks, in which the child supplies all needed information, reveal more about a child's writing than structured tasks in which the setting and characters are specified or in which the child retells a narrative. The latter types of tasks may be needed, however, for children with poor narrative skills. Older elementary school children or adolescents can provide expository writing samples.

Expository writing, the writing of the classroom, is of several genres: procedural, descriptive, opinion, cause-and-effect, and compare-and-contrast. Samples of each should be collected if possible. Although the focus changes by type of expository writing, clarity of ideas is important in each genre.

Executive function is best assessed within overall writing assessment or through dynamic assessment techniques mentioned in Chapter 3. There is a risk in separating the various functions and considering them separately from functional communication tasks (Fey, 1986).

Data Collection

Samples should be written in ink to allow the SLP to note revisions. The teacher or SLP should inform children that edits are fine and encourage children to do their best. It's helpful to allow children to plan and to write drafts. Paper can be provided for notes and plans and should be collected along with the finished product. These can be added to the portfolio mentioned previously. Whenever possible, the SLP can observe the writing process for evidence of planning and organizing, drafting, writing, revising, and editing.

Expository texts can be elicited by a number of procedures. For example, sequential/procedural texts can be elicited by asking the child, "Tell me how you make _____." With the cause-and-effect genre, the SLP might say, "Tell me what might happen if _____." Problem-solving genres can be encouraged with "How would you _____?" It is important to pose familiar and unfamiliar themes. Key words, such as *describe, compare, contrast, cause,* and *solve* can cue the child for the type desired.

Added information can be obtained if children read their paper aloud while being audiotaped. This procedure aids the SLP in interpreting garbled or poorly spelled words.

Data Analysis

Writing can be analyzed on several levels, including textual, linguistic, and orthographic (spelling). At a textual level, the SLP can note compositional length, an indication of the amount of effort; quality, a holistic rating on the nature of the task; and discourse structure, the way in which text is related to the global topic or comments support the topic (Berninger, 2000).

The child's writing can be photocopied for mark-up and analysis. Of interest are the total number of words, clauses, and T-units. The use of T-units can help to avoid long run-on sentences but does not reflect "grammatical accuracy," so further internal analysis must be performed (N. Nelson & Van Meter, 2002). These are outlined in Chapter 8. Writing conventions, such as capitalization and punctuation, plus the use of sentences and paragraphs, should be noted. Spelling can be analyzed as explained below.

Spelling Assessment

Although it may seem straightforward, spelling deficits are very complex and can be difficult to describe. Collection should be of sufficient quantity to allow for a broad-based analysis of error types.

Data Collection.   Spelling deficits should be assessed through both dictation and connected writing (Masterson & Apel, 2000). In dictation, either within standardized testing or from word inventories, the SLP or teacher reads words while the child writes them. Standardized tests include the Test of Written Language (Hammill & Larsen, 1996), Test of Written Spelling (Larson & Hammill, 1994), and the Wide Range Achievement Test—3 (Wilkinson, 1995).

Word inventories, either preselected—such as those found in Bear, Invernizzi, Templeton, and Johnston (2000)—or SLP-designed, should be developmental in nature and include several phoneme-grapheme variations, including, but not limited to, single consonants in various positions in words, blends, morphological inflections, diphthongs, digraphs such as "ch" and "sh," and complex derivations. The choice of words will vary with the age and functioning level of the child and should not be bizarre or totally unfamiliar to the child. The number of words must be sufficient to identify patterns of functioning. Using fifty to 100 words is probably adequate, although more is desirable (Masterson & Apel, 2000).

Single-word spelling may be of little real value because decontextualized spelling does not measure a child's ability in a real communicative context (Moats, 1995). Connected writing can be generated in response to pictures or narratives or provided through the portfolios mentioned previously. In a variation, the child can write an original sentence or narrative using representative words taken from word lists (Buchannan, 1989; Routman, 1991).

Testing tasks that require the child to select correctly spelled words may seen like a good assessment tool but may be of little actual value (Ehri, 2000). These tasks occur infrequently in the real world of the child and thus are not functional for either assessment or intervention.

Data from other areas of language functioning are also of interest. The SLP along with other team members should assess the child's reading, phonological awareness, and morphology use because of the close correlation of each of these areas with spelling.

Data Analysis.   Descriptive analysis should focus on orthographic patterns evident in the child's spelling (Bear et al., 2000). While individual errors are significant, error patterns are important for intervention. Of interest are the most frequent and the lowest level patterns.

The SLP tries to determine the type of error reflected in the child's spelling of each incorrect word. It's helpful to analyze base words (*teach*), inflected words (*teaches*), and derived words (*teacher*) separately to see if errors are related to any specific word form. Table 13.6 presents a classification system that can be helpful and relates to the developmental process described earlier.

Spelling is the result of segmenting a word into phonemic elements and selecting the appropriate graphemes. Unfortunately, for the beginning speller, not all phonemic components are readily appar-

TABLE 13.6 Levels of spelling analysis

Level	Description	Example
Preliterate	Unrecognizable symbols, some letters. Prephonetic spelling in which letters and sounds do not correspond.	υζT≈V●
Early letter name	Uses primarily letter names. Semi-phonetic spelling evidencing a few sound-letter relationships, but letters are missing, especially vowels.	T for *tea,* MT for *empty,* TP for *top*
Letter name	Spelling based on letter names and speech sounds. Consonant clusters usually reduced. Although many misspellings occur, the child has a notion of sound-letter associations.	JRAK, CHRAC, TRAC for *track*
Within-word pattern	Orthographic patterns, such as long and short vowel patterns used along with spelling by meaning, i.e., morphological inflections.	RATE, RAT, CONE, CON, and STOPS, WALKED, SINGING
Syllable juncture	Uses doubling principle and patterns in both stressed and unstressed syllables.	LITTLE, BUBBLE, STRAIGHT, VACATION
Derivational constancy	Uses roots and derivations consistently. Uses multiple strategies.	STARING and STARRING, NATURE and NATURAL

Based on Ehri (1986); Gentry (1982); Henderson (1990).

ent. Consonants often become lost in blends. In analyzing the spelling sample, the SLP should note consonant blends by location within the syllable and word and by the presence of other phonemes. Internal word consonants are omitted more than those at either end, thus *snack* might become *SAK.* The SLP should seek letter-name, phonemic, or morphologic explanations for error patterns (Bourassa & Treiman, 2001).

Phonological processing and spelling are related for elementary school children, less so for older students who use multiple spelling strategies (Berninger et al., 1994a). If the child uses an incorrect letter, the error most likely represents a problem in phonological awareness. Inserted or deleted letters may represent a speech perception problem (Moats, 1995).

In addition, the SLP should look at each error to determine the child's orthographic system knowledge. This includes letter selection and position constraints. For example, "ts" is an acceptable blend but is constrained by position and is not acceptable at the beginning of a word, with the exception of the Russian "tsar." Such knowledge addresses the question *Could this be a word?* Has the child's error violated acceptable English spelling or would the resultant word be an acceptable one? Orthographic constraints are presented in detail in Mersand, Griffith, and Griffith (1996).

Intervention for Writing Impairment

Intervention for writing may involve both general training and more specific techniques for narrative and expository forms. To learn to write, you must write, so intervention needs to focus on the actual writing process.

Executive function can be targeted within the writing process using a goal-plan-do-review format (Ylvisaker & Feeney, 1996; Ylvisaker & Szekeres, 1989; Ylvisaker, Szekeres, & Feeney, 1998).

There is little an SLP can do to alleviate the root causes of TBI, ADHD, or other impairments relative to executive function, but he or she can provide external support to enable children with these impairments to experience some level of success (Ylvisaker & DeBonis, 2000). This should not be interpreted to mean that the SLP acts as the child's executive function. In that situation, little changes for the child. SLPs give children the tools to facilitate their lives. SLPs change behaviors and processes. In the end, we cannot live our client's lives for them.

Instruction in handwriting is beyond the scope of speech and language services. If the child with LI uses a computer keyboard well, it might be advisable to use this method rather than handwriting to free working memory for text generation.

Intervention can begin by allowing children to select their own topics. This increases motivation and shifts the focus to ideas. Mechanics will come later. Topic selection works well with small groups of children and the sharing process often generates more ideas.

In the planning phase, the SLP and child can brainstorm ideas for inclusion in the writing (Troia, Graham, & Harris, 1999). Drawings and ideational maps or spider diagrams can help. For narratives, children might draw a few simple pictures and organize them in the appropriate order. Computer programs, such as The Amazing Writing Machine (Broderbund, 1999) and The Ultimate Writing and Creativity Center (The Learning Company), can also be helpful. It is also helpful for the child to focus on the potential audience. The SLP can ask questions such as the following (Graham & Harris, 1999):

Who will read this paper?
What do the readers know?
What do the readers need to know?
Why are you writing?

The SLP and child may prefer to use computers as an assistive technology for writing (MacArthur, 2000). Software, such as Inspiration (Inspirations Software, 1997), can aid text generation, and the result is easily modifiable by the child or teacher. Although the technology itself is unlikely to improve writing, it does remove the handwriting difficulties for some children. Typing can also detract from text development, and computer use can result in new burdens for working memory. Having said this, we should note that children with LD who receive training in executive function along with word processing make greater gains in the quality of their writing than children instructed only in executive function (MacArthur, Graham, Schwartz, & Schafer, 1995). Word processing experience alone, however, does not improve overall quality (MacArthur & Graham, 1987; MacArthur et al., 1995; Vace, 1987).

A word about spellcheckers and grammar checkers seems in order. Neither are foolproof, as I'm sure you know. Spellcheckers will be discussed in the following section on spelling. Grammar checkers miss many errors, especially if there are multiple spelling errors, and can easily confuse the writer who is left to figure out just what the error is. Some grammar checkers are very resistant, and only a strong writer can continue to insist on the structure desired. I sometimes have to change it back three times before I can override the system.

Word-prediction programs, such as *Co:Writer* (D. Johnston, 1998), *Write Away 2000* (Information Services, 1989), and *Clicker Plus* (Crick Software, 1997), are helpful, but mostly for spelling (MacArthur, 2000; Ylvisaker & DeBonis, 2000). Most have speech synthesis too. Inputs vary from spelling only to spelling plus grammar. It's important that the word-prediction program's vocabulary match the writing task of the child (MacArthur, 1999; Zhang, Brooks, Fields, & Redelfs, 1995). For example, *Co:Writer* incorporates the word frequency and topic of the writer. *Write Away 2000* allows the child or teacher to add vocabulary, and content-specific prompts can be added to expand the vocabulary. In contrast, *Clicker Plus* allows the child or teacher to download specific words.

Finally, speech recognition software allows children to compose by dictation, resulting in longer and higher quality papers by children with LLD (Graham, 1990). Children must be instructed to speak clearly in order to improve speech recognition and to dictate punctuation and formatting. Speech-recognition software cannot overcome oral language difficulties, although these can be moderated with the additional use of grammar checkers.

Narrative Writing

Narrative writing may require explicit instruction in story structure as outlined in Chapter 11. Story maps using pictures or story frames may be necessary initially but should be faded gradually as the child assumes more responsibility for the narrative. Story frames (Fowler, 1982) are written starters for each main-story grammar element. The child completes the sentence and continues with that portion of the narrative. Cards or checklists can also be used to remind the child of story grammar elements (Graves, Montague, & Wong, 1990; Montague, Graves, & Leavell, 1991).

During the writing process, the SLP can use story guides, prompts, and acronyms to aid the child. Story guides are questions that help the student construct the narrative, while prompts are story beginning and ending phrases (Graves et al., 1990; Montague et al., 1991; Thomas, Englert, & Morsink, 1984). Acronyms, such as SPACE for setting, problem, action, and consequent events, can also act as prompts for guiding writing (Harris & Graham, 1996). Children can be encouraged to write more with verbal prompts such as "Tell me more" or "What happened next?"

Feelings and motivations found in mature narratives are often missing from the stories of children with LI. These elements can be targeted with pictures and questions such as "How do you think she felt?" (Roth, 2000).

Expository Writing

Procedures for intervention with expository writing include collaborative planning; individual, independent writing; conferencing with the teacher/SLP and peers; individual, independent revising; and final editing (Wong, 2000). Whatever the expository genre involved, collaborative planning is important, including planning, writing, and revising. In the first step, the child should think aloud and solicit opinions. This is an opportunity for the child to hear alternative views and to reconcile these with his or her own.

For opinion papers, the child first needs to pick a topic. These might come from a prepared list, from the child, or from topics discussed in class. Once the topic is selected and discussed in small groups, with a peer, and/or with the SLP, the SLP can give the child a planning sheet to help organize her or his thoughts. It might include two columns: *What I believe* and *What someone else believes* (Wong, 2000). After the child has completed the sheet, either with help or working alone, the SLP can help the child form dyads of opposing views. This is a great time for verbal repartee, challenging, and helping the child clarify his or her views and prepare for independent writing.

Writing, although independent, can be fostered through the use of a prompt card containing key words for each major section of the paper (Wong, Butler, Ficzere, & Kuperis, 1996). Table 13.7 presents a sample prompt card.

After the child has completed the paper, he or she conferences with peers for feedback while the SLP mediates. The child revises the paper based on feedback.

TABLE 13.7   Sample prompt card for opinion writing

Section of Paper	Examples
Introduction	In my opinion… I believe… From my point of view,… I agree with… I disagree with… Supporting words: first, second, finally, for example, most important is…, consider, think about, remember
Counter Opinion	Although… However,… On the other hand,… To the contrary,… Even though…
Conclusion	In conclusion,… After considering both sides,… To summarize,…

Source: Adapted from Wong, B. Y., Butler, D. L., Ficzere, S. A., & Kuperis, S. (1996). Teaching low achievers and students with learning disabilities to plan, write, and revise opinion essays. *Journal of Learning Disabilities, 29* (2), 197–212.

At each stage in the process, the child should record progress on a checklist. In addition to providing a model for the writing process, the checklist can motivate the child as she or he finishes each step.

For compare-and-contrast writing, the planning process can be similar. Again, the topic—which entities are to be compared—can come from prepared lists, the child, or the curriculum. Through brainstorming, the child and SLP try to answer the question "How can we compare them?" SLPs should be prepared for some comparisons that are very "original," especially from children who have perceptual deficits and may view the world quite differently from adults.

Again, the child can be helped with writing prompts, such as the following (Ylsivaker & DeBonis, 2000):

> In this essay, I'm going to compare and contrast…
> I have chosen two (any number) features:…
> In conclusion,…

As mentioned previously, peer, teacher, and SLP review and feedback can help the child revise.

Intervention for Spelling

Words are the vehicles for teaching alphabetic and orthographic principles (Berninger et al., 1998b). The SLP is not the "spelling teacher." It is as inappropriate for the SLP to teach this week's spelling list as it is to teach this week's vocabulary.

Words selected for intervention should be individualized for each child and reflect both the curriculum and the child's desires (Graham, Harris, & Loynachan, 1994). Spelling intervention should be integrated into real writing and reading within the classroom. It is best if intervention can occur when the child is actually writing and he or she can be reminded of alphabetic and orthographic principles (Scott, 2000). Words misspelled in class can be analyzed by the SLP. Spelling strategies can be discussed with the child using these words.

Spelling can be taught within teaching of general executive function in which the child is taught to proofread, correct, and edit. Peer editing is also effective (Graham, 1999).

If needed, spelling intervention should begin with alphabetic principles, connecting sounds and letters. Targeted words can be taught as explained below but expanded into onset-rime training to facilitate overall spelling ability (Berninger et al., 1998b).

Children with LD benefit from multisensory input such as pictures, objects, or actions (Graham, 1999). Several multisensory study techniques have been proposed. In the 5-Step Study Strategy, the child (1) says the word, (2) writes it while saying it again, (3) checks spelling and, (4) if correct, traces it while saying it again, then finally, (5) writes the word and checks the spelling (Graham & Freeman, 1986).

In the Horn Method 2, the child focuses on the internal structure of the word (Horn, 1954). Words are pronounced carefully, followed by carefully looking at each part of the word. Letters are pronounced in sequence, then recalled. The child then writes the word, checks, and if incorrect, re-spells and checks again.

The 8-Step Method is designed for pencil or computer (Berninger et al., 1998a). First, the SLP sweeps his or her finger over the word and pronounces it out loud. Next, to call attention to the phoneme-grapheme correspondence, the SLP says the word again emphasizing sounds that correspond to colored letter groupings. For example, /b/-/i/-/d/ for "b"-"ea"-"d." On the third pass, the child names the letters as the SLP points to each in sequence. The child then closes his or her eyes and visualizes the word. In step five, while his or her eyes are closed, the child spells the word out loud. Following this step, the child writes the word, then compares it to the sample. In the final step, the SLP reinforces the child's correct spelling. If the child's spelling is incorrect, the SLP points out the difference between the sample and the child's attempt and repeats the previous steps.

Word analysis and sorting tasks can be used to strengthen the alphabetic principle (Scott, 2000). Patterns to be taught should be identified from the child's misspellings. Minimum pairs that differ on the bases of these processes can be used to demonstrate the lexical consequences of misspelling (Masterson & Crede, 1999). The SLP should use known and unknown words to facilitate generalization.

Sorting tasks will differ based on the spelling level of the child (Scott, 2000). At the letter-name level of development, words can be sorted or grouped by sounds and location, as in initial consonants or initial digraphs (two letters = one sound, "sh" = /ʃ/). Minimal pairs might contrast short vowels, long and short vowels, single consonants and blends, and one digraph with another. In contrast, with children at the within-word level, the SLP can sorted by orthographic patterns, such as vowel patterns, rimes, and homophones. In the later stages of syllable juncture and derivational constancy, words can be grouped by syllable juncture principles and meaning, including inflectional suffixes and simple prefixes and derivational suffixes, consonant doubling with open and closed syllables, compound words, changing final "y" to "i," and word roots. Minimal pairs may contrast variants of inflectional suffixes, such as "-s" and "-es," and base words with derivational suffixes, as in *teach/teacher.*

Computers are helpful and encourage editing, although spellcheckers are not foolproof and the child may learn little. In general, spellcheckers miss words in which the misspelling has inadvertently produced another word. Suggested spelling may also confound the child with poor word attack skills. In addition, suggested spellings may be far afield if the original word has multiple misspellings. Spellcheckers help only about 37 percent of the time for children with LD, a lower percentage than found among children developing typically (MacArthur, Graham, Haynes, & DeLaPaz, 1996).

On the other hand, word-prediction programs reduce spelling errors of children with LI by over half, although the user must get the initial letters correct for the program to work effectively (Newell, Booth, Arnott, & Beattie, 1992).

If children with LI are taught to spell phonetically when unsure of the correct spelling, spellcheckers generate more correct suggestions. Proofing and editing on a hard copy also seem to increase the number of correctly spelled words (McNaughton, Hughes, & Ofiesh, 1997). Internet searches can foster spelling learning because correct spelling is needed to complete searches successfully.

Conclusion

And so, we reach the end of this text. I hope that I have challenged your thinking along the way and that you'll use this book as a reference. Even in the area of literacy, functional communication is important. Using real reading and writing samples. Training for the kinds of reading and writing that the child is encountering in the classroom. And we have come full circle. Intervention in the classroom is about as close as an SLP in the schools can get to the actual use environment of the child. Other aspects of the model that we have discussed may also be present. For example, parents may be involved in their children's training. Cues and consequences should still be as natural as possible. Literacy being as functional as possible is especially important. Remember…

Decontextualized training routinely fails at the level of generalization…(Ylvisaker & DeBonis, 2000, p. 43).

Definitions of Illocutionary and Semantic Functions

Functions	Examples
Semantic	
Nomination—naming a person or object using a single- or multiword name or a demonstrative-plus as a name.	Doggie, Choo-choo, This horsie
Location—marking spatial relationships. Utterances may contain single-location words or two-word utterances containing an agent, action, or object plus a location word. The function can be demonstrated in response to *where* questions.	PARTNER: Where's Doggie? CHILD: Chair. Ball table, Doggie chair, Throw me, Throw here (*X* + locative)
Negation—marking of nonexistence, rejection, and denial using single negative words or a negative followed by another word (negative + *X*).	
Nonexistence generally develops first and marks the absence of a once-present object.	All gone (used as a single word), Away, No milk (child drank it), All gone car (the ride is over), No
Rejection marks an attempt to prevent or to stop an event.	PARTNER: Time for bed. CHILD: No (or No bed) Stop it, No milk (*pushes glass away*)
Denial marks rejection of a proposition.	PARTNER: See the bear? CHILD: No bear.

Continued

Functions	Examples
Semantic *(Continued)*	
Modification	
Possession—appreciating that an object belongs to or is frequently associated with someone. Single-word utterances signal the owner's name. In two-word utterances, stress is usually on the initial word, the possessor.	Mine, My dollie, Johnnie bike (modifier + head) Dollie (*child clutches doll*)
Attribution—using descriptors for properties not inherently part of the object.	Yukky, Big doggie, Little baby (modifier + head)
Recurrence—understanding that an object can reappear or an event can be reenacted.	More, More milk, 'Nuther cookie (modifier + head)
Notice—signaling that an object has appeared, an event has happened, or an attempt to gain attention.	Hi Mommy, Bye-bye, Look Jim, Hey man
State—signaling an internal emotion or feeling.	Hungry, I tired, Doggie sleepy
Action—marking an activity.	
Action—single-action words or expanded with addition of agent or action.	Jump, Eat, Mommy drink (agent + action)
Agent + Action—signal that an animate initiated an activity; expanded with addition of action.	Doggie Baby sleep, Mommy throw (agent + action)
Object—signal that an animate or inanimate object was the recipient of action; expanded with addition of action.	Cookie, Throw ball (action + object), Drink juice
Illocutionary	
Answer—child responds to questions. The questioner's behaviors are a cue for the child's response; the response probably would not be produced without this cue. The child's responses are cognitively related to the question, although they may be incorrect.	PARTNER (*holding doll*): What's this? CHILD: Baby. PARTNER: Is this a mirror? CHILD: No.
Question—child asks for information or verification by addressing the other person verbally. The child's behavior is a stimulus or cue and indicates that he expects an answer. The child can ask himself questions when engaged in egocentric play.	CHILD: (*picks up toy telephone*): Phone? CHILD: What this?
Reply—child makes meaningful response to the content of the other speaker's previous utterance, a verbal cue external to the child. The child may continue to build on the content and ignore the form of the utterance, such as responding to a word or thought in a question without answering the question. In many cases, the child will build on the content and respond with an appropriate form. This category does not include mere repetition.	PARTNER: Johnny, bring me the scissors. (command) CHILD: No. PARTNER: May I have the keys? (request) CHILD: In a minute. PARTNER: This is a cute dog. (declaration) CHILD: My doggie.

Functions	Examples
Illocutionary *(Continued)*	
Elicitation—child self-repeats in response to a request for repetition or clarification or in response to "Say *x*."	CHILD: Kitty go. (declaration) PARTNER: What? CHILD: Kitty go. PARTNER: Mary, say "ball." CHILD: Ball. Uh-huh, okay. I see, yes. What? Huh?
Continuant—child signals that he or she is listening and wants to continue the interchange or that he or she missed what was said.	
Declaration—child makes a statement that is situationally related and for communication but is not in response to another speaker. The utterance is more like a commentary. Cues are internal or situational but not verbal. This category also includes situationally related phonemic exclamations.	CHILD: (*playing game with mother and glances out*): It raining out. CHILD: (*playing with car*): Car go up. PARTNER: This is a cute doggie. CHILD: My doggie. (reply) He lives in a house. (declaration) PARTNER: This is a cute doggie. CHILD: My doggie. (reply) I have kitty, too. (declaration)
Practice—repeats or imitates in whole or part what she or he or another person says with no change in intonation that would indicate a change of intent. In addition, internal replay without added new information is considered *practice*. This category also includes counting, singing, babbling, or rhyming behaviors in which the child seems to be experimenting or rehearsing.	PARTNER: Ball. CHILD: Ball. PARTNER: See the red ball. CHILD: Red ball. PARTNER: See the red ball. CHILD: See ball. (practice) Ball, ball, ball. (practice)
Perseverative responses, even if the other person interjects an utterance between them, are considered *practice* as long as they do not mark discrete events or objects.	
Name—child labels an object or event that is present, but the label is not in response to a question. This verbal behavior usually is accomplished by pointing or nodding.	CHILD: (*picks up ball*): Ball. CHILD: (*points to ball*): That ball.
Suggestion, Command, Demand, Request—The primary function of the child's utterance is to influence another person's behavior by getting that person to do something or to give the child permission. The form may be imperative, declarative, or interrogative.	CHILD: Gimmie cookie. CHILD: Stop that. CHILD: Mommy. CHILD: Throw ball. (*parent throws*) Throw ball. (*parent throws*) Throw ball.

Source: Adapted from Owens (1982d).

B

Considerations for CLD Children

Most regional and ethnic dialects differ only slightly from the standard or are used by a limited number of individuals. Three ethnic dialects, however, represent rather large segments of the U.S. population and have some very important differences with Standard American English. These dialects are African American English, Latino English, and Asian English. African American English is used primarily by working-class African Americans in the urban northern United States and rural African Americans in the South. Not every African American uses African American English, and not everyone who uses it is African American.

Latino English and Asian English are probably misnomers. Latino English, as used here, is a composite of the English used by many speakers who are bilingual and learned English as a second language. Individual variations represent the age of learning and level of mastery, the Spanish dialect used, socioeconomic status, and where the person lives in the United States. Asian English is also a composite, but of bilingual speakers of Asian languages who learned English as a second language. As such, Asian English probably does not exist except to simplify our discussion. Asians speak many languages, and each has a different effect on the learning of English. In addition to the original language learned, other individual differences may reflect the same factors as those of Latino English. Each dialect is discussed in some detail. Where possible, information has been reduced to tables to aid presentation. Each dialect is compared with Standard American English, an idealized norm uninfluenced by the dialectal differences each person possesses.

African American English

African American English reflects the complex racial and economic history of the United States and the migration of African Americans from the rural South to the urban North after World War II. Regional differences exist to some degree. The major variations between Standard American English and African American English in phonology, syntax, and morphology are presented in Tables B.1 and B.2.

TABLE B.1 **Phonemic contrasts between African American English and Standard American English**

| SAE Phonemes | Position in Word | | |
	Initial	Medial	Final*
/p/		Unaspirated /p/	Unaspirated /p/
/n/			Reliance on preceding nasalized vowel
/w/	Omitted in specific words (*I 'as, too!*)		
/b/		Unreleased /b/	Unreleased /b/
/g/		Unreleased /g/	Unreleased /g/
/k/		Unaspirated /k/	Unaspirated /k/
/d/	Omitted in specific words (*I 'on't know*)	Unreleased /d/	Unreleased /d/
/ŋ/		/n/	/n/
/t/		Unaspirated /t/	Unaspirated /t/
/l/		Omitted before labial consonants (help-hep)	"uh" following a vowel (*Bill-Biuh*)
/r/		Omitted or /ə/	Omitted or prolonged vowel or glide
/θ/	Unaspirated /t/ or /f/	Unaspirated /t/ or /f/ between vowels	Unaspirated /t/ or /f/ (*bath-baf*)
/v/	Sometimes /b/	/b/ before /m/ and /n/	Sometimes /b/
/ð/	/d/	/d/ or /v/ between vowels	/d/, /v/, /f/
/z/		Omitted or replaced by /d/ before nasal sound (*wasn't-wud'n*)	

Blends
/str/ becomes /skr/
/ʃr/ becomes /str/
/θr/ becomes /θ/
/pr/ becomes /p/
/br/ becomes /b/
/kr/ becomes /k/
/gr/ becomes /g/

Final Consonant Clusters (second consonant omitted when these clusters occur at the end of a word)

/sk/	/nd/	/sp/
/ft/	/ld/	/dʒd/
/st/	/sd/	/nt/

*Note weakening of final consonants.

Source: Data drawn from Fasold & Wolfram (1970); Labov (1972); F. Weiner & Lewnau (1979); R. Williams & Wolfram (1977).

TABLE B.2 **Grammatical contrasts between African American English and Standard American English**

African American English Grammatical Structure	SAE Grammatical Structure
Possessive -*'s*	
Nonobligatory where word position expresses possession.	Obligatory regardless of position.
Get *mother* coat.	Get mother*'s* coat.
It be mother*'s*.	It's mother*'s*.
Plural -*s*	
Nonobligatory with numerical quantifier.	Obligatory regardless of numerical quantifier.
He got ten *dollar*.	He has ten dollar*s*.
Look at the cat*s*.	Look at the cat*s*.
Regular past -*ed*	
Nonobligatory; reduced as consonant cluster.	Obligatory.
Yesterday, I *walk* to school.	Yesterday, I walk*ed* to school.
Irregular past	
Case by case, some verbs inflected, others not.	All irregular verbs inflected.
I *see* him last week.	I *saw* him last week.
Regular present tense third-person singular -*s*	
Nonobligatory.	Obligatory.
She *eat* too much.	She eat*s* too much.
Irregular present tense third-person singular -*s*	
Nonobligatory.	Obligatory.
He *do* my job.	He *does* my job.
Indefinite *an*	
Use of indefinite *a*.	Use of *an* before nouns beginning with a vowel.
He ride in a airplane.	He rode in *an* airplane.
Pronouns	
Pronominal apposition: pronoun immediately follows noun.	Pronoun used elsewhere in sentence or in other sentence; not in apposition.
Momma *she* mad. She…	Momma is mad. *She*…
Future tense	
More frequent use of *be going to* (gonna).	More frequent use of *will*.
I *be going to* dance tonight.	I *will* dance tonight.
I *gonna* dance tonight.	I *am going to* dance tonight.
Omit *will* preceding *be*.	Obligatory use of *will*.
I *be* home later.	I *will* (I'll) *be* home later.
Negation	
Triple negative.	Absence of triple negative.
Nobody don't never like me.	*No* one ever likes me.
Use of *ain't*.	*Ain't* is unacceptable form.
I *ain't* going.	I'*m not* going.
Modals	
Double modals for such forms as *might, could,* and *should*.	Single modal use.
I *might could* go.	I *might be able to* go.

African American English Grammatical Structure	SAE Grammatical Structure
Questions	
Same form for direct and indirect.	Different forms for direct and indirect.
What *it is*?	What *is it*?
Do you know what *it is*?	Do you know what *it is*?
Relative pronouns	
Nonobligatory in most cases.	Nonobligatory with *that* only.
He the one stole it.	He's the one *who* stole it.
It the one you like.	It's the one (that) you like.
Conditional *if*	
Use of *do* for conditional *if*.	Use of *if*.
I ask *did* she go.	I asked *if* she went.
Perfect construction	
Been used for action in the distant past.	*Been* not used.
He *been* gone.	He left a long time ago.
Copula	
Nonobligatory when contractible.	Obligatory in contractible and uncontractible forms.
He sick.	He's sick.
Habitual or general state	
Marked with uninflected *be*.	Nonuse of *be;* verb inflected.
She *be* workin'.	She's *working* now.

Source: Data drawn from Fasold & Wolfram (1970); R. Williams & Wolfram (1977).

Latino English

Speakers who are bilingual may move back and forth between both languages in a process called *code switching.* The amount of code switching depends on the speaker's mastery of the two languages and on the audience being addressed. Of course, a great deal of code switching makes the speaker's English incomprehensible to the listener who is monolingual American English.

Most characteristics of Latino English reflect interference points, or points where the two languages differ, thus making learning somewhat more difficult. For example, the speaker of Latino English may continue to use the Spanish possessive form in which the owner is preceded by the entity owned, as in "the dress of Mary." The major variations between Standard American English and Latino English in phonology, syntax, and morphology are presented in Tables B.3 and B.4.

Asian English

Chinese culture and language have for centuries influenced all other Asian cultures and languages. Other cultures, such as that of the Indian subcontinents, have influenced nearby Asian neighbors. Colonial occupation, especially by the French in Indochina, also has influenced the culture and language of the affected region.

The most widely used languages—Chinese, Filipino, Japanese, Khmer, Korean, Laotian, and Vietnamese—represent only a portion of the languages of the area. Each language contains many

**TABLE B.3   Phonemic contrasts between Latino English
and Standard American English**

SAE Phonemes	Position in Word		
	Initial	**Medial**	**Final***
/p/	Unaspirated /p/		Omitted or weakened
/m/			Omitted
/w/	/hu/		Omitted
/b/			Omitted, distorted, or /p/
/g/			Omitted, distorted, or /k/
/k/	Unaspirated or /g/		Omitted, distorted, or /g/
/f/			Omitted
/d/		Dentalized	Omitted, distorted, or /t/
/ŋ/	/n/	/d/	/n/ (*sing-sin*)
/j/	/d*/		
/t/			Omitted
/ʃ/	/tʃ/	/s/, /tʃ/	/tʃ/ (*wish-which*)
/tʃ/	/ʃ/ (*chair-share*)	/ʃ/	/ʃ/ (*watch-wash*)
/r/	Distorted	Distorted	Distorted
/dʒ/	/d/	/j/	/ʃ/
/θ/	/t/, /s/ (*thin-tin, sin*)	Omitted	/ʃ/, /t/, /s/
/v/	/b/ (*vat-bat*)	/b/	Distorted
/z/	/s/ (*zip-sip*)	/s/ (*razor-racer*)	/s/
/ð/	/d/ (*then-den*)	/d/, /θ/, /v/ (*lather-ladder*)	/d/

Blends

/skw/ becomes /eskw/*

/sl/ becomes /esl/*

/st/ becomes /est/*

Vowels

/I/ becomes /i/ (*bit-beet*)

*Separates cluster into two syllables.

Source: Data drawn from J. Sawyer (1973); F. Weiner & Lewnau (1979); F. Williams, Cairns, & Cairns (1971).

dialects and has distinct linguistic features. It is therefore impossible to speak of an Asian English dialect. Instead, I shall attempt to describe the major overall differences between Asian English and Standard American English. These major or differences in phonology, syntax, and morphology are listed in Tables B.5 and B.6.

TABLE B.4   **Grammatical contrasts between Latino English and Standard American English**

Latino English Grammatical Structure	SAE Grammatical Structure
Possessive -'s	
Use post-noun modifier.	Post-noun modifier used only rarely.
This is the homework *of my brother.*	This is my brother*'s* homework.
Article used with body parts.	Possessive pronoun used with body parts.
I cut *the* finger.	I cut *my* finger.
Plural -s	
Nonobligatory.	Obligatory, excluding exceptions.
The *girl* are playing.	The *girls* are playing.
The *sheep* are playing.	The *sheep* are playing.
Regular past -ed	
Nonobligatory, especially when understood.	Obligatory.
I *talk* to her yesterday.	I *talked* to her yesterday.
Regular third-person singular present tense -s	
Nonobligatory.	Obligatory.
She *eat* too much.	She *eats* too much.
Articles	
Often omitted.	Usually obligatory.
I am going to store.	I am going to *the* store.
I am going to school.	I am going to school.
Subject pronouns	
Omitted when subject has been identified in the previous sentence.	Obligatory.
Father is happy. Bought a new car.	Father is happy. *He* bought a new car.
Future tense	
Use *go + to.*	Use *be + going to.*
I *go to* dance.	I *am going to* the dance.
Negation	
Use *no* before the verb.	Use *not* (preceded by auxiliary verb where appropriate).
She *no* eat candy.	She does *not* eat candy.
Question	
Intonation: no noun-verb inversion.	Noun-verb inversion usually.
Maria is going?	*Is Maria* going?
Copula	
Occasional use of *have.*	Use of *be.*
I *have* ten years.	I *am* ten years old.
Negative imperatives	
No used for *don't.*	*Don't* used.
No throw stones.	*Don't* throw stones.
***Do* insertion**	
Nonobligatory in questions.	Obligatory when no auxiliary verb.
You like ice cream?	*Do* you like ice cream?
Comparatives	
More frequent use of longer form (*more*).	More frequent use of shorter *-er.*
He is *more* tall.	He is tall*er.*

Source: Data drawn from Davis (1972); O. Taylor (1986a).

TABLE B.5 **Phonemic contrasts between Asian English and Standard American English**

SAE Phonemes	Position in Word		
	Initial	**Medial**	**Final**
/p/	/b/****	/b/****	Omission
/s/	Distortion*	Distortion*	Omission
/z/	/s/**	/s/**	Omission
/t/	Distortion*	Distortion*	Omission
/tʃ/	/ʃ/****	/ʃ/****	Omission
/ʃ/	/s/**	/s/**	Omission
/r/, /l/	Confusion***	Confusion***	Omission
/θ /	/s/	/s/	Omission
/dʒ/	/d/ or /z/***	/d/ or /z/***	Omission
/v/	/f/***	/f/***	Omission
	/w/**	/w/**	Omission
/ð/	/z/*	/z/*	Omission
	/d/***	/d/***	Omission

Blends

Addition of /ə/ between consonants***

Omission of final consonant clusters****

Vowels

Shortening or lengthening of vowels (seat-sit, it-eat*)

Difficulty with /I/, /ɔ/ and /æ/, and substitution of /e/ for /æ/**

Difficulty with /I/, /æ/, /ɔ/, and /ə/****

*Mandarin dialect of Chinese only

**Cantonese dialect of Chinese only

***Mandarin, Cantonese, and Japanese

****Vietnamese only

Source: Adapted from Cheng (1987).

TABLE B.6   Grammatical contrasts between Asian English and Standard American English

Asian English Grammatical Structure	SAE Grammatical Structure
Plural -s	
Not used with numerical adjective: *three cat*	Used regardless of numerical adjective: *three cats*
Used with irregular plural: *the sheeps*	Not used with irregular plural: *the sheep*
Auxiliaries *to be* and *to do*	
Omission: *I going home. She not want eat.*	Obligatory and inflected in the present progressive
Uninflected: *I is going. She do not want eat.*	form: *I am going home. She does not want to eat.*
Verb *have*	
Omission: *You been here.*	Obligatory and inflected: *You have been here. He*
Uninflected: *He have one.*	*has one.*
Regular past -ed	
Omission: *He talk yesterday.*	Obligatory, nonovergeneralization, and single-
Overgeneralization: *I eated yesterday.*	marking: *He talked yesterday. I ate yesterday. She*
Double-marking: *She didn't ate.*	*didn't eat.*
Interrogative	
Nonreversal: *You're late?*	Reversal and obligatory auxiliary: *Are you late? Do*
Omitted auxiliary: *You like ice cream?*	*you like ice cream?*
Perfect marker	
Omission: *I have write letter.*	Obligatory: *I have written a letter.*
Verb-noun agreement	
Nonagreement: *He go to school. You goes to school.*	Agreement: *He goes to school. You go to school.*
Article	
Omission: *Please give gift.*	Obligatory with certain nouns: *Please give the gift.*
Overgeneralization: *She go the school.*	*She went to school.*
Preposition	
Misuse: *I am in home.*	Obligatory specific use: *I am at home. He goes by*
Omission: *He go bus.*	*bus.*
Pronoun	
Subjective/objective confusion: *Him go quickly.*	Subjective/objective distinction: *He gave it to her.*
Possessive confusion: *It him book.*	Possessive distinction: *It's his book.*
Demonstrative	
Confusion: *I like those horse.*	Singular/plural distinction: *I like that horse.*
Conjunction	
Omission: *You I go together.*	Obligatory use between last two items in a series: *You and I are going together. Mary, John, and Carol went.*
Negation	
Double-marking: *I didn't see nobody.*	Single obligatory marking: *I didn't see anybody. He*
Simplified form: *He no come.*	*didn't come.*
Word order	
Adjective following noun (Vietnamese): *clothes new.*	Most noun modifiers precede noun: *new clothes.*
Possessive following noun (Vietnamese): *dress her.*	Possessive precedes noun: *her dress.*
Omission of object with transitive verb: *I want.*	Use of direct object with most transitive verbs: *I want it.*

Source: Adapted from Cheng (1987).

C

Forms for Reporting the Language Skills of CLD Children

TABLE C.1 Reporting language skills of CLD children

Assessment Instrument for Multicultural Clients

CLIENT'S NAME: _____
SEX: _____ SCHOOL GRADE: _____ AGE: _____
1. Evaluator of L1* _____ Date _____
(name of SLS or Interpreter)***

If Interpreter, check whether:
Family Member _____ Other _____
2. Evaluator of L2** _____ Date _____
(name of SLS)
3. Evaluator of Dialect _____ Date _____
(name of SLS)

Nonnative English Speaker
1. Spanish-influenced English _____
2. Asian-influenced English _____
3. Other _____

Nonstandard English Speaker
4. African-influenced English _____
5. Appalachian-influenced English _____
6. Other _____

UTILIZATION OF THE ASSESSMENT INSTRUMENT

1. The following assessment instrument can be used to evaluate the communicative proficiency of both LEP as well as nonstandard speakers of English. In particular, this model allows for the determination and recording of a client's (a) linguistic deficiencies *vs.* differences, (b) appropriate *vs.* inappropriate use of language, and (c) the quantity of normative or nonstandard English utterances.

2. At a minimum, obtain at least two relatively short language samples; if possible, obtain three samples in different situations.

3. Play back the language samples as frequently as is necessary in order to obtain the relevant information concerning the student's communication skills. As you do so, listen intently for each facet of the assessment instrument.

4. If necessary or desired, you may use a standard test, particularly an articulation test of your choice, to supplement the information obtained through the language samples.

AURAL/ORAL COMMUNICATIVE ASSESSMENTS

Check if Accomplished

_____ 1. Pragmatic Language Samples: Obtain samples of language usage in at least two different situations and, if possible, with two different testers in each of the situations. Note and discuss the following:

_____ A. Clinic: intelligibility of the sample................page 4a and the quantity of dialect/language differences.......page 4b

_____ B. Other: compare to clinic sample

_____ 2. Evaluate client's use of segmentals. By subjective or objective testing, note and discuss the phonological and morphosyntactic utterances you observe that are inappropriate for the language/dialect being assessed. See morphosyntactic summary..page 6

_____ 3. Evaluate client's use of suprasegmentals and body language..page 4c

_____ 4. Evaluate client's voice and fluency patterns..............page 4d

_____ 5. Evaluate client's auditory acuity and comprehension......page 5e

_____ 6. Use of Language in the Classroom (if appropriate).
Ascertain from teacher:........................page 7
(1) intelligibility of the speaker;
(2) amount of dialect/language differences used by child;
(3) his/her knowledge and use of standard language rules in the classroom;
(4) the child's auditory comprehension in L1 and L2

*L1 = Native Language
**L2 = Acquired Language/English
***SLS = Speech-Language Specialist

Continued

421

TABLE C.1 Continued

SUMMARY OF RESULTS

Circle the Appropriate Number

	NONNATIVE LANGUAGE SPEAKER		NONSTANDARD DIALECT SPEAKER
	Native Language _____ (specify)	English	_____ (specify)
1. Pragmatic Usage	1 2 3 4 5*	1 2 3 4 5	1 2 3 4 5
Intelligibility	1 2 3 4 5*	1 2 3 4 5	1 2 3 4 5
Quantity of Overall Language/Dialect Differences	1 2 3 4 5*	1 2 3 4 5	1 2 3 4 5
2. Segmentals Phonology	1 2 3 4 5*	1 2 3 4 5	1 2 3 4 5
Grammar	1 2 3 4 5*	1 2 3 4 5	1 2 3 4 5
Vocabulary	1 2 3 4 5*	1 2 3 4 5	1 2 3 4 5
3. Suprasegmentals and Body Language	1 2 3 4 5*	1 2 3 4 5	1 2 3 4 5
4. Voice and Fluency Patterns	1 2 3 4 5*	1 2 3 4 5	1 2 3 4 5

5. Audition

Acuity — passed screening _____ failed screening _____

Comprehension acceptable _____ unacceptable and below expectations _____

6. Use of Language in the Classroom (if school-aged child): acceptable _____ unacceptable and below expectations _____

* |___|___|___|___|
  1   2   3   4   5

1 = Appropriate or normal response; in the case of the quantity of language/dialect differences it refers to minimal or no differences.

5 = The most inappropriate or abnormal response—the most severe; in the case of the language/dialect differences it refers to the maximal difference.

FOR THE SPEECH-LANGUAGE SPECIALIST

Native Language (L1), Acquired English (L2), Nonstandard Dialect (D)

(a) INTELLIGIBILITY

	L1	L2	D
	——	——	——

1. Standard pronunciation, with no trace of "different" accent or dialect.
2. No conspicuous mispronunciations but would not be taken for a native speaker because of some subtle prosodic differences.
3. Marked accent and occasional mispronunciations that do not interfere with understanding.
4. Accent or prosody not appropriate to dialect/language being assessed and leading to occasional misunderstanding.
5. Frequent gross errors and a very heavy accent making understanding difficult.

(b) AMOUNT OF DIALECT/LANGUAGE DIFFERENCES NOTED WHEN SPEAKER IS USING "STANDARD" ENGLISH. Estimate the amount of dialect/language differences on the following scales (minimum or none to maximum). (Circle the appropriate number.)

```
 1   2   3   4   5      1   2   3   4   5      1   2   3   4   5      1   2   3   4   5      1   2   3   4   5
|___|___|___|___|      |___|___|___|___|      |___|___|___|___|      |___|___|___|___|      |___|___|___|___|
     Phonology               Grammar               Vocabulary             Prosody                Body Lang.             Over-all
```

(c) SUPRASEGMENTALS OR PROSODY

	L1	L2	D
	——	——	——

1. Appropriate
2. Stress pattern is unusual*
3. Intonation pattern is unusual
4. Inflection pattern is unusual
5. Loudness pattern is unusual
6. Pitch pattern is unusual
7. Other ——

BODY LANGUAGE

	L1	L2	D
	——	——	——

1. Appropriate
2. Eye contact pattern is unusual
3. Eye movement pattern is unusual
4. A body movement pattern is unusual
5. Spacial relationship is unusual
6. Other ——

(d) VOICE PATTERNS

	L1	L2	D
	——	——	——

1. Appropriate
2. Harshness seems to be abnormal*
3. Breathiness seems to be abnormal
4. Loudness seems to be abnormal
5. Pitch seems to be abnormal
6. Other ——

FLUENCY PATTERNS

	L1	L2	D
	——	——	——

1. Appropriate
2. Speech very slow and uneven
3. Speech more hesitant and jerky than a native speaker of the same age
4. Abnormal number of repetitions, prolongations, or stoppages in speech pattern
5. Other ——

*Whenever the terms *unusual* or *abnormal* are noted, discuss in detail the reasons for the notations. These terms suggest that the utterance is inappropriate for the language/dialect being assessed.

Continued

423

TABLE C.1 *Continued*

(e) AUDITORY ACUITY: passed screening _____ failed screening _____

(f) AUDITORY COMPREHENSION

L1	L2	D
___	___	___
___	___	___
___	___	___
___	___	___
___	___	___

1. Understands everything in both formal and colloquial speech expected of a native speaker of the same age.
2. Understands everything in conversation except for colloquial speech.
3. Understands somewhat simplified speech directed to him, with some repetition and rephrasing.
4. Understands only slow, very simple speech on concrete topics; requires considerably more repetition and rephrasing than would be expected of a native speaker of the same age.
5. Understands too little for the simplest type of conversations.

MORPHOSYNTACTIC ANALYSIS (from language sample)

Note the client's normative (acquired English) or nonstandard grammatical patterns; also rate the client on the accompanying grammar scale.

1. Morphological Problems

L1	L2	D	
___	___	___	**a.** noun forms
___	___	___	**b.** adjective
___	___	___	**c.** verb forms
___	___	___	**d.** adverb

2. Syntactic Problems

L1	L2	D	
___	___	___	**a.** word order
___	___	___	**b.** questions
___	___	___	**c.** negation
___	___	___	**d.** prepositions
___	___	___	**e.** pronouns
___	___	___	**f.** subject-verb
___	___	___	**g.** present for future

3. Grammar Scale:

L1	L2	D
___	___	___
___	___	___
___	___	___
___	___	___
___	___	___

1. Normal standard English grammar.
2. Few errors, with no patterns of failure, but still lacking full control over grammar that is expected of that age.
3. Occasional errors showing imperfect control of some grammatical patterns but no weakness that causes misunderstanding.
4. Frequent errors showing lack of control of some major patterns and causing more misunderstanding than would be expected for a native speaker of that age level.
5. Grammar almost entirely inaccurate except in common phrases.

FOR THE CLASSROOM TEACHER
Please Check and Discuss Any Information of Relevance

Child's Name _____ Age _____ Sex _____

Address _____

Grade Level _____

School _____

Address _____

CHILD IS:

Nonnative English Speaker
1. Spanish-influenced English _____
2. Asian-influenced English _____
3. Other _____

Nonstandard English Speaker
4. African-influenced English _____
5. Appalachian-influenced English _____
6. Other _____

Discuss:

Intelligibility (Understandability) of the Child

Amount of Dialect/Language Differences Used by Child in the Classroom

Estimate the amount of dialect/language differences (from minimal or none to maximum) on following scales.

1 2 3 4 5	1 2 3 4 5	1 2 3 4 5	1 2 3 4 5	1 2 3 4 5	1 2 3 4 5
Phonology or Articulation Usage	Grammar	Vocabulary	Prosody or Speech Rhythm	Body Lang. or Use of Body When Talking	Over-all

USE OF LANGUAGE IN THE CLASSROOM

____ 1. Appropriate.
____ 2. Opening or closing a conversation is unusual.
____ 3. Turn taking during conversations is unusual.
____ 4. Interruptions are unusual.
____ 5. Silence as a communicative device is unusual.
____ 6. Laughter as a communicative device is unusual.
____ 7. Appropriate types of conversation are unusual.
____ 8. Humor (and knowing when to use it) is unusual.
____ 9. Nonverbal behavior that accompanies conversation is unusual.
____ 10. Logical ordering of events during discourse is unusual.
____ 11. Other:

AUDITORY COMPREHENSION IN THE CLASSROOM

____ 1. Understands everything in both formal and colloquial speech expected of a native speaker of the same age.
____ 2. Understands everything in conversation except for colloquial speech.
____ 3. Understands somewhat simplified speech directed to him, with some repetition and rephrasing.
____ 4. Understands only slow, very simple speech on concrete topics; requires considerably more repetition and rephrasing than would be expected of a native speaker of the same age.
____ 5. Understands too little for the simplest type of conversations.

Source: Adler, S. (1991). Assessment of language proficiency in limited English proficient speakers: Implications for the speech-language pathologist. *Language, Speech, and Hearing Services in Schools, 22,* 12–18. Reprinted with permission.

TABLE C.2   The Adolescent Pragmatics Screening Scale (APSS)

Student information:

Name _____ Age _____ Grade _____ School _____ Date _____

1. Indicate the student's first language background. _____
2. Indicate the student's home language background if different from first language. _____
3. Indicate the student's English language proficiency level from 1 to 5 (1 = native-like, 2 = near native-like, 3 = medium, 4 = limited, 5 = very limited). _____
4. Indicate the student's cultural/ethnic background (e.g., Euro-American, African American, Hispanic, Asian American, Native American). _____
5. Indicate the number of years the student has been in schools in the United States. _____

Teacher/Rater information:

6. Indicate your professional background (speech-language pathologist, bilingual teacher, ESL teacher, regular education teacher, special education teacher, special education-classroom, psychologist). _____
7. Indicate your first language background. _____
8. Indicate your proficiency level from 1 to 5 in English (1 = native-like, 2 = near native-like, 3 = medium, 4 = limited, 5 = very limited). _____
9. Are you proficient in another language other than English? (Yes/No) _____
10. If yes, indicate what language. _____
11. Indicate your proficiency level from 1 to 5 in your other language (1 = native-like, 2 = near native-like, 3 = medium, 4 = limited, 5 = very limited). _____
12. Are you culturally knowledgeable or aware about another culture? _____
13. Indicate your cultural knowledge/awareness level of the other culture from 1 to 5 (1 = native-like, 2 = near native-like, 3 = medium, 4 = limited, 5 = very limited). _____
14. Indicate which culture or cultures. _____

Test score information:

Scoring: Mean Topic Scores (M.T.S.)

Topic 1   Sum of the individual behaviors _____ divided by 11 = _____ No. 1.
                                        M.T.S.
Topic 2   Sum of the individual behaviors _____ divided by 7 = _____ No. 2.
                                        M.T.S.
Topic 3   Sum of the individual behaviors _____ divided by 4 = _____ No. 3.
                                        M.T.S.
Topic 4   Sum of the individual behaviors _____ divided by 6 = _____ No. 4.
                                        M.T.S.
Topic 5   Sum of the individual behaviors _____ divided by 7 = _____ No. 5.
                                        M.T.S.
Topic 6   Sum of the individual behaviors _____ divided by 3 = _____ No. 6.
                                        M.T.S.

Sum of ALL the individual behaviors _____

Sum of ALL the individual behaviors _____ divided by 38 = _____ **Total Score (T.S.)**

15. Do you feel that this student's performance was influenced by the student's cultural background? _____ Yes _____ No

If the answer is **yes,** please indicate which behaviors led you to this conclusion by making a notation in the **Observation** section next to the corresponding behavior.

A. Performance Rating Scale

Please indicate the student's level of performance using the scale below.

1. Behavior is highly appropriate.
2. Behavior is moderately appropriate.
3. Behavior is borderline appropriate.
4. Behavior is moderately inappropriate.
5. Behavior is highly inappropriate.

B. Observations

This section is reserved for observations that you feel are pertinent to your rating.

	SCORE	OBSERVATIONS
1. Affects listener's behavior through language		
1. Asks for help (e.g., "I don't know how to do this problem" "Can you show me how to look up a word in the dictionary?" "How do you spell _____ ?")	**1.** _____	
2. Asks questions (e.g., "How many times does 9 go into 72?" "How does a president get elected?")	**2.** _____	
3. Attempts to persuade others (e.g., "I really think John is the best candidate because _____." "I don't think I should have to do this because _____.")	**3.** _____	
4. Informs another of important information (e.g., "Teacher, someone wrote some bad words on the wall outside." "I saw a snake in the boy's bathroom down the hall.")	**4.** _____	
5. Asks for a favor of a friend/classmate (e.g., "Can you give me a ride to school?" "Will you ask Sally out for Friday night for me?")	**5.** _____	
6. Asks for a favor of the teacher (e.g., "Can I redo the homework assignment?" "Can I get out of class 5 minutes early so I can catch the new bus?")	**6.** _____	
7. Asks for teachers' and/or adults' permission (e.g., going to the bathroom, asking to get a drink of water, asking to sharpen a pencil)	**7.** _____	
8. Asks for other student's permission (e.g., "Can I invite John to go with us?" "Can I ask your girlfriend for her phone number?")	**8.** _____	
9. Able to negotiate, give and take, in order to reach an agreement ("I'll give you a ride to school if you pay me five dollars a week for gas." "I'll help you with your algebra homework if you help me paint the signs for homecoming.")	**9.** _____	
10. Is able to give simple directions (e.g., telling how to find the Spanish teacher's classroom or how to find the bathroom)	**10.** _____	
11. Rephrases a statement (e.g., "You meant this, didn't you?" "Did you mean this _____?")	**11.** _____	

_____ **Topic 1. Sum of Scores**

	SCORE	OBSERVATIONS
2. Expresses self		
1. Describes personal feelings in an acceptable manner (e.g., says, "I wish that this English class wasn't so boring." "I'm feeling really frustrated by all the setbacks on my homework.")	**1.** _____	

Continued

TABLE C.2 *Continued*

	SCORE	OBSERVATIONS
2. Shows feelings in acceptable manner (e.g., taking audible breaths to contain one's anger or smiling with enthusiasm to show pleasure)	**2.** _____	
3. Offers a contrary opinion in class discussions (e.g., "I don't believe that Columbus was the first to discover America. Leif Ericson was said to have reached Greenland and Nova Scotia before Columbus." "I don't believe that the two-party system really offers a choice to voters.")	**3.** _____	
4. Gives logical reasons for opinions (e.g., "I believe that the two-party system offers a wider choice than the one-party system _____." "I think we should work on something else. We did something like this yesterday.")	**4.** _____	
5. Says that they disagree in a conversation (e.g., "I don't agree with you." "We can't agree on this one.")	**5.** _____	
6. Stays on topic for an appropriate amount of time	**6.** _____	
7. Switches response to another mode to suit the listener (e.g., speaks differently when addressing the principal than when addressing a friend; speaks differently to a younger child of 2–3 years than when addressing peers of the same age)	**7.** _____	

_____ **Topic 2. Sum of Scores**

3. Establishes appropriate greetings

	SCORE	OBSERVATIONS
1. Establishes eye contact when saying hello or greeting	**1.** _____	
2. Smiles when meeting friends	**2.** _____	
3. Responds to an introduction by other similar greeting	**3.** _____	
4. Introduces self to others ("Hi, I'm_____" "My name is_____, what's yours?")	**4.** _____	

_____ **Topic 3. Sum of Scores**

4. Initiates and maintains conversation

	SCORE	OBSERVATIONS
1. Displays appropriate response time	**1.** _____	
2. Asks for more time (e.g., "I'm still thinking." "Wait a second." "Give me some more time.")	**2.** _____	
3. Notes that the listener is not following the conversation and needs clarification or more information (e.g., "There's a thing down there, down there, I mean there's a snake down in the boy's bathroom down the hall.")	**3.** _____	
4. Talks to others with appropriate pitch and loudness levels of voice (e.g., uses appropriate levels for the classroom, physical education, the lunchroom, or after school)	**4.** _____	
5. Answers questions relevantly (e.g., "Nine goes into 72 8 times." "The President gets elected by the people.")	**5.** _____	
6. Waits for appropriate pauses in conversation before speaking.	**6.** _____	

_____ **Topic 4. Sum of Scores**

	SCORE	OBSERVATIONS

5. Listens actively

1. Asks to repeat what has been said for better understanding (e.g., "Could you say that again?" "What do you mean?")   1. _____

2. Looks at teacher when addressed (e.g., through occasional glances or maintained eye contact)   2. _____

3. Listens to others in class (e.g., head is up, leaning toward the speaker, eyes on the speaker)   3. _____

4. Changes activities when asked by the teacher (e.g., is able to put away his or her paper and pencil or close a book or pull out something different without having to be told personally)   4. _____

5. Acknowledges the speaker verbally (e.g., Says "Uh-huh, yeah, what else?")   5. _____

6. Acknowledges the speaker nonverbally (e.g., looks at the speaker through occasional glances, maintains eye contact, or nodding)   6. _____

7. Differentiates between literal and figurative language (e.g., knows that the expression "John is sharp as a tack" actually means that John is very smart, or that if "Sally's leg is killing her," it does not mean that Sally will die)   7. _____

_____ **Topic 5. Sum of Scores**

6. Cues the listener regarding topic shifts

1. Waits for a pause in the conversation before speaking about something else (waits for a pause of approximately 3–5 seconds at the end of a thought or sentence)   1. _____

2. Looks away to indicate loss of interest in conversation (looks away and maintains this look for approximately 3–5 seconds)   2. _____

3. Makes easy transitions between topics (e.g., the listener does not question what they are talking about)   3. _____

_____ **Topic 6. Sum of Scores**

Source: Brice, A., & Montgomery, J. (1996). Adolescent pragmatic skills: A comparison of Latino students in English as a second language and speech and language programs. *Language, Speech, and Hearing Services in Schools, 27,* 68–81. Reprinted with permission.

APPENDIX **D**

Language Analysis
Methods

Assigning Structural Stage/Complex Sentence Development

In Assigning Structural Stage, Miller (J. Miller, 1981) proposes a three-tiered analysis that includes MLU, percentage correct of Brown's 14 morphemes, and sentence analysis. These three measures enable the SLP to determine the stage of development and to describe the forms used. Although less precise than Developmental Sentence Scoring (DSS) (L. Lee, 1974), Assigning Structural Stage is more descriptive and prescriptive in nature. After determining the child's stage of language development, the SLP can target linguistic forms in the next stage (Prutting, 1979).

Analysis begins by collecting a language sample. The SLP collects 50 to 100 utterances or 15 minutes of conversation, whichever is larger, from the child for analysis. Unlike for DSS, these utterances do not have to be sentences. First, the SLP calculates MLU to determine the stage of development and the approximate language age of the child. MLU calculation is discussed in Chapter 7.

After determining MLU, the SLP decides on the analysis method to follow. He or she may choose Assigning Structural Stage and/or Complex Sentence Development. If the MLU of the child is below 3.0, the SLP uses only Assigning Structural Stage. If the child's MLU is above 4.5, the SLP uses only Complex Sentence Development. For MLUs of 3.0 to 4.5, the SLP uses both procedures.

In Assigning Structural Stage, the SLP calculates the percentage correct for Brown's 14 morphemes. A minimum number of occurrences or possibilities of occurrence are needed before the SLP can decide on consistency or inconsistency of use or nonuse. The child should attempt a morpheme at least four times before a percentage correct figure is calculated.

The percentage correct value is determined by dividing the number of correct appearances by the total number of obligatory contexts. After calculating the percentage correct, the SLP again can attempt to describe the child's stage of language development.

Next, the SLP analyzes each utterance within four possible categories of noun phrase, verb phrase, and negative and interrogative development. Utterances are divided into noun and verb phrases where applicable, and each phrase is assigned to the stage of development that best describes its structures. Negative or interrogative utterances are further assigned to stages representing their level of development.

The SLP should be familiar with the information Miller (1981) presents for each stage of development. Some of this information is presented in Table 7.16, although Miller presents a great deal more. The analysis process is demonstrated here by using some of the information in Table 7.16. Consider the child's utterance, "Want a big doggie." The noun phrase *a big doggie* has been expanded by the addition of an article and an adjective to the noun. This noun phrase occurs in the object position of the sentence. Expansion of the noun phrase only in the object position is an example of Stage II (see intrasentence column of Table 7.16). Therefore, this sentence represents noun phrase development characteristic of Stage II. The verb phrase is unelaborated, and no subject is present. This represents Stage I development.

Complex Sentence Development is used similarly, but different samples and categories are used for analysis. Analysis is based on a 15-minute sample of the child's communication, rather than on 50 utterances. For children with MLUs between 3.0 and 4.5, these samples can overlap. Five aspects of complex sentences are noted: percentage of both conjoined and embedded sentences within the sample, type of embedding, conjoining, conjunctions, and the number of different conjunctions. At each stage, development is described by the forms exhibited by 50 to 90 percent and by greater than 90 percent of the children.

Limited data from Complex Sentence Development are incorporated into Table 7.16. By post-Stage V, 90 percent of children should be using *and* within a 15-minute sample. To complete a full analysis, the SLP should consult Complex Sentence Development (J. Miller, 1981).

Each sentence is analyzed by using Assigning Structural Stage and/or Complex Sentence Development, and the data are summarized. Most likely, the child will exhibit language forms in each stage of development. Now, the SLP must use his or her skill.

Even mature language users occasionally use language forms that are characteristic of less mature learning. Adults use many one-word utterances everyday. These forms are not the most characteristic forms, however, and the SLP must gather a summary of overall language form to determine most accurately the user's abilities. It is the same with the child with language impairment. The SLP determines those behaviors that are most characteristic of the child. These might be behaviors at a particular stage that the child uses most frequently or behaviors that represent the highest attainment level. The SLP must make this determination.

All data from the two analysis methods—Assigning Structural Stage and Complex Sentence Development—are combined to place the child's language form within a stage or stages of development and to describe the child's language form. The child functioning well below age expectancy may need intervention.

Developmental Sentence Scoring

Developmental Sentence Scoring, the process discussed in *Developmental Sentence Analysis* (L. Lee, 1974), is one of the most widely used and popular methods for assessing children's syntactic and morphological development. Even so, DSS requires considerable study by the SLP to score language samples correctly. Although the instructions are explicit and straightforward, they require a thorough understanding of English syntax and morphology. Because the scale does not evaluate many aspects of children's language, it should be only one aspect of an evaluation battery.

TABLE D.1   Developmental sentence scoring categories and point values

Score	Indefinite Pronouns or Noun Modifiers	Personal Pronouns	Main Verbs	Secondary Verbs
1	it, this, that	1st and 2nd person: I, me, my, mine, you, your(s)	**A.** Uninflected verb: I *see* you. **B.** Copula, is or 's: *It's* red. **C.** is + verb + ing: He *is coming*.	
2		3rd person: he, him, his, she, her, hers	**A.** -s and -ed: *plays, played* **B.** Irregular past: *ate, saw* **C.** Copula: *am, are, was, were* **D.** Auxiliary: *am, are, was, were*	Five early-developing infinitives: I wan*na see* (want *to see*) I'm gon*na see* (going *to see*) I got*ta see* (got *to see*) Lem*me [to] see* (let me [*to*] *see*) Let's [*to*] *play* (let us [*to*] *play*)
3	**A.** no, some, more, all, lot(s), one(s), two (etc.), other(s), another **B.** something, somebody, someone	**A.** Plurals: we, us, our(s), they, them, their **B.** these, those		Noncomplementing infinitives: I stopped *to play.* I'm afraid *to look.* It's hard *to do that.*
4	nothing, nobody, none, no one		**A.** can, will, may + verb: *may go* **B.** Obligatory do + verb: *don't go* **C.** Emphatic do + verb: I *do see.*	Participle, present or past: I see a boy *running.* I found the toy *broken.*

In the following section I discuss the primary aspects of DSS and its most common problems. This survey cannot take the place of a thorough reading of DSS procedures and actual practice with the instrument.

To rate a sample of child language, the SLP collects 50 different consecutive *sentences.* No speaker uses full sentences all the time. Therefore, utterances that do not qualify as sentences simply are omitted, and the remainder is collected until 50 consecutive sentences are amassed. DSS analysis should not be undertaken if less than 50 percent of the child's utterances are sentences.

Because the sample should include 50 different consecutive sentences, repeated sentences are discarded unless some change occurs. Run-on sentences of several independent clauses joined by *and* are segmented so that no more than two independent clauses are joined. For example, the following run-on should be divided as noted:

[We went to the zoo, and I saw monkeys,] [(and) we had a picnic, and I ate a hot dog,] [(and) I fed pigeons, and we came home on the bus.]

Score	Negatives	Conjunctions	Interrogative Reversals	Wh-Questions
1	it, this, that + copula or auxiliary is, 's, + not: It's *not* mine. This is *not* a dog. That *is not* moving.		Reversal of copula: *Isn't it* red? *Were they* there?	
2				**A.** who, what, what + noun: *Who* am I? *What is* he eating? *What book* are you reading? **B.** where, how many, how much, what…do, what…for: *Where* did it go? *How much* do you want? *What* is he *doing*? What is a hammer *for*?
3		and		
4	can't, don't		Reversal of auxiliary be: *Is he* coming? *Isn't he* coming? *Was he* going? *Wasn't he* going?	

Continued

The *and* at the beginning of each sentence ("[*and*] we had…, [*and*] I fed…") would not be scored. A sentence may have more than one *and* if the word does not link clauses, but rather is used for compound subjects, verbs, or objects, for example:

Jorge, Maria, *and* Shanisa were throwing *and* kicking beach balls *and* soccer balls.

Sentences that begin with a conjunction, such as "Because I fell down," are included in the sample, but the conjunction itself should not be scored because it does not link clauses.

Each sentence is rated on the basis of eight grammatical categories and assigned a score of 1 to 8 points in the applicable categories. The categories and point values are given in Table D.1. Each structure demonstrated in the sentence is scored each time it occurs. For example, sentence 1 in Table D.2, "I don't know what I like," contains the word *I* twice. Therefore, the word receives a score of 1 twice under personal pronouns, in addition to other points.

TABLE D.1 *Continued*

Score	Indefinite Pronouns or Noun Modifiers	Personal Pronouns	Main Verbs	Secondary Verbs
5		Reflexives: myself, yourself, himself, herself, itself, themselves		**A.** Early infinitival complements with differing subjects in kernels: I want you *to come.* Let him [*to*] *see.* **B.** Later infinitival complements: I had *to go.* I told him *to go.* I tried *to go.* He ought *to go.* **C.** Obligatory deletions: Make it [*to*] *go.* I'd better [*to*] *go.* **D.** Infinitive with wh-word: I know what *to get.* I know how *to do* it.
6		**A.** Wh- pronouns: who, which, whose, whom, what, that, how many, how much: I know *who* came. That's *what* I said. **B.** Wh- word + infinitive: I know *what* to do. I know *who*(*m*) to take.	**A.** could, would, should, might + verb: *might come, could be* **B.** Obligatory does, did + verb **C.** Emphatic does, did + verb	

Sentences that would be acceptable mature forms are given an additional point called a *sentence point.* The sentence point should only be awarded when the sentence is syntactically and semantically correct by mature standards. The following would not receive a sentence point:

Carol and me went to the store.
Nobody didn't go.
I got six pencils in my desk.

In Table D.2, sentence 2, "What you like?" receives a score of 4; it does not receive a sentence point because it is not an acceptable mature sentence. Sentence 3, "I don't know," does receive the sentence point.

Attempt markers and incomplete markers may be awarded for structures. An *attempt marker*— a line or hyphen in place of a score—is awarded when a structure is attempted but incorrect. Naturally, as in sentence 4, "He bes happy," the sentence cannot receive a sentence point. Surface struc-

Score	Negatives	Conjunctions	Interrogative Reversals	Wh-Questions
5	isn't, won't	**A.** but **B.** so, and so, so that **C.** or, if		when, how, how + adjective: *When* shall I come? *How* do you do it? *How big* is it?
6		because	**A.** Obligatory do, does, did: *Do they* run? *Does it* bite? *Didn't it* hurt? **B.** Reversal of modal: *Can you* play? *Won't it* hurt? *Shall I* sit down? **C.** Tag question: It's fun, *isn't it*? It isn't fun, *is it*?	

Continued

tures that are conversationally appropriate but incomplete receive the incomplete marker *inc* in place of a score. If the structure is conversationally acceptable, it receives a sentence point. For example, in the following exchange, the child's response would receive an incomplete for the main verb, but would receive a sentence point.

SLP: Who let the guinea pig out?

Child: I didn't. (I didn't [let him out].)

Attempt and incomplete markers are difficult to use and confusing for those not familiar with DSS. They do not affect the score and are meant to aid the SLP in deciding where to begin intervention. This decision can be made on the basis of other data.

    The point value of each sentence is totaled and added to the value for every other sentence. This overall total is divided by the number of sentences (usually 50) to yield a score. The SLP must remember that this value is a DSS score, not an MLU. The two values are very different.

TABLE D.1   *Continued*

Score	Indefinite Pronouns or Noun Modifiers	Personal Pronouns	Main Verbs	Secondary Verbs
7	**A.** any, anything, anybody, anyone **B.** every, everything, everybody, everyone **C.** both, few, many, each, several, most, least, much, next, first, last, second (etc.)	(his) own, one, oneself, whichever, whoever, whatever Take *whatever* you like.	**A.** Passive with *get,* any tense Passive with *be,* any tense **B.** must, shall + verb: *must come* **C.** have + verb + en: *I've eaten* **D.** have got: *I've got* it.	Passive infinitival complement: With *get:* I have *to get dressed.* I don't want to *get hurt.* With *be:* I want *to be pulled.* It's going *to be locked.*
8			**A.** have been + verb + ing had been + verb + ing **B.** modal + have + verb + -en: *may have eaten* **C.** modal + be + verb + -ing: *could be playing* **D.** Other auxiliary combinations: *should have been sleeping*	Gerund: *Swinging* is fun. I like *fishing.* He started *laughing.*

The SLP then applies the DSS score to a table of ages and scores to compare the child's performance with that of other children at that age. Figure D.1 shows the average scores (50th percentile) for each age and the scores for the 10th, 25th, 75th, and 90th percentiles. For example, an average score for a 4-year-old would be approximately 7.3. Only the highest 10 percent of 4-year-olds would receive a score of 9.0 (90th percentile).

According to the instructions, children whose scores place them below the 10th percentile should be considered for therapy. Therefore, a 4-year-old who scores below 4.7 should be considered for therapy.

Score	Negatives	Conjunctions	Interrogative Reversals	Wh Questions
7	All other negatives **A.** Uncontracted negatives: I can *not* go. He has *not* gone. **B.** Pronoun-auxiliary or pronoun-copula contraction: I'm *not* coming. He's *not* here. **C.** Auxiliary-negative or copula-negative contraction: He *wasn't* going. He *hasn't* been seen. It *couldn't* be mine. They *aren't* big.			why, what if, how come, how about + gerund: *Why* are you crying? *What if* I won't do it? *How come* he is crying? *How about* coming with me?
8		**A.** where, when, how, while, whether (or not), till, until, unless, since, before, after, for, as, as + adjective + as, as if, like, that, than: I know *where* you are. Don't come *till* I call. **B.** Obligatory deletions: I run faster *than* you [run]. I'm *as big as* a man [is big]. It looks *like* a dog [looks]. **C.** Elliptical deletions (score 0): That's *why* [I took it]. I know *how.* [*I can do it*]. **D.** Wh- words + infinitive: I know how to do it.	**A.** Reversal of auxiliary have: *Has he* seen you? **B.** Reversal with two or three auxiliaries: *Has he been* eating? *Couldn't he have* waited? *Could he have been* crying? *Wouldn't he have been* going?	whose, which, which + noun: *Whose* cat is that? *Which book* do you want?

An age equivalent for the child placing below the 10th percentile can be determined by noting the point at which the horizontal line for the child's score crosses the diagonal 50th-percentile line. At this age, the child's score is an average score. For example, the child aged 5½ who receives an average score of 5.0 points is well below the 10th percentile for that age and needs intervention. The age equivalent would be found by following the 5.0 line to the left until it intersects the diagonal 50th-percentile line. This occurs at an age of 3 years. Thus, the child has received a score that would be expected at approximately 3 years of age.

TABLE D.2 Language sample analysis using developmental sentence scoring

Developmental sentence scoring form

Name:
D.O.B.:
D.O.K.:
C.A.:
Score:

Sentence	Indefinite Pronouns	Personal Pronouns	Main Verbs	Secondary Verbs	Negatives	Conjunctions	Interrogative Reversals	Wh-Questions	Sentence Point	Total
I don't know what I like.		1,1,6	4,1		4				1	18
What you like?		1	1					2		4
I don't know.		1	4		4				1	10
He bes happy.		2	inc							2
I want to go home.		1	1	2					1	5
What's that?			1				1	2	1	5
I can't go now.		1	4		4				1	10

438

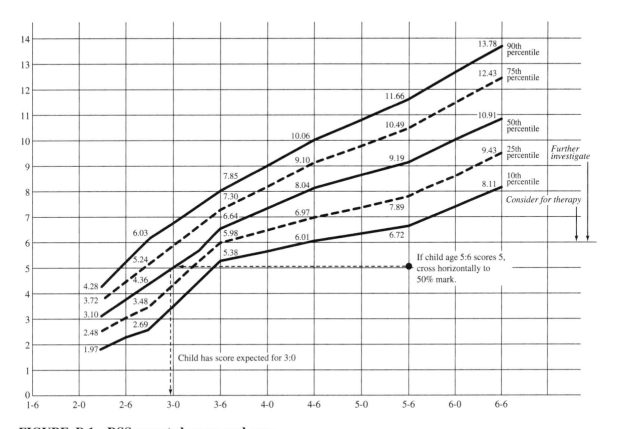

FIGURE D.1   DSS expected scores and ages.

Source: Lee, L. (1974). *Developmental sentence analysis.* Evanston, IL: Northwestern University Press. Reprinted with permission.

Age equivalence, if needed, can be found in the same way for children, such as those with mental retardation, who may exceed the age-norm ceiling of 6½ years. Obviously, the percentile values are not relevant.

Language delay in years can be determined by subtracting the age equivalent from the child's chronological age. In the previous example, the child's language delay is approximately 2½ years. Although this value means little for the direction of therapy, it does provide a score for those people, such as administrators, who demand such data, and it can be used as an index of change over time. The same precautions for such statistics given in Chapter 3 apply.

The most common problems encountered with DSS are associated with determination of grammatical units and with scoring (Lively, 1984). These problems are discussed briefly in the following section. Readers can refer to Lively (1984) and Hughes, Fey, and Long (1992) for a more thorough discussion.

Scoring Adverbs as Indefinite Pronouns/Noun Modifiers.   Words such as *first, last,* and *everywhere* that tell the manner or place of an action are adverbs ("Let's do this *first*") and should not be scored as indefinite pronoun/noun modifiers. In contrast, other words, especially numbers, should be scored when they do function as indefinite pronoun/noun modifiers, as in the following:

Can I have *one*?
I have *two* dolls.
No one don't like me.

Personal Pronoun/*wh*- Conjunction/*wh*- Question Confusion.   *Wh*- words may be used as personal pronouns (score 6) or as conjunctions (score 8). The distinction can be clarified by remembering that a complete clause will follow the conjunction.

I want the one *that* talks.	(Pronoun, because "talks" is not a complete clause)
He told us *that* we could shovel his driveway.	(Conjunction, because "we could shovel his driveway" is a complete clause)
I know *what* you want.	(Pronoun, because "you want" is not a complete clause)
What do you want?	(Wh- question)

Main Verbs.   All uninflected or unmarked verbs receive a score of 1. Regular and irregular inflected verbs receive some other score.

I *like* ice cream.	(Uninflected = 1)
She *likes* ice cream.	(Inflected = 2)
She *ate* ice cream.	(Inflected = 2)

Incorrect attempts, such as using *got* for *have*, receive an attempt score. The verb *do* as a main verb receives a 1 or 2. As an auxiliary, it receives a 4 if uninflected and a 6 if inflected. The modal auxiliary verbs *can, will*, and *may* are scored in the same manner.

Do it for me.	(Uninflected main verb = 1)
I *did* my homework.	(Inflected main verb = 2)
I *do* like ice cream.	(Uninflected auxiliary = 4)
I *did* like ice cream.	(Inflected auxiliary = 6)
He *does* like ice cream.	(Inflected auxiliary = 6)
I *can* swim.	(Uninflected modal = 4)
I *could* swim.	(Inflected modal = 6)

In contrast, the modal auxiliaries *must* and *shall* are always scored as 7. The perfect tense forms of *have* + *verb* (*-en*) also receive a 7. All sentences with two or more auxiliaries, as in "He could have gone," receive an 8.

Passive sentences present a special case, and SLPs should refer to L. Lee (1974).

Compound sentences can be very difficult, especially if material is omitted. With compound verbs, each is scored. If the auxiliary is omitted, both verbs still should receive the full score.

I *was singing* and *dancing.*	(The second "was" is omitted and understood, so each verb receives a score of 2.)

If, on the other hand, the main verb is omitted, only the complete form is scored and the other abbreviated or elliptical form receives an incomplete score.

I *did* complete my lesson, but Carol *didn't.*	(The second "did" receives an incomplete score, whereas the first received a 6.)

Secondary Verbs. The chief error in this category is in identifying the infinitive. Often the signal word *to* is omitted. If the child uses *gonna, wanna, gotta, lemme,* or *let's,* the infinitive is scored as 2. Other infinitives receive a 5 if the subject of the infinitive is different from the subject of the main verb.

I wanna go.	(Score as 2)
I want to go.	(Score as 2)
I want her to go.	(Different subjects = 5)
Make the car (to) go.	(The subject is understood to be "you," and car is "to go," so score the infinitive as 5.)

The form *be + verb(-en)* in the present tense is scored as copula plus adjective unless the agentive prepositional is explicit. In the past form *was/were + verb(-en),* it is scored as passive as long as it makes sense when the agentive phrase is added.

The door is broken.	(Score as 1)
The glass is broken by the cat.	(Score as 7)
The glass was broken (by the cat).	(Score as 7)
The girl was lost.	(Score as 2)

Negatives. The only negative to receive a score of 1 is the *this/that/it + is/'s not* form. All other forms of this combination receive a higher score. Any other subject or auxiliary verb receives a score of 7.

It is not yours.	("It is not" = 1)
It's not yours.	("It's not" = 1)
It isn't yours.	("It isn't" = 5)
You *can't* do it.	("Can't" = 7)

Conjunctions. Score the conjunction *then* as 3 for *and then,* even though the *and* is omitted, as long as two independent clauses are joined.

Interrogative Reversals. SLPs often overlook interrogative reversals when scoring *wh-* questions. Tag questions, except those ending in *huh, okay, eh,* and the like, receive a score of 6.

Sentence Point.   If the child *has been interrupted* in mid-sentence but has produced the subject and the predicate of the sentence and this stem is grammatically acceptable, the partial sentence should be scored and given a sentence point.

Obviously, Developmental Sentence Scoring is a very complex analysis system, not to be attempted without a thorough knowledge of both English syntax and DSS procedures. Unfortunately, the child's score offers little direction for intervention, although Lee suggests appropriate places at which to begin intervention based primarily on the percentage of correct production. The hierarchy presented in Table D.1 offers only limited guidance and omits many important structures. This type of problem seems inherent in any analysis system that reduces complex behavior to point values.

Modification for CLD Children

The nature of the DSS makes it an inappropriate tool to use for assessing the language abilities of CLD children. Some advances have been made in this area. Black English Sentence Scoring (BESS) is a promising attempt to maintain the DSS format while measuring African American English usage. The scoring criteria, a sample scoring, and means and standard deviations are listed in Tables D.3, D.4, and D.5 respectively.

Summary

DSS is a good quantitative measure, although no data are available on the relationship of DSS scores to the type and extent of a child's LI (Hughes et al., 1992). Even when matched with peers on the basis of MLU, children with LI tend to have more difficulty with the main verb and pronoun categories and may have difficulty with secondary verbs, negatives, and conjunctions. DSS has shown great resiliency and has been modified for speakers of Black English, expanded to 6- to 10-year-olds, and converted to a computerized version (Hughes, Low, Fey, & Alsop, 1990; Long & Fey, 1991; N. Nelson & Hyter, 1990; Stephens, Dallman, & Montgomery, 1988).

Language Assessment, Remediation, and Screening Procedure (LARSP)

The Language Assessment, Remediation, and Screening Procedure (LARSP) (Crystal et al., 1976) is used more widely in England, Canada, and Australia than in the United States. More psycholinguistic in nature than the other methods included in this appendix, LARSP analyzes language on the basis of phrase and sentence structure and on the number of elements found in the child's utterances. These values relate to seven stages of language development, mostly in the preschool years.

The SLP collects 30 minutes of the child's speech from two different 15-minute activities. In the first, the child plays with a familiar adult; in the second, the child and the adult participate in a dialogue.

All utterances are included in the analysis, describing what the child can or cannot do. Therefore, all utterances are transcribed with intonations and pauses indicated. Important nonlinguistic information is included to aid analysis. The SLP uses the following markers when transcribing:

( )	Parentheses, placed around unintelligible speech, may be left blank, may signal the possible number of syllables, or may guess at the unintelligible portion by placing words within.

?	A question mark is placed before any word for which the transcriptional accuracy is in doubt. This occurs when two listeners disagree.
*	Asterisks are placed around speakers' words that overlap.
(())	Double parentheses are placed around interjections or repairs that do not disturb the flow of communication.

Analysis is accomplished on a worksheet and transferred to the Profile Chart shown in Table D.6. First, synchronic analysis is accomplished in Sections A, B, and C. In-depth analysis is accomplished by using the developmental stage portion of the chart. The authors recommend that the total analysis be completed by using eight separate scans of the transcript.

In Scan 1, the SLP removes for later analysis all utterances that cannot be analyzed. These are of two types: unanalyzed and problematic. Unanalyzed utterances may be wholly unintelligible, may consist of symbolic noise, such as truck or airplane sounds, or may be *deviant* sentences. Deviant sentences are utterances that are structurally inadmissible in adult grammar and are not part of the expected grammatical development of children developing normally. Problematic utterances include incomplete sentences that do not represent expected grammatical development, and ambiguous sentences that may be interpreted in two different ways on the basis of the communication situation. The number of utterances within each category is tallied and placed in Section A of the Profile Chart. With these utterances identified, the subsequent scans are less problematic.

Scan 2, recorded in Sections B and C, establishes the proportion of spontaneous to responsive utterances and analyzes the type of each. The type of response depends on the type of stimulus sentence. LARSP distinguishes between question stimuli and others.

Normal responses may be classified as *elliptical major sentences,* in which shared information is omitted; *full major sentences;* or *minor sentences* consisting of single word answers, such as *yes/no.* In addition, elliptical sentences are rated by the number of elements included in each. Abnormal responses may demonstrate either structural deviance, in which a mismatch occurs between the expected structural pattern of the response and the one produced, or *zero response,* in which a response is expected but not received. Other responses are classified as *repetitions* of the other speaker or *problems.* The problems category is an *other* category for those utterances that do not fit anywhere else. The number of each type of response is recorded in Section B in the type of response column and in the stimulus row.

Spontaneous utterances are divided into *novel* sentences and *full self-repetitions.* The number of utterances within each category is recorded in the appropriate space on the Profile Chart.

Scan 3 is for sentence connectivity. Each type is tabulated and counted. The four types include *intonation,* in which emphasis or stress indicates old or contrasting information; *vocabulary replacement,* in which a word other than a pronoun replaces the old information; *commonsense semantic connection,* in which sequencing provides connectivity; and *grammatical links,* such as adverbs, cross-referenced articles and pronouns, and ellipses.

Scans 4 through 7 are more grammatical in nature and include coordination and subordination, clause structure, phrase structure, and word structure, respectively. Scans 5, 6, and 7 provide the most information on structure. Information regarding the number of each type of structure is recorded under the most appropriate stage next to the structures listed. Clausal and phrasal structure coding is listed in Table D.7. The stages represent seven theoretical levels of development of syntax and should not be confused with Brown's stages of development. Approximate ages for each stage are given in Table D.8. Crystal et al. (1976) provide descriptions and examples of each stage.

TABLE D.3   Black English sentence scoring categories and point values

	Indefinite Pronouns or Noun Modifiers	Personal Pronouns	Main Verbs	Secondary Verbs
1	• these/this: *these* many	• mine's/my, you/your: That *you* book? • y'all (plural *you*) • me/I (in compound subj.): Me and my brother went in it.	• Ø copula is, am, are: That boy my friend. Or hypercorrect: *I'm is* six. • Ø aux. be + -ing: The girl singin'. • Locational go or existential it's: Here *go* some lights. *It's* two dimes stuck on the table. • *got* as uninflected have: You gotta take it home.	
2		• he, she (in apposition): My brother, *he* bigger than you. • they/he: They my uncle. • he, he's/his: He's name is Terry. • she, she's/her	• Third-person singular and regular past tense markers deleted • have/has: It *have* money on it. • Regularization of -s and -ed: Trudy and my sister hide*s*. (hypercorrect) • Aux. was/were: We *was gon'* rob some money. • Irreg. past tense–Uninflected: He *find* the money. Past form as participle: We *have went*. Participle as past form: He *done* it first.	• *I'm, I'mon, I'ma* pronunciation of I'm gonna + V: *I'm* play. *I'ma* be tired. • *go* pronunciation of gonna: His nose go bleed. • fixin' to (used like gonna): I'm *fixin' to* take him to jail.
3	• *no* (when 2nd or 3rd neg. marker): He don't like me *no* more.	• we, they (in apposition): The boys, *they* got in trouble. • they/their: *They* name is Tanya and Bryan. • them/they or their: I know what *them* is. One of *'em* name is Caesar. • them/those: *them* kids		

	Negatives	Conjunctions	Interrogative Reversal	Wh- Questions
1	• it, this, that + Ø copula/ aux. + not/ain't: That *not* mine. It *ain't* on?		• rising intonation with deleted or unreversed copula: You my friend? Where the gas at? What this is? • is/are: Derrick, is you?	
2				• who, what, what + noun (with deleted aux. or copula) • where, how many, how much, what… do, what…for (with deleted aux. or copula): Where the man? • wh- Qs formed without interrogative reversal: What that is?
3		• and plus • Ø and (when intonation makes sentence combination clear): He pointed his finger at him (with rising intonation); he pointed his finger at him (with falling intonation).		

Continued

TABLE D.3   *Continued*

Indefinite Pronouns or Noun Modifiers	Personal Pronouns	Main Verbs	Secondary Verbs
4 • nothing, nobody, none, no one (when 2nd or 3rd neg. marker): Ain't *nobody* got *none*.		• Ø modal will or 'll: I be five when my birthday come. • don't + verb (3rd pers. sing.): My mama, she don't like it. • do uninflected: *Do* he still have it? (Score inc. in My sister *do*.) • Ø do in Qs: You still have it? • ain't (as copula or aux.): *Ain't* no dirt in it. Nobody *ain't* got no more. • can't, don't, won't as preposed neg. aux.: *Can't nobody* do it. • could/can: He *could* climb that tree.	• Participal with deleted -en: I found the toy broke. (morphological difference)
5	• personal datives me, him, her: I'm gonna buy *me* some candy. He make *him* a lot of 'em. • reflexives: hisself, theirselves, themself, theyselves.		• deleted to in infinitival complements: My grandma tell me stay away from him. I like go shopping. My mommy used do it.
6	• what (in apposition): My voice gonna come out of here *what* I said on that book? • what/that or who: He's the one *what* I told you about. • Deleted relative pronoun: I saw a little girl was on the street.	• did + -n't + verb (when 2nd or 3rd neg. marker: Nobody *didn't* do it. • could, would, should + -n't + verb (preposed neg. aux.): *Couldn't nobody do* it. • Ø contracted could or would (phonol. deletions): You('d) burn your head off. • might/will: Who *might* be the baby?	

	Negatives	Conjunctions	Interrogative Reversal	Wh- Questions
4	• don't (with 3rd pers. sing. as 2nd or 3rd neg. marker): He *don't* want none. No, nobody *don't* live with me. • can't, don't (as pre-posed aux.): *Can't* nobody make me. • Ø copula/aux. + not + V: My mama *not* gonna pick me up today. He *not* a baby. • ain't (as negative copula or aux. *be*): He *ain't* my friend.		• Ø auxiliary be: My voice gonna come out of here? You gonna tell my mama? • was/were: *Was* you throwin' rocks?	
5	• won't (as preposed aux.): *Won't* nobody help him.	• for/so: The dog make too much noise for they won't catch many fish. • conditional and: You do that *and* I'm gonna smack you. • if with phrase deletions: He lookin' *if* he see the money. • aux. inversion in indi-rect Qs (instead of if): She ask me *do he want* some more.		• when, how (with deleted aux., copula, or do): How you do this?
6		• or either, or neither (as disjunctives): He will go *or either* he will stay. He told her that he wouldn't be bad *or neither* get in trouble. • preposed why phrase (with because): *Why* he's in here, *cause* baby scared the dog.	• Ø do: You know that one with the tractor? Where you work? You got blue eyes? • do (with 3rd pers. sing.) *Do* he still have it? • Ø or unreversed modal: Now, what else *I be* doin? Why *you can't* talk on that? • Tag question with ain't: It gonna be fun, *ain't it?*	

Continued

TABLE D.3 *Continued*

	Indefinite Pronouns or Noun Modifiers	Personal Pronouns	Main Verbs	Secondary Verbs
7	• many a: *Many a* people likes to give him a nickel		• passive verb + en with *getting* (aux deleted): Leroy *getting* dressed. • passive verb ± be ± en: One *is name* Brick. They *named* Chief and JoJo. • done + verb + en (completive aspect): *I done tried.* • ± (neg.) aux. + supposed: He *don't supposed* to do it. What toy you *supposed* to play with? • ± have ± verb ± en: We *seen* him already. He *have made* him mad.	• passive with phonological deletions: I'm *be dressed up* real cute. *I'ma be* tired. She *gonna be surprise,* ain't she? I want it cut on.
8			• invariant be: My daddy know I skip school 'cause I *be* home with him. He *be* mad when somebody leave him home. • double modals: We *might could* come. • other expanded aux forms: He *be done jumped* out the tub. He *been going. (have* has undergone phonological deletion) You *shouldn't did* that. • remote past aspect: She *been whuptin'* the baby. I *been wanted* this.	• gerund with go to, got to, start to: When I cry, she *goes to whipping* me. He *started to crying.* He *got to thinking.*

	Negatives	Conjunctions	Interrogative Reversal	Wh- Questions
7	• ain't (for have + not) ± uninflected V: I *ain't* taste any. • ain't (for did + not) ± uninflected V: Yesterday, he *ain't* go to school. I *ain't* found Marge in the school. • couldn't, wouldn't, shouldn't (as preposed aux) • wasn't/weren't: The brakes *wasn't* workin' right. • weren't/wasn't: There *weren't no* money. • uncontracted, uninflected neg. aux.: Lester *do not* like it.			• why, what if, how come (with deleted or unreversed aux. copula or do, or with got): *Why she* turn that way? Hey, *why you got* a dress on mama?
8		• less'n (for unless) • to/till: I didn't get to sleep *to* I had to come in the morning. • ± as + adjective + as: He sock Leroy in the arm *hard as* he could.	• deleted have: He seen it? How you been? What you been doing? • have with 3rd pers. sing.: *Have he* seen you?	• whose, which, which + noun (with deleted aux. copula or do) • who/whose: *Who* this bed? *Who* baby is that?

Source: Nelson, N. W., & Hyter, Y. D. (1990). *Black English Sentence Scoring: Development and Use as a tool for nonbiased assessment* Unpublished manuscript. Western Michigan University, Kalamazoo. Copyright 1990 by N. W. Nelson. Reprinted by permission.

TABLE D.4 Language sample analysis using Black English sentence scoring

Name ___Eric___
Age ___4:0___
Date ___May 31, 1993___ DSS ___3.73___ BESS ___6.55___

	Indef. Pron.	Pers. Pron.	Prim. Verb	Sec. Verb	Neg.	Conj.	Inter. Rev.	Wh-Ques.	Sent. Point	Total
1. That the food that grandma ate.	1	6	1 -,2						1[c] 0	11[b] 9[a]
2. I goin' to nursery school.		1	1 -						1 0	3 1
3. I putting my sister on a motorcycle.		1,1	1 -						1 0	4 2
4. I listening.		1	1 -						1 0	3 1
5. I watched him yesterday.		1,2	2						1	6
6. I like these.		1,3	1						1	6
7. I push all these buttons, ok?	3	1,3	4 -						1 0	12 7
8. They try catch me.		3,1	2 -	5 -					1 0	12 4
9. I had a spoon.		1	2						1	4
10. Who this on the phone?	1		1 -				1 -	2 -	1 0	6 1
11. Where the gun?			1 -				1 -	2 -	1 0	5 0

Total DSS for this partial sample:
41 divided by 11 = 3.73

Total BESS for this partial sample:
72 divided by 11 = 6.55

[a]Sentence total for DSS.

[b]Sentence total for BESS.

[c]Point earned for BESS but not DSS. (Numbers above DSS attempt markers (—) represent credit awarded for BESS but not DSS.)

Source: Nelson, N. W., & Hyter, Y. D. (1990). *Black English sentence scoring: Development and and use as a tool for nonbiased assessment.* Unpublished manuscript. Western Michigan University, Kalamazoo. Reprinted by permission.

450

TABLE D.5   Means and standard deviations for DSS and BESS

Age Range	N	Mean DSS	SD	Mean Bess	SD
3:0–3:6	8	5.63	0.91	7.44	1.15
3:6–4:0	8	5.73	1.04	7.71	0.98
4:0–4:6	8	7.47	1.58	9.33	1.26
4:6–5:0	8	7.51	1.68	8.85	1.48
5:0–5:6	8	8.86	1.93	10.79	1.92
5:6–6:0	8	8.31	2.04	10.02	2.16
6:0–6:6	8	9.12	2.43	11.08	1.61
6:6–7:0	8	9.47	1.72	11.17	2.17

Source: Nelson, N. W., & Hyter, Y.D. (1990). *Black English Sentence Scoring: Development and and use as a tool for nonbiased assessment.* Unpublished manuscript. Western Michigan University, Kalamazoo. Reprinted by permission.

Morphological markers, or *word-structure patterns,* also are recorded on the right-hand side of the Profile Chart. These are not related to any specific stage. The coding for these markers is given in Table D.9.

Scan 8 involves only the utterances that are problems because of structural abnormalities. These may provide a key to disordered language.

Finally, three additional items of information are computed: the total number of sentences, the mean number of sentences per turn, and the mean sentence length in words. The total number of sentences includes all utterances, even repetitions, except for unanalyzed and problem utterances. The mean number of utterances per turn is found by combining the totals in Sections B and C and dividing this amount by the total of the conversational partner's stimulus types, found in Section B.

Conclusion

Although somewhat more specific than Assigning Structural Stage/Complex Sentence Development (J. Miller, 1981), LARSP is more theoretical and based on older, more psycholinguistic models of language development. Although LARSP avoids the pitfalls of phrase structure-based grammars, it still adheres to the notion of elements added one at a time. It might be best to ignore the stage information but incorporate a portion of the analysis methodology, especially the phrasal and sentential structures. Responsive versus spontaneous data and the mean number of sentences per turn are also valuable.

Crystal et al. (1976) provide some interpretation of the results with regard to specific language impairments. Sketchy intervention programs are suggested for the patterns exhibited in the samples.

Systematic Analysis of Language Transcripts

Systematic Analysis of Language Transcripts (SALT for Windows, Version 6.1) (J. Miller & Chapman, 2003) is one of the most promising computer analysis methods available. Based on Assigning Structural Stage/Complex Sentence Development (J. Miller, 1981), SALT is designed for use with the IBM PCs and Macintosh computers. Within limits, SALT analyzes morphemic, syntactic, and semantic aspects of a language sample.

TABLE D.6   LARSP profile chart

Name			Age		Sample date		Type	

A   Unanalyzed
1 Unintelligible	2 Symbolic Noise	3 Deviant	**Problematic** 1 Incomplete	2 Ambiguous	3 Stereotypes

B   Responses

					Normal Response				Abnormal		
					Major						
				Elliptical							
Stimulus Type	Totals	Repetitions	1	2	3+	Reduced	Full	Minor	Structural	θ	Problems
☐ Questions											
Others											

C   Spontaneous

D   Reactions

	General	Structural	θ	Other	Problems

Stage I (0:9–1:6)

Minor	Responses		Vocatives		Other	Problems	
Major	*Comm.*	*Quest.*	*Statement*				
	"V"	"Q"	"V"	"N"	Other	Problems	

Stage II (1:6–2:0)

Conn.			Clause		Phrase		Word
	V*X*	Q*X*	SV	A*X*	DN	VV	-ing
			SO	VO	Adj N	V part	pl
			SC	VC	NN	Int *X*	-ed
			Neg *X*	Other	PrN	Other	

Stage III (2:0–2:6)

X + S:NP	*X* + V:VP	*X* = C:NP	*X* + O:NP	*X* + A:AP		-en
V*XY*	Q*XY*	SVC	VCA	D Adj N	Cop	3s
		SVO	VOA	Adj Adj N	Aux$_O^M$	gen
let XY	VS(*X*)	SVA	VO$_d$O$_i$	Pr DN	Other	n't
do XY		Neg *XY*	Other	Pron$_O^P$		

Stage IV (2:6–3:0)

XY + S:NP	*XY* + V:VP	*XY* + C:NP	*XY* + O:NP	*XY* + A:AP		cop
+ S	QVS	SVOA	AA*XY*	NP Pr NP	Neg V	aux
	Q*XY*+	SVCA	Other	Pr D Adj N	Neg *X*	-est
V*XY*+	VS(*X*+)	SVO$_d$O$_i$		c*X*	2 Aux	
	tag	SVOC		*X*c*X*	Other	

Stage V (3:0–3:6)

and	Coord.	Coord.	Coord.	1	1+	Postmod. clause 1	1+	-er
c	Other	Other	Subord. A	1	1+			-ly
s			S	C	O			
Other			Comparative			Postmod. phrase 1+		

Stage VI (3:6–4:6)

(+)							(−)						
NP	VP	Clause	Conn.	Clause			Phrase						Word
				Element	NP			VP			N	V	
Initiator	Complex	Passive	*and*	Ø	D	Pr	Pron^P	Aux^M	Aux^O	Cop	*irreg*	
Coord.		Complement	c	⇄	DØ	PrØ						
		how	s	Concord	D⇄	Pr⇄	Ø		Ø		*reg*	
		what										
Other						Ambiguous						

Stage VII (4:6 +)

Discourse		*Syntactic Comprehension*	
A Connectivity	*it*		
Comment Clause	*there*		
Emphatic Order	Other	Style	
Total No. Sentences	Mean No. Sentences Per Turn		Mean Sentence Length

Source: Crystal, D., Fletcher, P., & Garman, M. (1976, revised 1981). *The grammatical analysis of language disability.* New York: Elsevier. Reprinted with permission.

TABLE D.7   LARSP clausal and phrasal structure coding

V	Verb
Q	Question word (*What, where*)
N	Noun
X	All elements that may co-occur with another element
S	Subject
C/O	Complement/object
A	Adverb (Usually location)
Neg	Negative word (*No, not*)
D	Demonstrative (Including possessive pronouns)
Adj	Adjective
Pr	Preposition
Part	Particle (*Out* as in *Come out*)
Y	Used with X to indicate any **two** elements of clause structure
NP	Noun phrase
VP	Verb phrase
Cop	Copula
Aux	Auxiliary verb (Not just *be*)
Pron	Pronoun
O_d	Direct object
O_i	Indirect object
Z	Use with X and Y to indicate any **three** elements of clause structure
c	Coordinating conjunction
s	Subordinating conjunction

TABLE D.8   LARSP stages and approximate ages

Stage I	9 mos.–1 yr. 6 mos.
Stage II	1 yr. 6 mos.–2 yrs.
Stage III	2 yrs.–2 yrs. 6 mos.
Stage IV	2 yrs. 6 mos.–3 yrs.
Stage V	3 yrs.–3 yrs. 6 mos.
Stage VI	3 yrs. 6 mos.–4 yrs. 6 mos.
Stage VII	4 yrs. 6 mos.–9 yrs.

TABLE D.9   LARSP word-structure pattern codes

-ing	Present progressive *-ing*
pl	Plural *-s* marker
-ed	Past-tense *-ed*
-en	Past participle *-en*
3s	Third-person singular *-s*
gen	Possessive *-'s*
n't	Contracted negative (is*n't*)
'cop	Contracted form of the copula (She*'s* happy)
'aux	Contracted form of the auxiliary *be* (He*'s* eating)
-est	Superlative *-est*
-er	Comparative *-er*
-ly	Adverbial suffix *-ly*

The transcript is typed in standard English orthography. Time is critical for calculation of duration and pause times and must be noted. Each feature to be analyzed is signaled with a different marker. Therefore, it takes approximately 7 minutes for even the skilled user to enter each minute of conversation into the transcription format.

The SLP can accomplish several types of analyses by using SALT. These types include utterance type; turn overlap and distribution; pause duration and number; utterances per minute and words per utterance; frequency of verbal and nonverbal data of interest, such as past tense; utterance length; type-token ratio; MLU; Brown's stages of development; expected age range of development; word and category lists; and other user-designated analysis.

Conclusion

SALT is a very promising and versatile analysis method that is easy for the SLP to use after becoming familiar with entering the transcript into the computer. As with other computer analysis methods, however, it is not the great panacea. At present, most results are a calculation of those features signaled by the SLP when he or she enters the data. Thus, special care is required to ensure that features are signaled accurately.

E

Selected English Morphological Prefixes and Suffixes

TABLE E.1   Prefixes and suffixes

Derivational		Inflectional
Prefixes	Suffixes	
a- (in, on, into, in a manner)	-able (ability, tendency, likelihood)	-ed (past)
bi- (twice, two)	-al (pertaining to, like, action, process)	-ing (at present)
de- (negative, descent, reversal)	-ance (action, state)	-s (plural)
ex- (out of, from, thoroughly)	-ation (denoting action in a noun)	-s (third person marker)
inter- (reciprocal between, together)	-en (used to form verbs from adjectives)	-'s (possession)
mis- (ill, negative, wrong)	-ence (action, state)	
out- (extra, beyond, not)	-er (used as an agentive ending)	
over- (over)	-est (superlative)	
post- (behind, after)	-ful (full, tending)	
pre- (to, before)	-ible (ability, tendency, likelihood)	
pro- (in favor of)	-ish (belonging to)	
re- (again, backward motion)	-ism (doctrine, state, practice)	
semi- (half)	-ist (one who does something)	
super- (superior)	-ity (used for abstract nouns)	
trans- (across, beyond)	-ive (tendency or connection)	
tri- (three)	-ize (action, policy)	
un- (not, reversal)	-less (without)	
under- (under)	-ly (used to form adverbs)	
	-ment (action, product, means, state)	
	-ness (quality, state)	
	-or (used as an agentive ending)	
	-ous (full of, having, like)	
	-y (inclined to)	

F

Indirect Elicitation Techniques

There is an infinite variety of indirect elicitation techniques, although we tend to rely on two old favorites:

Tell me what you see.
Tell me in a whole sentence.

Here are a few conversational techniques that came to mind one day. The list is not exhaustive, merely illustrative.

Technique	Target	Example
The emperor's new clothes	Negative statements	CLINICIAN: Oh, Shirley, what beautiful yellow boots! CHILD: I'm not wearing boots!
Pass it on	Requests for information	CLINICIAN: John, do you know where Linda's project is? CHILD: No. CLINICIAN: Oh, see if she does? CHILD: Linda, where's your project?
Violating routines ("Silly rabbit")	Imperatives, directives	CLINICIAN: Here's your sandwich. CHILD: Nothing in it. CLINICIAN: Oh, you must like different sandwiches than I do. What do you want? CHILD: Peanut butter. CLINICIAN: How do I do it? (There's your opener)

Continued

Technique	Target	Example
Nonblabbermouth	Requests for information	CLINICIAN: (Place interesting object in front of child) "Boy, is this neat." CHILD: What is it? CLINICIAN: A flibbideejibbit. (Now STOP. Don't give any more info) CHILD: What's it do?
What I have	Request for action	CLINICIAN: Oh, I can't wait to show you what I have in this bag. It's really neat. (Wait child out)
Guess what I did	Request for information, past tense verbs	CLINICIAN: Guess what I did yesterday in the park. CHILD: Jogged? Picked flowers? Had a picnic?
Mumble	Contingent query	At height of an interesting story or punchline of a joke, clinician should mumble so that child does not receive message. If needed, increase pressure by asking questions on what was just said.
Ask someone else	Request for information	CLINICIAN: What do you need? CHILD: Sugar. CLINICIAN: I don't know where it is. Why don't you ask Sally where the sugar is.
Rule giving	Requests for objects	CLINICIAN: I have the athletic equipment for recess. If you need some, just ask me. CHILD: I want jump rope.
Request for assistance	Initiating conversation	CLINICIAN: John, can you ask Keith to help me?
Modeling with meaningful intent	I want _____	CLINICIAN: We have lots of colored paper for our project. Now let's see who needs some. I want a green one. (Take one and wait) CHILD: I want blue.
"Screw up" #1	Locatives, prepositions	CLINICIAN: Can you help me dress this doll? (Place shoe on doll's head) How's that? CHILD: No. The shoe goes *on* the doll's foot. CLINICIAN: But now the foot's all gone. CHILD: No. It's *in* the shoe.
"Screw up" #2	Negative statements	CLINICIAN: Here's your snack. (Give child a pencil) CHILD: That's not a snack.
Requests for topic	Statements	CLINICIAN: Now let's talk about your birthday party. (Not shared information)
Expansion of child utterance into desired form	Infinitives	CHILD: I want paste crayon. CLINICIAN: You want crayon to *sing with?* CHILD: No, to color. CLINICIAN: What? CHILD: I want crayon to color.

G

Intervention Activities and Language Targets

FIGURE G.1 Activities and targets.

Activities	Nouns	Plurals	Verb tensing	Adjectives/descriptive words	Adverbs	Pronouns	Articles and/or demonstrations	Prepositions/spatial terms	Requests for objects	Requests for assistance	Requests for information	Negatives	Interrogatives	Following directions	Giving directions	Sequencing	Turn taking	Topic introduction and maintenance	Categorization	Register	Presupposition	Conversational repair	Variety of pragmatic features	Auditory processing and memory	Word association	Vocabulary
Barrier tasks	X													X	X	X					X			X		
Body tracing			X	X				X		X				X	X	X										X
Colorforms			X	X			X	X																		
*Cooking		X	X	X	X		X		X	X	X		X	X	X				X							X
Describes pictures that others cannot see	X	X		X			X														X					
Dolls, clothing, and furniture	X	X		X				X						X	X					X						X
Dressing	X	X																								
Dress-up			X	X		X	X	X	X																	
Explaining "how-to"				X				X				X			X	X	X	X		X	X	X				
Farm or zoo play	X	X		X								X							X							
Guiding others through an activity								X						X	X	X		X			X		X			
Treasure Hunt—"You're getting warmer"										X				X	X						X					
Interviewing				X					X		X		X							X		X			X	
"I see something that's...."						X	X	X	X		X	X	X												X	
Jeopardy				X							X		X					X							X	
Kitchen play	X		X	X	X			X		X	X			X	X	X	X	X					X			X
*Making things			X	X				X		X				X	X		X									X
Map following											X	X	X	X		X		X								
Mime														X							X					

460

Activity																			
My "ME" book			X	X													X			
Music and action songs		X	X									X	X	X					X	X
Nature or science activity								X	X	X	X	X		X						
Obstacle course		X	X					X	X	X										
Planning an activity		X	X	X	X			X					X		X		X		X	X
Planting seeds		X	X	X						X	X									
Playhouse		X	X	X										X	X	X				
Playing teacher					X				X				X	X	X	X				
Pretend shopping	X	X				X	X	X		X	X		X	X					X	X
Puppet show												X		X	X					
Putting objects in order		X	X	X		X					X		X	X		X			X	X
"Safety Town" (Safety curriculum for preschool and kindergarten)		X	X	X		X	X	X	X		X		X	X		X				
Simon Says								X	X	X									X	
Simulated restaurant					X		X	X				X	X	X	X	X				X
Sorting clothing	X	X				X	X					X		X						
Story-telling (true or make-believe)		X			X		X	X	X	X		X	X	X	X	X	X			
Telephone play		X	X	X		X	X	X	X	X		X	X	X	X	X	X	X	X	X
TV commercials		X	X				X	X	X	X		X	X	X	X		X	X	X	X
"Twenty questions" variations																				
Washing dishes	X	X	X		X	X		X	X	X										
"What am I?"		X	X	X		X		X	X	X		X	X	X	X		X		X	X
"What did you do....?"	X	X	X	X	X	X		X	X	X		X	X	X	X		X		X	X

*See third page of table

Continued

FIGURE G.1   *Continued*

*Possible cooking activities:

1. Cookies, cupcakes, muffins
2. Cornbread and butter
3. Edible honeybees—Mix 1/2 cup peanut butter, 1 T. plus 1/3 cup honey, 2 T. sesame seeds, and 2 T. toasted wheat germ. Roll into balls. Make stripes on the bee by dipping a toothpick in cocoa powder and pressing into ball. Use slivered almonds for wings.
4. English muffin pizzas
5. Fruit salad—Use a few vegetables just to confuse the issue and to elicit some language.
6. Ice cream sundaes
7. Instant pudding
8. Milkshakes—Lots of variations here, such as vanilla, chocolate, and banana (use real ones in the blender).
9. Peanut butter and jelly sandwiches.
10. Peanut butter balls—Mix 1/2 cup honey, 1/2 cup peanut butter, 1 cup dry milk, and 1 cup oatmeal. Roll into balls. Refrigerate.
11. Peanut butter "face" sandwiches—Make faces on the bread with a peanut butter base using raisins (eyes), peanut (nose), chocolate chips (mouth), and carrot slivers or coconut (hair).
12. Picnic lunch
13. Popcorn and popcorn balls

**Things to make:

1. Cereal box instrument—Use a strong cereal box with a circular hole cut in the face similar to the hole in a guitar. Stretch various size rubber bands around the box and tack them into wooden blocks that act as bridges.
2. Costumes from grocery bags—Cut eye holes or a hole for face. Cut arm holes if desired. Decorate bag. Slip over child.
3. Cowgirl and cowboy outfits from grocery bags—Bags can easily be cut to resemble vests and yokes. Be sure to fringe them. Add a bandanna and you have the outfit.
4. Decorate a shoebox "room" with scraps of wallpaper.
5. Food sculptures—Use shredded coconut or lettuce, raisins, peanuts, M&Ms, hot cinnamon candies, cheese strips, fruit halves, celery and carrot sticks, olives, marshmallows, gum drops, and toothpicks.
6. Holiday cards
7. Kites
8. Paper bag puppets
9. Paper butterflies
10. Paper flowers
11. Playdough—Mix 2 cups flour, 1 cup water, 1 T. salad oil, 1 cup salt, and food coloring.
12. Potato and sponge prints
13. Sachets—Cloves and crumbled bay leaves and cinnamon sticks in square of cloth. Pull ends of cloth together and tie with a ribbon.
14. Snowmen and snowwomen—Use styrofoam balls, pipecleaners, cloves, and toothpicks.
15. Stained glass windows—Cut out a cardboard mold. Tape aluminum foil over one side of the cut-out sections. Place this side down. Fill the holes with Elmer's glue. Swirl in food coloring. Allow to dry thoroughly. Peel foil. Hang in sunny window.

Note: A variety of language features can be elicited within these activities by using the indirect elicitation techniques in Appendix F and the nonlinguistic strategies in Chapter 10.

Analyzing Classroom Communication Breakdown

The following questions can serve as a guideline to the teacher in determining where students are failing in formal communicative interactions in the classroom. Several different interactions should be analyzed to get an overall perspective of the child's linguistic abilities, cognitive status, and communicative competence.

Language

Phonological System

Has the child acquired the rules that govern the sounds of the language being used? (e.g., Does Jim make different articulation errors each time he speaks?)

How successful is the child in understanding spoken utterances? (e.g., Does Mary know that *cat* and *rat* are two different words?)

How successful is the child in producing spoken utterances? (e.g., To what degree is the child unintelligible?)

Semantic System

Is the child familiar with the vocabulary being used by the teacher? Has she or he heard these words before in similar situations? In different situations? (e.g., Does Joan know this is an angle without someone pointing to it?)

Do the vocabulary items have meaning for the child? Do the words have meaning only in specific contexts, or does the child understand the words in all contexts? (e.g., Does Keesha know what an angle is?)

Does the child have word-finding difficulties for familiar vocabulary items? For new words? (e.g., Are there hesitations or word substitutions when Jackie speaks?)

Syntactic System

Has the child acquired the rules that govern word order and other aspects of grammar? (e.g., Does Rang understand subject-verb agreement?)

Is the child familiar with the grammatical form being used by the teacher? Has she or he heard this form in similar situations? In different situations? (e.g., Does Diego know who is doing the hitting in the sentence "Mary was hit by Tom"?)

Is the grammatical form that is being used meaningful to the child? Does the child understand the relationships that exist among the lexical items in the utterance? (e.g., Does Maria know why the sentence "The desk stepped on my toes" is anomalous?)

Does the child have access to the grammatical form needed to express his response? (e.g., How adequately does Tommy express himself on a topic of his interest?)

Pragmatics—Functional Use or Intent?

Does the child know the rules for communicative intent that govern social interaction at home? At school? (e.g., Who talks when and under what conditions?)

Does the child know the rules for politeness?

Does the child know when to make eye contact?

Does the child know how close it is permissible to stand when talking with another person?

Does the child know when to raise his hand for recognition?

Does the child know that it is helpful to the learning process to request clarification of new information?

Does the child know how to interpret both direct and indirect requests?

Thinking

Information Processing

Is the child's attention span long enough to attend to a stimulus utterance or event? (e.g., Does Juwan watch the teacher when she holds up a pencil?)

Does the child attend to so many environmental stimuli that she or he is unable to focus on a single one? (e.g., Is Junko constantly turning to look when noises or movements occur?)

Is the child's sensory input reduced or distorted?

What is the length of the child's short-term memory? Is it long enough for the child to hold the utterance to decode it? (e.g., Can Mai-Ling remember a list of things to buy at the play store?)

Does the child spontaneously rehearse or use mnemonic devices to aid short-term memory? If the child does not rehearse spontaneously, can she or he be taught to use such strategies?

Does the child have a backlog of experiences against which to judge new information? (e.g., "Kay, have you ever been to a farm to see a cow?")

Is the child's long-term memory functionally accessible? (e.g., "Do you remember your phone number, Tim?")

Does the child form associations between new and previously stored information? Is the new information integrated with the old? (e.g., "What does this new ball look like? Isn't it just like the one we saw at the soccer game?)

Is retrieval from long-term memory impaired?

Does the child spontaneously evaluate the quality of the information received and the response being formulated?

Conceptual Information

Has the child had enough previous experience to interpret conceptual notions correctly? (e.g., Has the child had experience with blocks of different shapes before being asked to classify them?)

If not, has the previous experience been deficient in the quantity of experiences or in the appropriateness or variety of concept instances?

Does the child have difficulty expressing the conceptual relationships required by the situation? (e.g., Has the child been given the language to use to talk about squares and rectangles?)

Integration and Association of Information

Is the child able to integrate new information into old, previously stored information?

Is the child able to make use of integrated or associated information provided by the teacher? (e.g., Can the child use analogies provided by the teacher?)

Is the child able to formulate a response that demonstrates that integration of information has taken place?

The consequence of going through an analysis of this sort is having the information needed to modify classroom interactions to make them better situations for learning. Modifications might be in teacher language, topics or content, and the context of the interaction. The assessment by the teacher can be developed into an ongoing activity that provides continuing feedback on the success of interactions as learning situations. For children with language disorders, such interactive assessment in the classroom setting provides the opportunity for linguistic experience appropriate to the level of functioning and in an amount that is not possible under traditional models of intervention.

Source: Vetter, D. (1982). Language Disorders and Schooling. *Topics in Language Disorders, 2*(4), 13–19. Reprinted with permission of Aspen Publishers, Inc. Copyright 1982.

I

Use of Children's Literature in Preschool Classrooms

Book	Language Use	Theme
Aardema, *Oh, Kojo! How could you!* (M)	Predicting, cause and effect	
Aardema, *Bring the rain to Kapiti Plain* (M)	Rhyming, predicting, past tense, plosives, chanting	WEATHER
Adler, *Bunny Rabbit Rebus*	Word play	
Agee, *Flapsticks*	Rhyming	
Ahlberg, *Jolly postman*	Predicting	
Ahlberg, *Each peach pear plum*	Rhyming, predicting, visual discrimination, "I spy" with prepositions	SENSES
Albert, *Where does the trail lead?*	Predicting, chanting	
Alborough, *Where's my teddy?*	Rhyming	
Allard, *Miss Nelson has a field day*	Predicting, cause and effect, emotions	
Allard, *Miss Nelson is missing*	Predicting, cause and effect, reasoning	
Allard, *Miss Nelson is back*	Predicting, cause and effect	
Allard, *The Stupids die*	Verbal absurdities	
Allard, *The Stupids have a ball*	Verbal absurdities	
Allard, *The Stupids step out*	Verbal absurdities	
Allen, *A lion in the night*	Predicting, present progressive and future tense, sequencing	ANIMALS
Allen, *Who sank the boat?*	Predicting, chanting, interrogative structures	TRANSPORTATION
Anholt & Anholt, *Here come the babies*	Rhyming, naming, /b/ words	
Anno, *Anno's counting house*	Numbers, counting, observational skills	COUNTING

Book	Language Use	Theme
Appelt, *Elephants aloft*	Locative prepositions	ANIMALS
Arnold, *Green Wilma*	Past tense, noticing the ridiculous	
Arnold, *The simple people*	Past tense, /s/ words, emotions	FEELINGS
Asch, *Just like daddy* (Surprise ending)	Chanting	FAMILY
Asch, *The last puppy*	First/last	ANIMALS
Ash, *Little fish, big fish* (Visual interest)	Big/little contrast	
Avery, *Everybody has feelings (Todos tenemos sentimientos)* (M)	Emotions, discussion	FEELINGS
Aylesworth, *The good night kiss*	Predicting, fill-ins	BEDTIME
Aylesworth, *The old black fly* (A little grim)	Creative alphabet, chanting, initial /ʃ/ words	COLORS
Baer, *Thump, thump, rat-a-tat-tat*	Chanting, making sounds	
Bang, *Ten, nine, eight* (M)	Counting, rhyming	COUNTING
Baker, *Hide and Snake*	Observational skills, elicited descriptions	
Baker, *The third-story cat*	Prepositions, past tense	ANIMALS
Baker, *White rabbit's coloring book*	Adjectives, predicting	COLORS
Banchek, *Snake in, snake out*	Prepositions	
Barret, *Animals should definitely not act like people*	Word play, illiteration, absurdity	
Barrett, *Cloudy with a chance of meatballs*	Metaphors, if/then conditional sentences, "s" words, humor	WEATHER
Barton, *Airplanes*	Vocabulary, noun-verb agreement, categories	TRANSPORTATION
Barton, *Airport*	Vocabulary, noun-verb agreement, categories, relating experiences	TRANSPORTATION
Barton, *Boats*	Vocabulary, noun-verb agreement, categories, relating experiences	TRANSPORTATION
Barton, *Harry is a scaredy-cat*	Present progressive tense, initial /k/ words, /sk/ blends, discussion	FEELINGS
Bennett & Cooke, *One cow moo moo*	Chanting, auditory memory	ANIMALS, COUNTING
Berger, *Grandfather Twilight*	Final consonants, night vs. day	BEDTIME
Borden, *Caps, hats, socks, and mittens*	Final /ts, ps/ blends	AUTUMN
Boyd, *Black dog, red house*	Colors	COLORS
Boynton, *A is for angry*	Alphabet with animals and adjectives	
Brown, *A dark dark tale*	Sequencing, prepositions, adjectives	
Brown, *Arthur's nose*	Possessive /-'s/ marker, pronouns	SENSE
Brown, *Big red barn*	Initial /r/ words	ANIMALS
Brown, *Goodnight moon*	Predicting, noun-verb agreement, plurals	BEDTIME
Brown, *If at first you do not see*	Observation, imaginative language	FEELINGS
Brown, *The noise book*	Auditory discrimination	SENSES
Brown, *Old MacDonald had a farm*	Singing, /f/ words	ANIMALS
Brown, *The runaway bunny*	Prepositions, pronouns, present progressive tense	ANIMALS

Book	*Language Use*	*Theme*
Buckley & Carle, *The foolish tortoise*	Sequencing, discussion ("Why it's good to be me")	SELF-ESTEEM
Burningham, *Hey! Get off our train*	Chanting	TRANSPORTATION
Burningham, *Jingle, twang*	Present progressive tense, word play	
Burningham, *Mr. Gumpy's outing*	Predicting, narratives and interrogatives	TRANSPORTATION
Burningham, *Skip, trip*	Verb vocabulary, use to elicit SVO structures	
Burningham, *Sniff, shout*	Verb vocabulary, use to elicit SVO structures	
Burningham, *Would you rather?*	Basis for *why not* discussions	ANIMALS
Butterworth & Inkpen, *Nice or nasty: A book of opposites*	Antonyms	
Byars, *Go and hush the baby*	Predicting	
Calmenson, *It begins with an A*	Initial sounds, auditory attending, and synthesis, word play	
Capucilli, *Inside a barn in the country*	Chanting, /s/ blends	ANIMALS
Carle, *The grouchy ladybug*	Pragmatics, emotions, chanting	
Carle, *A house for a hermit crab*	Initial /s/ and /s/ blends	
Carle, *The secret birthday message*	Word play, prepositions, vocabulary	BIRTHDAY
Carle, *The tiny seed*	Sequencing	SEASONS
Carle, *The very busy spider*	Predicting, initial /sp/ blends, initial /v/ words	
Carle, *The very hungry caterpillar*	Sequencing, auditory memory, present progressive tense	SENSES
Carle, *The very quiet cricket*	Predicting, initial /kw, k/ blends, initial /s/ words	
Carlson, *I like me*	Final /k/ words, initial /l/ words	SELF-ESTEEM
Carlstrom, *Goodbye geese*	Body parts	WINTER
Carlstrom, *How do you say it today, Jesse Bear?*	General speech, chanting, seasons	MANNERS
Cauley, *Goldilocks and the three bears*	Predicting	ANIMALS
Cauley, *Jack and the beanstalk*	Predicting	
Charles, *What am I?*	Colors, visual recognition, question-answer	COLORS
Charlip, *Fortunately*	Predicting emotions, past tense, adverbs, initial /f/ words	BIRTHDAY, FEELINGS
Cheltenham, *Kindergarteners, we are all alike...we are all different* (M)	Descriptors, same/different discussion	SELF-ESTEEM
Chorao, *Kate's box*	Pronouns, possessive /-'s/ marker, prepositions, present progressive & past tense	
Christelow, *Five little monkeys jumping on the bed*	Chanting, counting, initial /l/ words	COUNTING
Cole, *Monster manners*	Pragmatic past tense	MANNERS
Collington, *The midnight circus*	Sequencing, describing, cohesion	
Corey, *Everyone takes turns*	Pragmatics	MANNERS
Crews, *Freight trains*	Blends, colors, two-word semantic rules	TRANSPORTATION, COLORS

Book	Language Use	Theme
Dabkovich, *Sleepy bear*	Predicting, verb tensing	BEDTIME
Davol, *Black, white, just right* (M)	Descriptors, verb person markers	SELF-ESTEEM
Day, *Good dog, Carl*	Sequencing, narratives, descriptors	
Day, *Carl goes to daycare*	Sequencing, narratives, descriptors	COMMUNITY
Day, *Carl goes shopping*	Sequencing, narratives, descriptors	COMMUNITY
Day, *Carl's afternoon in the park*	Sequencing, narratives, descriptors	COMMUNITY
Deming, *Who is tapping at my window?*	Chanting, rhyming	
DePaola, *Charlie needs a cloak*	Sequencing, vocabulary (words defined at end), past tense	CLOTHES
DePaola, *I love you, mouse*	Imagining, if…then	ANIMALS, FEELING
DePaola, *The knight and the dragon*	Present progressive & past tense, vocabulary	
DePaola, *Pancakes for breakfast*	Predicting, storytelling, sequencing, present progressive tense, final /k/ words	SENSES
deRegniers, *Going for a walk*	Chanting, rhyming, predicting	FEELINGS
deRegniers, *It does not say meow*	Auditory attending and processing, adjectives, problem solving	ANIMALS
Dunrea, *Deep down underground*	Chanting, counting, initial /g, s, b, r, d/ words	ANIMALS, COUNTING
Ehlert, *Planting a rainbow*	Initial /r/ words	COLORS
Ehlert, *Red leaf, yellow leaf*	Regular plurals, regular past, seasons	AUTUMN, COLORS
Emberley, *Go away, big green monster*	Predicting, chanting	FEELINGS
Ets, *In the forest*	Singular/plural contrasts, present progressive & past tense	ANIMALS
Ets, *Play with me*	Past tense, discussion	ANIMALS
Evans, *Hunky Dory found it*	Chanting, predicting	ANIMALS
Everitt, *Frida the wondercat*	Predicting, past tense	ANIMALS
Fleming, *In the tall, tall grass*	Final /ʃ/ words	
Fox, *Hattie and the fox*	Predicting, chanting, auditory memory	ANIMALS
Fox, *Shoes from grandpa*	Predicting, chanting, rhyming	CLOTHES
Ga'g, *Millions of cats*	Predicting	ANIMALS
Galdone, *Henny penny*	Predicting	ANIMALS
Galdone, *The teeny-tiny woman*	Initial /t/ words, fill-ins	
Galdone, *The three billy goats gruff*	Initial /g/ words	ANIMALS
Gantos, *Greedy greeny*	Initial /g/ words	MANNERS
Gelman, *I went to the zoo*	Present progressive tense, chanting, acting out	ANIMALS, FEELINGS
Geisert, *Oink, oink*	Sequencing, narrating, descriptors	ANIMALS
Gibbons, *The season of Arnold's apple tree*	Regular plural, possessive -*'s,* third-person -*s*	AUTUMN, WINTER, SPRING
Gill, *The spring hat*	Sequencing, narrating, descriptors	CLOTHES, SPRING

Book	Language Use	Theme
Ginsburg, *Good morning, Chick*	Past tense, chanting, predicting, demonstratives (*this, that*)	ANIMALS
Glassman, *The wizard next door*	Imagining, descriptors	
Goffe, *Ma, you're driving me crazy*	Chanting, predicting	FEELINGS
Goode, *Where's our mama?*	Chanting, questions-answers in unison	
Graham, *Full moon soup or the fall of the Hotel Splendide*	Narrating, observing, descriptors, questioning, answering	
Graham, *I love you mouse*	Predicting, chanting	ANIMALS, FEELINGS
Guarino, *Is your mama a llama?*	Guessing, chanting, descriptors	ANIMALS, FAMILY
Guarino, *Tu mama es una llama?*	Guessing, chanting, descriptors	ANIMALS, FAMILY
Grindley, *Knock, knock! Who's there*	Questioning, chanting, if-then	FAMILY
Gwynne, *A chocolate moose for dinner*	Figurative language, absurdities	
Gwynne, *A king who rained*	Figurative language, absurdities	
Hale, *Mary had a little lamb*	Initial /l/ words	ANIMALS
Hayes, *The grumpalump*	Chanting, auditory memory, past tense	FEELINGS
Hempworth, *Antics*	Prereading skills	
Henck, *Pony and bear are friends*	Prereading skills	FEELINGS
Henrietta, *A mouse in the house*	Observing	BIRTHDAY
Hill, *Spot's birthday party*	Prepositions	BIRTHDAY
Hines, *Daddy makes the best spaghetti*	Sequencing, relating experiences	FAMILY
Hines, *It's just me, Emily*	Predicting, chanting	
Hoban, *Exactly the opposite*	Descriptors, opposites	
Hoban, *Is it rough, is it smooth, is it shiny?*	Adjectives, antonyms	
Hoban, *Is it larger? Is it smaller?*	Singular/plural contrast (regular & irregular), descriptors, comparative	
Hudson, *Jamal's busy day* (M)	Discussion (importance of school)	COMMUNITY
Hudson & Ford, *Bright eyes, brown skin* (M)	Descriptors	SELF-ESTEEM
Hutchins, *Don't forget the bacon*	Auditory memory, word play, initial /f/ words, chanting	COMMUNITY
Hutchins, *The doorbell rang*	Predicting, conversational skills, simple practical math, initial /g, k, r/ words	
Hutchins, *Goodnight owl*	Predicting, chanting, regular past tense	
Hutchins, *I hunter*	Observing, counting	COUNTING
Hutchins, *Rosie's walk*	Prepositions, present progressive & past tense, sequencing	ANIMALS
Hutchins, *The surprise party*	Predicting, auditory memory	BIRTHDAY
Hutchins, *The very worst monster*	Present progressive, adjectives	MANNERS
Janovitz, *Look out, bird*	Chanting, initial /f, t, s, b/d/ words	
Johnson, *The girl who wore snakes* (M)	Initial /s/ words	
Johnson, *When I am old with you* (M)	Imagining, discussion	FAMILY

Book	Language Use	Theme
Johnson, *Never babysit the hippopotamuses*	Noticing the ridiculous, initial /p/ words, absurdities	
Jonas, *Reflections*	Descriptors	
Jonas, *The 13th clue*	Descriptors, predicting, visual searching	
Jonas, *The trek*	Descriptors, visual searching	
Jonas, *This old man*	Accompanies song, rhyming, singing	
Jonas, *Where can it be?*	Descriptors, visual searching, initial /g, k/ words	
Joslin & Sendak, *What do you say dear*	Predicting	MANNERS
Kandoian, *Molly's seasons*	Plurals, rhyming, descriptors, seasons	AUTUMN, WINTER, SPRING
Keats, *Over in the meadow*	Singular/plural contrast, present progressive & past tense	COUNTING
Keats, *Peter's chair*	Present progressive & past tense, possessive -'s, adjectives, discussion	FEELINGS
Keats, *The snowy day*	Initial /sn/ blends, relating experiences	WEATHER, WINTER
Keller, *Geraldine's blanket*	Retelling with present possessive, relating experiences	FEELINGS
Kent, *There's no such thing as a dragon*	Initial /b/ words, past tense	
Kennedy & Hague, *The teddy bears' picnic*	Initial /s/ words	
King, *Gus is gone*	Vocabulary	
King, *Lucy is lost*	Vocabulary	
Klamath County YMCA Family Preschool, *The land of many colors* (M)	Colors, emotions	COLORS, FEELINGS
Knowlton, *Why do cowboys sleep with their boots on?*	Regular and irregular past tense, initial /k/	CLOTHES
Krahn, *The creepy thing* (no words)	Following a theme/story line, descriptors	
Krahn, *Robot-Bot-Bot* (no words)	Following a theme/story line, descriptors	
Kraus, *Bears*	Vocabulary, prepositions, present progressive tense	ANIMALS
Kraus, *Leo the late bloomer*	Predicting, emotions, initial /l/ words	
Kraus, *Milton the early riser*	Chanting, initial /s/ words	
Kraus, *Whose mouse are you?*	Possessive -'s, interrogative sentences	FAMILY, FEELINGS
Krauss, *A hole is to dig*	Expression, make own definitions	
Krauss, *The carrot seed*	Past tense, present progressive tense, sequencing	SENSES
Lacome, *Walking through the jungle*	Chanting, predicting	
Lear, *The owl and the pussycat*	Present progressive & past tense, rhyming	
Lehrman, *Loving the earth*	Discussion, if…then	ANIMALS, COMMUNITY
LeSaux, *Daddy shaves*	Verbs, third-person -*s*	FAMILY
Lester, *Clive eats alligators*	Verbs, following a theme/story line, third-person -*s*	SELF-ESTEEM
Lester, *It wasn't my fault*	Chanting, describing	SELF-ESTEEM

Book	Language Use	Theme
Lewin, *Jafta*	Similes	FEELINGS
Lewin, *Jafta's mother* (M)	Emotions, initial "s" words, noun-verb agreement	FAMILY
Lillie, *Everything has a place*	In & on	
Little, DeVries, & Gilman, *Once upon a golden apple*	Noticing the ridiculous, responding, chanting	
Lionni, *A color of his own*	Regular plural, /l/ in all positions	FEELINGS, COLORS
London, *Froggy gets dressed*	Regular & irregular past, body parts	CLOTHING, WINTER
London, *Let's go, froggy!*	Prepositions, regular & irregular past	
Loomis, *In the diner*	Verbs, third-person -*s*	
Lotz, *Snowsong shistling*	Rhyming, present progressive	AUTUMN, WINTER
Lukesova, *Julian in the Autumn Woods*	Regular plurals, emotions	AUTUMN, FEELINGS
Lyon, *Together*	Rhyming, chanting, verbs	FEELINGS
Macauley, *Black and white*	Following a theme/story line	
Maccarone, *Itchy, itchy chicken pox*	Final /tʃ/ words	
Martin, *Brown bear, brown bear, what do you see?*	Sequencing, present progressive, categorization, rhyming, chanting, adjectives	ANIMALS, COLORS, SENSES
Martin, *The happy hippopotami*	Rhyming	
Martin, *Polar bear, polar bear, what do you hear?*	Sequencing, present progressive, categorization, initial /p, b, l/ words, rhyming, chanting	ANIMALS, COLORS, SENSES
Martin, *When dinosaurs go visiting*	Verbs, adjectives	
Martin & Archambault, *Here are my hands*	Body parts, present progressive	
Marzolla & Pinkney, *Pretend you're a cat*	Verbs, adjectives, questions	ANIMALS
Marzollo & Wick, *I spy*	"I spy" game, vocabulary, descriptors	SENSES
Marzolla & Wick, *I spy mystery*	"I spy" game, vocabulary, descriptors	SENSES
Mayer, *Ah-choo* (No words)	Sequencing, descriptors, predicting	
Mayer, *A boy, a dog, a frog and a friend* (No words)	Sequencing, descriptors	
Mayer, *Frog goes to dinner* (No words)	Sequencing, descriptors, predicting, following a theme/story line	
Mayer, *Frog on his own* (No words)	Sequencing, descriptors, predicting, following a theme/story line	
Mayer, *The great cat chase* (No words)	Sequencing, descriptors, predicting, following a theme/story line	
Mayer, *Hiccup* (No words)	Sequencing, descriptors	MANNERS
Mayer, *Just my friend and me*	Pronouns, verbs, sequencing	FEELINGS
Mayer, *Just me and my little sister*	Pronouns, present progressive & past tense	FAMILY
Mayer, *One monster after another*	Initial /g, b/ words	
Mayer, *There's an alligator under my bed*	Sequencing, predicting, present progressive & past tense, prepositions	FEELINGS

Book	Language Use	Theme
McCarthy, *Happy hiding hippos*	Initial /h, s/ words	FEELINGS
McCauley, *Why the chicken crossed the road*	Problem solving, inference, cause and effect, idioms and metaphors, temporal markers	
McCully, *Picnic* (No words)	Descriptors, following a theme/story line	
McGilvray, *Don't climb out of the window tonight*	Predicting, causal events	
McNaughten, *Guess who just moved in next door*	Predicting, descriptors	COMMUNITY
McPhail, *Emma's pet*	Descriptors	
Meddaugh, *Martha speaks*	Pragmatics	
Morninghouse, *Nightfeathers*	Poetry	
Munsch, *The paper bag princess*	Predictable patterning, inference, logical sequencing, life skills, initial /th/ words, final consonant blends	CLOTHES, SELF-ESTEEM
Murphy, *What next, baby bear!*	Predicting, sequencing	
Novak, *Elmer Blunt's open house*	Sequencing descriptors	
Noll, *Jiggle, wiggle, prance*	Present progressive tense, vocabulary, prepositions	
Numeroff, *Dogs don't wear sneakers*	Negatives, verbs, noticing the ridiculous	ANIMALS
Numeroff, *If you give a mouse a cookie*	Sequencing, auditory and visual memory, cause and effect, temporal markers, idioms	
Numeroff, *If you give a moose a muffin*	Sequencing, auditory and visual memory, cause and effect, temporal markers, idioms	
Neitzel, *The jacket I wear in the snow*	Sequencing, chanting, auditory memory	WINTER, CLOTHES
Offen, *The sheep made a leap*	Following directions, verbs	
O'Malley, *Bruno, you're late for school* (No words)	Sequencing, descriptors	
Oxenbury, *The car trip*	Initial /k/ words	
Patron, *Dark Cloud, strong breeze*	Rhyming, following a theme/story line	
Peek, *Mary wore her red dress*	Predicting, color words, modifiers, initial /r/ words, initial and final /l/ words, chanting, visual detail, sequencing	COLORS, CLOTHES
Peppe, *Odd one out*	Visual attending, present progressive & past tense, vocabulary	
Piper, *Little engine that could*	Predicting	TRANSPORTATION
Philpot, *Amazing Anthony ant*	Creative rhyming, visual search	
Polushkin, *Mother, mother, I want another*	Noticing the ridiculous, rhyming, predicting	BEDTIME
Porter-Gaylord, *I love my daddy because*	Causal phrase, discussion	FAMIILY
Preston, *The temper tantrum book*	Discussion ("I hate it when…")	FEELINGS
Raskin, *Nothing ever happens on my block*	Sequencing, predicting, descriptors	
Raschka, *Yo! Yes?*	Question-answers, chanting, descriptors, inflection	FEELINGS
Rathman, *Good night, gorilla*	Sequencing, predicting, descriptors	BEDTIME

Book	Language Use	Theme
Reiss, *Colors*	Vocabulary, adjectives	COLORS
Riddell, *The trouble with elephants*	Noticing the ridiculous, discussion ("if...then")	
Rockwell, *Big wheels*	Vocabulary, adjectives, categories, relating experiences	TRANSPORTATION
Rockwell, *First comes spring*	Present progressive tense	SPRING
Rockwell, *The first snowfall*	Initial /st/ blends	WINTER
Rockwell, *My kitchen*	Vocabulary, categories	
Rockwell, *Things that go*	Vocabulary	TRANSPORTATION
Rockwell, *Things to play with*	Vocabulary	
Rockwell & Rockwell, *At the beach*	Present progressive tense, vocabulary, relating experiences	SUMMER
Roddie & Cony, *Hatch egg hatch*	Final /g, tʃ/ words	
Roe, *All I am*	Descriptors, discussion (All that you are)	SELF-ESTEEM
Roffey, *Look, there's my hat*	Pronouns	CLOTHES
Rosen & Oxenbury, *We're going on a bear hunt*	Initial /g, k, f/ blends	
Rosen & Robins, *Little rabbit foo foo*	Initial /g, k, f/ words	
Ross, *I'm coming to get you*	Predicting, discussion about fear and monsters	FEELINGS
Ruschak, *One hot day*	Superlatives, regular & irregular past tense	SUMMER
Russo, *The great treasure hunt*	Descriptors, visual searching	
Ryder, *Chipmunk song*	Imagining	
Ryder, *The snail's spell*	Imagining, blends	ANIMALS
Schecter, *When will the snow trees grow?*	"When...and" sentences	AUTUMN
Scheer, *Rain makes applesauce*	Predicting, noticing the ridiculous, chanting	
Schories, *Mouse around* (No words)	Descriptors, following a theme/story line	
Scieszka, *The true story of the three little pigs*	Predicting, regular & irregular past tense, compare to other versions	
Scott & Coalson, *Hi*	Initial /m/ words,...but sentences	MANNERS, COMMUNITY
Sendak, *Alligators all around*	Present progressive tense, noun-verb agreement	
Sendak, *Chicken soup with rice*	Predicting, months, chanting	
Sendak, *Pierre*	Chanting, negative, /k/ words	MANNERS
Seuss, *Hop on Pop*	Rhyming, initial and final /p/ words	
Shaw, *It looked like spilt milk*	Predicting, chanting, initial /l/ words, verbal expression	SENSES
Shaw, *Sheep in a shop*	Initial /ʃ/ and final /p/ words, verbs	COMMUNITY, BIRTHDAY
Shaw, *Sheep on a ship*	Initial /ʃ/ and final /p/ words, verbs	TRANSPORTATION
Shaw, *Sheep out to eat*	Initial /ʃ/ and final /p/ words, verbs	COMMUNITY
Silverstein, *Who wants to buy this cheap rhinoceros?*	Imagination	MANNERS

Book	Language Use	Theme
Slepian & Seidler, *The hungry thing returns*	Noticing the ridiculous, word & sound play	
Slobodkina, *Caps for sale*	Final /ps/ blends	CLOTHES
Small, *Imogene's antlers*	Imagination, discussion (What if . . .)	
Smalls-Hector, *Jonathan and his mommy* (M)	Verbs, following directions	FAMILY, COMMUNITY
Spier, *Dreams* (No words)	Imagining, descriptors	SUMMER
Stickland & Stickland, *Dinosaur roar!*	Rhyming, chanting	
Stinson, *Red is best*	Initial /r/ words	COLORS
Tafuri, *This is the farmer*	Third-person -*s* marker	
Teague, *Pigsty*	Noticing the ridiculous, initial /p/ words	ANIMALS
Tojhurst, *Somebody and the three Blairs*	Predicting (twist on The Three Bears), /b/ and b blends, past tense	
Turkle, *Deep in the forest* (No words)	Predicting, sequencing, following a theme/story line	
Vagin & Asch, *Here comes the cat!*	Predicting, chanting	TRANSPORTATION
Van Laan, *Possum come a-knockin'*	Present progressive tense	
Viorst, *Alexander and the terrible, horrible, no good, very bad day*	Categorization, inference, feelings, modifiers, functional vocabulary	FEELINGS
Viorst, *My mama says*	Adjectives, /k/ words	FEELINGS
Waddell & Oxenbury, *Father Duck*	Final /k/ words	
Wells, *Noisy Nora*	Present progressive & past tense, relating experiences	SENSES, MANNERS
Westcott, *The lady with the alligator purse*	Verbs, prepositions	
Wheeler, *Marmalade's yellow leaf*	Colors, prepositions	AUTUMN
Wildsmith, *The lazy bear*	Discussion	FEELINGS, MANNERS
Wildsmith, *What the moon saw*	Antonyms	
Williams, *The little old lady who was not afraid of anything*	Predicting, chanting	FEELINGS, CLOTHES, AUTUMN
Wolf, *And then what?*	Chanting, "and then . . ." sentences	
Wood, *King Bidgood's in the tub*	Predicting, /g/ words	
Wood, *The napping house*	Present progressive tense, adjectives, synonyms, cause and effect, descriptors, rhyming	BEDTIME
Wood, *Quick as a cricket*	Initial /l/ words	SELF-ESTEEM
Wood, *Silly Sally*	Initial /s/ relative clauses, chanting	
Yabuuchi, *Whose footprints?*	Posessive -'*s* marker, categories, vocabulary	ANIMALS
Young, *Golden bear* (M)	Verbs	
Zolotow, *Do you know what I'll do?*	Predicting, future tense, discussion	
Zolotow, *Some things go together*	Predicting, word associations, categorization	
Zolotow, *Someday*	Predicting, future tense, initial /s/ words	FEELINGS
Zolotow, *When I have a little boy*	Discussion	FAMILY

Book	Language Use	Theme
Zolotow, *When I have a little girl*	Discussion	FAMILY
Zukman & Edelman, *It's a good thing*	Verbal expression, discussion, "because…" structures	
(M) Denotes multicultural titles that feature minority characters.		

Source: Owens, R. E., & Robinson, L. A. (1997). Once upon a time: Use of children's literature in the preschool classroom. *Topics in Language Disorders, 17*(2), 19–48. Reprinted with permission.

Publications to Assist in Classroom Use of Books

Charner, K. (1993). *The Giant Encyclopedia of Theme Activities.* Mt. Rainier, MD: Gryphon House.

Gebers, J. (1990). *Books are for talking, too! A sourcebook for using children's literature in speech and language remediation.* Tucson, AZ: Communication Skill Builders.

Jett-Simpson, M. (Ed.). (1989). *Adventures with books: A booklist fore pre-K–grade 6.* Urbana, IL: National Council of Teachers of English.

Lockhart, B. (1992). *Read to me, Talk with me (Revised): Language activities based on children's favorite literature.* Tucson, AZ: Communication Skill Builders.

Raines, S. C., & Canady, R. J. (1989) *Story s-t-r-e-t-c-h-e-r-s: Activities to expand children's favorite books.* Mt. Rainier, MD: Gryphon House.

Trelease, J. (1989). *The new read-aloud handbook.* New York: Penguin.

J

Thematic Unit on Listening*

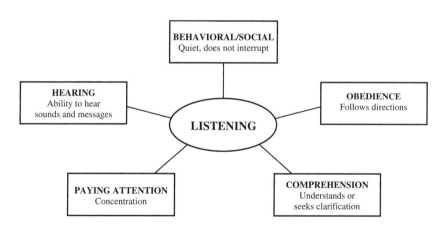

FIGURE J.1 **Semantic map for thematic unit on LISTENING, based on dimensions children used in their definitions of a "good listener."**

*Reprinted with permission of Mavis Donahue, University of Illinois at Chicago, and Carol Duggleby, Art Institute of Phoenix. Model of "good listening" adapted from Karen Czarnik, St. Xavier University, Chicago, Illinois.

HEARING DIMENSIONS

The Way We Hear

EARS ARE FOR HEARING

THE FIVE SENSES—HEARING

Study a model of the ear and different parts.

Study how sound changes through different mediums.

Make telephones from strings and cans.

Graph the number of ear infections each child has had.

Discuss balance.

  Do balance beam activities.

  Play statue with the children on the playground.

Sounds

TEACH ME ABOUT LISTENING

WHAT WAS THAT?

WHO SAID MEOW?

Take the children to a museum and visit an echo chamber.

Tape record different sounds and play games.

Hold inflated balloon and play loud music to feel vibrations.

Tape-record children's stories, describing the effect of loud and soft.

Have children discriminate between different animal sounds. It can be specific, such as animals of the ocean.

Make wind chimes from different media, such as tin lids, poker chips, PVC pipe, bamboo sticks.

Hearing Difficulties

A BUTTON IN HER EAR

THE MYSTERY OF THE BOY NEXT DOOR

Have an audiologist come in and test students' hearing. Graph the results.

Have children think about different kinds of occupations that might cause hearing loss, e.g., being a mechanic, a groundsperson for the airlines, a construction worker using jack hammers or heavy machinery.

*Have students interview a grandparent or older person about hearing devices.

Discuss how people with hearing difficulties "hear" a doorbell, alarms, and telephone.

Bring in a closed caption device for students to view.

Barriers

WHY MOSQUITOES BUZZ IN PEOPLE'S EARS

THE CAT WHO WORE A POT ON HER HEAD

Discuss the effects of not having the sun rise.

Play math games using story characters (e.g., adding the number of legs on the iguana and the fly).

*Interview parents about what they think causes poor listening. Graph results.

*home component

BEHAVIORAL/SOCIAL DIMENSIONS

Listen!

THE LISTENING WALK

Children go on a nature walk, keeping track of sounds. Be alert to noisy and quiet sounds. Graph the results.

WE'RE GOING ON A BEAR HUNT

Have the children use their imaginations on the bear hunt and think of other places and sounds. Draw a map or wall mural of the route.

THREE BILLY GOATS GRUFF

Design an obstacle course, having the children role-play the goats. They can only maneuver their way during the troll's snoring (drum beating).

Play Silence Game. Whisper children's names. They move silently to a line or another part of the room only when their name is whispered.

WILLY CAN COUNT

Make additional games of objects seen on the listening walk.

No Interruptions! I Can't Think

MARTHA SPEAKS

TOO MUCH NOISE

Martha speaks after eating alphabet soup. Read a series of scrambled letters to students that will form words.

*Students design posters of listening rules practiced in their homes.

*home component

Quiet Is Nice

TOO MUCH NOISE

A QUIET MOTHER AND THE NOISY BOY

*Make a list of noises that are at school/home. Graph results.

WISE OWL'S BOOK OF SOUNDS

What makes noises frightening? Write a spooky story.

HORTON HEARS A WHO

Why didn't the others hear a Who? Were they interrupting or talking? Discuss how Horton must have felt. Make a miniature village, using specific dimensions for the trees, roads, buildings, and so forth.

Socially Appropriate

OH BOTHER, NO ONE'S LISTENING

Two children read two different stories simultaneously. Have children give a synopsis of stories and discuss how hard the task was.

While practicing good listening, plan a picnic. Assign students different duties. Figure food portions, supplies, and costs. Students make all preparations, including food.

LITTLE MISS CHATTERBOX

Have students brainstorm about when it is necessary to talk very quietly and times to be very noisy.

TACKY THE PENGUIN

Re-enact the story and discuss the moral of the story. Poor social skills do not mean you're not a good "penguin."

OBEDIENCE DIMENSIONS

Following Directions

A POCKET FOR CORDUROY

BERENSTAIN BEARS AND THE SLUMBER PARTY

BERENSTAIN BEARS AND THE TRUTH

Discuss the consequences of not following directions. Students write stories of a specific time that they did not obey their parents.

STREGA NONA

Students prepare menus for restaurants. Specific directions on the types of food that are served in each restaurant are given. Using addition, subtraction, and money skills, students compute various costs of different foods.

*Students map their diet from dinner one evening. (e.g., pasta from Italy, potatoes from Idaho, etc.).

Strega Nona uses magic to make pasta. Listening to Anno's *MAGIC SEEDS,* let students discover how numbers greatly increase by calculating the number of seeds Anno has after 1 day, 5 days, etc.

*Students prepare a pasta luncheon for grandparents. They must follow directions in their preparations. Also, discuss the relationship of the volume of dried foods and cooked foods.

In addition to *STREGA NONA,* read *CLOUDY WITH A CHANCE OF MEATBALLS.* What listening skills are used? Give directions to children to monitor temperature, windspeed, and rainfall. (The wind and rain gauges can be made.) Compute averages and graph.

THE GINGERBREAD MAN

Discuss morals of stories. Students write stories with a moral. They also can do a wall mural or creative dramatics with this story.

Following Directions or Disobeying

PINKERTON, BEHAVE!

JUST ME AND MY BABYSITTER

JUST ME AND MY LITTLE SISTER

JUST ME AND MY PUPPY

Discuss the discrepancy between the directions and the listeners' responses. What are the listeners' intentions? Write stories using opposites. For example, "I am so hot that I need to put on my jacket."

*home component

PAYING ATTENTION DIMENSIONS

Paying Attention

THE CONVERSATION CLUB

Students must pick topics in which they are experts. They prepare a presentation or demonstration. Students ask questions and give constructive feedback on the presentation.

After reading *THE CONVERSATION CLUB,* the students write spooky stories on large rolls of paper. Make a TV from a large box. The students roll their stories on dowels and read to classmates.

BIGMOUTH

In *BIGMOUTH,* Bunny does not pay attention. What problems arise? Have students form groups, write a small play about not paying attention, and perform for younger grades.

Bunny is excited about moving to London. Pick historic landmarks and do replications of these with a report.

While reading, skip a key word and see if students can predict what it might be.

Write a group story, and erase certain words. Have students rewrite the story.

Have the students read a sentence from a book orally. Their partner must repeat the sentence. Use addition and subtraction to find the total number of words that a student can repeat correctly and the number of mistakes. Graph the results of the class.

NATE THE GREAT AND THE BORING BEACH BALL

Nate is a type of a detective. Have the students make maps of treasures that they have hidden.

Students develop "I Spy" game. Other students can have 10 turns to guess.

NOBODY LISTENS TO ME

MY MOTHER NEVER LISTENS TO ME

*Have students interview parents. Make a list of responses to "When is it easy and when is it hard to get parents' attention?"

*home component

COMPREHENSION DIMENSIONS

Misunderstandings Due to Lack of Shared Knowledge/Experiences

JUNE B. JONES AND THE STUPID SMELLY BUS

NEVER SPIT ON YOUR SHOES

THE PRINCIPAL FROM THE BLACK LAGOON

THE GYM TEACHER FROM THE BLACK LAGOON

Discuss why new experiences can be frightening or confusing. Write a journal article describing a new, yet scary experience.

YOU DON'T NEED WORDS

People in different cultures may use different gestures and sayings to express their thoughts. In groups, have students create a gesture system, such as crossing your fingers to say please. Determine the length of time it takes for other class members to break the code.

GOSSIP

Have students play "Through the Grapevine," where an initial student whispers a message in the next person's ear, and so on. See how distorted the message becomes.

FISH IS FISH

MOUSE SOUP

*In *FISH IS FISH* and *MOUSE SOUP*, the grass appears greener on the other side. These characters decide home is best. Have students interview parents or grandparents probing for the answers to: "Are there immigrants in our family? Why did they leave their homeland?"

In writing, have students write stories around an adage, such as "That's the pot calling the kettle black" or "You don't change horses in the middle of the stream."

GILA MONSTERS MEET YOU AT THE AIRPORT

Students design a travel agency. They determine the costs for tickets, food, and transportation. Students will be given a travel allowance to spend however they choose. Also, they must investigate what preparations would be necessary before traveling.

Words May Mean Different Things

THE KING WHO RAINED

THE SIXTEEN HAND HORSE

THE CHOCOLATE MOOSE

THE CASE OF THE DUMB BELLS

Students will write books using similes and metaphors, such as "She eats like a bird" or "It's raining cats and dogs." Have students illustrate their books.

Discuss humor. There's always an element of surprise. Have class compose a book similar to *WHEN YOU LICK A SLUG, YOUR TONGUE GOES NUMB.*

AMELIA BEDELIA SERIES

Amelia Bedelia gets out of jams by cooking. Students can make a sponge cake following oral directions. They can also make cakes in art using different mediums such as styrofoam packing pellets. For math, have students figure out problems using paper cakes, such as "if one large cake feeds six people, a medium feeds three, and a cupcake feeds one, how many different combinations will feed the class?"

ARABELLA AND MR. CRACK

Mr. Crack devises his own language system to run his household. Have students write a story with an invented language to see if classmates can crack the code.

*home component

Why Didn't I Ask Questions?

A MOOSE IS NOT A MOUSE

WELL WHY DIDN'T YOU SAY SO

Most of the time confusion can be cleared up by asking questions. Have students do a referential communication task using geometric shapes. This involves directing the students' placement of the shapes to a preconceived pattern. Have students do this with partners. First, do this task with the rule that the listener cannot ask questions. Then, do it again without that rule. Discuss the differences in the listener's ability to copy the pattern.

*Have students direct younger siblings, if possible, on how to make a peanut butter sandwich.

A FLY WENT BY

FOOLISH RABBIT'S BIG MISTAKE

WHY MOSQUITOES BUZZ IN PEOPLE'S EARS

Discuss the characters who FINALLY saved the day. What qualities did they possess?

In these books, a chain of negative events was caused by not questioning. Come up with ways to set into motion positive chains.

Draw a mural of the characters or do creative dramatics with students acting out the story.

Listening for Feelings

KASSIM'S SHOES

Kassim's tears were misinterpreted for tears of joy. Students journal how their feelings have been hurt.

COMMUNICATION

COMMUNICATION uses cartoons to illustrate the different ways a person can make comments, one hurting the listener's feelings, such as "You look different in your new glasses." Have students design their own cartoons.

DIFFERENT, NOT DUMB

LIAR, LIAR, PANTS ON FIRE

LOUDMOUTH GEORGE AND THE FISHING TRIP

Students can write and perform skits with an emphasis on social skills. Possible topics could include how to help kids understand when communication breaks down, how to become included in a game, how to solve a conflict, etc.

BARTHOLOMEW THE BOSSY

Bartholomew the Bossy formed a club. Have the students in your classroom discuss unfair practices and rules within the club. Provide a suggestion box as an avenue to discuss possible problems as they arise. In a similar vein, form a pen pal club or a club to save an endangered animal. Set goals for fundraising and purchases.

THE QUARRELING BOOK

PIGGYBOOK

*Do (or say) something nice for a parent in the morning. At the end of the day, ask the parent, "How was your day?" Keep results to see if this has any effect.

*home component

Glossary

AAC Method of communication that supplements or complements speech with other methods, such as signs, gestures, communication boards, or electronic signals.

ADHD Characterized by overactivity and an inability to attend for more than short periods of time. Although related to LD, the disorder does not manifest itself in severe perceptual and learning difficulties.

Anaphoric reference Linguistic device of referring to previously identified information, as in the use of pronouns to refer to previously introduced nouns.

Asperger's syndrome A mild form of pervasive development disorder in which the child exhibits LI and some autistic-like characteristics without the extreme "aloneness" found in many children with ASD.

Associative strategies A memory and retrieval strategy in which words are linked so that one aids recall of the other as in *red, white, and* _____.

Coda The ending part of a rime and can consist of up to three consonants.

Code switching The shifting from one language to another within and/or across different utterances.

Collaborative teaching An educational method that combines consultation, team teaching, direct individual intervention, and side-by-side teaching in which the teacher and speech-language pathologist share the same goals for individual children.

Communication event An entire conversation and/or the topic or topics included therein.

Conjunction A word that joins together sentences, clauses, phrases, or words.

Construct validity Accuracy with which or extent to which a measure describes or measures some trait or construct.

Content validity Faithfulness with which a sample or measure represents some attribute or behavior.

Contrast training Training method that teaches a child to discriminate between structures and situations that obligate use of the feature being trained and those features that do not.

Criterion validity Effectiveness or accuracy with which a measure predicts success.

Culture A shared framework of meanings within which a population shapes its way of life. Culture is what one needs to know or believe to function in a manner acceptable to a particular group. It includes, but is not limited to, history and the explanation of natural phenomenon; societal roles; rules for interactions, decorum, and discipline; family structure; education; religious beliefs; standards of health, illness, hygiene, appearance, and dress; diet; perceptions of time and space; definitions of work and play; artistical and musical values; life expectations; and aspirations; and communication and language use.

C-unit Nonclausal response to a question in which ellipsis or one main clause plus any attached or embedded subordinate clause or nonclausal structure (T-unit) is evident.

Deixis Process of using the speaker's perspective as a reference.

Dynamic assessment Assessment tasks suggested for children with limited English proficiency (LEP) that emphasize ability to communicate and learn language rather than ability to use grammar. Typical tasks are narration, conversation, or teach-test paradigms.

Dysgraphia A writing disorder characterized by letter reversal, misspellings, and word transposition due to no known emotional, environmental, intellectual, perceptual, or obvious neurological problem.

Dyslexia A reading disorder, characterized by word recognition and/or reading comprehension abilities two years below the expected level but not due to any known emotional, environmental, intellectual, perceptual, or obvious neurological problem.

Echolalia Immediate or delayed whole or partial repetition of previous utterances of others with the same intonational pattern.

Ellipsis Omission of known or shared information in subsequent utterances in which it would be redundant.

Figure-ground perception Perceptual ability to isolate a stimulus against a background.

Functional language intervention A client-based, communication-first assessment and intervention method that employs language as it is actually used as the vehicle for change.

Hyperactivity A motor difficulty of overactivity often associated with learning disabilities and accompanied by attention problems.

Hyperlexia A variety of Pervasive Developmental Disorder characterized by spontaneous early reading ability and an intense preoccupation with letters and words but little real reading comprehension.

Illocutionary function Intention(s) of a speaker.

Inclusive schooling An educational philosophy that proposes one integrated educational system—versus the two-tiered system, with regular and special education—based on each classroom becoming a supportive environment for all its members.

Interference The influence of one language on the learning and use of another.

Interjudge reliability The probability of two judges scoring a child's performance on a test in the same manner.

Interlanguage A combination of the rules of two languages plus ad hoc rules from neither or both languages.

Internal consistency Degree of relationship among items and the overall test.

Jargon Meaningless combination of words and sounds with the international pattern of speech.

Language impairment A heterogeneous group of developmental and/or acquired disorders and/or delays principally characterized by deficits and/or immaturities in the use of spoken or written language for comprehension and/or production purposes that may involve the form, content, and/or function of language in any combination.

Limited English Proficiency Proficiency in another language but not in English. The term is typically used for those who are not truly bilingual because of poor English language skills.

Maze Language segments that disrupt, confuse, and slow conversational movements. Mazes may consist of silent pauses, fillers, repetitions, and revisions.

Mediational strategies A memory and retrieval strategy in which a word or symbol, such as a category name, is used, as in "types of clothing" or "things that go in the kitchen."

Normed test A standardized test that has been given to a sample of individuals that supposedly represents all individuals for whom the test was designed. Scores are used to determine the typical performance expected for the entire population from whom the sample was drawn.

Onset The initial phonemes in a word consisting of up to three consonants, usually prior to the vowel.

PDD-NOS Pervasive Developmental Disorder—Not Otherwise Specified is mild form of PDD lacking the extreme characteristics of ASD.

Perseveration Repetition of the same behavior with a seeming inability to shift to another behavior or to stop.

Phonics Sound-letter correspondence used as the basis for most reading instruction.

Phonological awareness Literacy knowledge of the sounds and the sound and syllable structure of words. Better phonological awareness is related to better reading and spelling skills are to better phonological production.

Presupposition The speaker's assumption about the knowledge level of the listener, or what the listener knows and needs to know.

Print awareness Literacy knowledge that includes knowing the direction in which reading proceeds across a page and through a book, being interested in print, recognizing letters, knowing that words are discrete units, and using literacy terminology, such as *letter, work,* and *sentence.*

Prognosis Estimate of the rate and extent of recovery from illness or injury.

Recast Changed form of a child's utterance that maintains the same relation and immediately follows the child's utterance.

Referential communication Speaker selects and verbally identifies attributes of an entity, thereby enabling the listener to identify the entity accurately.

Reliability Repeatability of a measure, based on the accuracy or precision with which a sample, at one time, represents performance based on either a different but similar sample or the same sample at a different time.

Rime The part of a word that follows the onset and consists of a nucleus or vowel and a coda.

Script Basic sequential notion of familiar events.

Semantic networking A method of improving reading comprehension, writing cohesion, retention, and recall by teaching organization of information around a central theme or sequence.

Sensory integration Interpretation and synthesis of information received from two or more senses, such as hearing and vision.

Social disinhibition Inability to inhibit "acting out" behaviors often seen with traumatic brain injury.

Standard error of measure (SEm) The statistical error inherent in a score, representing the range that a score may indicate.

Standardized test Test in which items are presented, cued, and consequated in a prescribed manner.

Story grammar Organizational pattern of narratives.

Strategy-based intervention model Training that teaches the child information processing and problem-solving strategies.

Systems model Intervention that targets the child's interactive systems or contexts.

Topic The subject matter about which the speaker is either providing or requesting information.

T-units (minimal terminal units) A main clause plus any attached or embedded subordinate clause or nonclausal structure.

Type-token ratio Ratio of the number of different words to the total number of words, used as a measure of vocabulary and word retrieval.

Validity Effectiveness of a test in representing, describing, or predicting an attribute. A test's ability to assess what it purports to measure.

Working memory Memory in which information is kept active while processed.

References

Abbeduto, L., Davies, B., Solesby, S., & Furman, L. (1991). Identifying the referents of spoken messages: Use of context and clarification requests by children with and without mental retardation. *American Journal on Mental Retardation, 95,* 551–562.

Abbeduto, L., Furman, L., & Davies, B. (1989). Relation between the receptive language and mental age of persons with mental retardation. *American Journal on Mental Retardation, 93,* 535–545.

Abbeduto, L., Short-Meyerson, K., Benson, G., & Dolish, J. (1997). Signaling of noncomprehension by children and adolescents with mental retardation: Effects of problem type and speaker identity. *Journal of Speech, Language, and Learning Research, 40,* 20–32

Abkarian, G., Jones, A., & West, G. (1992). Young children's idiom comprehension: Trying to get the picture. *Journal of Speech and Hearing Research, 35,* 580–587.

Acevedo, M. A. (1986). Assessment instruments for minorities. In F. H. Bess, B. S. Clark, & H. R. Mitchell (Eds.), *Concerns for minority groups in communication disorders* (pp. 46–51). Rockville, MD: American Speech-Language-Hearing Association.

Ackerman, P., Dykman, R., & Gardner, M. (1990). Counting rate, naming rate, phonological sensitivity, and memory span: Major factors in dyslexia. *Journal of Learning Disabilities, 23,* 325–327.

Adams, M. (1990). *Beginning to read: Thinking and learning about print.* Cambridge: MIT Press.

Adamson, L. B., Romski, M. A., Deffenbach, K., & Sevik, R. A. (1992). Symbol vocabulary and the focus of conversations: Augmenting language development for youth with mental retardation. *Journal of Speech and Hearing Research, 35,* 1333–1343.

Adler, S. (1988). A new job description and a new task for the public school clinician: Relating effectively to the nonstandard dialect speaker. *Language, Speech, and Hearing Services in Schools, 19,* 28–33.

Adler, S. (1990). Multicultural clients: Implications for the speech-language pathologist. *Language, Speech, and Hearing Services in Schools, 21,* 135–139.

Adler, S. (1991). Assessment of language proficiency in limited English proficient speakers: Implications for the speech-language specialist. *Language, Speech, and Hearing Services in Schools, 22,* 12–18.

Allen, J. B., & Mason, J. M. (1989). *Risk makers, risk takers, risk breakers: Reducing the risks for young literacy learners.* Portsmouth, NH: Heinemann.

Allen, R. E., & Wasserman, G. A. (1985). Origins of language delay in abused children. *Child Abuse and Neglect, 9,* 333–338.

Alpert, C., & Rogers-Warren, A. (1984). *Mothers as incidental language trainers of their language-disordered children*. Unpublished manuscript, University of Kansas, Lawrence.

American Association on Mental Retardation (AAMR). (1992). *Mental retardation: Definition, classification, and systems of support* (9th ed.). Washington, DC: Author.

American Psychiatric Association (APA). (1996). *Diagnostic and statistical manual of mental disorders* (DSM-IV-R; 4th ed. rev.). Washington, DC: Author.

American Speech-Language-Hearing Association (ASHA). (1983). Position of the American Speech-Language-Hearing Association on social defects. *Asha, 25*(9), 23–25.

American Speech-Language-Hearing Association. (2001). *Roles and responsibilities of speech-language pathologists with respect to reading and writing in children and adolescents* (position paper, technical report, and guidelines). Rockville, MD: Author.

Anderson, G., & Nelson, N. (1988). Integrating language intervention and education in an alternate adolescent language classroom. *Seminars in Speech and Language, 9,* 341–353.

Anderson, N. B. (1991). Understanding cultural diversity. *American Journal of Speech-Language Pathology, 1*(3), 9–10.

Anderson, N. B. (1992). Understanding cultural diversity. *American Journal of Speech-Language Pathology, 1*(2), 11–12.

Anderson, R. C., & Davison, A. (1988). Conceptual and empirical bases of readability formulas. In G. Green & A. Davison (Eds.), *Linguistic complexity and text comprehension* (pp. 23–54). Hillsdale, NJ: Lawrence Erlbaum.

Anderson, R. C., Hiebert, E., Scott, J. A., & Wilkenson, J. A. (1985). *Becoming a nation of readers*. Washington, DC: National Institute of Education.

Anderson, R. T. (1996). Assessing the grammar of Spanish-speaking children: A comparison of two procedures. *Language, Speech, and Hearing Services in Schools, 27,* 333–344.

Andrews, J., Andrews, M., & Shearer, W. (1989). Parents' attitudes toward involvement in speech-language services. *Language, Speech, and Hearing Services in Schools, 20,* 391–399.

Anselmi, D., Tomasello, M., & Acunzo, M. (1986). Young children's responses to neutral and specific contingent queries. *Journal of Child Language, 13,* 135–144.

Applebee, A. N. (1978). *The child's concept of story.* Chicago: University of Chicago Press.

Aram, D. M. (1988). Language sequelae of unilateral brain lesions in children. In F. Plumb (Ed.), *Language, com-munication, and the brain* (pp. 171–197). New York: Raven.

Aram, D. M. (1991). Comments on specific language impairment as a clinical category. *Language, Speech, and Hearing Services in Schools, 22,* 84–87.

Aram, D. M. (1997). Hyperlexia: Reading without meaning in young children. *Topics in Language Disorders, 17*(3), 1–13.

Aram, D. M., & Eisele, J. A. (1994). Limits to a left hemisphere explanation of specific language impairment. *Journal of Speech and Learning Research, 37,* 824–830.

Aram, D. M., & Ekelman, B. L. (1987). Unilateral brain lesions in children: Performance on the Revised Token Test. *Brain and Language, 32,* 137–158.

Aram, D. M., & Ekelman, B. L. (1988). Scholastic aptitude and achievement among children with unilateral brain lesions. *Neuropsychologia, 26,* 903–916.

Aram, D. M., Ekelman, B. L., & Whitaker, H. A. (1986). Spoken syntax in children with acquired unilateral hemispheric lesions. *Brain and Language, 27,* 75–100.

Aram, D. M., Ekelman, B. L., & Whitaker, H. A. (1987). Lexical retrieval in left and right brain lesioned children. *Brain and Language, 31,* 61–87.

Aram, D. M., Morris, R., & Hall, N. (1993). Clinical and research congruence in identifying children with specific language impairment. *Journal of Speech and Hearing Research, 36,* 580–591.

Armbuster, B. B., Anderson, T. H., & Ostertag, J. (1987). Does text structure/summarization instruction facilitate learning from expository text? *Reading Research Quarterly, 22,* 331–346.

ASHA Position Paper. (1985, June). Clinical management of communicatively handicapped minority language populations. *Asha, 27*(6), 29–32.

Astington, J. (1990). Narrative and the child's theory of mind. In B. K. Britton & A. D. Pelligrini (Eds.), *Narrative thought and narrative language* (pp. 151–171). Hillsdale, NJ: Erlbaum.

Atkinson, R. H., & Longman, D. G. (1985). Sniglets: Give a twist to teenage and adult vocabulary instruction. *Journal of Reading, 29,* 103–105.

Atlas, J. A., & Lapadis, L. B. (1988). Symbolization levels in communicative behaviors of children showing pervasive developmental disorders. *Journal of Communication Disorders, 21,* 75–84.

Audet, L. R., & Hummel, L. J. (1990). A framework for assessment and treatment of language-learning disabled children with psychiatric disorders. *Topics in Language Disorders, 10*(4), 57–74.

Baddeley, A. (1996). Exploring the central executive. *Quarterly Journal of Experimental Psychology: A Human Experimental Psychology, 49A*(1), 5–28.

Bailet, L. L. (1990). Spelling rule usage among students with learning disabilities and normally achieving students. *Journal of Learning Disabilities, 18,* 162–165.

Bain, B., Olswang, L., & Johnson, G. (1992). Language sampling for repeated measures with language impaired preschoolers: Comparison of two procedures. *Topics in Language Disorders, 12*(2), 13–27.

Baker, J. G., Ceci, S. J., & Hermann, D. (1987): Semantic structure and processing: Implications for the learning disabled child. In H. L. Swanson (Ed.), *Memory and learning disability: Advances in learning and behavioral disabilities.* Greenwich, CT: JAI Press.

Baker, L., & Brown, A. L. (1984). Metacognitive skills and reading. In P. D. Pearson, M. Kamil, R. Barr, & P. Moesenthal (Eds.), *Handbook of reading research* (pp. 353–394). New York: Longman.

Balota, D. A., & Duchek, J. (1989). Age-related differences in lexical access, spreading activation, and simple pronunciation. *Psychology and Aging, 3,* 84–93.

Barrow, I. M., Holbert, D., & Rastatter, M. P. (2000). Effect of color on developmental picture-vocabulary naming of 4-, 6-, and 8-year-old children. *American Journal of Speech-Language Pathology, 9,* 310–318.

Bashir, A. S. (1989). Language intervention and the curriculum. *Seminars in Speech and Language, 10*(3), 181–191.

Basil, C. (1992). Social interaction and learned helplessness in severely disabled children. *Augmentative and Alternative Communication, 8,* 188–199.

Bass, P. M. (1988, November). *Attention deficit disorder/Management in preschool, adolescent, and adult populations.* Paper presented at the Annual Conference of the American Speech-Language-Hearing Association, Boston.

Bates, E., Bretherton, I., & Snyder, L. (1988). *From first words to grammar: Individual differences and dissociable mechanisms.* New York: Cambridge University Press.

Bates, E., O'Connell, B., & Shore, C. (1987). Language and communication in infancy. In J. Osofsky (Ed.), *Handbook of infant development* (pp. 149–203). New York: John Wiley.

Battle, D. (1990, March). *Black dialects.* Paper presented at the Spring Workshop of the Genesee Valley Speech-Language-Hearing Association, Rochester, NY.

Battle, D. E. (1993). *Communication disorders in multicultural populations.* Boston: Andover Medical Publishers.

Bauer, N. M., & Sapona, R. H. (1988). Facilitating communication as a basis for intervention for students with severe behavior disorders. *Journal of the Council for Children with Behavior Disorders, 13,* 280–287.

Bauer, S. (1995a). Autism and the pervasive developmental disorders: Part I. *Pediatrics in Review, 16*(4), 130–136.

Bauer, S. (1995b). Autism and the pervasive developmental disorders: Part II. *Pediatrics in Review, 16*(5), 168–176.

Bear, D., Invernizzi, M., Templeton, S., & Johnston, F. (2000). *Words their way: Word study for phonics, vocabulary, and spelling instruction* (2nd ed.). Upper Saddle River, NJ: Prentice Hall.

Beastrom, S., & Rice, M. (1986, November). *Comprehension and production of the articles "a" and "the."* Paper presented at the Convention of the American Speech-Language-Hearing Association, Detroit.

Beck, A.R., & Dennis, M. (1997). Speech-language pathologists and teachers' perceptions of classroom-based interventions. *Language, Speech, and Hearing Services in Schools, 28,* 146–153.

Beck, I. L., McKeown, M. G., & Omanson, R. C. (1987). The effects and uses of diverse vocabulary instructional techniques. In M. G. McKeown & M. E. Curtis (Eds.), *The nature of vocabulary acquisition* (pp. 147–164). Hillsdale, NJ: Lawrence Erlbaum.

Bedore, L. M., & Leonard, L. B. (1998). Specific language impairment and grammatical morphology: A discriminant function analysis. *Journal of Speech, Language, and Hearing Research, 41,* 1185–1192.

Bedore, L. M., & Leonard, L. B. (2001). Grammatical morphology deficits in Spanish-speaking children with specific language impairment. *Journal of Speech, Language, and Hearing Research, 44,* 905–924.

Bedrosian, J. L. (1982). *A sociolinguistic approach to communication skills: Assessment and treatment methodology for mentally retarded adults.* Unpublished doctoral dissertation, University of Wisconsin.

Bedrosian, J. L. (1985). An approach to developing conversational competence. In D. N. Ripich & R. M. Spinelli (Eds.), *School discourse problems* (pp. 231–255). San Diego: College-Hill.

Bedrosian, J. L. (1988). Adults who are mildly to moderately mentally retarded: Communicative performance, assessment, and intervention. In S. Calculator & J. Bedrosian (Eds.), *Communication assessment and intervention for adults with mental retardation* (pp. 265–307). San Diego: College-Hill.

Bedrosian, J. L. (1993). Making minds meet: Assessment of conversational topic in adults with mild to moderate mental retardation. *Topics in Language Disorders, 13*(3), 36–46.

Bedrosian, J. L., & Willis, T. (1987). Effects of treatment on the topic performance of a school-age child. *Language, Speech, and Hearing Services in Schools, 18,* 158–167.

Beeghly, M., Jernberg, E., & Burrows, E. (1989). *Validity of the Early Language Inventory (ELI) for use with 25-month-olds.* Paper presented at the Biennial Meeting of the Society for Research in Child Development.

Bell, D. (1995). Speech-language pathologists respond to inclusion: Survey and study results. *Advance for Speech-Language Pathologists and Audiologists, 5*(21).

Ben-Yishay, Y. (1985). *Rehabilitation of cognitive and perceptual deficits in persons with chronic brain damage: A comparative study. Annual progress report.* New York: New York University, Medical and Research Training Center for Head Trauma and Stroke.

Berninger, V. W. (2000). Development of language by hand and its connections with language by ear, mouth, and eye. *Topics in Language Disorders, 20*(4), 65–84.

Berninger, V. W., Abbott, R., Rogan, L., Reed, L., Abbott, S., Brooks, A., Vaughan, K., & Graham, S. (1998a). Teaching spelling to children with specific learning disabilities: The mind's ear and eye beats the computer and pencil. *Learning Disability Quarterly, 21,* 106–122.

Berninger, V. W., Cartwright, A., Yates, C., Swanson, H. L., & Abbott, R. (1994). Developmental skills related to writing and reading acquisition in the intermediate grades: Shared and unique variance. *Reading and Writing: An Interdisciplinary Journal, 6,* 161–196.

Berninger, V. W., & Swanson, H. L. (1994). Modifying Hayes & Flower's model of skilled writing to explain beginning and developing writing. In E. Butterfield (Ed.), *Children's writing: Toward a process theory of development of skilled writing* (pp. 57–81). Greenwich, CT: JAI Press.

Berninger, V. W., Vaughan, K., Abbott, R., Brooks, A., Abbott, S., Reed, E., Rogan, L., & Graham, S. (1998b). Early intervention for spelling problems: Teaching spelling units of varying size within a multiple connections framework. *Journal of Educational Psychology, 90,* 587–605.

Bernstein, D. (1986). The development of humor: Implications for assessment and intervention. *Topics in Language Disorders, 1*(4), 47–58.

Bernstein, D. (1989). Assessing children with limited English proficiency: Current prospectives. *Topics in Language Disorders, 9*(3), 15–20.

Beukelman, D. R., Jones, R., & Rowan, M. (1989). Frequency of word usage by non-disabled peers in integrated preschool programs. *Augmentative and Alternative Communication, 5,* 243–248.

Beukelman, D. R., McGinnis, J., & Morrow, D. (1991). Vocabulary selection in augmentative and alternative communication. *Augmentative and Alternative Communication, 7,* 171–185.

Biber, D. (1986). Spoken and written textual dimensions in English: Resolving the contradictory findings. *Language, 62,* 384–414.

Bird, J., Bishop, D. V., & Freeman, N. H. (1995). Phonological awareness and literacy development in children with expressive phonological impairments. *Journal of Speech and Hearing Research, 38,* 446–462.

Bishop, D. V. (1982). Comprehension of spoken, written, and signed sentences in childhood language disorders. *Journal of Child Psychology and Psychiatry, 23,* 1–20.

Bishop, D. V. (1985). Automated LARSP [Computer program]. Manchester, England: University of Manchester.

Bishop, D. V., & Adams, C. (1992). Comprehension problems in children with specific language impairments: Literal and inferential meaning. *Journal of Speech and Hearing Research, 35,* 119–129.

Bishop, D. V., & Bishop, S. J. (1998). "Twin language": A risk factor for language impairment? *Journal of Speech, Language, and Hearing Research, 41,* 150–160.

Bishop, D. V., North, T., & Donlan, C. (1996). Nonword repetition as a behavioral marker in inherited language impairment: Evidence from a twin study. *Journal of Child Psychology and Psychiatry, 37,* 391–403.

Bjork, R. A., & Bjork, E. L. (1992). A new theory of disuse and an old theory of stimulus fluctuation. In A. F. Healy, S. M. Kosslyn, & R. M. Shiffrin (Eds.), *From learning processes to cognitive processes: Essays in honor of William K. Estes* (Vol. 2, pp. 35–67). Hillsdale, NJ: Lawrence Erlbaum.

Blachman, B. (1984). Relationship of rapid naming ability and language analysis skills in kindergarten and first grade reading achievement. *Reading Research Quarterly, 13,* 223–253.

Blalock, J., & Johnson, D. (1987). *Adults with learning disabilities: Clinical studies.* New York: Grune & Stratton.

Blank, M., & Marquis, A. (1987). *Directing discourse: 80 situations for teaching meaningful conversations to children.* Tucson, AZ: Communication Skill Builders.

Bleile, K. M., & Wallach, H. (1992). A sociolinguistic investigation of the speech of African American preschoolers. *American Journal of Speech-Language Pathology, 1*(2), 54–62.

Bliss, L. S. (1987). "I can't talk any more: My mouth doesn't want to." The developmental and clinical applications of modal auxiliaries. *Language, Speech, and Hearing Services in Schools, 18,* 72–79.

Bliss, L. S. (1989). Selected syntactic usage by language impaired children. *Journal of Communication Disorders, 22,* 277–289.

Bliss, L. S. (1992). A comparison of tactful messages by children with and without language impairments. *Language, Speech, and Hearing Services in Schools, 23,* 343–347.

Bloom, L., & Lahey, M. (1978). *Language development and language disorders.* New York: John Wiley.

Bloom, L., Lahey, M., Hood, L., Lifter, K., & Fiess, K. (1980). Complex sentences: Acquisition of syntactic connectives and the semantic relations they encode. *Journal of Child Language, 7,* 235–261.

Bloomberg, K., Karlan, G., & Lloyd, L. (1990). The comparative translucency of initial lexical items represented in five graphic symbol systems and sets. *Journal of Speech and Hearing Research, 33,* 717–725.

Borgh, K., & Dickson, W. P. (1986, April). *The effects on children's writing of adding speech synthesis to a word processor.* Paper presented at the Annual Meeting of the American Educational Research Association, San Francisco.

Borsch, J. C., & Oaks, R. (1992). Effective collaboration at Central Elementary School. *Language, Speech, and Hearing Services in Schools, 23,* 367–368.

Bosman, A., & van Orden, G. (1997). Why spelling is more difficult than reading. In C. Perfetti, L. Riebert, & M. Fayol (Eds.), *Learning to spell: Research, theory, and practice across languages* (pp. 173–194). Mahwah, NJ: Lawrence Erlbaum.

Boudreau, D. M., & Chapman, R. S. (2000). The relationship between event representation and linguistic skill in narratives of children and adolescents with Down syndrome. *Journal of Speech, Language, and Hearing Research, 43,* 1146–1159.

Boudreau, D. M., & Hedberg, N. L. (1999). A comparison of early literacy skills in children with specific language impairment and their typically developing peers. *American Journal of Speech-Language Pathology, 8,* 249–260.

Bourassa, D. C., & Treiman, R. (2001). Spelling development and disability: The importance of linguistic factors. *Language, Speech, and Hearing Services in Schools, 32*(3), 172–181.

Bowers, P. G., Steffy, R. A., & Swanson, L. B. (1986). Naming speed, memory, and visual processing in reading disability. *Canadian Journal of Behavioral Science, 18,* 209–223.

Bowers, P. G., & Swanson, L. B. (1991). Naming speed deficits in reading disability: Multiple measures of a singular process. *Journal of Experimental Child Psychology, 51,* 195–219.

Bowey, J., & Hansen, J. (1994). The development or orthographic rimes as units of word recognition. *Journal of Experimental Psychology, 58,* 465–488.

Bowman, S. (1984). A review of referential communication skills. *Australian Journal of Human Communication Disorders, 12,* 93–112.

Boyce, N., & Larson, V. L. (1983). *Adolescents' communication: Development and disorders.* Eau Claire, WI: Thinking Publications.

Bracken, B. (1988). Rate and sequence of positive and negative poles in basic concept acquisition. *Language, Speech, and Hearing Services in Schools, 19,* 410–417.

Bradley, L., & Bryant, P. (1985). *Rhyme and reason in reading and spelling.* Ann Arbor: University of Michigan Press.

Bradshaw, M. L., Hoffman, P. R., & Norris, J. A. (1998). Efficacy of expansions and cloze procedures in the development of interpretations by preschool children exhibiting delayed language development. *Language, Speech, and Hearing Services in Schools, 29,* 85–95.

Brandel, D. (1992). Collaboration: Full steam ahead with no prior experience! *Language, Speech, and Hearing Services in Schools, 23,* 369–370.

Braten, I. (1994). *Learning to spell.* Oslo, Norway: Scandanavian University Press.

Brice, A., & Montgomery, J. (1996). Adolescent pragmatic skills: A comparison of Latino students in English as a second language and speech and language programs. *Language, Speech, and Hearing Services in Schools, 27,* 68–81.

Bricker, D. D. (1986). *Early education of at-risk and handicapped infants, toddlers, and preschool children.* Glenview, IL: Scott, Foresman.

Brinton, B., & Fujiki, M. (1982). A comparison of request-response sequences in the discourse of normal and language-disordered children. *Journal of Speech and Hearing Disorders, 47,* 57–62.

Brinton, B., & Fujiki, M. (1989). *Conversational management with language-impaired children: Pragmatic assessment and intervention.* Rockville, MD: Aspen.

Brinton, B., & Fujiki, M. (1992). Setting the context for conversational language sampling. *Best Practices in School Speech Language Pathology, 2,* 9–19.

Brinton, B., Fujiki, M., & Higbee, L. M. (1998). Participation in cooperative learning activities by children with specific language impairment. *Journal of Speech, Language, and Hearing Research, 41,* 1193–1206.

Brinton, B., Fujiki, M., & McKee, L. (1998). Negotiating skills of children with specific language impairment. *Journal of Speech, Language, and Hearing Research, 41,* 927–940.

Brinton, B., Fujiki, M., & Sonnenberg, E. (1988). Responses to requests for clarification by linguistically normal and language-impaired children in conversation. *Journal of Speech and Hearing Disorders, 53,* 383–391.

Brinton, B., Fujiki, M., Winkler, E., & Loeb, D. (1986). Responses to requests for clarification in linguistically normal and language-impaired children. *Journal of Speech and Hearing Disorders, 51,* 370–378.

Briscoe, J., Gathercole, S. E., & Marlow, N. (1998). Short-term memory and language outcomes after extreme prematurity at birth. *Journal of Speech, Language, and Hearing Research, 41,* 654–666.

Bristol, M. (1985). Designing programs for young developmentally disabled children: A family systems approach to autism. *Remedial and Special Education, 6*(4), 46–53.

Bristol, M. (1988). Impact of autistic children on families. In B. Prizant & B. Schaechter (Eds.), *Autism: The emotional and social dimensions.* Boston: The Exceptional Parent.

Broen, P. A., & Westman, M. J. (1990). Project parent: A preschool speech program implemented through parents. *Journal of Speech and Hearing Disorders, 55,* 495–502.

Brown, A. L., & Palincsar, A. S. (1982). Inducing strategic learning from texts by means of informed, self-control training. *Topics in Learning and Learning Disabilities, 2,* 1–17.

Brown, J. (1989). The truth about scores children achieve on tests. *Language, Speech, and Hearing Services in Schools, 20,* 366–371.

Brown, L., Shiraga, B., Rogan, P., York, J., Zanella Albright, K., McCarthy, E., Loomis, R., & Van-Deventer, P. (1988). The "why" question in instruction programs for people who are severely intellectually disabled. In S. Calculator & J. Bedrosian (Eds.), *Communication assessment and intervention for adults with mental retardation* (pp. 139–153). San Diego: College-Hill.

Brown, R. (1973). *A first language: The early stages.* Cambridge, MA: Harvard University Press.

Browne, K., & Sagi, S. (1988). Mother-infant interaction and attachment in physically abusing families. *Journal of Reproductive and Infant Psychology, 6,* 163–182.

Bruck, M., & Waters, G. (1990). An analysis of the component spelling and reading skills of good readers-good spellers, good readers-poor spellers, and poor readers-poor spellers. In T. Carr & B. Levy (Eds.), *Reading and its development* (pp. 161–206). San Diego, CA: Academic Press.

Bryen, D., Goldman, A., & Quinlisk-Gill, S. (1988). Sign language with students with severe/profound mental retardation: How effective is it? *Education and Training in Mental Retardation, 23,* 129–137.

Bryen, D., & Joyce, D. (1985). Language intervention with the severely handicapped: A decade of research. *Journal of Special Education, 19,* 7–39.

Bryen, D., & McGinley, V. (1991). Sign language input to community residents with mental retardation. *Education and Training in Mental Retardation, 26,* 207–214.

Buchannan, E. (1989). *Spelling for whole-language classrooms.* Winnipeg, Canada: Whole Language Consultants.

Bunce, B. (1989). Using a barrier game format to improve children's referential communication skills. *Journal of Speech and Hearing Disorders, 54,* 33–43.

Bunce, B., Ruder, K., & Ruder, C. (1985). Using the miniature linguistic system in teaching syntax: Two case studies. *Journal of Speech and Hearing Disorders, 50,* 247–253.

Burke, A. E., Crenshaw, D. A., Green, J., Schlosser, M. A., & Strocchia-Rivera, L. (1989). Influence of verbal ability on the expression of aggression in physically abused children. *Journal of the American Academy of Child and Adolescent Psychiatry, 28,* 215–218.

Butkowsky, I. S., & Willows, D. M. (1980). Cognitive-motivational characteristics of children varying in reading ability: Evidence for learned helplessness in poor readers. *Journal of Educational Psychology, 72,* 408–422.

Butler, K. (1986). *Language disorders in children.* Austin, TX: Pro-Ed.

Butler, K. (1993, November). *Toward a model of dynamic assessment: Application to speech.* Paper presented at the Annual Convention of the American Speech-Language-Hearing Association, Anaheim, CA.

Butler-Hinz, S., Caplan, D., & Waters, G. (1990). Characteristics of syntactic comprehension deficits following closed head injury versus left cerebrovascular accident. *Journal of Speech and Hearing Research, 33,* 269–280.

Buttrill, J., Niizawa, J., Biemer, C., Takahashi, C., & Hearn, S. (1989). Serving the language learning disabled adolescent: A strategies-based model. *Language, Speech, and Hearing Services in Schools, 20,* 185–204.

Buzock, K., & League, R. (1978). *Receptive Expressive Emergent Language Test.* Austin, TX: Pro-Ed.

Buzolich, M., King, J., & Baroody, S. (1991). Acquisition of the commenting function among system users. *Augmentative and Alternative Communication, 7,* 88–99.

Buzolich, M., & Wiemann, J. (1988). Turn-taking in atypical conversations: The case of the speaker-augmented communicator dyad. *Journal of Speech and Hearing Research, 31,* 3–18.

Calandrella, A. M., & Wilcox, M. J. (2000). Predicting language outcomes for young prelinguistic children with developmental delay. *Journal of Speech, Language, and Hearing Research, 43,* 1061–1071.

Calculator, S. (1985). Describing and treating discourse problems in mentally retarded children: The myth of mental retardese. In D. Ripich & F. Spinelli (Eds.), *School discourse problems* (pp. 125–147). San Diego: College-Hill.

Calculator, S. N. (1988a). Exploring the language of adults with mental retardation. In S. Calculator & J. Bedrosian (Eds.), *Communication assessment and intervention for adults with mental retardation* (pp. 95–106). San Diego: College-Hill.

Calculator, S. N. (1988b). Promoting the acquisition and generalization of conversational skills by individuals with severe disabilities. *Augmentative and Alternative Communication, 4,* 94–103.

Calculator, S. N. (1988c). Teaching functional communication skills to adults with mental retardation. In S. Calculator & J. Bedrosian (Eds.), *Communication assessment and intervention for adults with mental retardation* (pp. 309–338). San Diego: College-Hill.

Calculator, S. N., & Delaney, D. (1986). Comparison of nonspeaking and speaking mentally retarded adults' clarification strategies. *Journal of Speech and Hearing Research, 51,* 252–259.

Calculator, S. N., & Dollaghan, C. (1982). The use of communication boards in a residential setting: An evaluation. *Journal of Speech and Hearing Disorders, 47,* 281–287.

Calculator, S. N., & Jorgensen, C. M. (1991). Integrating AAC instruction into regular education settings: Expounding on best practices. *Augmentative and Alternative Communication, 7,* 204–214.

Calfee, R., & Calfee, K. (1981). *Interactive reading assessment systems.* Unpublished manuscript, Stanford University. (Available from authors)

Calvert, M. B., & Murray, S. L. (1985). Environmental Communication Profile: An assessment procedure. In C. S. Simon (Ed.), *Communication skills and classroom success: Assessment of language-learning disabled students* (pp. 135–165). Austin, TX: Pro-Ed.

Camarata, S. M., Hughes, C., & Ruhl, K. (1988). Mild/moderate behaviorally disordered students: A population at risk for language disorders. *Language, Speech, and Hearing Services in Schools, 19,* 191–200.

Camarata, S. M., Nelson, K., & Camarata, M. (1994). Comparison of conversational-recasting and imitative procedures for training grammatical structures in children with specific language impairment. *Journal of Speech and Hearing Research, 37,* 1414–1423.

Camarata, S. M., Nelson, K. E., Welsh, J., Butkowski, L., Harmer, M., & Camarata, M. (1991, October). The effects of treatment procedures on normal language acquisition [abstract]. *Asha,* p. 152.

Campbell, C. R., & Jackson, S. T. (1995). Transparency of one-handed Amer-Ind hand signals to unfamiliar viewers. *Journal of Speech and Hearing Research, 38,* 1284–1289.

Campbell, L. R. (1993). Maintaining the integrity of home linguistic varieties: Black English vernacular. *American Journal of Speech-Language Pathology, 2*(1), 11–12.

Campbell, L. R., & Champion, T. (1996, November). *Bridging the gap between home and school cultures.* Paper presented at the annual convention of the American Speech-Language-Hearing Association, Seattle.

Campbell, S. B. (1985). Hyperactivity in preschoolers: Correlates and prognostic implications. *Clinical Psychology Review, 5,* 405–428.

Campbell, T., Dollaghan, C., Needleman, H., & Janosky, J, (1997). Reducing bias in language assessment: Processing-dependent measures. *Journal of Speech, Language, and Hearing Research, 40,* 519-525.

Campbell, T. F., & Dollaghan, C. A. (1990). Expressive language recovery in severely brain-injured children and adolescents. *Journal of Speech and Hearing Disorders, 55,* 567–581.

Campbell, T. F., & Dollaghan, C. A. (1992). A method for obtaining listener judgments of spontaneously produced language: Social validation through direct magnitude estimation. *Topics in Language Disorders, 12*(2), 42–55.

Carlisle, J. F. (1988). Knowledge of derivational morphology and spelling ability in fourth, sixth, and eighth graders. *Applied Psycholinguistics, 9,* 247–266.

Carlson, J., & Wiedl, K. H. (1992). Use of testing-the-limits procedures in the assessment of intellectual capabilities in children with learning difficulties. *American Journal of Mental Deficiency, 82,* 559–564.

Carlson, V., Cicchetti, D., Barnett, D., & Braunwald, K. B. (1989). The development of disorganized/disoriented attachment in maltreated infants. *Developmental Psychology, 25,* 525–531.

Caro, P, & Snell, M. (1989). Characteristics of teaching communication to people with moderate and severe disabilities. *Education and Training in Mental Retardation, 29,* 63–77.

Carpenter, A., & Strong, J. (1988). Pragmatic development in normal children: Assessment of a testing protocol. *National Student Speech-Language-Hearing Association Journal, 12,* 40–49.

Carr, E., & Durand, V. (1985). Reducing behavior problems through functional communication training. *Journal of Applied Behavior Analysis, 18,* 111–126.

Casby, M. (1992). An intervention approach for naming problems in children. *American Journal of Speech-Language Pathology, 1*(3), 35–42.

Casby, M. W. (1997) Symbolic play of children with language impairment: A critical review. *Journal of Speech, Language, and Hearing Research, 40,* 468–479.

Catts, H. W. (1986). Speech production/phonological deficits in reading-disordered children. *Journal of Learning Disabilities, 19,* 504–508.

Catts, H. W. (1996). Defining dyslexia as a developmental language disorder: An expanded view. *Topics in Language Disorders, 16*(2), 14–29.

Catts, H. W. (1997). The early identification of language-based reading disabilities. *Language, Speech, and Hearing Services in Schools, 28,* 86–89.

Catts, H. W., & Kamhi, A. G. (1986). The linguistic basis of reading disorders: Implications for the speech-language pathologist. *Language, Speech, and Hearing Services in Schools, 17,* 329–341.

Catts, H. W., & Kamhi, A. G. (1987). Intervention for reading disabilities. *Journal of Childhood Communication Disorders, 2*(1), 67–80.

Catts, H., & Kamhi, A. (Eds.). (1999). *Language and reading abilities.* Boston: Allyn and Bacon.

Chafe, W. (1970). *Meaning and the structure of language.* Chicago: University of Chicago Press.

Chamberlain, P., & Medinos-Landurand, P. (1991). Practical considerations for the assessment of LEP students with special needs. In E. V. Hamayan & J. S. Damico (Eds.), *Limiting bias in the assessment of bilingual students* (pp. 112–156). Austin, TX: Pro-Ed.

Chaney, C. (1992). Language development, metalinguistic skills, and print awareness in 3-year-old children. *Applied Psycholinguistics, 13,* 485–514.

Channell, R., & Ford, C. (1991). Four grammatical completion measures of language ability. *Language, Speech, and Hearing Services in Schools, 22,* 211–218.

Chapman, K., & Terrell, B. (1988). "Verb-alizing": Facilitating action word usage in young language-impaired children. *Topics in Language Disorders, 8*(2), 1–13.

Chapman, R. L. (1987). *A new dictionary of American slang.* New York: Harper & Row.

Chapman, R. S. (1981). Exploring children's communicative intents. In J. Miller (Ed.), *Assessing language production in children* (pp. 22–25). Baltimore: University Park Press.

Chapman, R. S., Kay-Raining Bird, E., & Schwartz, S. E. (1990). Fast mapping of words in event contexts by children with Down syndrome. *Journal of Speech and Hearing Disorders, 55,* 761–770.

Chapman, R. S., Schwartz, S. E., & Kay-Raining Bird, E. (1988, November). *Predicting comprehension of children with Down syndrome.* Paper presented at the Annual Convention of the American Speech-Language-Hearing Association, Boston.

Chapman, S. B. (1997). Cognitive-communication abilities in children with closed head injury. *American Journal of Speech-Language Pathology, 6*(2), 50–58.

Chapman, S. B., Levin, H. S., Matejka, J., Harward, H. N., & Kufera, J. (1995). Discourse ability in head-injured children: Considerations of linguistic psychosocial, and cognitive factors. *Journal of Head Trauma Rehabilitation, 10,* 36–54.

Chapman, S. B., Watkins, R., Gustafson, C., Moore, S., Levin, H., & Kufera, J. A. (1997). Narrative discourse in children with closed head injury, children with language impairment, and typically developing children. *American Journal of Speech-Language Pathology, 6*(2), 66–76.

Charlop, M. (1986). Setting effects on the occurrence of autistic children's immediate echolalia. *Journal of Autism and Development Disorders, 16,* 473–483.

Charlop, M., Schreibman, L., & Thebodeau, M. (1985). Increasing spontaneous verbal responding in autistic children using time delay. *Journal of Applied Behavior Analysis, 18,* 155–166.

Cheng, L. (1987). Cross-cultural and linguistic considerations in working with Asian populations. *Asha, 29*(6), 33–38.

Chi, M., & Ceci, S. (1987). Content knowledge in memory development. *Advances in Child Development and Behavior, 20,* 91–143.

Cicchetti, D. (1987). Developmental psychopathology in infancy: Illustration from the study of maltreated youngsters. *Journal of Consulting and Clinical Psychology, 55,* 837–845.

Cicchetti, D., & Lynch, M. (1993) Toward an ecological/transactional model of community violence and child maltreatment: Consequences for children's development. *Psychiatry, 56,* 131–153.

Cimorell, J. (1983). *Language facilitation, a complete cognitive therapy program.* Baltimore: University Park Press.

Cirrin, F. M., & Rowland, C. M. (1985). Communicative assessment of nonverbal youths with severe/profound mental retardation. *Mental Retardation, 23,* 52–62.

Clahsen, H. (1989). The grammatical characterization of developmental aphasia. *Linguistics, 27,* 897–920.

Clark, G., & Seifer, R. (1982). Facilitating mother-infant communication: A treatment model for high risk and developmentally delayed infants. *Infant Mental Health Journal, 4*(2), 67–81.

Clark, J. O. (1990). *Harrup's dictionary of English idioms.* London: Harrup.

Clarke, S. (1987). *An evaluation of the relationship between receptive speech and manual sign language with mentally handicapped children.* Unpublished doctoral dissertation, University of Southampton, UK.

Clay, M. M. (1979). *The early detection of reading difficulties: A diagnostic survey with recovery procedures.* Exeter, NH: Heinemann.

Cleave, P. L., & Fey, M. E. (1997). Two approaches to the facilitation of grammar in children with language impairments: Rationale and description. *American Journal of Speech-Language Pathology, 6*(1), 22–32.

Cochran, P. S., & Bull, G. L. (1991). Integrating word processing into language instruction. *Topics in Language Disorders, 11*(2), 31–49.

Cochrane, R. (1983). Language and the atmosphere of delight. In H. Winitz (Ed.), *Treating language disorders: For clinicians by clinicians* (pp. 143–162). Baltimore: University Park Press.

Coelho, C. A., Liles, B. Z., & Duffy, R. J. (1991). *Conversational patterns of aphasic, closed head injured, and normal speakers.* Paper presented at the 21st Annual Clinical Aphasiology Conference, Destin, FL.

Coggins, T. (1991). Bringing context back into assessment. *Topics in Language Disorders, 11*(4), 43–54.

Coggins, T., & Olswang, L. B. (1987). The pragmatics of generalization. *Seminars in Speech and Language, 8,* 283–302.

Coggins, T., Olswang, L., & Guthrie, J. (1987). Assessing communicative intents in young children: Low structured observation or elicitation tasks? *Journal of Speech and Hearing Disorders, 52,* 44–49.

Cohen, S. (1991). Adapting educational programs for students with head injuries. *Journal of Head Trauma Rehabilitation, 6,* 56–64.

Cole, K. N., & Dale, P. (1986). Direct language instruction and interactive language instruction with language-delayed preschool children: A comparison study. *Journal of Speech and Hearing Research, 29,* 206–217.

Cole, K. N., Coggins, T. E., & Vanderstoep, C. (1999). The influence of language/cognitive profile on discourse intervention outcome. *Language, Speech, and Hearing Services in Schools, 30,* 61–67.

Cole, K. N., Mills, R., & Dale, P. (1989). Examination of test-retest and split-half reliability for measures derived from language samples of young handicapped children. *Language, Speech, and Hearing Services in Schools, 20,* 259–268.

Coleman, M., & Gillberg, C. (1985). *The biology of the autistic syndrome.* New York: Praeger.

Coley, J., & Gelman, S. (1989). The effect of object orientation and object type on children's interpretation of the word "big." *Child Development, 60,* 372–380.

Condus, M. M., Marshall, K. L., & Miller, S. R. (1986). Effects of reference keyword mnemonic strategy on vocabulary acquisition and maintenance of learning-disabled children. *Journal of Learning Disabilities, 19,* 609–613.

Confal, K. L. (1993). Collaborative consultation for speech-language pathologists. *Topics in Language Disorders, 14*(1), 1–14.

Connell, P. J. (1982). On training language rules. *Language, Speech, and Hearing Services in Schools, 13,* 231–240.

Connell, P. J. (1986a). Acquisition of semantic role by language-disordered children: Differences between production and comprehension. *Journal of Speech and Hearing Research, 29,* 366–374.

Connell, P. J. (1986b). Teaching subjecthood to language-disordered children. *Journal of Speech and Hearing Research, 29,* 481–493.

Connell, P. J. (1987a). A comparison of modeling and imitation teaching procedures on language-disordered children. *Journal of Speech and Hearing Research, 30,* 105–113.

Connell, P. J. (1987b). An effect of modeling and imitation teaching procedures on children with and without language impairment. *Journal of Speech and Hearing Research, 30,* 105–113.

Connell, P. J. (1987c). Teaching language rules as solutions to language problems: A baseball analogy. *Language, Speech, and Hearing Services in Schools, 18,* 194–205.

Connell, P. J., & Stone, C. (1992). Morpheme learning of children with specific language impairments under controlled conditions. *Journal of Speech and Hearing Research, 35,* 844–852.

Connell, P. J., & Stone, C. A. (1994). The conceptual basis for morpheme learning problems in children with specific language impairment. *Journal of Speech and Learning Research, 37,* 389–398.

Constable, C. M. (1983). Creating communicative context. In H. Winitz (Ed.), *Treating language disorders: For clinicians by clinicians* (pp. 97–120). Baltimore: University Park Press.

Constable, C. M. (1986). The application of scripts in the organization of language intervention contexts. *Event Knowledge, 10,* 205–230.

Constable, C. M. (1992, March). *What can classroom ethnography do for clinical intervention?* Paper presented at the Conference on Pragmatics: From Theory to Therapy, State University of New York, Buffalo.

Conti-Ramsden, G. (1990). Material recasts and other contingent replies to language-impaired children. *Journal of Speech and Hearing Disorders, 55,* 262–274.

Conti-Ramsden, G., & Friel-Patti, S. (1987). Situational variability in mother-child conversations. In K. E. Nelson & A. van Kleeck (Eds.), *Children's language* (Vol. 6, pp. 43–63). Hillsdale, NJ: Lawrence Erlbaum.

Conti-Ramsden, G., Hutcheson, G. D., & Grove, J. (1995). Contingency and breakdown: Children with SLI and their conversations with mothers and fathers. *Journal of Speech and Learning Research, 38,* 1290–1302.

Cooper, D. C., & Anderson-Inman, L. (1988). Language and socialization. In M. A. Nippold (Ed.), *Later language development: Ages nine through nineteen* (pp. 225–245). Austin, TX: Pro-Ed.

Cooper, J., & Flowers, C. (1987). Children with a history of acquired aphasia: Residual language and academic impairments. *Journal of Speech and Hearing Disorders, 52,* 251–262.

Cosaro, J. (1989). Activities to enhance listening skills. *Language, Speech, and Hearing Services in Schools, 20,* 433–435.

Coster, W. J., & Cicchetti, D. (1993). Research on the development of maltreated children: Clinical implications. *Topics in Language Disorders, 13*(4), 25–38.

Coster, W. J., Gersten, M. S., Beeghly, M., & Cicchetti, D. (1989). Communicative functioning in maltreated toddlers. *Developmental Psychology, 25,* 1020–1029.

Courchesne, E. (1988). Hypoplasia of cerebellar vermal lobules VI and VII in autism. *New England Journal of Medicine, 318,* 1349–1354.

Cowan, N. (1995). *Attention and memory: An integrated framework.* New York: Oxford University Press.

Cox, M., & Richardson, J. (1985). How do children describe spatial relationships? *Journal of Child Language, 12,* 611–620.

Crago, M. B.,, & Eriks-Brophy, A. (1992, March). *Culture, conversation, and the co-construction of interaction: Implications for intervention.* Paper presented at the Conference on Pragmatics: From Theory to Therapy, State University of New York, Buffalo.

Craig, H. K. (1983). Applications of pragmatic language models for intervention. In T. Gallagher & C. Prutting (Eds.), *Pragmatic assessment and intervention issues in language* (pp. 101–127). San Diego: College-Hill.

Craig, H. K. (1993). Social skills of children with specific language impairment: Peer relationships. *Language, Speech, and Hearing Services in Schools, 24,* 206–215.

Craig, H. K., & Evans, J. (1989). Turn exchange characteristics of SLI children's simultaneous and nonsimultaneous speech. *Journal of Speech and Hearing Disorders, 54,* 334–347.

Craig, H. K., & Evans, J. (1992). Language sample collection and analysis: Interview compared to freeplay assessment contexts. *Journal of Speech and Hearing Research, 35,* 343–353.

Craig, H. K., & Evans, J. L. (1993). Pragmatics and SLI: Within-group variations in discourse behaviors. *Journal of Speech and Hearing Research, 36,* 777–789.

Craig, H. K., & Washington, J. (1986). Children's turn-taking behaviors: Social-linguistic interactions. *Journal of Pragmatics, 10,* 173–197.

Craig, H. K., & Washington, J. A. (1993). Access behaviors of children with specific language impairment. *Journal of Speech and Hearing Research, 36,* 322–337.

Craig, H. K., & Washington, J. A. (2002). Oral language expectations for African American preschoolers and kindergarteners. *American Journal of Speech-Language Pathology, 11,* 59–70.

Craig, H. K., Washington, J. A., & Thompson-Porter, C. (1998). Average C-unit lengths in the discourse of African American children from low-income urban homes. *Journal of Speech, Language, and Hearing Research, 41,* 433–444.

Crais, E. R. (1987). Fast mapping of novel words in oral story context. *Papers and Reports in Child Language Development, 26,* 40–47.

Crais, E. R. (1990). World knowledge to word knowledge. *Topics in Language Disorders, 10*(3), 45–62.

Crais, E. R. (1991). Moving from "parent involvement" to family-centered services. *American Journal of Speech-Language Pathology, 1*(1), 5–8.

Crais, E. R. (1992, April). *Family-centered assessment and collaborative goal-setting.* Paper presented at the Annual Convention of the New York State Speech-Language-Hearing Association, Kiamesha Lake.

Crais, E. R., & Chapman, R. (1987). Story recall and inferencing skills in language-learning disabled and nondisabled children. *Journal of Speech and Hearing Disorders, 52,* 50–55.

Crais, E. R., & Roberts, J. (1991). Decision making in assessment and early intervention planning. *Language, Speech, and Hearing Services in Schools, 22,* 19–30.

Creaghead, N. A. (1984). Strategies for evaluating and targeting pragmatic behaviors in young children. *Seminars in Speech and Language, 5,* 241–251.

Creaghead, N. A. (1992). Classroom interactional analysis/script analysis. *Best Practices in School Speech Language Pathology, 2,* 65–72.

Creech, R. (1989). Incorporating prefixes and suffixes into words strategy. *Fourth Annual Minspeak Conference.* St. Louis, MO: Prentke Romich.

Crites, L. S., Fischer, K. L., McNeish-Stengel, M., & Siegel, C. J. (1992). Working with families of drug-exposed children: Three model programs. *Infant-Toddler Intervention: The Transdisciplinary Journal, 2*(1), 13–23.

Crittenden, P. M. (1988). Relationships at risk. In J. Belsky & T. Nazwarski (Eds.), *Clinical implications of attachment* (pp. 136–174). Hillsdale, NJ: Lawrence Erlbaum.

Crowhurst, M., & Piche, G. L. (1979). Audience and mode of discourse effects on syntactic complexity in writing at two grade levels. *Research in the Teaching of English, 13,* 101–109.

Crumrine, L., & Lonegan, H. (1998). *Pre-Literacy Skills Screening.* Chicago: Applied Symbolix.

Crystal, D. (1982). *Profiling linguistic disability.* London, UK: Edward Arnold.

Crystal, D. (1987). Towards a "bucket" theory of language disability: Taking account of interaction between linguistic levels. *Clinical Linguistics and Phonetics, 1,* 7–22.

Crystal, D., Fletcher, P., & Garman, R. (1976). *The grammatical analysis of language disability.* New York: Elsevier.

Culatta, B. (1992, March). *Replica play, role play, and story enactments: A format for language therapy.* Paper presented at the Conference on Pragmatics: From Theory to Therapy, State University of New York, Buffalo.

Culatta, B., Horn, D., Theadore, G., & Sutherland, D. (1993, November). *Scripted play: Enhancing language and literacy in diverse learners.* Paper presented at the Annual Convention of the American Speech-Language-Hearing Association, Anaheim, CA.

Culp, R. E., Watkins, R. V., Lawrence, H., Letts, D., Kelly, D. J., & Rice, M. (1991). Maltreated children's language and speech development: Abused, neglected, and abused and neglected. *First Language, 11,* 337–389.

Cummins, J. (1986). Empowering minority students: A framework for intervention. *Harvard Educational Review, 58,* 18–39.

Cupples, L., & Iacono, T. (2000). Phonological awareness and oral reading skill in children with Down syndrome. *Journal of Speech, Language, and Hearing Research, 43,* 595–608.

Curtis, M. E. (1987). Vocabulary testing and vocabulary instruction. In M. G. McKeown & M. E. Curtis (Eds.), *The nature of vocabulary acquisition* (pp. 37–51). Hillsdale, NJ: Lawrence Erlbaum.

Curtiss, S., Kutz, W., & Tallal, P. (1992). Delay versus deviance in the language acquisition of language-impaired children. *Journal of Speech and Hearing Research, 35,* 373–383.

Dale, P. S. (1991). The validity of a parent report measure of vocabulary and syntax at 24 months. *Journal of Speech and Hearing Research, 34,* 565–571.

Dale, P. S., Bates, E., Reznick, J. S., & Morisset, C. (1989). The validity of a parent report instrument of child language at 20 months. *Journal of Child Language, 16,* 239–249.

Dale, P. S., & Cole, K. (1991). What's normal? Specific language impairment in an individual differences perspective. *Language, Speech, and Hearing Services in Schools, 22,* 80–83.

Damico, J. S. (1985a). Clinical discourse analysis: A functional approach to language assessment. In C. Simon (Ed.), *Communication skills and classroom success* (pp. 165–206). San Diego: College-Hill.

Damico, J. S. (1985b). *The effectiveness of direct observation as a language assessment technique.* Unpublished doctoral dissertation, University of New Mexico, Albuquerque.

Damico, J. S. (1987). Addressing language concerns in the schools: The SLP as a consultant. *Journal of Childhood Communication Disorders, 11*(1), 17–40.

Damico, J. S. (1988). The lack of efficacy in language therapy: A case study. *Language, Speech, and Hearing Services in Schools, 19,* 51–66.

Damico, J. S. (1991a). Clinical Discourse Analysis: A functional language assessment technique. In C. S. Simon (Ed.), *Communication skills and classroom success: Assessment and therapy methodologies for language and learning disabled students* (pp. 125–150). Eau Claire, WI: Thinking Publications.

Damico, J. S. (1991b). Descriptive assessment of communicative ability in LEP students. In E. V. Hamayan & J. S. Damico (Eds.), *Limiting bias in the assessment of bilingual students* (pp. 157–218). Austin, TX: Pro-Ed.

Damico, J. S. (1993). Language assessment in adolescents: Addressing critical issues. *Language, Speech, and Hearing Services in Schools, 24,* 29–35.

Damico, J. S., & Oller, J. (1985). *Spotting language problems.* San Diego: Los Amigos Research Associates.

Damico, J. S., Secord, W. A., & Wiig, E. H. (1992). Descriptive language assessment at school: Characteristics and design. *Best Practices in School Speech Language Pathology, 2,* 1–8.

Danserean, D. (1987). Transfer from cooperative to individual studying. *Journal of Reading, 30,* 614–619.

Davis, A. (1972). *English problems of Spanish speakers.* Urbana, IL: National Council of Teachers of English.

Davis, H., Stroud, A., & Green, L. (1988). Maternal language environment of children with mental retardation. *American Journal of Mental Retardation, 93,* 144–153.

Denner, P. R., & Pehrsson, R. S. (1987, April). *A comparison of the effects of episodic organizers and traditional notetaking on story recall.* Paper presented at the Annual Meeting of the American Educational Research Association, Washington, DC.

Dennis, M. (1992). Word finding in children and adolescents with a history of brain injury. *Topics in Language Disorders, 13*(1), 66–82.

Dennis, M., & Barnes, M. A. (1990). Knowing the meaning, getting the point, bridging the gap, and carrying the message: Aspects of discourse following closed head injury in children and adolescents. *Brain and Language, 39,* 428–446.

DeSpain, A., & Simon, C. (1987). Alternative to failure: A junior high school language development-based curriculum. *Journal of Childhood Communication Disorders, 11*(1), 139–179.

deVilliers, L., & deVilliers, P. (1978). *Language acquisition.* Cambridge, MA: Harvard University Press.

Diana v. Board of Education. (1991). 186 W.Va. 141; 411 S.E.2d 466; 1991 W.Va. LEXIS 168.

Dickinson, D. K., & DeTemple, J. (1998). Putting parents in the picture: Maternal reports of preschoolers' literacy as a predictor of early reading. *Early Childhood Research Quarterly, 13,* 241–261.

Dobe, L. (1989). *A study of interaction styles and patterns of mothers of preverbal children.* Unpublished master's thesis, Ohio State University, Columbus.

Dodge, E., & Mallard, A. (1992). Social skills training using a collaborative service delivery model. *Language, Speech, and Hearing Services in Schools, 23,* 130–135.

Dollaghan, C. A. (1987a). Comprehension monitoring in normal and language-impaired children. *Topics in Language Disorders, 7*(2), 45–60.

Dollaghan, C. A. (1987b). Fast mapping in normal and language-impaired children. *Journal of Speech and Hearing Disorders, 52,* 218–222.

Dollaghan, C. A., & Campbell, T. (1998). Nonword repetition and child language impairment. *Journal of Speech, Language, and Hearing Research, 41,* 1136–1146.

Dollaghan, C. A., & Campbell, T. F. (1992). A procedure for classifying disruptions in spontaneous language samples. *Topics in Language Disorders, 12*(2), 56–68.

Dollaghan, C. A., Campbell, T., & Tomlin, R. (1990). Video narration as a language sampling context. *Journal of Speech and Hearing Disorders, 55,* 582–590.

Dollaghan, C. A., & Kaston, N. (1986). A comprehension monitoring program for language-impaired children. *Journal of Speech and Hearing Disorders, 51,* 264–271.

Dollaghan, C. A., & Miller, J. (1986). Observational methods in the study of communicative competence. In R. Schiefelbusch (Ed.), *Language competence: Assessment and intervention* (pp. 99–129). San Diego: College-Hill.

Donahue, M. (1983). Language-disabled children as conversational partners. *Topics in Language Disorders, 4,* 15–27.

Donahue, M. (1984). Learning disabled children's conversational competence: An attempt to activate an inactive listener. *Applied Psycholinguistics, 5,* 21–36.

Donahue, M. (1985). Communicative style in learning disabled children: Some implications for classroom discourse. In D. Ropich & F. Spinelli (Eds.), *School discourse problems* (pp. 97–124). San Diego: College-Hill.

Donahue, M., & Bryan, T. (1984). Communicative skills and peer relations of learning-disabled adolescents. *Topics in Language Disorders, 4*(2), 10–21.

Donnellan, A. M., Mirenda, P. L., Mesaros, R., & Fassbender, L. (1984). Analyzing the communicative functions of aberrant behavior. *Journal of the Association for Persons with Severe Handicaps, 9,* 210–222.

Dore, J. (1974). A pragmatic description of early language development. *Journal of Psycholinguistic Research, 3,* 343–350.

Dore, J. (1986). The development of conversational competence. In R. Schiefelbusch (Ed.), *Language competence: Assessment and intervention* (pp. 3–60). San Diego: College-Hill.

Douglas, D., & Selinker, L. (1985). Principles for language tests within the "discourse domains" theory of interlanguage. *Language Testing, 2,* 205–226.

Downing, J. (1987). Conversational skills training: Teaching adolescents with mental retardation to be verbally assertive. *Mental Retardation, 25,* 147–155.

Downing, J., & Siegel-Causey, E. (1988). Enhancing the nonsymbolic communicative behavior of children with multiple impairments. *Language, Speech, and Hearing Services in Schools, 19,* 338–348.

Dromi, E., Leonard, L. B., Adam, G., & Zadunaisky-Ehrlich, S. (1999). Verb agreement morphology in Hebrew-speaking children with specific language impairment. *Journal of Speech, Language, and Hearing Research, 42,* 1414–1431.

Duchan, J. F. (1982a). The elephant is soft and mushy: Problems in assessing children's language. In N. Lass, L. McReynolds, J. Northern, & D. Yoder (Eds.), *Speech, language, and hearing: Vol. 2. Pathologies of speech and language* (pp. 741–760). Philadelphia: W. B. Saunders.

Duchan, J. F. (1984). Clinical interactions with autistic children: The role of theory. *Topics in Language Disorders, 4*(4), 62–71.

Duchan, J. F. (1986a). Language intervention through sense-making and fine tuning. In R. Schiefelbusch (Ed.), *Language competence: Assessment and intervention* (pp. 187–212). San Diego: College-Hill.

Duchan, J. F. (1986b). Learning to describe events. *Topics in Language Disorders, 6*(4), 27–36.

Duchan, J. F. (1997). A situated pragmatics approach for supporting children with severe communication disorders. *Topics in Language Disorders, 17*(2), 1–18.

Duchan, J. F., & Waltzman, M. M. (1992). Then as an indicator of deictic discontinuity in adults' oral descriptions of a film. *Journal of Speech and Hearing Research, 35,* 1367–1375.

Duchan, J. F., & Weitzner-Lin, B. (1987). Nurturant-naturalistic intervention for language-impaired children: Implications for planning lessons and tracking progress. *Asha, 29*(7), 45–49.

Dudley-Marling, C. (1987). The role of SLPs in literacy learning. *Journal of Childhood Communication Disorders, 2*(1), 81–90.

Dudley-Marling, C., & Rhodes, L. (1987). Pragmatics and literacy. *Language, Speech, and Hearing Services in Schools, 18,* 41–52.

Dunham, J. (1989). The transparency of manual signs in a linguistic and an environmental non-linguistic context. *Augmentative and Alternative Communication, 5,* 214–225.

Dunn, M., Flax, J., Sliwinski, M., & Aram, D. (1996). The use of spontaneous language measures as criteria for identifying children with specific language impairment: An attempt to reconcile clinical and research incongruence. *Journal of Speech and Hearing Research, 39,* 643–654.

Dunst, C., Lowe, L., & Bartholomew, P. (1990). Contingent social responsiveness, family ecology and infant communicative competence. *NSSLHA Journal, 17,* 39–49.

Durand, V., & Kishi, G. (1986). *Reducing severe behavior problems among persons with dual sensory impairments: An evaluation of a technical assistance model.* Unpublished manuscript, State University of New York, Albany.

Dyer, K., Santarcangelo, S., & Luce, S. (1987). Developmental influences in teaching language forms to individuals with developmental disabilities. *Journal of Speech and Hearing Disorders, 52,* 335–347.

Dyer, K., Williams, L., & Luce, S. (1991). Training teachers to use naturalistic communication strategies in classrooms for students with autism or other severe handicaps. *Language, Speech, and Hearing Services in Schools, 22,* 313–321.

Ecklund, S., & Reichle, J. (1987). A comparison of normal children's ability to recall symbols from two logographic systems. *Language, Speech, and Hearing Services in Schools, 18,* 34–40.

Edmaiston, R. (1988). Preschool Literacy Assessment. *Seminars in Speech and Hearing, 9,* 27–36.

Edmonston, N. K., & Thane, N. L. (1990, April). *Children's concept comprehension: Acquisition, assessment, intervention.* Paper presented at the Annual Convention of the New York State Speech-Language-Hearing Association, Kiamesha Lake.

Edmonston, N. K., & Thane, N. L. (1992). Children's use of comprehension strategies in response to relational words: Implications for assessment. *American Journal of Speech-Language Pathology, 1*(2), 30–35.

Edwards, J., & Lahey, M. (1998). Nonword repetitions of children with specific language impairment: Exploration of some explanations for their inaccuracies. *Applied Psycholinguistics, 19,* 279–309.

Ehren, B. J. (2000). Maintaining a therapeutic focus and sharing responsibility for student success: Keys to in-classroom speech-language services. *Language, Speech, and Hearing Services in Schools, 31,* 219–229.

Ehren, B. J., & Mullins, B. (1988). *Contextualized adolescent language learning (CALL) curriculum.* West Palm Beach, FL: School Board of Palm Beach County, Florida.

Ehri, L. C. (1986). Sources of difficulty in learning to read and spell. In M. L. Wolraich & D. Routh (Eds.), *Advances in developmental and behavioral pediatrics* (Vol. 7, pp. 121–195). Greenwich, CT: JAI Press.

Ehri, L. C. (1992). Reconceptualizing the development of sight word reading and its relationship to recoding. In P.

Gough, L. Ehri, & R. Treiman (Eds.), *Reading acquisition* (pp. 107–143). Hillsdale, NJ: Lawrence Erlbaum.

Ehri, L. C. (2000). Learning to read and learning to spell: Two sides of a coin. *Topics in Language Disorders, 20*(3), 19–36.

Ehri, L. C., & Wilce, L. (1987). Does learning to spell help beginners learn to read words? *Reading Research Quarterly, 22,* 47–65.

Eisenberg, S. L., McGovern Fersko, T., & Lundgren, C. (2001). The use of MLU for identifying language impairment in preschool children: A review. *American Journal of Speech-Language Pathology, 10,* 323–342.

Elbert, M., & McReynolds, L. (1985). The generalization hypothesis: Final consonant deletion. *Language and Speech, 28,* 281–294.

Ellis, N., Deacon, J., & Wooldridge, P. (1985). On the nature of short-term memory deficit in mentally retarded persons. *American Journal of Mental Deficiency, 89,* 393–402.

Ellis, N., Woodley-Zanthos, P., & Dulaney, C. (1989). Memory for spatial location in children, adults, and mentally retarded persons. *American Journal of Mental Retardation, 93,* 521–527.

Ellis Weismer, S. E. (1991). Hypothesis-testing abilities of language-impaired children. *Journal of Speech and Hearing Research, 34,* 1329–1338.

Ellis Weismer, S. (1994). *Factors influencing novel word learning and linguistic processing in children with specific language impairment.* Paper presented at the 15th Annual Symposium on Research in Children with Language Disabilities, Madison, WI.

Ellis Weismer, S., & Evans, J. L. (2002). The role of processing limitations in early identification of specific language impairment. *Topics in Language Disorders, 22*(3), 15–29

Ellis Weismer, S., Evans, J., & Hesketh, L. J. (1999). An examination of verbal working memory capacity in children with specific language impairment. *Journal of Speech, Language, and Hearing Research, 42,* 1249–1260.

Ellis Weismer, S., & Hesketh, L. (1996). Lexical learning by children with specific language impairments: Effects of linguistic input presented at varying speaking rates. *Journal of Speech, Language, and Hearing Research, 39,* 177–190.

Ellis Weismer, S., & Hesketh, L. J. (1998). The impact of emphatic stress on novel word learning by children with specific language impairment. *Journal of Speech, Language, and Hearing Research, 41,* 1444–1458.

Ellis Weismer, S., Tomblin, J. B., Zhang, X., Buckwalter, P., Chynoweth, J. G., & Jones, M. (2000). Nonword repetition performance in school-age children with and without language impairment. *Journal of Speech, Language, and Hearing Research, 43,* 865–878.

Elshout-Mohr, M., & van Daalen-Kapteijns, M. M. (1987). Cognitive processes in learning word meanings. In M. G. McKeown & M. E. Curtis (Eds.), *The nature of vocabulary acquisition* (pp. 53–71). Hillsdale, NJ: Lawrence Erlbaum.

Emerick, L., & Haynes, W. (1986). *Diagnosis and evaluation in speech pathology* (3rd ed.). Englewood Cliffs, NJ: Prentice-Hall.

Englert, C., Raphael, T., Fear, K., & Anderson, L. (1988). Students' metacognitive knowledge about how to write informational texts. *Learning Disability Quarterly, 11,* 18–46.

Englert, C. S., & Thomas, C. C. (1987). Sensitivity to text structure in reading and writing: A comparison of learning disabled and nonhandicapped students. *Learning Disability Quarterly, 10,* 93–105.

Ertmer, D. J. (1986). Language Carnival [Computer program]. Moline, IL: LinguiSystems.

Ervin-Tripp, S. (1977). Wait for me roller skate. In S. Ervin-Tripp & C. Mitchell-Kerner (Eds.), *Child discourse* (pp. 165–188). New York: Academic Press.

Espin, C. A., & Sindelar, P. T. (1988). Auditory feedback and writing: Learning disabled and nondisabled students. *Exceptional Children, 55*(1), 45–51.

Ewing-Cobbs, L., Fletcher, J. M., & Levin, H. S. (1985). In M. Ylvisaker (Ed.), *Head injury rehabilitation: Children and adolescents* (pp. 71–89). Austin, TX: Pro-Ed.

Ewing-Cobbs, L., Levin, H. S., Eisenberg, H. M., & Fletcher, J. M. (1987). Language functions following closed-head injury in children and adolescents. *Journal of Clinical and Experimental Neuropsychology, 9,* 575–592.

Ezell, H., & Goldstein, H. (1991). Comparison of idiom comprehension of normal children and children with mental retardation. *Journal of Speech and Hearing Research, 34,* 812–819.

Fagundes, D. D., Haynes, W. O., Haak, N.J., & Moran, M. J. (1998). Task variability effects on the language test performance of southern lower socioeconomic class African American and caucasian five-year-olds. *Language, Speech, and Hearing Services in Schools, 29,* 148–157.

Falvey, M. A. (1986). *Community-based curriculum: Instructional strategies for students with severe handicaps.* Baltimore: Paul H. Brookes.

Falvey, M. A., Bishop, K., Grenot-Scheyer, M., & Coots, J. (1988). Issues and trends in mental retardation. In S. Calculator & J. Bedrosian (Eds.), *Communication assessment and intervention for adults with mental retardation* (pp. 45–65). San Diego: College-Hill.

Falvey, M. A., McLean, D., & Rosenberg, R. L. (1988). Transition from school to adult life: Communication strategies. *Topics in Language Disorders, 9*(1), 82–86.

Farber, J., Denenberg, M. E., Klyman, S., & Lachman, P. (1992). Language resource room level of service: An urban school district approach to integrative treatment. *Language, Speech, and Hearing Services in Schools, 23,* 293–299.

Farber, J. G., & Klein, E. R. (1999). Classroom-based assessment of a collaborative intervention program with kindergarten and first-grade students. *Language, Speech, and Hearing Services in Schools, 30,* 83–91.

Farrier, L., Yorkston, K., Marriner, N., & Beukelman, D. (1985). Conversational control in non-impaired speakers using an augmentative communication System. *Augmentative and Alternative Communication, 1,* 65–73.

Fasold, R. W. (1990). *The sociolinguistics of language.* Cambridge, UK: Basil Blackwell.

Fasold, R. W., & Wolfram, W. (1970). Some linguistic features of Negro dialect. In R. Fasold & R. Shuy (Eds.), *Teaching standard English in the inner city* (pp. 41–86). Washington, DC: Center for Applied Linguistics.

Fazio, B. B. (1996). Serial memory in children with specific language impairment: Examining specific content areas for assessment and intervention., *Topics in Language Disorders 17*(1), 56–71.

Fazio, B. B., (1998). The effect of presentation rate on serial memory in young children with specific language impairment. *Journal of Speech, Language, and Hearing Research, 41,* 1375–1383.

Fazio, B. B., Naremore, R. C., & Connell, P. J. (1996). Tracking children from poverty at risk for specific language impairment: A 3-year longitudinal study. *Journal of Speech and Hearing Research, 39,* 611–624.

Feagans, L., & Short, E. (1986). Referential communication and reading performance in learning disabled children over a 3-year period. *Developmental Psychology, 22,* 177–183.

Felsenfeld, S., Broen, P. A., & McCue, M. (1992). A 23-year follow-up of adults with a history of moderate phonological disorder: Linguistic and personality results. *Journal of Speech and Hearing Research, 35,* 1114–1125.

Felton, R., & Brown, I. S. (1990). Phonological processes as predictors of specific reading skills in children at risk for reading failure. *Reading and Writing: An Interdisciplinary Journal, 2,* 39–59.

Ferguson, M. L. (1992a). Implementing collaborative consultation: An introduction. *Language, Speech, and Hearing Services in Schools, 23,* 361–362.

Ferguson, M. L. (1992b). The transition to collaborative teaching. *Language, Speech, and Hearing Services in Schools, 23,* 371–372.

Feuerstein, R., Rand, Y., Jensen, M. R., Kaniel, S., & Tzuriel, D. (1987). Prerequisites for assessment of learning potential: The LPAD model. In C. Schneider Lidz (Ed.), *Dynamic assessment: An interactional approach to evaluating learning potential* (pp. 35–51). New York: Guilford.

Fey, M. E. (1986). *Language intervention with young children.* San Diego: College-Hill.

Fey, M. E. (1988). Generalization issues facing language interventionists: An introduction. *Language, Speech, and Hearing Services in Schools, 19,* 272–281.

Fey, M. E., Cleave, P. L., & Long, S. H. (1997). Two models of grammar facilitation in children with specific language impairments: Phase 2. *Journal of Speech, Language, and Hearing Research, 40,* 5–19.

Fey, M. E., Cleave, P. L., Long, S. H., & Hughes, D. L. (1993). Two approaches to the facilitation of grammar in children with language impairment: An experimental evaluation. *Journal of Speech and Hearing Research, 36,* 141–157.

Fey, M. E., & Frome Loeb, D. (2002). An evaluation of the facilitative effects of inverted yes-no questions on the acquisition of auxiliary verbs. *Journal of Speech, Language, and Hearing Research, 45,* 160–174.

Fey, M. E., Krulik, T. E., Frome Loeb, D., & Proctor-Williams, K. (1999). Sentence recast use by parents of children with typical language and children with specific language impairment. *American Journal of Speech-Language Pathology, 8,* 273–286.

Fey, M. E., & Leonard, L. (1983). Pragmatic skills of specific language impairment. In T. Gallagher & C. Prutting (Eds.), *Pragmatic assessment and intervention issues in language* (pp. 65–82). San Diego: College-Hill.

Fey, M. E., & Leonard, L. (1984). Partner age as a variable in the conversational performance of specifically language-impaired and normal-language children. *Journal of Speech and Hearing Research, 27,* 413–424.

Fey, M. E., Leonard, L., & Wilcox, K. (1981). Speech-style modifications of language-impaired children. *Journal of Speech and Hearing Disorders, 46,* 91–97.

Fey, M. E., Long, S. H., & Cleave, P. L. (1994). Reconsiderations of IQ criteria in the definition of specific language impairment. In R. V. Watkins & M. L. Rice (Eds.), *Specific language impairment in children* (pp. 161–178). Baltimore, MD: Paul H. Brookes.

Fey, M. E., Warr-Leeper, G., Webber, S., & Disher, L. (1988). Repairing children's repairs: Evaluation and facilitation of children's clarification requests and responses. *Topics in Language Disorders, 8*(2), 63–84.

Fillmore, C. (1968). The case for case. In E. Bach & R. Harmas (Eds.), *Universals in linguistic theory* (pp. 1–90). New York: Holt, Rinehart & Winston.

Fisher, F. W., Shankweiler, D., & Liberman, I. Y. (1985). Spelling proficiency and sensitivity to word structure. *Journal of Memory and Language, 24,* 423–441.

Fitch, J. L. (1986). *Clinical applications of microcomputers in communication disorders.* New York: Academic Press.

Fivush, R., & Slackman, E. (1986). The acquisition and development of scripts. In K. Nelson (Ed.), *Event Knowledge: Structure and function in development.* Hillsdale, NJ: Lawrence Erlbaum.

Fleming, J., & Forester, B. (1997). Infusing language enhancement into the reading curriculum for disadvantaged adolescents. *Language, Speech, and Hearing Services in Schools, 28,* 177–180.

Folger, J., & Chapman, R. (1978). A pragmatic analysis of spontaneous imitations. *Journal of Child Language, 5,* 25–38.

Foster, S. (1985). The development of discourse topic skills in infants and young children. *Topics in Language Disorders, 5*(2), 31–45.

Fowler, G. (1982). Developing comprehension skills in primary students through the use of story frames. *Reading Teacher, 36,* 176–179.

Fox, L., Long, S. H., & Langlois, A. (1988). Patterns of language comprehension deficit in abused and neglected children. *Journal of Speech and Hearing Disorders, 53,* 239–244.

Foxx, R., Kyle, M., Faw, G., & Bittle, R. (1988). Cue-pause-point training and simultaneous communication to teach the use of signed labeling repertoires. *American Journal on Mental Retardation, 93,* 305–311.

Francik, E., & Clark, H. (1985). How to make requests that overcome obstacles to compliance. *Journal of Memory and Language, 24,* 560–568.

French, L. A., & Nelson, K. (1985). *Young children's knowledge of relational terms.* New York: Springer Verlag.

Fried-Oken, M. (1987). Qualitative examination of children's naming skills through test adaptations. *Language, Speech, and Hearing Services in Schools, 18,* 206–216.

Friel-Patti, S. (1999). Specific language impairment: Continuing clinical concerns. *Topics in Language Disorders, 20*(1),1–13.

Friend, T., & Channell, R. (1987). A comparison of two measures of receptive vocabulary. *Language, Speech, and Hearing Services in Schools, 18,* 231–237.

Frome Loeb, D., & Leonard, L. B. (1991). Subject case marking and verb morphology in normally developing and specifically language-impaired children. *Journal of Speech and Hearing Research, 34,* 340–346.

Fuchs, D., & Fuchs, L. (1989). Effects of examiner familiarity on black, Caucasian, and Hispanic children: A meta-analysis. *Exceptional Children, 55*(4), 303–308.

Fujiki, M., & Brinton, B. (1987). Elicited imitation revisited: A comparison with spontaneous language production. *Language, Speech, and Hearing Services in Schools, 18,* 301–311.

Fujiki, M., Brinton, B., Isaacson, T., & Summers, C. (2001). Social behavior of children with language impairment on the playground: A pilot study. *Language, Speech, and Hearing Services in Schools, 32,* 101–113.

Fujiki, M., Brinton, B., Morgan, M., & Hart, C. H. (1999). Withdrawal and sociable behavior of children with language impairment. *Language, Speech, and Hearing Services in Schools, 30,* 183–195.

Fujiki, M., & Brinton, B., Todd, C. M. (1996). Social skills of children with specific language impairment. *Language, Speech, and Hearing Services in Schools, 27,* 195–202.

Fujiki, M., & Willbrand, M. (1982). A comparison of four informal methods of language evaluation. *Language, Speech, and Hearing Services in Schools, 13,* 42–52.

Furman, L. N., & Walden, T. A.. (1989, April). *The effect of script knowledge on children's communicative interactions.* Paper presented at the meeting of the Society for Research in Child Development, Kansas City, MO.

Galaburda, A. M. (1989). Ordinary and extraordinary brain development: Anatomical variation in developmental dyslexia. *Annals of Dyslexia, 39,* 67–80.

Garcia, S. B., & Ortiz, A. A. (1988). Preventing inappropriate referrals of language minority students to special education. *New Focus: Occasional Papers in Bilingual Education, 5,* 1–12.

Gardner, H. (1989). An investigation of material interaction with phonologically disabled children as compared to two groups of normally developing children. *British Journal of Disorders of Communication, 24,* 41–59.

Garnett, K. (1986). Telling tales: Narratives and learning disabled children. *Topics in Language Disorders, 6*(2), 44–56.

Gavin, W. J., & Giles, L. (1996). Size effects on temporal reliabilty of language sample measures of preschool children. *Journal of Speech and Hearing Research, 39,* 1258–1262.

Gee, J. P. (1986). Units in production of narrative discourse. *Discourse Processes, 9,* 391–422.

Gee, J. P. (1989). Two styles of narrative construction and their linguistic and educational implications. *Discourse Processes, 12,* 287–307.

Genesee, F. (1987). *Learning through two languages: Studies of immersion and bilingual education.* Cambridge, MA: Newbury House.

Genesee, F. (1988). Bilingual language development in preschool children. In D. Bishop & K. Mogford (Eds.), *Language development in exceptional circumstances* (pp. 62–79). London: Churchill Livingstone.

Gentry, J. R. (1982). An analysis of developmental spelling in GNYS AT WRK. *The Reading Teacher, 36,* 192–200.

Gerber, M. M. (1986). Generalization of spelling strategies by LD students as a result of contingent imitation/modeling and mastery criteria. *Journal of Learning Disabilities, 19,* 530–537.

German, D. J. (1982). Word-finding substitutions in children with learning disabilities. *Language, Speech, and Healing Services in Schools, 13,* 223–230.

German, D. J. (1984). Diagnosis of word-finding disorders in children with learning disabilities. *Journal of Learning Disabilities, 17,* 353–359.

German, D. J. (1986/89). National College of Education Test of Word Finding (TWF). Allen, TX: DLM Teaching Resources.

German, D. J. (1987). Spontaneous language profiles of children with word-finding problems. *Language, Speech, and Hearing Services in Schools, 18,* 217–230.

German, D. J. (1990). National College of Education Test of Adolescent/Adult Word Finding (TAWF). Allen, TX: DLM Teaching Resources.

German, D. J. (1992). Word-finding intervention for children and adolescents. *Topics in Language Disorders, 13*(1), 33–50.

German, D. J., & Simon, E. (1991). Analysis of children's word-finding skills in discourse. *Journal of Speech and Hearing Research, 34,* 309–316.

Gersten, M., Coster, W. J., Schneider-Rosen, K., Carlson, V, & Cicchetti, D. (1986). The socio-emotional basis of communicative functioning: Quality of attachment, language development, and early maltreatment. In M. Lamb, A. L. Brown, & B. Rogoff (Eds.), *Advances in developmental psychology* (Vol. 4, pp. 105–151). Hillsdale, NJ: Lawrence Erlbaum.

Gertner, B. L., Rice, M. L., & Hadley, P. A. (1994). Influence of communicative competence on peer preferences in a preschool classroom. *Journal of Speech and Hearing Research, 37,* 913–923.

Gibbons, J., Anderson, D. R., Smith, R., Field, D. E., & Fischer, C. (1986). Young children's recall and reconstruction of audio and audiovisual narratives. *Child Development, 57,* 1014–1023.

Gibbs, R. W. (1987). Linguistic factors in children's understanding of idioms. *Journal for Child Language, 14,* 569–586.

Gibbs, R. W. (1991). Semantic analyzability in children's understanding of idioms. *Journal of Speech and Hearing Research, 34,* 613–620.

Gillam, R. B. (1999). Computer-assisted language intervention using *Fast ForWord:* Theoretical and empirical considerations for clinical decision-making. *Language, Speech, and Hearing Services in Schools, 30,* 363–370.

Gillam, R. B., & Bedore, L. M. (2000). Language science. In R. B. Gillam, T. P. Marquardt, & F. R. Martin (Eds.), *Communication sciences and disorders: From science to clinical practice* (pp. 385–408). San Diego, CA: Singular.

Gillam, R. B., & Carlile, R. M. (1997). Oral reading and story retelling of students with specific language impairment. *Language, Speech, and Hearing Services in Schools, 28,* 30–42.

Gillam, R. B., Cowan, N., & Day, L. (1995) Sequential memory in children with and without language impairment. *Journal of Speech, Language, and Hearing Research, 38,* 393–402.

Gillam, R. B., Hoffman, L. M., Marler, J. A., & Wynn-Dancy, M. L. (2002) Sensitivity to increased task demands: Contributions from data-driven and conceptually driven information processing deficits. *Topics in Language Disorders, 22*(3), 30–48.

Gillam, R. B., & Johnston, J. R. (1985). Development of print awareness in language-disordered preschoolers. *Journal of Speech and Hearing Research, 28,* 521–526.

Gillam, R. B., & Johnston, J. R. (1992). Spoken and written language relationships in language/learning-impaired and normal achieving school-age children. *Journal of Speech and Hearing Research, 35,* 1303–1315.

Gillam, R. B., Peña, E. D., & Miller, L. (1999). Dynamic assessment of narrative and expository discourse. *Topics in Language Disorders, 20*(1), 33–47.

Girolometto, L. E. (1988). Improving the social-conversational skills of developmentally delayed children: An intervention study. *Journal of Speech and Hearing Disorders, 53,* 156–167.

Girolometto, L. E., Pearce, P. S., & Weitzman, E. (1996). Interactive focused stimulation for toddlers with expressive vocabulary delays. *Journal of Speech and Hearing Research, 39,* 1274–1283.

Girolometto, L. E., Weitzman, E., Wiigs, M., & Steig Pierce, P. (1999). The relationship between maternal language measures and language development in toddlers with expressive vocabulary delays. *American Journal of Speech-Language Pathology, 8,* 364–374.

Glass, A. L., & Holyoak, S. (1986). *Cognition* (2nd ed.). New York: Random House.

Glenn, C., & Stein, N. (1980). *Syntactic structures and real world themes in stories generated by children* (Technical report). Urbana: University of Illinois, Center for the Study of Reading.

Gobbi, L., Cipani, E., Hudson, C., & Lapenta-Neudeck, R. (1986). Developing spontaneous requesting among children with severe mental retardation. *Mental Retardation, 24,* 357–364.

Goetz, L., Gee, K., & Sailor, W. (1985). Using a behavior chain interruption strategy to teach communication skills to students with severe disabilities. *Journal of the Association for Persons with Severe Handicaps, 10,* 21–30.

Goetz, L., & Sailor, W. (1988). New directions: Communication development in persons with severe disabilities. *Topics in Language Disorders, 8*(4), 41–54.

Goffman, L., & Leonard, J. (2000). Growth of language skills in preschool children with specific language impairment. *American Journal of Speech-Language Pathology, 9,* 151–161.

Golder, C., & Coirier, P. (1994). Argumentative text writing: Developmental trends. *Discourse Processes, 18,* 187–210.

Goldman, S., & McDermott, R. (1987). The culture of competition in American schools. In G. Spindler (Ed.), *Education and cultural process* (2nd ed., pp. 282–299). Prospect Heights, IL: Waveland.

Goldstein, H. (1985). Enhancing language generalization using matrix and stimulus equivalence training. In S. F. Warren & A. K. Rogers-Warren (Eds.), *Teaching functional language: Generalization and maintenance of language skills* (pp. 225–250). Baltimore: UPP.

Goldstein, H., English, K., Shafer, K., & Kaczmarek, L. (1997). Interaction among preschoolers with and without disabilities: Effects of across-the-day peer intervention. *Journal of Speech, Language, and Hearing Research, 40,* 33–48.

Goldstein, H., & Ferrell, D. (1987). Augmenting communicative interaction between handicapped and nonhandicapped preschool children. *Journal of Speech and Hearing Disorders, 52,* 200–211.

Goldstein, H., & Strain, P. S. (1988). Peers as communication intervention agents: Some new strategies and research findings. *Topics in Language Disorders, 9*(1), 44–59.

Goldstein, H., & Wickstrom, S. (1986). Peer intervention effects on communicative interaction among handicapped and nonhandicapped preschoolers. *Journal of Applied Behavior Analysis, 19,* 209–214.

Goldstein, H., Wickstrom, S., Hoyson, M., Jamieson, B., & Odom, S. (1988). Effects of sociodramatic play training on social and communicative interaction. *Education and Treatment of Children, 11,* 97–117.

Goodluck, H. (1986). Children's knowledge of prepositional phrase structure: An experimental test. *Journal of Psycholinguistic Research, 15,* 177–188.

Goodman, J., & Remington, B. (1993). Acquisition of expressive signing: Comparison of reinforcement strategies. *Augmentative and Alternative Communication, 9,* 26–35.

Goosens, C., & Kraat, A. (1985). Technology as a tool for conversation and language learning for the physically disabled. *Topics in Language Disorders, 6,* 56–70.

Gordon, C., & Braun, C. (1985). Metacognitive processes: Reading and writing narrative discourse in D. Forrest-Pressley, G. MacKinnon, & T. Waller (Eds.), *Metacognition, cognition, and human performance* (Vol. 2, pp. 1–75). New York: Academic Press.

Goswami, U. C. (1988) Children's use of analogy in learning to spell. *British Journal of Developmental Psychology, 6,* 1–22.

Gottschalk, M. E., Prelock, P. A., Weiler, E. M., & Sandman, D. (1997). Metapragmatic awareness of explanation adequacy II: Follow-up. *Language, Speech, and Hearing Services in Schools, 28,* 108–114.

Graham, S. (1990). The role of production factors in learning disabled students' compositions. *Journal of Educational Psychology, 82,* 781–791.

Graham, S. (1999). Handwriting and spelling instruction for students with learning disabilities: A review. *Learning Disability Quarterly, 22,* 78–98.

Graham, S., & Freeman, S. (1986). Strategy training and teacher- vs. student-controlled study conditions: Effects on LD students' performance. *Learning Disability Quarterly, 9,* 15–22.

Graham, S., & Harris, K. R. (1996). Addressing problems in attention, memory, and executive functioning: An example from self-regulated strategy development. In G.

Reid Lyon & N. A. Krasnegor (Eds.), *Attention, memory, and executive function* (pp. 349–365). Baltimore, MD: Paul H. Brookes.

Graham, S., & Harris, K. R. (1997). Self-regulation and writing: Where do we go from here? *Contemporary Educational Psychology, 22,* 102–114.

Graham, S., & Harris, K. R. (1999). Assessment and intervention in overcoming writing difficulties: An illustration from the self-regulation strategy development model. *Language, Speech, and Hearing Services in Schools, 30,* 255–264.

Graham, S., Harris, K., & Loynachan, C. (1994). The spelling for writing list. *Journal of Learning Disability, 27,* 210–217.

Graham, S., Harris, K., MacArthur, C. A., & Schwartz, S. S. (1991). Writing and writing instruction for students with learning disabilities: A review of a program of research. *Learning Disability Quarterly, 14,* 89–114.

Graves, A., Montague, M., & Wong, Y. (1990). The effects of procedural facilitation on the composition of learning disabled students. *Learning Disabilities Research, 5,* 88–93.

Graves, M. F. (1987). The roles of instruction in fostering vocabulary development. In M. G. McKeown & M. E. Curtis (Eds.), *The nature of vocabulary acquisition* (pp. 165–184). Hillsdale, NJ: Lawrence Erlbaum.

Greenberg, D., Ehri, L., & Perin, D. (1997). Is word reading processed the same or different in adult literacy students and third through fifth graders matched for reading level? *Journal of Educational Psychology, 89,* 262–275.

Greene, J. F. (1996). Psycholinguistic assessment: The clinical base for identity of dyslexia. *Topics in Language Disorders, 16*(2), 45–72.

Greenhalgh, K. S., & Strong, C. J. (2001). Literate language features in spoken narratives of children with typical language and children with language impairments. *Language, Speech, and Hearing Services in Schools, 32,* 114–126.

Greenspan, S. (1988). Fostering emotional and social development in infants with disabilities. *Zero to Three, 8,* 8–18.

Greenspan, S. I., & Wieder, S. (1997). Developmental patterns and outcomes in infants and children with disorders relating and communicating: A chart review of 200 cases of children with autism spectrum diagnoses. *Journal of Developmental and Learning Disorders, 1,* 87–141.

Grey, S., Plante, E., Vance, R., & Henrichsen, M. (1999). The diagnostic accuracy of four vocabulary tests administered to preschool-age children. *Language, Speech, and Hearing Services in Schools, 30,* 196–206.

Griffith, D. R. (1988). *Caring for crack cocaine babies.* Chicago: National Association for Perinatal Addiction Research and Education.

Griffith, P. (1991). Phonemic awareness helps first graders invent spellings and third graders remember correct spelling. *Journal of Reading Behavior, 23,* 215–233.

Griffith, P. L., Ripich, D. N., & Dastoli, S. L. (1986). Story structure, cohesion, and propositions in story recalls by learning-disabled and nondisabled children. *Journal of Psycholinguistic Research, 15*(6), 539–555.

Gruenewald, L., & Pollack, S. (1984). *Language interaction in teaching and learning.* Baltimore: University Park Press.

Guess, D., & Helmsteter, E. (1986). Skill cluster instruction and individualized curriculum sequencing model. In R. Horner, L. Meyers, & H. Fredericks (Eds.), *Education of learners with severe handicaps: Exemplary service strategies* (pp. 221–248). Baltimore: Paul H. Brookes.

Guevremont, D., Osnes, R., & Stokes, T. (1986a). Preparation for effective self-regulation: The development of generalized verbal control. *Journal of Applied Behavior Analysis, 19,* 99–104.

Guevremont, D., Osnes, R., & Stokes, T. (1986b). Programming maintenance after correspondence training interventions with children. *Journal of Applied Behavior Analysis, 19,* 215–219.

Guilford, A. M., & Nawojczyk, D. C. (1988). Standardization of the Boston Naming Test at the kindergarten and elementary school levels. *Language, Speech, and Hearing Services in Schools, 19,* 395–400.

Gulland, D. M., & Hinds-Howell, D. G. (1986). *The Penguin dictionary of English idioms.* London: Penguin.

Gullo, F., & Gullo, J. (1984). An ecological language intervention approach with mentally retarded adolescents. *Language, Speech, and Hearing Services in Schools, 15,* 182–191.

Gummersall, D. M., & Strong, C. J. (1999). Assessment of complex sentence production in a narrative context. *Language, Speech, and Hearing Services in Schools, 30,* 152–164.

Guralnick, M. J. (1990). Peer interactions and the development of handicapped children's social and communicative competence. In H. C. Foot, M. J. Morgan, & R. H. Shute (Eds.), *Children helping children* (pp. 275–305). New York: John Wiley.

Gutierrez-Clellan, V. F., & Heinrichs-Ramos, L. (1993). Referential cohesion in the narratives of Spanish-speaking children: A developmental study. *Journal of Speech and Hearing Research, 36,* 559–567.

Gutierrez-Clellan, V. F., & Iglesias, A. (1992). Causal coherence in the oral narratives of Spanish-speaking children. *Journal of Speech and Hearing Research, 35,* 363–372.

Gutierrez-Clellan, V. F., & McGrath, A. (1991, November). *Syntactic complexity in Spanish narratives: A developmental study.* Paper presented at the Annual Convention of the American Speech-Language-Hearing Association, Atlanta.

Gutierrez-Clellan, V. F., & Peña, E. D. (2001). Dynamic assessment of diverse children: A tutorial. *Language, Speech, and Hearing Services in Schools, 32,* 212–224.

Gutierrez-Clellan, V. F., Peña, E., & Quinn, R. (1995). Accommodating cultural differences in narrative style: A multicultural perspective. *Topics in Language Disorders, 15*(4), 54–67.

Gutierrez-Clellan, V. F., & Quinn, R. (1993). Assessing narratives of children from diverse cultural-lingual groups. *Language, Speech, and Hearing Services in Schools, 24,* 2–9.

Gutierrez-Clellen, V. F., Restrepo, M. A., Bedore, L., Pena, E., & Anderson, R. (2000). Language sample analysis in Spanish-speaking children: Methodological considerations. *Language, Speech, and Hearing Services in Schools, 31,* 88–98.

Gutowski, W., & Chechile, R. (1987). Encoding, storage, and retrieval components of associative memory deficits of mildly mentally retarded adults. *American Journal of Mental Deficiency, 92,* 85–93.

Haaf, R., Duncan, B., Skarakis-Doyle, E., Carew, M., & Kapitan, P. (1999). Computer-based language assessment software: The effects of presentation and response format. *Language, Speech, and Hearing Services in Schools, 30,* 68–74.

Haas, A., & Owens, R. (1985, November). *Preschoolers' pronoun strategies: You and me make us.* Paper presented at the Annual Convention of the American Speech-Language-Hearing Association, Washington, DC.

Hadley, P. A. (1998a). Early verbal-related vulnerability among children with specific language impairment. *Journal of Speech, Language, and Hearing Research, 41,* 1384–1397.

Hadley, P. A. (1998b). Language sampling protocols for eliciting test-level discourse. *Language, Speech, and Hearing Services in Schools, 29,* 132–147.

Hadley, P. A. (1999). Validating a rate-based measure of early grammatical abilities: Unique syntactic types. *American Journal of Speech-Language Pathology, 8,* 261–272.

Hadley, P. A., & Rice, M. L. (1991). Conversational responsiveness of speech- and language-impaired preschool-

ers. *Journal of Speech and Hearing Research, 34,* 1308–1317.

Hadley, P. A., & Schuele, C. M. (1998). Facilitating peer interaction: Socially relevant objectives for preschool language intervention. *American Journal of Speech-Language Pathology, 7*(4), 25–36.

Haelsig, P., & Madison, C. (1986). A study of phonological processes exhibited by 3-, 4-, and 5-year-old children. *Language, Speech, and Hearing Services in Schools, 17,* 107–114.

Hale-Benson, J. E. (1986). *Black children: Their roots, culture, and learning styles* (rev. ed.). Baltimore: Johns Hopkins University Press.

Hale-Benson, J. E. (1990a). Visions for children: Afro-American early childhood education programs. *Early Childhood Research Quarterly, 5,* 199–213.

Hale-Benson, J. E. (1990b). Visions for children: Educating Black children in the context of their culture. In K. Lomotry (Ed.), *Going to school: The Afro-American experience* (pp. 209–222). Albany: State University of New York.

Haley, K. L., Camarata, S. M., & Nelson, K. E. (1994). Social valence in children with specific language impairment during imitation-based and conversation-based intervention. *Journal of Speech and Learning Research, 37,* 378–388.

Hall, R. (1984). *Sniglets (Snig'lit): Any word that doesn't appear in the dictionary, but should.* New York: Macmillan.

Halle, J. W. (1987). Teaching language in the natural environment: An analysis of spontaneity. *Journal of the Association of Persons with Severe Handicaps, 12,* 28–37.

Halle, J. W. (1988). Adopting the natural environment as the context of training. In S. Calculator & J. Bedrosian (Eds.), *Communication assessment and intervention for adults with mental retardation* (pp. 155–185). San Diego: College-Hill.

Halliday, M.A., & Hasan, R. (1976). *Cohesion in English.* London: Longman.

Hamayan, E., & Damico, J. (1991). Developing and using a second language. In E. Hamayan & J. Damico (Eds.), *Limiting bias in the assessment of bilingual students* (pp. 40–75). Austin, TX: Pro-Ed.

Hambly, C., & Riddle, L. (2002, April). *Phonological awareness training for school-age children.* Paper presented at the annual convention of the New York State Speech-Language-Hearing Association, Rochester.

Hamman, S., & Squire, L. (1996). Levels of processing effects in word-completion priming: A neuropsychological study. *Journal of Experimental Psychology: Learning, Memory and Cognition, 22,* 933–947.

Hamman, S., & Squire, L. (1997). Intact perceptual memory in the absence of conscious memory. *Behavioral Neuroscience, 111,* 850–854.

Hammill, D., & Larson, S. (1996). *Test of Written Language-3.* Austin, TX: Pro-Ed.

Handekman, J., Harris, S., Kristoff, B., Fuentes, F., & Alessandri, M. (1991). A specialized program for preschool children with autism. *Language, Speech, and Hearing Services in Schools, 22,* 107–110.

Haring, T., Neetz, J., Lovinger, L., Peck, C., & Semmel, M. (1988). Effects of four modified incidental teaching procedures to create opportunities for communication. *Journal of the Association for Persons with Severe Handicaps, 12,* 218–226.

Haring, T., Roger, B., Lee, M., Breen, C., & Gaylord-Ross, R. (1986). Teaching social language to moderately handicapped students. *Journal of Applied Behavior Analysis, 19,* 159–171.

Harris, K. R., & Graham, S. (1996). Improving learning disabled students' composition skills: Self-control strategy training. *Learning Disability Quarterly, 8,* 27–36.

Harris, P., Morris, J., & Terwogt, M. (1986). The early acquisition of spatial adjectives: A cross-linguistic study *Journal of Child Language, 13,* 335–352.

Harris Wright, H., & Newhoff, M. (2001). Narration abilities of children with language-learning disabilities in response to oral and written stimuli. *American Journal of Speech-Language Pathology, 10,* 308–319.

Hart, B. (1985). Naturalistic language training techniques. In S. Warren & A. Rogers-Warren (Eds.), *Teaching functional language* (pp. 63–88). Baltimore: University Park Press.

Hart, B., & Risley, T. R. (1995). *Meaningful differences in the everyday experience of young American children.* Baltimore, MD: Paul H. Brookes.

Haynes, W., & Moran, M. (1989). A cross-sectional developmental study of final consonant production in southern Black children: from preschool through third grade. *Language, Speech, and Hearing Services in Schools, 20,* 400–406.

Hazel, E. (1990). Peer-assisted carryover alternatives. *Language, Speech, and Hearing Services in Schools, 21,* 185–187.

Hazen, N. L., & Black, B. (1989). Preschool peer communication skills: The role of social status and interaction context. *Child Development, 60,* 867–876.

Heath, S. B. (1983). *Ways with words: Language, life, and work in communities and classrooms.* London: Cambridge University Press.

Heath, S. B. (1986a). Separating "things of the imagination" from life: Learning to read and write. In W. Teale & E. Sulzby (Eds.), *Emergent literacy* (pp. 156–172). Norwood, NJ: Ablex.

Heath, S. B. (1986b). Taking a cross-cultural look at narratives. *Topics in Language Disorders, 7*(1), 84–94.

Heberle, D. (1992, April). *Effective instructional strategies.* Paper presented at LEP/ESL Conference, State University of New York, Geneseo.

Hedberg, N.L., & Stoel-Gammon, C. (1986). Narrative analysis: Clinical procedures. *Topics in Language Disorders, 7,* 58–69.

Heimlich, J., & Pittelman, S. (1986). *Semantic mapping: Classroom applications.* Newark, DE: International Reading Association.

Helmstetter, E., & Guess, D. (1987). Application of individualized curriculum sequencing model to learners with severe sensory impairments. In L. Goetz, D. Guess, & K. Stremel-Campbell (Eds.), *Innovative program design for individuals with sensory impairments* (pp. 255–282). Baltimore: Paul H. Brookes.

Helzer, J. R., Champlin, C. A., & Gillam, R. B. (1996) Auditory temporal resolution in specific language-impaired and age-matched children. *Perceptual & Motor Skills, 83*(3, pt 2), 1171–1181.

Hemphill, L., Uccelli, P., Winner, K., Chang, C., & Bellinger, D. (2002). Narrative discourse in young children with histories of early corrective heart surgery. *Journal of Speech, Language, and Hearing Research, 45,* 318–331.

Henderson, E. H. (1990). *Teaching spelling* (2nd ed.). Boston: Houghton Mifflin.

Henry, F. M., Reed, V. A. & McAllister, L. L. (1995). Adolescents' perceptions of the relative importance of selected communication skills in their positive peer relations. *Language, Speech, and Hearing Services in Schools, 26,* 263–272.

Henry, M. (1990). *Words.* Los Gatos, CA: Lex.

Hess, C., Haug, H., & Landry, R. (1989). The reliability of type-token ratios for the oral language of school age children. *Journal of Speech and Hearing Research, 32,* 536–540.

Hess, C., Sefton, K., & Landry, R. (1986). Sample size and type-token ratios for oral language of preschool children. *Journal of Speech and Hearing Research, 29,* 129–134.

Hess, L. J., & Fairchild, J. L. (1988). Model, analyze, practice (MAP): A language therapy modle for learning-disabled adolescents. *Child Language Teaching and Therapy, 4,* 325–338.

Hewitt, L. E., (1992, March). *Facilitating narrative comprehension: The importance of subjectivity.* Paper presented at the Conference on Pragmatics: From Theory to Therapy, State University of New York, Buffalo.

Hewitt, L. E., & Duchan, J. F. (1995). Subjectivity in children's fictional narratives. *Topics in Language Disorders, 15*(4), 1–15.

Higginbotham, D. (1992). Evaluation of keystroke savings across five assistive communication technologies. *Augmentative and Alternative Communication, 8,* 258–272.

Hill, S., & Haynes, W. (1992). Language performance in low-achieving elementary school students. *Language, Speech, and Hearing Services in Schools, 23,* 169–175.

Hixson, P. K. (1985). DSS Computer Program [Computer program]. Omaha, NE: Computer Language Analysis.

Hobbs, M., & Bacharach, V. (1990). Children's understanding of big buildings and big cars. *Child Study Journal, 20,* 1–18.

Hoffman, L. P. (1993, May). Language in the school context: What is least restrictive. *Proceedings of contemporary issues in language and learning: Toward the year 2000* (pp. 16–18). Rockville, MD: American Speech-Language-Hearing Association.

Holton, J. (1987). *Parent interaction strategies with handicapped children: Evaluation of a new assessment scale through measurement over intervention.* Unpublished master's thesis, Ohio State University, Columbus.

Holzhauser-Peters, L., & Andrin-Husemann, D. (1990). Alternate service delivery: What are our options? *Hearsay: Journal of the Ohio Speech and Hearing Association,* Fall/Winter, 91–96.

Horn, E. (1954). *Teaching spelling.* Washington, DC: American Education Research Association.

Hoskins, B. (1987). *Conversations: Language intervention for adolescents.* Allen, TX: DLM Teaching Resources.

Houghton, J., Bronicki, G., & Guess, D. (1987). Opportunities to express preferences and make choices among students with severe disabilities in classroom settings. *Journal of the Association for Persons with Severe Handicaps, 12,* 18–27.

Huang, R., Hopkins, J., & Nippold, M. A. (1997). Satisfaction with standardized language testing: A survey of speech-language pathologists. *Language, Speech, and Hearing Services in School, 28,* 12–29.

Hughes, D., Fey, M., & Long, S. (1992). Developmental sentence scoring: Still useful after all these years. *Topics in Language Disorders, 12*(2), 1–12.

Hughes, D., Low, W., Fey, M. E., & Alsop, W. (1990). Computer-Assisted Tutorial for Learning Developmental Sentence Scoring, Version 2.0 [Computer program]. Mt. Pleasant: Central Michigan University, Department of Communication Disorders.

Hughes, M., & Searle, D. (1997). *The violet E and other tricky sounds: Learning to spell from kindergarten to grade 6.* York, ME: Stenhouse.

Hunt, P., Alwell, M., & Goetz, L. (1988). Acquisition of conversational skills and the reduction of inappropriate social interactional behaviors. *Journal of the Association of Persons with Severe Handicaps, 13*(1), 20–27.

Hunt, P., Alwell, M., & Goetz, L. (1991). Interacting with peers through conversation turntaking with a communication book adaptation. *Augmentative and Alternative Communication, 7,* 117–126.

Hunt, P., & Goetz, L. (1988). Teaching spontaneous communication in natural settings through interrupted behavior chains. *Topics in Language Disorders, 9*(1), 58–71.

Hunt, P., Goetz, L., Alwell, M., & Sailor, W. (1986). Using an interrupted behavior chain strategy to teach generalized communication responses. *Journal of the Association for Persons with Severe Handicaps, 11,* 196–204.

Hyltenstam, K. (1985). Second language variable output and language teaching. In K. Hyltenstam & M. Pienemann (Eds.), *Modeling and assessing second language acquisition* (pp. 113–136). Clevedon, Avon: Multilingual Matters.

Hynd, G. W., Marshall, R., & Gonzalez, J. (1991). Learning disabilities and presumed central nervous system dysfunction. *Learning Disabilities Quarterly, 14,* 283–296.

Iacono, T., Mirenda, P., & Beukelman, D. (1993). Comparison of unimodal and multimodal AAC techniques for children with intellectual disabilities. *Augmentative and Alternative Communication, 9,* 83–94.

Iglesias, A. (1986, May). *The cultural-linguistic minority student in the classroom: Management decisions.* Workshop presented at the State University College at Buffalo, NY.

Iglesias, A., Gutierrez-Clellan, V. F., & Marcano, M. (1986, November). *School discourse: Cultural variations.* Short course presented to the American Speech-Language-Hearing Association, Detroit, MI.

Ingram, D. (1991). Toward a theory of phoneme acquisition. In J. Miller (Ed.), *Research on child language disorders: A decade of progress* (pp. 55–72). Austin, TX: Pro-Ed.

Irwin, J. W. (1988). Linguistic cohesion and the developing reader/writer. *Topics in Language Disorders, 8*(3), 14–23.

Irwin, J. W., & Moe, A. (1986). Cohesion, coherence, and comprehension. In J. W. Irwin (Ed.), *Understanding and teaching cohesion comprehension.* Newark, DE: International Reading Association.

Isaacs, G. J. (1996). Persistence of non-standard dialect in school-age children. *Journal of Speech and Hearing Research, 39*, 434–441.

Isaacson, S. (1987). Effective instruction in written language. *Focus on Exceptional Children, 19*, 1–12.

Jackson, S. C., & Roberts, J. E. (2001). Complex syntax production of African American preschoolers. *Journal of Speech, Language, and Hearing Research, 44*, 1083–1096.

Jacobson, R. (1985). Uncovering the covert bilingual: How to retrieve the hidden home language. In E. E. Garcia & R. V. Padilla (Eds.), *Advances in bilingual education research* (pp. 150–180). Tucson: University of Arizona Press.

James, S. (1989). Assessing children with language disorders. In D. Bernstein & E. Tiegerman (Eds.), *Language and communication disorders in children* (2nd ed., pp. 157–207). New York: Merrill/Macmillan.

Jankovic, J. (2001). Tourette's syndrome. *The New England Journal of Medicine, 345*, 1184–1192.

Jarrold, C., Baddeley, A. D., & Phillips, C. E. (2002). Verbal short-term memory in Down syndrome: A problem of memory, audition, or speech? *Journal of Speech, Language, and Hearing Research, 45*, 531–544.

Jerome, A. C., Fujiki, M., Brinton, B., & James, S. L. (2002). Self-esteem in children with specific language impairment. *Journal of Speech, Language, and Hearing Research, 45*, 700–714.

Jimenez, B., & Iseyama, D. (1987). A model for training and using communication assistants. *Language, Speech, and Hearing Services in Schools, 18*, 168–171.

Johnson, A., Johnston, E., & Weinrich, B. (1981, November). *I say yes—but I mean no: Pragmatic therapy ideas.* Paper presented at the Annual Convention of the American Speech-Language-Hearing Association, Los Angeles.

Johnson, A., Johnston, E., & Weinrich, B. (1984). Assessing pragmatic skills in children's language. *Language, Speech, and Hearing Services in Schools, 15*, 2–9.

Johnson, B., McGonigel, M., & Kaufman, R. (1989). *Guidelines and recommended practices for the individualized family service.* Chapel Hill, NC: Frank Porter Graham Child Development Center.

Johnson, C. J., Ionson, M. E., & Torreiter, S. M. (1997). Assessing children's knowledge of multiple meaning words. *American Journal of Speech-Language Pathology, 6*(1), 77–86.

Johnston, J. (1982b). Narratives: A new look at communication problems in older language disordered children. *Language, Speech, and Hearing Services in Schools, 13*, 144–145.

Johnston, J. (1984). Acquisition of locative meanings: *Behind* and *in front of. Journal of Child Language, 11*, 407–422.

Johnston, J. (1988a). Generalization: The nature of change. *Language, Speech, and Hearing Services in Schools, 19*, 314–329.

Johnston, J. (1988b). Specific language disorders in the child. In N. Lass, L. McReynolds, J. Northern, & D. Yoder (Eds.), *Handbook of speech-language pathology and audiology* (pp. 685–715). Philadelphia: B. C. Decker.

Johnston, J. (1991). The continuing relevance of cause: A reply to Leonard's "Specific language impairment as a clinical category." *Language, Speech, and Hearing Services in Schools, 22*, 75–79.

Johnston, J., & Kamhi, A. (1984). The same can be less: Syntactic and semantic aspects of the utterances of language impaired children. *Merrill-Palmer Quarterly, 30*, 65–86.

Johnston, J., & Smith, L. (1989). Dimensional thinking in language impaired children. *Journal of Speech and Hearing Research, 32*, 33–38.

Johnston, J. R. (1995). Cognitive abilities of children with language impairments. In R. Watkins & M. Rice (Eds.), *Specific language impairment in children* (pp. 91–106). Baltimore, MD: Paul H. Brookes.

Johnston, J. R. (2001). An alternative MLU calculation: Magnitude and variability of effects. *Journal of Speech, Language, and Hearing Research, 44*, 156–164.

Johnston, P. H., & Winograd, P. N. (1985). Passive failure in reading. *Journal of Reading Behavior, 4*, 279–301.

Jones, C., & Adamson, L. (1987). Language used in mother-child and mother-child-sibling interactions. *Child Development, 58*, 356–366.

Jordan, F., Murdock, B., & Buttsworth, D. (1991). Closed-head injured children's performance on narrative tasks. *Journal of Speech and Hearing Research, 34*, 572–582.

Jordan, F. M., Ozanne, A. O., & Murdoch, B. E. (1988). Long-term speech and language disorders subsequent to closed head injury in children. *Brain Injury, 2*, 179–185.

Juel, C. (1988). Learning to read and write: A longitudinal study of 54 children from first through fourth grades. *Journal of Educational Psychology, 80*, 437–447.

Justice, L. M., & Ezell, H. K. (2000). Enhancing children's print and word awareness through home-based parent intervention. *American Journal of Speech-Language Pathology, 9*, 257–269.

Justice, L. M., & Ezell, H. K. (2002). Use of storybook reading to increase print awareness in at-risk children. *American Journal of Speech-Language Pathology, 11*, 17–29.

Justice, L. M., Invernizzi, M. A., & Meier, J. D. (2002). Designing and implementing an early literacy screening protocol: Suggestions for the speech-language pathologist. *Language, Speech, and Hearing Services in Schools, 33,* 84–101.

Justice, L. M., Weber, S. E., Ezell, H. K., & Bakeman, R. (2002). A sequential analysis of children's responsiveness to parental print references during shared book-reading interactions. *American Journal of Speech-Language Pathology, 11,* 30–40.

Kaderavek, J. N., & Sulzby, E. (1998, November). *Low versus high orientation towards literacy in children.* Paper presented at the annual convention of the American Speech-Language-Hearing Association, San Antonio, TX.

Kail, R. (1984). *The development of memory in children* (2nd ed.). San Francisco: Freeman.

Kail, R., Hale, C., Leonard, L., & Nippold, M. (1984). Lexical storage and retrieval in language-impaired children. *Applied Psycholinguistics, 5,* 37–50.

Kail, R., & Leonard, L. B. (1986). Word-finding abilities in language-impaired children. *ASHA Monographs Number 25.* Rockville, MD: American Speech-Language-Hearing Association.

Kaiser, A. P., & Hester, P. P. (1994). Generalization effects of enhanced milieu teaching. *Journal of Speech and Hearing Research, 37,* 1320–1340.

Kameenui, E. J., Dixon, R. C., & Carnine, D. W. (1987). Issues in the design of vocabulary instruction. In M. G. McKeown & M. E. Curtis (Eds.), *The nature of vocabulary acquisition* (pp. 129–146). Hillsdale, NJ: Lawrence Erlbaum.

Kamhi, A. G. (1984). Problem solving in child language disorders: The clinician as clinical scientist. *Language, Speech, and Hearing Services in Schools, 15,* 226–234.

Kamhi, A. G. (1987). Metalinguistic abilities in language-impaired children. *Topics in Language Disorders, 7*(2), 1–12.

Kamhi, A. G. (1988). A reconceptualization of generalization and generalization problems. *Language, Speech, and Hearing Services in Schools, 19,* 304–313.

Kamhi, A. G. (1993). Assessing complex behaviors: Problems with reification, quantification, and ranking. *Language, Speech, and Hearing Services in Schools, 24,* 110–113.

Kamhi, A. (1998). Trying to make sense of developmental language disorders. *Language, Speech, and Hearing Services in Schools, 29,* 35–44.

Kamhi, A. G., Gentry, B., Mauer, D., & Gholson, B. (1990). Analogical learning and transfer in language-impaired children. *Journal of Speech and Hearing Disorders, 55,* 140–148.

Kamhi, A. G., & Hinton, L. N. (2000). Explaining individual differences in spelling ability. *Topics in Language Disorders, 20*(3), 37.

Kamhi, A. G., Minor, J., & Mauer, D. (1990). Content analysis and intratest performance profiles on the Columbia and the TONI. *Journal of Speech and Hearing Research, 33,* 375–379.

Kamhi, A. G., & Nelson, L. (1988). Early syntactic development: Simple clause types and grammatical morphology. *Topics in Language Disorders, 8*(2), 26–43.

Kangas, K., & Lloyd, L. (1988). Early cognitive skills as prerequisites to augmentative and alternative communication use: What are we waiting for? *Augmentative and Alternative Communication, 4,* 211–221.

Kaufman, S. S., Prelock, P. A., Weiler, E. M., Creaghead, N. A., & Donnelly, C. A. (1994). Metapragmatic awareness of explanation adequacy: Developing skills for academic success from a collaborative communication skills unit. *Language, Speech, and Hearing Services in Schools, 25,* 174–180.

Kay-Raining Bird, E., & Chapman, R. S. (1994). Sequential recall in individuals with Down syndrome. *Journal of Speech and Learning Research, 37,* 1369–1380.

Kay-Raining Bird, E., & Vetter, D. K. (1994). Storytelling in Chippewa-Cree children. *Journal of Speech and Learning Research, 37,* 1354–1368.

Kaye, K., & Charney, R. (1981). Conversational asymmetry between mothers and children. *Journal of Child Language, 8,* 35–49.

Keefe, K., Feldman, H., & Holland, A. (1989). Lexical learning and language abilities in pre-schoolers with perinatal brain damage. *Journal of Speech and Hearing Disorders, 54,* 395–402.

Keller-Cohen, D. (1987). Context and strategy in acquiring temporal connectives. *Journal of Psycholinguistic Research, 16,* 165–183.

Kelly, D., & Rice, M. (1986). A strategy for language assessment of young children: A combination of two approaches. *Language, Speech, and Heating Services in Schools, 17,* 83–94.

Kemper, S., & Edwards, L. (1986). Children's expression of causality and their construction of narratives. *Topics in Language Disorders, 7*(1), 11–20.

Keogh, J., & Sugden, D. (1985). *Motor skill development.* New York: Macmillan.

Keogh, W. J., & Reichle, J. (1985). Communication and intervention for the "difficult-to-teach" severely handicapped.

In S. Warren & A. Rogers-Warren (Eds.), *Teaching functional language: Generalization and maintenance of language skills* (pp. 157–194). Baltimore: University Park Press.

Kernan, K. (1990). Comprehension of syntactically indicated sequence by Down's syndrome and other mentally retarded adults. *Journal of Mental Deficiency Research, 34,* 169–178.

Kiernan, B., & Gray, S. (1998). Word learning in a supported-learning context by preschool children with specific language impairment. *Journal of Speech, Language, and Hearing Research, 41,* 161–171.

Kiernan, B., Snow, D., Swisher, L., & Vance, R. (1997). Another look at nonverbal rule induction in children with specific language impairment: Testing a flexible reconceptualization hypothesis. *Journal of Speech, Language, and Learning Research, 40,* 75–82.

Kiernan, B., & Swisher, L. (1990). The initial learning of novel English words: Two single-subject experiments with minority-language children. *Journal of Speech and Hearing Research, 33,* 707–716.

Kim, Y., & Lombardino, L. (1991). The efficacy of script contexts in language comprehension intervention with children who have mental retardation. *Journal of Speech and Hearing Research, 34,* 845–857.

King, T. (1991). A signalling device for non-oral communicators. *Language, Speech, and Hearing Services in Schools, 22,* 277–282.

Kintsch, W. (1998). *Comprehension. A paradigm for cognition.* New York: Cambridge University Press.

Klecan-Aker, J. (1985). Syntactic abilities in normal and language deficient middle school children. *Topics in Language Disorders, 5*(3), 46–54.

Klecan-Aker, J. S., & Carrow-Woolfolk, E. (1987). Elicited imitation and spontaneous language sampling as tools in language assessment and intervention. *Tejas, XIII,* 34–39.

Klecan-Aker, J., & Hamburg, E. (1991). *An investigation of the stories of normal and language-disordered second- and fourth-grade children.* Unpublished manuscript.

Klecan-Aker, J. S., Swank, P. R., & Johnson, D. L. (1991, November). *A reliability and validity study of children's stories.* Paper presented at the Annual Convention of the American Speech-Language-Hearing Association, Atlanta.

Klee, T. (1992). Developmental and diagnostic characteristics of quantitative measures of children's language production. *Topics in Language Disorders, 12*(2), 28–41.

Klee, T., Carson, D. K., Gavin, W. J., Hall, L., Kent, A., & Reece, S. (1998). Concurrent and predictive validity of an early language screening program. *Journal of Speech, Language, and Hearing Research, 41,* 627–641.

Klee, T., & Fitzgerald, M. (1985). The relation between grammatical development and mean length of utterance in morphemes. *Journal of Child Language, 12,* 251–269.

Klee, T., Schaffer, M., May, S., Membrino, I., & Mougey, K. (1989). A comparison of the age-MLU relationship in normal and specifically language impaired preschool children. *Journal of Speech and Hearing Disorders, 54,* 226–233.

Klein, H. (1984). Procedure for maximizing phonological information from single-word responses. *Language, Speech, and Hearing Services in Schools, 15,* 267–274.

Klein, M. D., & Briggs, M. H. (1987). *Observation of communicative interactions.* Los Angeles: California State University, Mother-Infant Communication Project.

Klink, M., Gerstman, L., Raphael, L., Schlanger, B., & Newsome, L. (1986). Phonological process usage by young EMR children and nonretarded preschool children. *American Journal of Mental Deficiency, 91,* 190–195.

Koegel, R., Dyer, K., & Bell, L. (1987). The influence of child-preferred activities on autistic children's social behavior. *Journal of Applied Behavior Analysis, 20,* 243–252.

Koegel, R., & Johnson, J. (1989). Motivating language use in autistic children. In G. Dawson (Ed.), *Autism: Nature, diagnosis, and treatment.* New York: Guilford.

Koenig, L., & Biel, C. (1989). A delivery system of comprehensive language services in a school district. *Language, Speech, and Hearing Services in Schools, 20,* 338–365.

Kohl, F. (1981). Effects of motoric requirements on the acquisition of manual sign responses by severely handicapped students. *American Journal of Mental Deficiency, 85,* 396–403.

Kohler, F., & Fowler, S. (1985). Training prosocial behaviors to young children: An analysis of reciprocity with untrained peers. *Journal of Applied Behavior Analysis, 18,* 187–200.

Kohnert, K. J., & Bates, E. (2002). Balancing bilinguals II: Lexical comprehension and cognitive processing in children learning Spanish and English. *Journal of Speech, Language, and Hearing Research, 45,* 347–359.

Kouri, T. A. (1994). Lexical comprehension in young children with developmental delays. *American Journal of Speech-Language Pathology, 3*(1), 79–87.

Kovarsky, D. (1992). Ethnography and language assessment: Toward the contextualized description and interpretation of communicative behavior. *Best Practices in School Speech-Language Pathology, 2,* 115–122.

Kovarsky, D., & Duchan, J. (1997). The interactional dimensions of language therapy. *Language, Speech, and Hearing Services in Schools, 28,* 297–307.

Kovarsky, D., & Maxwell, M. (1997). Rethinking the context of language in the schools. *Language, Speech, and Hearing Services in Schools, 28,* 219–230.

Kozleski, E. S. (1991). Expectant delay procedure for teaching requests. *Augmentative and Alternative Communication, 7,* 11–19.

Kraat, A. W. (1985). *Communicative interaction between aided and natural speakers: An IPCAS study report.* Toronto: Canadian Rehabilitation Council for the Disabled.

Krashen, S. D., & Biber, D. (1988). *On course.* Sacramento: California Association for Bilingual Education.

Kroll, B. M. (1981). Developmental relationships between speaking and writing. In B. M. Kroll & R. J. Vann (Eds.), *Exploring speaking-writing relationships: Connections and contrasts* (pp. 32–54). Champaign, IL: National Council of Teachers of English.

Kunze, L., Lockhart, S., Didow, S., & Caterson, M. (1983). Interactive model for the assessment and treatment of the young child. In H. Winits (Ed.), *Treating language disorders: For clinicians by clinicians* (pp. 19–96). Baltimore: University Park Press.

Kurth, R. J. (1988, April). *Process variables in writing instruction using word processing, word processing with voice synthesis, and no word processing in second grade.* Paper presented at the Annual Meeting of the American Educational Research Association, New Orleans.

Kwiatkowski, J., & Shriberg, L. D. (1992). Intelligibility assessment in developmental phonological disorders: Accuracy of caregiver gloss. *Journal of Speech and Hearing Research, 35,* 1095–1104.

Labov, W. (1972). *Language in the inner city.* Philadelphia: University of Pennsylvania Press.

Lahey, M. (1988). *Language disorders and language development.* New York: Macmillan.

Lahey, M. (1990). Who shall be called language disordered? Some reflections and one perspective. *Journal of Speech and Hearing Disorders, 55,* 612–620.

Lahey, M. (1992). Lingual and cultural diversity: Further problems for determining who shall be called language disordered. *Journal of Speech and Hearing Research, 35,* 638–639.

Lahey, M. (1994). Grammatical morpheme acquisition: Do norms exist? *Journal of Speech and Hearing Research, 37,* 1192–1194.

Lahey, M., & Edwards, J. (1995). Specific language impairment: Preliminary investigation of factors assessed with family history and with patterns of language performance. *Journal of Speech and Hearing Research, 38,* 643–657.

Lahey, M., & Silliman, E. (1987, April). *In other words, how do you put it? Narrative development and disorders.* Paper presented at the Annual Convention of the New York State Speech-Language-Hearing Association, Kiamesha Lake.

LaMarre, J., & Holland, J. (1985). The functional independence of mands and tacts. *Journal of Experimental Analysis of Behavior, 43,* 5–19.

Landry, S. H., & Chapieski, M. L. (1990). Joint attention of six-month-old Down syndrome and preterm infants: I. Attention to toys and mother. *American Journal of Mental Retardation, 94,* 488–498.

Langdon, H. W. (1989). Language disorder or difference? Assessing the language skills of Hispanic students. *Exceptional Children, 56,* 37–45.

Langenfield, K. K., & Coltrane, C. (1991, November). *Preschool phonological classroom: A pilot program.* Paper presented at the Annual Convention of the American Speech-Language-Hearing Association, Atlanta.

Lapadat, J. C. (1991). Pragmatic language skills of students with language and/or learning disabilities: A quantitative synthesis. *Journal of Learning Disabilities, 24,* 147–158.

Larry P. v. Riles. (1984). 793 F.2d 969; 1984 U.S. App. LEXIS 26195. Amended June 25, 1986.

Larson, S., & Hammill, D. (1994). *Test of Written Spelling-3.* Austin, TX: Pro-Ed.

Larson, V. L., & McKinley, N. L. (1987). *Communication assessment and intervention strategies for adolescents.* Eau Claire, WI: Thinking Publications.

Larson, V. L., & McKinley, N. L. (1993). Adolescent language: An introduction. *Language, Speech, and Hearing Services in Schools, 24,* 19–20.

Larson, V. L., & McKinley, N. L. (1998). Characteristics of adolescents' conversations: A longitudinal study. *Clinical Linguistics and Phonetics, 12,* 183–203.

Larson, V. L., McKinley, N. L., & Boley, D. (1993). Service delivery models for adolescents with language disorders. *Language, Speech, and Hearing Services in Schools, 24,* 36–42.

Lau v. Nichols, 411 U.S. 563 (1974).

Laughton, J., & Hasenstab, M. (1986). *The language learning process: Implications for management of disorders.* Rockville, MD: Aspen.

Lawrence, C. (1992). Assessing the use of age-equivalent scores in clinical management. *Language, Speech, and Hearing Services in Schools, 23,* 6–8.

Lazar, R. T., Warr-Leeper, G. A., Nicholson, C. B., & Johnson, S. (1989). Elementary school teachers' use of multiple meaning expressions. *Language, Speech, and Hearing Services in Schools, 20,* 420–430.

Lee, L. (1974). Developmental Sentence Analysis. Evanston, IL: Northwestern University Press.

Lee, R. F., & Kamhi, A. G. (1990). Metaphoric competence in children with learning disabilities. *Journal of Learning Disabilities, 23,* 476–482.

Lehnert, W., & Vine, E. (1987). The role of affect in narrative structure. *Cognition and Emotion, 1,* 299–322.

Lehr, E. (1989). Community integration after traumatic brain injury: Infants and children. In P. Bach-y-Rita (Ed.), *Traumatic brain injury.* New York: Demos.

Lennox, C., & Siegel, L. S. (1996). The development of phonological rules and visual strategies in average and poor spellers. *Journal of Experimental Child Psychology, 62,* 60–83.

Leonard, L. B. (1981). Facilitating language skills in children with specific language impairment: A review. *Applied Psycholinguistics, 2,* 89–118.

Leonard, L. B. (1986). Conversational replies in children with specific language impairment. *Journal of Speech and Hearing Research, 29,* 114–119.

Leonard, L. B. (1987). Is specific language impairment a useful construct? In S. Rosenberg (Ed.), *Advances in applied psycholinguistics* (Vol. 1, pp. 1–39). Cambridge, UK: Cambridge University Press.

Leonard, L. B. (1988). Lexical development and processing in specific language impairment. In R. L. Schiefelbusch & L. L. Lloyd (Eds.), *Language perspectives: Acquisition, retardation, and intervention* (2nd ed., pp. 69–87). Austin, TX: Pro-Ed.

Leonard, L. B. (1989). Language learnability and specific language impairment in children. *Applied Psycholinguistics, 10,* 179–202.

Leonard, L. B. (1990). Language disorders in preschool children. In G. H. Shames & E. H. Wiig (Eds.), *Human communication disorders: An introduction* (3rd ed., pp. 159–192). New York: Merrill/Macmillan.

Leonard, L. B. (1991). Specific language impairment as a clinical category. *Language, Speech, and Hearing Services in Schools, 22,* 66–68.

Leonard, L. B. (1998). *Children with specific language impairment.* Cambridge, MA: MIT Press.

Leonard, L. B., McGregor, K. K., & Allen, G. D. (1992). Grammatical morphology and speech perception in children with specific language impairments. *Journal of Speech and Hearing Research, 35,* 1076–1085.

Leonard, L. B., Miller, C. A., Deevy, P., Rauf, L., Gerber, E., & Charest, M. (2002). Production operations and the use of nonfinite verbs by children with specific language impairment. *Journal of Speech, Language, and Hearing Research, 45,* 744–758.

Leonard, L. B., Sabbadini, L., Leonard, J., & Volterra, V. (1987). Specific language impairments in children: A cross-lingual study. *Brain and Language, 32,* 233–252.

Leonard, L. B., Sabbadini, L., Volterra, V., & Leonard, J. (1988). Some influences on the grammar of English and Italian-speaking children with specific language impairments. *Applied Psycholinguistics, 9,* 39–57.

Lesar, S. (1992). Prenatal cocaine exposure: The challenge to education. *Infant-Toddler Intervention: The Transdisciplinary Journal, 2*(1), 37–52.

Leslie, L., & Caldwell, J. (2000). *Qualitative Reading Inventory-III.* New York: Longman.

Levine, M. (1987). *Developmental variation and learning disorders.* Cambridge, MA: Educators Publishing Service.

Lewis, B. A., O'Donnell, B., Freebairn, L. A., & Taylor, H. G. (1998). Spoken language and written expression—Interplay of delays. *American Journal of Speech-Language Pathology, 7*(3), 77–84.

Lewis, L., Duchan, J., & Lubinski, R. (1985, November). *Assessing aspect through videotape procedures.* Paper presented at the Annual Convention of the American Speech-Language-Hearing Association, Washington, DC.

Lewy, A. L., & Dawson, G. (1992). Social stimulation and joint attention in young autistic children. *Journal of Abnormal Child Psychology, 20,* 555–556.

Liberman, I. Y. (1983). A language-oriented view of reading and its disorders. In H. Myklebust (Ed.), *Progress in learning disabilities* (Vol. 5, pp. 81–102). New York: Grune & Stratton.

Liberman, I. Y., Rubin, H., Duques, S., & Carlisle, J. (1985). Linguistic abilities and spelling proficiency in kindergartners and adult poor spellers. In D. B. Gray & J. F. Kavanaugh (Eds.), *Biobehavioral measures of dyslexia* (pp. 163–176). Parkton, MD: York.

Liberman, I. Y., & Shankweiler, D. (1985). Phonology and problems of learning to read and write. *RASE Remedial and Special Education, 6,* 8–17.

Lidz, C. S. (1987). Historical perspectives. In C. S. Lidz (Ed.), *Dynamic assessment: An interactional approach to evaluating learning potential* (pp. 3–34). New York: Guilford.

Lidz, C. S., & Peña, E. D. (1996). Dynamic assessment: The model, its relevance as a nonbiased approach, and its application to Latino American preschool children.

Language, Speech, and Hearing Services in Schools, 27, 367–372.

Lieberman, P., Meskill, R. H., Chatillon, M., & Schupack, H. (1985). Phonetic speech perception deficits in dyslexia. *Journal of Speech and Hearing Research, 20,* 480–486.

Lieberman, R., Heffron, A., West, S., Hutchinson, E., & Swem, T. (1987). A comparison of four adolescent language tests. *Language, Speech, and Hearing Services in Schools, 18,* 250–266.

Lieberman, R., & Michael, A. (1986). Content relevance and content coverage in tests of grammatical ability. *Journal of Speech and Language Disorders, 51,* 71–81.

Lieven, E. (1984). Interactional style and children's language learning. *Topics in Language Disorders, 4*(4), 15–23.

Light, J. (1988). Interaction involving individuals using augmentative and alternative communication systems: State of the art and future directions. *Augmentative and Alternative Communication, 2,* 98–107.

Light, P., Remington, B., Clarke, S., & Watson, J. (1989). Signs of language? In I. Leudar, M. Beveridge, & G. Conti-Ramsden (Eds.), *Language and communication in the mentally handicapped* (pp. 56–79). London: Chapman & Hall.

Liles, B. (1985a). Cohesion in the narratives of normal and language disordered children. *Journal of Speech and Hearing Research, 28,* 1213–133.

Liles, B. (1985b). Production and comprehension of narrative discourse in normal and language disordered children. *Journal of communication disorders, 18,* 409–427.

Liles, B. (1987). Episode organization and cohesive conjunctives in narratives of children with and without language disorder. *Journal of Speech and Hearing Research, 30,* 185–196.

Liles, B. (1990, April). *Clinical implications for narrative production.* Paper presented at the Annual Convention of the New York State Speech-Language-Hearing Association, Kiamesha Lake.

Liles, B., Coelho, C., Duffy, R., & Zalagens, M. (1989). Effects of elicitation procedures on the narratives of normal and closed-head-injured adults. *Journal of Speech and Hearing Disorders, 54,* 356–366.

Liles, B., Duffy, R. J., Merritt, D. D., & Purcell, S. L. (1995). Measurement of narrative discourse ability in children with language disorders. *Journal of Speech and Hearing Research, 38,* 415–425.

Lilius, B. (1993). Personal correspondence.

Lindamood, C., & Lindamood, R. (1979). Lindamood Auditory Conceptualization Test. Allen, TX: DLM Teaching Resources.

Lively, M. (1984). Developmental sentence scoring: Common scoring errors. *Language, Speech, and Hearing Services in Schools, 15,* 154–168.

Lockhart, R., & Craik, F. (1990). Levels of processing: A retrospective commentary on a framework for memory research. *Canadian Journal of Psychology, 44,* 87–112.

Loeb, D., & Leonard, L. B. (1988). Specific language impairment and parameter theory. *Clinical Linguistics and Phonetics, 2,* 317–327.

Lomax, R. G., & McGee, L. M. (1987). Young children's concepts about print and reading: Toward a model of word acquisition. *Reading Research Quarterly, 22,* 237–256.

Lombardino, L. J., Bedford, T., Fortier, C., Carter, J., & Brandi, J. (1997). Invented spelling: Developmental patterns in kindergarten children and guidelines for early literacy intervention. *Language, Speech, and Hearing Services in Schools, 28,* 333–343.

Long, S. H. (1991). Integrating microcomputer applications into speech and language assessment. *Topics in Language Disorders, 11*(2), 1–17.

Long, S. H., & Fey, M. E. (1988). Computerized Profiling Version 6.1 (Apple II series) [Computer program]. Ithaca, NY: Ithaca College.

Long, S. H., & Fey, M. E. (1989). Computerized Profiling Version 6.2 (Macintosh and MS-DOS series) [Computer program]. Ithaca, NY: Ithaca College.

Long, S. H., & Fey, M. E. (1991). Computerized Profiling, Version 1.0 (Macintosh) (Computer program]. Ithaca, NY: Ithaca College, Department of Speech Pathology and Audiology.

Long, S. H., & Masterson, J. J. (1993). Computer technology: Use in language analysis. *Asha, 35*(8), 40–41, 51.

Longhurst, T. (1984). The scope of normative language assessment. In K. Ruder & M. Smith (Eds.), *Developmental language intervention: Psycholinguistic applications* (pp. 21–55). Baltimore: University Park Press.

Lonigan, C. J., Burgess, S. R., Anthony, J. S., & Barker, T. A. (1998). Development of phonological sensitivity in 2- to 5-year-old children. *Journal of Educational Psychology, 90,* 294–311.

Lord, C. (1985). Autism and the comprehension of language. In E. Schopler & G. Mesibov (Eds.), *Communication problems in autism* (pp. 257–282). New York: Plenum.

Lord, C. (1988). Enhancing communication in adolescents with autism. *Topics in Language Disorders, 9*(1), 72–81.

Lord, C., & Magill, J. (1988). Observing social behavior in an asocial population: Methodological and clinical issues. In G. Dawson (Ed.), *Autism: New perspectives on diagnosis, nature, and treatment* (pp. 46–66). New York: Guilford.

Lord, C., Rutter, M. L., Goode, S., Heemsbergen, J., Jordan, H., Mawhood, L., & Schoplar, E. (1989). Autism Diagnostic Observation Schedule: A standardized observation of communication and social behavior. *Journal of Autism and Developmental Disabilities, 19,* 185–212.

Love, R. J., & Webb, W. G. (1986). *Neurology for the speech-language psychologist.* Stoneham, MA: Butterworth.

Loveland, K., Landry, S., Hughes, S., Hall, S., & McEvoy, R. (1988). Speech acts and the pragmatic deficits of autism. *Journal of Speech and Hearing Research, 31,* 593–604.

Lovett, M., Dennis, M., & Newman, J. (1986). Making reference: The cohesive use of pronouns in the narrative discourse of hemidecorticate adolescents. *Brain and Language, 29,* 224–251.

Lucariello, J. (1990). Freeing talk from the here-and-now: The role of event knowledge and maternal scaffolds. *Topics in Language Disorders, 10*(3), 14–29.

Lucariello, J., Kyratzis, A., & Engel, S. (1986). Event representations, context, and language. *Event Knowledge, 7,* 136–160.

Lucas, E. (1980). *Semantic and pragmatic language disorders.* Rockville, MD: Aspen.

Lund, N. J., & Duchan, J. F. (1993). *Assessing children's language in naturalistic contexts.* Englewood Cliffs, NJ: Prentice-Hall.

Lutzer, V. D. (1988). Comprehension of proverbs by average children and children with learning disorders. *Journal of Learning Disabilities, 21,* 104–108.

Lynch, E. W., & Hanson, M. J. (1992). *Developing cross-cultural competence: A guide for working with young children and their families.* Baltimore: Paul H. Brookes.

Lyytinen, P., Poikkeus, A., Laakso, M., Eklund, K., & Lyytinen, H. (2001). Language development and symbolic play in children with and without familial risk of dyslexia. *Journal of Speech, Language, and Hearing Research, 44,* 873–885.

MacArthur, C. A. (1988). The impact of computers on the writing process. *Exceptional Children, 54,* 536–542.

MacArthur, C. A. (1999). Word processing with speech synthesis and word prediction: Effects on the dialogue journal writing of students with learning disabilities. *Learning Disability Quarterly, 21,* 1–16.

MacArthur, C. A. (2000). New tools for writing: Assistive technology for students with writing difficulties. *Topics in Language Disorders, 20*(4), 85–104.

MacArthur, C. A., & Graham, S. (1987). Learning disabled students' composing under three methods of text production: Handwriting, word processing, and dictation. *Journal of Special Education, 21*(3), 22–42.

MacArthur, C. A., Graham, S., Haynes, J. A., & DeLaPaz, S. (1996). Spelling checkers and students with learning disabilities: Performance comparisons and impact on spelling. *Journal of Special Education, 30,* 35–57.

MacArthur, C. A., Graham, S., Schwartz, S. S., & Schafer, W. (1995). Evaluation of a writing instruction model that integrated a process approach, strategy instruction, and word processing. *Learning Disability Quarterly, 18,* 278–291.

MacArthur, D., & Adamson, L. B. (1996). Joint attention in preverbal children: Autism and developmental language disorders. *Journal of Autism and Developmental Disorders, 26,* 481–496.

MacDonald, C. C. (1992). Perinatal cocaine exposure: Predictor of an endangered generation. *Infant-Toddler Intervention: The Transdisciplinary Journal, 2*(1), 1–12.

MacDonald, J. (1978a). Environmental Language Inventory. San Antonio: Psychological Corp.

MacDonald, J. (1978b). OLIVER: Parent-Administered Communication Inventory. San Antonio: Psychological Corp.

MacDonald, J. (1985). Language through conversation: A model for intervention with language-delayed persons. In S. Warren & A. Rogers-Warren (Eds.), *Teaching functional language* (pp. 89–122). Baltimore: University Park Press.

MacDonald, J. (1989). *Becoming partners with children: From play to conversation.* Chicago: Riverside.

MacDonald, J., & Carroll, J. (1992a). Communication with young children: An ecological model for clinicians, parents, collaborative professionals. *American Journal of Speech-Language Pathology, 1*(4), 39–48.

MacDonald, J., & Carroll, J. (1992b). A social partnership model for assessing early communication development: An interaction model for preconversational children. *Language, Speech, and Hearing Services in Schools, 23,* 113–124.

MacDonald, J., & Gillette, Y. (1982). *A conversational approach to language delay: Problems and solutions.* Columbus, OH: Nisonger Center.

MacDonald, J., & Gillette, Y. (1986). Communicating with persons with severe handicaps: Roles of parents and professionals. *Journal of the Association for Persons with Severe Handicaps, 11,* 255–265.

MacLachlan, B. G., & Chapman, R. S. (1988). Communication breakdowns in normal and language-learning-disabled children's conversation and narration. *Journal of Speech and Hearing Disorders, 53,* 2–9.

Maclean, M., Bryant, P., & Bradley, L. (1987). Rhymes, nursery rhymes, and reading in early childhood. *Merrill-Palmer Quarterly, 33,* 255–282.

Madrid, D. L., & Garcia, E. E. (1985). The effect of language transfer on bilingual proficiency. In E. E. Garcia & R. V. Padilla (Eds.), *Advances in bilingual education research* (pp. 53–70). Tucson: University of Arizona Press.

Magill, J. (1986). *The nature of social deficits of children with autism.* Unpublished doctoral dissertation, University of Alberta, Edmonton.

Mahoney, G., & Powell, A. (1986). *Transactional intervention program: Teacher's guide.* Farmington: University of Connecticut, Health Center, Pediatric Research and Training Center.

Mahoney, G., & Weller, E. (1980). An ecological approach to language intervention. *New Directions for Exceptional Children, 2,* 17–32.

Manning Kratcoski, A. (1998). Guidelines for using portfolios in assessment and evaluation. *Language, Speech, and Hearing Services in Schools, 29,* 3–10.

Manolson, A. (1985). *It takes two to talk: Hanen early language parent guidebook.* Toronto: Hanen Resource Center.

Marcell, M., & Weeks, S. (1988). Short-term memory difficulties and Down's syndrome. *Journal of Mental Deficiency Research, 32,* 153–162.

Markman, E. (1981). Comprehension monitoring. In W. P. Dickson (Ed.), *Children's oral communication skills* (pp. 61–84). New York: Academic Press.

Marler, J. A. (2000). *Precortical and cortical contributions to backward masking in children with language-learning impairment.* Unpublished doctoral dissertation, University of Texas at Austin.

Marler, J. A., Champlin, C. A., & Gillam, R. B. (2001). *Prephonemic auditory memory in children with language impairment.* Paper presented at the 22nd Annual Symposium for Research in Child Language Disorders, Madison, WI.

Marsh, H. W., Cairns, L., Relich, J., Barnes, J., & Debus, R.L. (1984). The relationship between dimensions of self-attribution and dimensions of self-concept. *Journal of Educational Psychology, 76,* 3–32.

Marvin, C. (1987). Consultation services: Changing roles for SLP'S. *Journal of Childhood Communication Disorders, 11*(1), 1–16.

Marvin, C. A., & Wright, D. (1997). Literacy socialization in the homes of preschool children. *Language, Speech, and Hearing Services in Schools, 28,* 154–163.

Masterson, J. J. (1993a). Classroom-based phonological intervention. *American Journal of Speech-Language Pathology, 2*(1), 5–10.

Masterson, J. J. (1993b). The performance of children with language learning disabilities on two types of cognitive tasks. *Journal of Speech and Hearing Research, 36,* 1026–1036.

Masterson, J. J., & Apel, K. (2000). Spelling assessment: Charting a path to optimal intervention. *Topics in Language Disorders, 20*(3), 50–65.

Masterson, J. J., & Crede, L. A. (1999). Learning to spell: Implications for assessment and intervention. *Language, Speech, and Hearing Services in Schools, 30,* 243–354.

Masterson, J. J., Evans, L. H., & Aloia, M. (1993). Verbal analogical reasoning in children with language learning disorders. *Journal Speech and Hearing Research, 36,* 76–82.

Masterson, J. J., & Kamhi, A. G. (1991). The effects of sampling conditions on sentence production in normal, reading-disabled, and language-learning-disabled children. *Journal of Speech and Hearing Research, 34,* 549–558.

Masterson, J. J. & Perrey, C. D. (1994). A program for training analogical reasoning skills in children with language disorders. *Language, Speech, and Hearing Services in Schools, 25,* 268–270.

Masterson, J. J., & Perrey, C. D. (1999) Training analogical reasoning skills in children with language disorders. *American Journal of Speech-Language Pathology, 8,* 53–61.

Matsuda, M. (1989). Working with Asian parents: Some communication strategies. *Topics in Language Disorders, 9*(3), 45–53.

Mattes, L. (1982). The elicited language analysis procedure: A method for scoring sentence imitation tasks. *Language, Speech, and Hearing in Schools, 13,* 37–41.

Mattes, L. J., & Omark, D. R. (1984). *Speech and language assessment for the bilingual handicapped.* Austin, TX: Pro-Ed.

Mayer, M. (1969). *Frog, where are you?* New York: Penguin Putnam.

Mayer, M., & Mayer, M. (1975). *One frog too many.* New York: Penguin Putnam.

McCabe, A., & Peterson, C. (1990). *Keep them talking: Parental styles of interviewing and subsequent child narrative skill.* Paper presented at the 5th International Congress for the Study of Child Language, Budapest.

McCabe, A., & Rollins, P. R. (1994). Assessment of preschool narrative skills. *American Journal of Speech Language Pathology, 3*(1), 45–56.

McCaleb, P., & Prizant, B. (1985). Encoding of new versus old information by autistic children. *Journal of Speech and Hearing Disorders, 50,* 230–240.

McCauley, R., & Swisher, L. (1984a). Psychometric review of language and articulation tests for preschool children. *Journal of Speech and Hearing Disorders, 49,* 34–42.

McCauley, R., & Swisher, L. (1984b). Use and misuse of norm-referenced tests in clinical assessment: A hypothetical case. *Journal of Speech and Hearing Disorders, 49,* 338–348.

McCauley, R., & Swisher, L. (1987). Are maltreated children at risk for speech and language impairment? An unanswered question. *Journal of Speech and Hearing Disorders, 52,* 301–303.

McCauley, R. J. (1996). Familiar strangers: Criterion-referenced measures in communication disorders. *Language, Speech, and Hearing Services in Schools, 27,* 122–131.

McCormick, L. (1986). Keeping up with language intervention trends. *Teaching Exceptional Children, 18,* 123–129.

McDade, H. L., & Varnedoe, D. (1987). Training parents to be language facilitators. *Topics in Language Disorders, 7*(3), 19–30.

McFadden, T. U. (1996). Creating language impairments in typically achieving children: The pitfall for "normal" normative sampling. *Language, Speech, and Hearing Services in Schools, 27,* 3–9.

McFadden, T. U. (1998). Sounds and stories: Teaching phonemic awareness in interactions around text. *American Journal of Speech-Language Pathology, 7*(2), 5–13.

McFadden, T. U., & Gillam, R. B. (1996). An examination of the quality of narratives produced by children with language disabilities. *Language, Speech, and Hearing Services in Schools, 27,* 48–56.

McGregor, G., Young, J., Gerak, J., Thomas, B., & Vogelsberg, R. T (1992). Increasing functional use of an assistive communication device by a student with severe disabilities. *Augmentative and Alternative Communication, 8,* 243–250.

McGregor, K., & Leonard, L. (1989). Facilitating word finding skills of language-impaired children. *Journal of Speech and Hearing Disorders, 54,* 141–147.

McGregor, K. K. (1994). Use of phonological information in a word-finding treatment for children. *Journal of Speech and Hearing Research, 37,* 1381–1393.

McGregor, K. K. (2000). The development and enhancement of narrative skills in a preschool classroom: Towards a solution to clinician-client mismatch. *American Journal of Speech-Language Pathology, 9,* 55–71.

McGregor, K. K., & Windsor, J. (1996). Effects of priming on the naming accuracy of preschoolers with word-finding deficits. *Journal of Speech and Hearing Research, 39,* 1048–1058.

McKeown, M. G., & Curtis, M. E. (Eds.). (1987). *The nature of vocabulary acquisition.* Hillsdale, NJ: Lawrence Erlbaum.

McKinley, N., & Lord-Larson, V. (1985). Neglected language-disordered adolescents: A delivery model. *Language, Speech, and Hearing Services in Schools, 16,* 2–15.

McKinley, N., & Schwartz, L. (1987). *Referential communication: Barrier activities for speakers and listeners, Part 2.* Eau Claire, WI: Thinking Publications.

McLean, J. E., & Snyder-McLean, L. K. (1987). Form and function of communicative behaviour among persons with severe developmental disabilities. *Australia and New Zealand Journal of Developmental Disabilities, 13*(2), 83–98.

McLean, J. E., & Snyder-McLean, L. K. (1988b, September). *Assessment and treatment of communicative competencies among clients with severe/profound developmental disabilities.* Workshop presented for Craig Developmental Disabilities Service Office and State University of New York, Geneseo.

McLean, J. E., Snyder-McLean, L. K., Brady, N. C., & Etter, R. (1991). Communication profiles of two types of gesture using nonverbal persons with severe to profound mental retardation. *Journal of Speech and Hearing Research, 34,* 294–308.

McLeod, S., Hand, L., Rosenthal, J. B., & Hayes, B. (1994). The effect of sampling condition on children's productions of consonant clusters. *Journal of Speech and Hearing Research, 37,* 868–882.

McMorrow, M., Foxx, R., Faw, G., & Bittle, E. (1987). Cues-pause-point language training: Teaching echolalics functional use of their verbal labeling repertoires. *Journal of Applied Behavior Analysis, 20,* 11–22.

McNamara, M., Carter, A., McIntosh, B., & Gerken, L. (1998). Sensitivity to grammatical morphemes in children with specific language impairment. *Journal of peech, Language, and Hearing Research, 41,* 1147–1157.

McNaughton, D., Hughes, C., & Ofiesh, N. (1997). Proofreading for students with learning disabilities: Integrating computer use and strategic use. *Learning Disabilities Research and Practice, 12,* 16–28.

McNaughton, D., & Light, J. (1989). Teaching facilitators to support the communication skills of an adult with severe cognitive disabilities: A case study. *Augmentative and Alternative Communication, 5,* 35–41.

McWilliams, P. J., & Winton, P. (1990). *Brass tacks: A self-rating of family-focused practices in early intervention. Part II: Individual interactions.* Chapel Hill, NC: Frank Porter Graham Child Development Center.

Meline, T., & Brackin, S. (1987). Language-impaired children's awareness of inadequate messages. *Journal of Speech and Hearing Disorders, 52,* 263–270.

Mentis, M., & Lundgren, K. (1995). Effects of prenatal exposure to cocaine and associated risk factors on language development. *Journal of Speech and Hearing Research, 38,* 1303–1318.

Mentis, M., & Prutting, C. A. (1987). Cohesion in the discourse of normal and head-injured adults. *Journal of Speech and Hearing Research, 30,* 88–98.

Mentis, M., & Prutting, C. A. (1991). Analysis of topic as illustrated in a head-injured and a normal adult. *Journal of Speech and Hearing Research, 34,* 583–595.

Menyuk P., Chesnick, M., Liebergott, J., Korngold, B., D'Agostino, R., & Belanger, A. (1991). Predicting reading problems in at-risk children. *Journal of Speech and Hearing Research, 34,* 893–903.

Merrell, A. W., & Plante E. (1997). Norm-referenced test interpretation in the diagnostic process. *Language, Speech, and Hearing Services in Schools, 28,* 50–58.

Merrill, E. (1985). Differences in semantic processing speed of mentally retarded and nonretarded persons. *American Journal of Mental Deficiency, 90,* 71–80.

Merrill, E., & Bilsky, L. (1990). Individual differences in the representation of sentences in memory. *American Journal on Mental Retardation, 95,* 68–76.

Merritt, D., & Liles, B. (1985, November). *Story recall and comprehension in older language disordered children.* Paper presented at the Annual Convention of the American Speech-Language-Hearing Association, San Francisco.

Merritt, D., & Liles, B. (1987). Story grammar ability in children with and without language disorder: Story generation, story retelling, and story comprehension. *Journal of Speech and Hearing Research, 30,* 539–552.

Merritt, D., & Liles, B. (1989). Narrative analysis: Clinical applications of story generation and story retelling. *Journal of Speech and Hearing Disorders, 54,* 438–447.

Mersand, J., Griffith, F., & Griffith, K. O. (1996). *Spelling the easy way* (3rd ed.). Hauppauge, NY: Barron's Educational Series.

Mervis, C. B. (1988). Early lexical development: Theory and application. In L. Nadel (Ed.), *The psychobiology of Down's syndrome* (pp. 104–144). Cambridge: MIT Press.

Mervis, C. B. (1990). Early conceptual development of children with Down syndrome. In D. Cicchetti & M. Beeghly

(Eds.), *Children with Down syndrome: A developmental perspective* (pp. 252–301). Cambridge, UK: Cambridge University Press.

Messick, C. (1988). Ins and outs of the acquisition of spatial terms. *Topics in Language Disorders, 8*(2), 14–25.

Meyer, A., & Rose, D. (1987, October). Word processing: A new route around old barriers. *The Exceptional Parent,* pp. 26–29.

Meyer, L. F., & Evans, J. (1986). Modification of excess behavior: An adaptive and functional approach for educational and community settings. In R. Horner, L. Meyer, & H. Fredericks (Eds.), *Education of learners with severe handicaps* (pp. 315–350). Baltimore: Paul H. Brookes.

Meyers, L. F., & Fogel, P. (1985). Representational Play [Computer program]. Santa Monica, CA: Peal Software.

Miall, D. (1989). Beyond the schema given: Affective comprehension of literary narratives. *Cognition and Emotion, 3,* 55–78.

Michaels, S. (1986). Narrative presentations: An oral preparation for literacy with first graders. In J. Cook-Gumperz (Ed.), *The social construction of literacy* (pp. 94–116). Cambridge, UK: Cambridge University Press.

Middleton, J. (1989). Annotation: Thinking about head injuries in children. *Journal of Child Psychology and Psychiatry, 30,* 663–670.

Miles, S., & Chapman, R. S. (2002). Narrative content as described by individuals with Down syndrome and typically developing children. *Journal of Speech, Language, and Hearing Research, 45,* 175–189.

Miller, C. A., Kail, R., Leonard, L. B., & Tomblin, J. B. (2001). Speed of processing in children with specific language impairment. *Journal of Speech, Language, and Hearing Research, 44,* 416–433.

Miller, G. A., & Gildea, P. M. (1987). How children learn words. *Scientific American, 257,* 94–99.

Miller, J., & Chapman R. S. (2003). SALT for Windows, Version 6.1.

Miller, J., Sedey, A. L., & Miolo, G. (1995). Validity of parent report measures of vocabulary development for children with Down syndrome. *Journal of Speech and Hearing Research, 38,* 1037–1044.

Miller, J. F. (1981). *Assessing language production in children: Experimental procedures.* Baltimore: University Park Press.

Miller, J. F. (1991). Quantitative productive language disorders. In J. Miller (Ed.), *Research on child language disorders: A decade of progress.* Austin, TX: Pro-Ed.

Miller, J. F., & Chapman, R. (1985). Systematic Analysis of Language Transcripts (SALT) Version 1.3 (MS-DOS)

[Computer program]. Madison, WI: Language Analysis Laboratory, Waisman Center on Mental Retardation and Human Development.

Miller, J. F., Freiberg, C., Rolland, M., & Reeves, M. A. (1992). Implementing computerized language sample analysis in the public school. *Topics in Language Disorders, 12*(2), 69–82.

Miller, L. (1984). Problem solving and language disorders. In G. P. Wallach & K. G. Butler (Eds.), *Language learning disabilities in school-age children* (pp. 199–229). Baltimore: Williams & Wilkins.

Miller, L. (1989). Classroom-based language intervention. *Language, Speech, and Hearing Services in Schools, 20,* 153–169.

Miller, L. (1993). Testing and the creation of disorder. *American Journal of Speech-Language Pathology, 2*(1), 13–16.

Miller, L. (1999a). *Two friends.* New York: Smart Alternatives.

Miller, L. (1999b). *Bird and his ring.* New York: Smart Alternatives.

Milosky, L. (1990). The role of world knowledge in language comprehension and language intervention. *Topics in Language Disorders, 10*(3), 1–13.

Minami, M., & McCabe, A. (1991). Haiku as a discourse regulation device: A stanza analysis of Japanese children's personal narratives. *Language in Society, 20,* 577–599.

Mineo, B. A., & Goldstein, H. (1990). Generalized learning of receptive and expressive action-object responses by language-delayed preschoolers. *Journal of Speech and Hearing Disorders, 55,* 665–678.

Miniutti, A. (1991). Language deficiencies in inner-city children with learning and behavioral problems. *Language, Speech, and Hearing Services in Schools, 22,* 31–38.

Mire, S., & Chisholm, R. (1990). Functional communication goals for adolescents and adults who are severely and moderately mentally handicapped. *Language, Speech, and Hearing Services in Schools, 21,* 57–58.

Mirenda, P., & Donnellan, A. (1986). Effects of adult interaction style on conversational behavior in students with severe communication problems. *Language, Speech, and Hearing Services in Schools, 17,* 126–141.

Mirenda, P, & Locke, P. (1989). A comparison of symbol transparency in nonspeaking persons with intellectual disabilities. *Journal of Speech and Hearing Disorders, 54,* 131–140.

Mirenda, P., & Schuler, A. L. (1988). Augmentative communication for persons with autism: Issues and strategies. *Topics in Language Disorders, 9*(1), 24–43.

Mistry, J., & Lange, G. (1985). Children's organization and recall of information in scripted narratives. *Child Development, 56,* 953–961.

Mizuko, M. (1987). Transparency and ease of learning of symbols represented by Blissymbolics, PCS, and Picsyms. *Augmentative and Alternative Communications, 3,* 129–136.

Moats, L. (1995). *Spelling development, disability, and instruction.* Baltimore, MD: York.

Moats, L. C., & Smith, C. (1992). Derivational morphology: Why it should be included in language assessment and instruction. *Language, Speech, and Hearing Services in Schools, 23,* 312–319.

Moeller, M., Osberger, M., & Eccarius, M. (1986). Cognitively based strategies for use with hearing impaired students with comprehension deficits. *Topics in Language Disorders, 6*(4), 37–50.

Montague, M., Graves, A., & Leavell, A. (1991). Planning procedural facilitation, and narrative composition of junior high students with learning disabilities. *Learning Disabilities Research and Practice, 6,* 219–224.

Montgomery, J. W. (1992a, May). *Collaborating within the classroom: Using whole language to remediate speech and language disorders in school-age children.* Genesee Valley Speech-Language-Hearing Association Spring Workshop, Rochester, NY.

Montgomery, J. W. (1992b). Perspectives from the field: Language, speech, and hearing services in schools. *Language, Speech, and Hearing Services in Schools, 23,* 363–364.

Montgomery, J. W. (1995). Sentence comprehension in children with specific language impairment: The role of phonological working memory. *Journal of Speech and Hearing Research, 38,* 187–199.

Montgomery, J. W. (2000a). Relation of working memory to off-line and real-time sentence processing in children with specific language impairment. *Applied Psycholinguistics, 21,* 117–148.

Montgomery, J. W. (2000b). Verbal working memory and sentence comprehension in children with specific language impairment. *Journal of Speech, Language, and Hearing Research, 43,* 293–308.

Montgomery, J. W. (2002a). Information processing and language comprehension in children with specific language impairment. *Topics in Language Disorders, 22*(3), 62–86.

Montgomery, J. W. (2002b). Understanding the language difficulties of children with specific language impairments: Does verbal working memory matter? *American Journal of Speech-Language Pathology, 11,* 77–91.

Montgomery, J. W., & Leonard, L. B. (1998). Real-time inflectional processing by children with specific language impairment: Effects of phonetic substance. *Journal of Speech, Language, and Hearing Research, 41,* 1432–1443.

Mooney, M. (1988). *Developing life-long readers.* Wellington, New Zealand: Department of Education.

Moore-Brown, B. (1991). Moving in the direction of change: Thoughts for administrators and speech language pathologists. *Language, Speech, and Hearing Services in Schools, 22,* 148–149.

Moran, M., Money, S., & Leonard, D. (1984). Phonological process analysis of the speech of mentally retarded adults. *American Journal of Mental Deficiency, 89,* 304–306.

Mordecai, D. R., Palin, M. W., & Palmer, C. B. (1985). Lingquest 1 [Computer program]. Columbus, OH: Macmillan.

Morris, D., & Perney, J. (1984). Developmental spelling as a predictor of first grade reading achievement. *Elementary School Journal, 84,* 441–457.

Morris, S., & Klein, M. (1987). *Pre-Feeding Skills.* Tucson, AZ: Therapy Skill Builders.

Morrow, D. R., Mirenda, P., Beukelman, D. P., & Yorkston, K. M. (1993). Vocabulary selection for augmentative communication systems: A comparison of three techniques. *American Journal of Speech-Language Pathology, 2*(2), 19–30.

Moses, N., & Maffei, L. (1989, April). *Classroom language intervention for communication-oriented preschools.* Paper presented at the Annual Convention of the New York State Speech-Language-Hearing Association, Liberty.

Mosisset, C. E., Barnard, K. E., Greenberg, M. T., Booth, C. L., & Spicker, S. J. (1990). Environmental influences on early language development: The context of social risk. *Development and Psychopathology, 2,* 127–149.

Muma, J. (1983). Speech-language pathology: Emerging clinical expertise in language. In T. Gallagher & C. Prutting (Eds.), *Pragmatic assessment and intervention issues in language* (pp. 195–205). San Diego: College-Hill.

Muma, J. (1986). *Language acquisition: A functional perspective.* Austin, TX: Pro-Ed.

Mundy, P., Kasari, C., Sigman, M., & Ruskin, E. (1995) Nonverbal communication and early language acquisition in children with Down syndrome and in normally developing children. *Journal of Speech and Learning Research, 38,* 157–167.

Murray-Branch, J., Udavari-Solner, A., & Bailey, B. (1991). Textural communication systems for individuals with severe intellectual and dual sensory impairments. *Language, Speech, and Hearing Services in Schools, 22,* 260–268.

Musselwhite, C. (1983). Pluralistic assessment in speech-language pathology: Use of dual norms in the placement process. *Language, Speech, and Hearing Services in Schools, 14,* 29–37.

Nagy, W. E., Anderson, R. C., & Herman, P. A. (1987). Learning word meanings from context during normal reading. *American Educational Research Journal, 24,* 237–270.

Nagy, W. E., Anderson, R. C., Schommer, M., Scott, J. A., & Stallman, A. C. (1989). *Reading Research Quarterly, 24,* 262–283.

Nagy, W. E., & Herman, P. A. (1987). Breadth and depth of vocabulary knowledge: Implications for acquisition and instruction. In M. G. McKeown & M. E. Curtis (Eds.), *The nature of vocabulary acquisition* (pp. 19–35). Hillsdale, NJ: Lawrence Erlbaum.

Nagy, W. E., Herman, P. A., & Anderson, R. C. (1985). Learning words from context. *Reading Research Quarterly, 20,* 233–253.

Nakayama, M. (1987). Performance factors in subject-auxiliary inversion in children. *Journal of Child Language, 14,* 113–127.

Naremore, R. C. (2001). *Narrative frameworks and early literacy.* Seminar presentation by Rochester Hearing and Speech Center and Nazareth College, Rochester, NY.

Nation, K., & Hulme, C. (1997). Phonemic segmentation, not onset-rime segmentation, predicts early reading and spelling skills. *Reading Research Quarterly, 32,* 154–167.

National Council of Teachers of English (NCTE) (1976). *Language development: Kindergarten through grade twelve.* Urbana, IL: National Council of Teachers of English.

National Joint Committee on Learning Disabilities. (1991). Learning disabilities: Issues on definition (A position paper). *Asha, 33,* (Suppl. 5), 18–20.

National Reading Panel. (2000). *National Reading Panel Progress Report.* Bethesda, MD: Author.

Neeley, P. M., Tipton, C., & Neeley, R. A. (1994, November). *Improvement of functional language using a scripted play paradigm.* Paper presented at the annual convention of the American Speech-Language-Hearing Association, New Orleans.

Nelson, C. D. (1991). *Practical procedures for children with language disorders.* Austin, TX: Pro-Ed.

Nelson, K. (1973). *Structure and strategy in learning to talk.* Society for Research in Guild Development monograph. Chicago: University of Chicago Press.

Nelson, K. (1981a). Acquisition of words by first-language learners. *Annals of the New York Academy of Sciences, 379,* 148–159.

Nelson, K. (1985). *Making sense: The acquisition of shared meaning.* New York: Academic Press.

Nelson, K. (Ed.) (1986). *Event knowledge: Structure and function in development.* Hillsdale, NJ: Lawrence Erlbaum.

Nelson, K., Camarata, S. M., Welsh, J., Butkovsky, L., & Camarata, M. (1996). Effects of imitative and conversational recasting treatment on the acquisition of grammar in children with specific language impairment and younger language-normal children. *Journal of Speech and Hearing Research, 39,* 850–859.

Nelson, K., Welsh, J., Camarata, S., Butkovsky, L., & Camarata, M. (1995). Available input for language-impaired children and younger children of matched language levels. *First Language, 43,* 1–18.

Nelson, L., Kamhi, A. G., & Apel, K. (1987). Cognitive strengths and weaknesses in language-impaired children: One more look. *Journal of Speech and Hearing Disorders, 52,* 36–43.

Nelson, N. W. (1985). Teachers talk and children listen—Fostering a better match. In C. Simon (Ed.), *Communication skills and classroom success: Assessment of language-learning disabled students* (pp. 65–104). San Diego: College-Hill.

Nelson, N. W. (1986a). Individual processing in classroom settings. *Topics in Language Disorders, 6*(2), 13–27.

Nelson, N. W. (1986b). What is meant by meaning (and how can it be taught)? *Topics in Language Disorders, 6*(4), 1–14.

Nelson, N. W. (1988a). The consultant model. *ASHA Audioteleconference.* Rockville, MD: ASHA.

Nelson, N. W. (1989). Curriculum-based language assessment and intervention. *Language, Speech, and Hearing Services in Schools, 20,* 170–184.

Nelson, N. W. (1992). Targets of curriculum-based language assessment. *Best Practices in School Speech-Language Pathology, 2,* 73–86.

Nelson, N. W. (1993). *Childhood language disorders in context: Infancy through adolescence.* New York: Macmillan.

Nelson, N. W. (1994). Curriculum-based language assessment and intervention across grades. In G. P. Wallach & K. G. Butler (Eds.), *Language learning disabilities in school-age children and adolescents* (pp. 104–131). Boston: Allyn and Bacon.

Nelson, N. W. (1998). *Childhood language disorders in context: Infancy through adolescence* (2nd ed.). Boston: Allyn and Bacon.

Nelson, N. W., & Hyter, D. (1990). *Black English Sentence Scoring: Development and use as a tool for nonbiased assessment.* Unpublished manuscript, Western Michigan University, Kalamazoo.

Nelson, N. W., & Schwentor, B. A. (1990). Reading and writing. In D. R. Beukelman & K. M. Yorkston (Eds.), *Communication disorders following traumatic brain injury: Management of cognitive, language, and motor impairments* (pp. 191–249). Austin, TX: Pro-Ed.

Nelson, N. W., & Van Meter, A. M. (2002). Assessing curriculum-based reading and writing samples. *Topics in Language Disorders, 22*(2), 35–59.

Newell, A. F., Arnott, J. L., Booth, L., Beattie, W., Brophy, B., & Ricketts, I. W. (1992). Effect of the "PAL" word prediction system on the quality and quantity of text generation. *Augmentative and Alternative Communication, 8,* 304–311.

Newell, A. F., Booth, L., Arnott, J., & Beattie, W. (1992). Increasing literacy levels by the use of linguistic prediction. *Child Language Teaching and Therapy, 8,* 138–187.

Newman, J., Lovett, M., & Dennis, M. (1986). The use of discourse analysis in neurolinguistics: Some findings from the narratives of hemidecorticate adolescents. *Topics in Language Disorders, 7*(1), 31–44.

Newman, S., Fields, H., & Wright, S. (1993). A developmental study of specific spelling disability. *British Journal of Educational Psychology, 63,* 287–296.

Nicholas, M., Obler, L. K., Albert, M. L., & Helm-Estabrooks, N. (1985). Empty speech in Alzheimer's disease and fluent aphasia. *Journal of Speech and Hearing Research, 28,* 405–410.

Nippold, M. (1985). Comprehension of figurative language in youth. *Topics in Language Disorders, 5*(3), 120.

Nippold, M. A., (1988a). Figurative language. In M. A. Nippold (Ed.), *Later language development: Ages nine through nineteen* (pp. 179–210). Austin, TX: Pro-Ed.

Nippold, M. A. (1990). *Idioms in textbooks for kindergarten through eighth grade students.* Unpublished manuscript.

Nippold, M. A. (1991). Evaluating and enhancing idiom comprehension in language-disordered students. *Language, Speech, and Hearing Services in Schools, 22,* 100–106.

Nippold, M. A. (1992). The nature of normal and disordered word finding in children and adolescents. *Topics in Language Disorders, 13*(1), 1–14.

Nippold, M. A. (1993). Developmental markers in adolescent language: Syntax, semantics, and pragmatics. *Language, Speech, and Hearing Services in Schools, 24,* 21–28.

Nippold, M. A. (1995). School-age children and adolescents: Norms for word definition. *Language, Speech, and Hearing Services in Schools, 26,* 320–325.

Nippold, M. A. (2000). Language development during the adolescent years: Aspects of pragmatics, syntax, and semantics. *Topics in Language Disorders, 20*(2), 15–28.

Nippold, M. A., Erskine, B., & Freed, D. (1988). Proportional and functional analogical reasoning in normal and language-impaired children. *Journal of Speech and Hearing Disorders, 53,* 440–449.

Nippold, M. A., & Haq, F. S. (1996). Proverb comprehension in youth: The role of concreteness and familiarity. *Journal of Speech and Hearing Research, 39,* 166–176.

Nippold, M. A., & Martin, S. T. (1989). Idiom interpretation in isolation versus context: A developmental study with adolescents. *Journal of Speech and Hearing Research, 32,* 59–66.

Nippold, M. A., Moran, C., & Schwarz, I. E. (2001). Idiom understanding in preadolescents: Synergy in action. *American Journal of Speech-Language Pathology, 10,* 169–179.

Nippold, M. A., & Rudzinski, M. (1993). Familiarity and transparency in idiom explanation: A developmental study of children and adolescents. *Journal of Speech and Hearing Research, 36,* 728–737.

Nippold, M. A., Schwarz, I. E., & Lewis, M. (1992). Analyzing the potential benefit of the microcomputer use for teaching figurative language. *American Journal of Speech-Language Pathology, 1*(2), 36–43.

Nippold, M. A., Schwarz, I. E., & Undlin, R. A. (1992). Use and understanding of adverbial conjuncts: A developmental study of adolescents and young adults. *Journal of Speech and Hearing Research, 35,* 108–118.

Nippold, M. A., Scott, C. M., Norris, J. A., & Johnson, C.J. (1993, November). *School-age children and adolescents: Establishing language norms, Part 2.* Paper presented at the Annual Convention of the American Speech-Language-Hearing Association, Anaheim, CA.

Norris, J. (1989). Providing language remediation in the classroom: An integrated language-to-reading intervention model. *Language, Speech, and Hearing Services in Schools, 20,* 205–218.

Norris, J. A. (1997). Functional language intervention in the classroom: Avoiding the tutor trap. *Topics in Language Disorders, 17*(2), 49–68.

Norris, J. A., & Bruning, R. (1988). Cohesion in the narratives of good and poor readers. *Journal of Speech and Hearing Disorders, 53,* 416–424.

Norris, J. A., & Damico, J. S. (1990). Whole language in theory and practice: Implications for language intervention. *Language, Speech, and Hearing Services in Schools, 21,* 212–220.

Norris, J. A., & Hoffman, P. R. (1990a). Comparison of adult-initiated vs. child-initiated interaction styles with handicapped prelanguage children. *Language, Speech, and Hearing Services in Schools, 21,* 28–36.

Norris, J. A., & Hoffman, P. R. (1990b). Language intervention within naturalistic environments. *Language, Speech, and Hearing Services in Schools, 21,* 72–84.

Norris, M., Juarez, M., & Perkins, M. (1989). Adaptation of a screening test for bilingual and bidialectal populations. *Language, Speech, and Hearing Services in Schools, 20,* 381–390.

Nugent, P., & Mosley, J. (1987). Mentally retarded and nonretarded individuals' attention allocation and capacity. *American Journal of Mental Deficiency, 91,* 598–605.

Nye, C., Foster, S., & Seaman, D. (1987). Effectiveness of language intervention with the language/learning disabled. *Journal of Speech and Hearing Disorders, 52,* 348–357.

O'Brien, M., & Nagel, K. (1987). Parents' speech to toddlers: The effect of play context. *Journal of Child Language, 14,* 269–279.

O'Connor, L., & Schery, T. K. (1989). *Using microcomputers to develop communication skills in young severely handicapped children* (Unpublished final project report, Grant No. G0087300283). Washington, DC: U. S. Department of Education.

Odom, S., Hoyson, M., Jamieson, B., & Strain, P. (1985). Increasing handicapped preschoolers' peer social interactions: Cross-setting and component analysis. *Journal of Applied Behavior Analysis, 18,* 3–16.

Oetting, J. B., & Morohov, J. E. (1997). Past-tense marking by children with and without specific language impairment. *Journal of Speech, Language, and Hearing Research, 40,* 62–74.

Ogletree, W. (1993, April). *Communication assessment and intervention for persons with severe-to-profound mental retardation.* Paper presented at the Annual Convention of the New York State Speech-Language-Hearing Association, Rochester.

Oller, J. W. (1983). *Issues in language testing research.* Rowley, MA: Newbury House.

Olswang, L. B., & Bain, B. (1991). Intervention issues for toddlers with specific language impairment. *Topics in Language Disorders, 11*(4), 69–84.

Olswang, L. B., & Bain, B. A. (1996). Assessing information for predicting upcoming change in language production. *Journal of Speech and Hearing Research, 39,* 414–423.

Olswang, L. B., Bain, B., & Johnson, G. (1990). Using dynamic assessment with children with language disorders. In S. Warren & J. Reichle (Eds.), *Causes and effects in communication and language intervention* (pp. 187–215). Baltimore: Paul H. Brookes.

Olswang, L. B., Coggins, T. E., & Timler, G. R. (2001) Outcome measures of school-age children with social communication. *Topics in Language Disorders, 22*(1), 50–73.

Olswang, L. B., Kriegsmann, E., & Mastergeorge, A. (1982). Facilitating functional requesting in pragmatically impaired children. *Language, Speech, and Hearing Services in Schools, 13,* 202–222.

Olswang, L. B., Rodriguez, B., & Timler, G. (1998). Recommending intervention for toddlers with specific language learning difficulties: We may not have all the answers but we know a lot. *American Journal of Speech-Language Pathology, 7*(1), 23–32.

Oram, J., Fine, J., Okamoto, C., & Tannock, R. (1999). Assessing the language of children with attention deficit hyperactivity disorder. *American Journal of Speech-Language Pathology, 8,* 72–80.

Orelove, F., & Sobsey, D. (1987). *Educating children with multiple disabilities: A transdisciplinary approach.* Baltimore: Paul H. Brookes.

Orum, L. (1986). *The education of Hispanics: Status and implications.* Washington, DC: National Council of La Raza.

Owens, R. (1978). *Speech acts in the early language of nondelayed and retarded children: A taxonomy and distributional study.* Unpublished doctoral dissertation, Ohio State University, Columbus.

Owens, R. (1982a). Caregiver Interview and Environmental Observation. San Antonio: Psychological Corp.

Owens, R. (1982b). Developmental Assessment Tool. San Antonio: Psychological Corp.

Owens, R. (1982c). Diagnostic Interactional Survey (DIS). San Antonio: Psychological Corp.

Owens, R. (1982d), *Program for the acquisition of language with the severely impaired (PALS).* San Antonio: Psychological Corp.

Owens, R. (1989). Cognitive and language in the mentally retarded population. In M. Beveridge, G. Couti-Ramsden, & I. Leudar (Eds.), *Language and communication in mentally handicapped people.* New York: Chapman & Hill.

Owens, R. (1997). Mental retardation. In D. Bernstein & E. Tiegerman (Eds.), *Language and communication disorders in children* (pp. 457–523). Boston: Allyn and Bacon.

Owens, R., & MacDonald, J. (1982). Communicative uses of the early speech of nondelayed and Down syndrome children. *American Journal of Mental Deficiency, 86,* 503–510.

Owens, R., McNerney, C., Bigler-Burke, L., & Lepre-Clark, C. (1987, June). Language facilitators with residential retarded populations. *Topics in Language Disorders, 7*(3), 47–63.

Owens, R., & Robinson, L. A. (1997). Once upon a time: Use of children's literature in the preschool classroom. *Topics in Language Disorders, 17*(2), 19–48.

Owens, R., & Rogerson, B. (1988). Adults at the presymbolic level. In S. Calculator & J. Bedrosian (Eds.), *Communication assessment and intervention for adults with mental retardation* (pp. 189–230). San Diego: College-Hill.

Palincsar, A. S., & Brown, A. L. (1986). Interactive teaching to promote independent learning from text. *The Reading Teacher, 39,* 771–777.

Papanicolaon, A. C., DiScenna, A., Gillespie, L., & Aram, D. M. (1990). Probe-evoked potential findings following unilateral left hemisphere lesions in children. *Archives of neurology, 47,* 562–566.

Paratore, J. R. (1995). Assessing literacy: Establishing common standards in portfolio assessment. *Topics in Language Disorders, 16*(1), 67–82.

Parente, R., & Hermann, D. (1996). Retraining memory strategies. *Topics in Language Disorders, 17*(1), 45–57.

Paris, S. G., & Oka, E. (1986). Children's reading strategies, metacognition, and motivation. *Developmental Review, 6,* 25–56.

Parnell, M., & Amerman, J. (1983). Answers to *wh-* questions: Research and application. In T. Gallagher & C. Prutting (Eds.), *Pragmatic assessment and intervention issues in language* (pp. 129–150). San Diego: College-Hill.

Parnell, M., Amerman, J., & Harting, R. (1986). Responses of language-disordered children to *wh-* questions. *Language, Speech, and Hearing Services in Schools, 17,* 95–106.

Patterson, J. L. (1998). Expressive vocabulary development and word combinations of Spanish-English bilingual toddlers. *American Journal of Speech-Language Pathology, 7*(4), 46–56.

Patterson, J. L. (2000). Observed and reported expressive vocabulary and word combinations in bilingual toddlers. *Journal of Speech, Language, and Hearing Research, 43,* 121–128.

Paul, R. (1989a, June). *Outcomes of early expressive language delay: Age three.* Paper presented at the Symposium for Research in Child Language Disorders, University of Wisconsin, Madison.

Paul, R. (1989b). *Profiles of toddlers with delayed expressive language development.* Paper presented at the Biennial Meeting of the Society for Research in Child Development, Kansas City, MO.

Paul, R. (1990). Comprehension strategies: Interactions between world knowledge and the development of sentence comprehension. *Topics in Language Disorders, 10*(3), 63–75.

Paul, R. (1996). Clinical implications of the natural history of slow expressive language development. *American Journal of Speech-Language Pathology, 5*(2), 5–22.

Paul, R., Fisher, M., & Cohen, D. (1988). Comprehension strategies in children with autism and specific language disorders. *Journal of Autism and Developmental Disorders, 18,* 669–679.

Paul, R., Looney, S., & Dahm, P. (1991). Communication and socialization skills at age 2 and 3 in "late-talking" young children. *Journal of Speech and Hearing Research, 34,* 858–865.

Pearson, D. (1988). A group therapy idea for new clinicals in the school setting: Keep little hands busy. *Language, Speech, and Hearing Services in Schools, 19,* 432.

Pease, D. M., Gleason, J. B., & Pan, B. A. (1989). Gaining meaning: Semantic development. In J. B. Gleason (Ed.), *The development of language* (2nd ed., pp. 101–134). New York: Merrill/Macmillan.

Peck, C., & Schuler, A. (1987). Assessment of social/communicative behavior for students with autism and severe handicaps: The importance of asking the right questions. In T. Layton (Ed.), *Language and treatment of autistic and developmentally disordered children.* Springfield, IL: Charles C. Thomas.

Pecyna-Rhyner, P., Lehr, D., & Pudlas, K. (1990). An analysis of teacher responsiveness to communicative initiations of preschool children with handicaps. *Language, Speech, and Hearing Services in Schools, 21,* 91–97.

Pehrsson, R. S., & Denner, P. R. (1985). *Assessing silent reading during the process: An investigation of the opin procedure.* Paper presented at the Annual Meeting of the Northern Rocky Mountain Educational Research Association, Jackson, WY.

Pehrsson, R. S., & Denner, P. R. (1988). Semantic organizers: Implications for reading and writing. *Topics in Language Disorders, 8*(3), 24–37.

Pehrsson, R. S., & Robinson, H. A. (1985). *The semantic organizer approach to writing and reading instruction.* Rockville, MD: Aspen.

Pellegrini, A. D. (1985). Relations between symbolic play and literate behavior. In L. Galda & A. Pellegrini (Eds.), *Play, language, and stories: The development of children's literate behavior* (pp. 79–97). Norwood, NJ: Ablex.

Pellegrini, A. D., & Galda, L. (1990). Children's play, language, and early literacy. *Topics in Language Disorders, 10*(3), 76–88.

Pellegrini, A. D., & Perlmutter, J. (1989). Classroom contextual effects on children's play. *Developmental Psychology, 25,* 289–296.

Peña, E. D. (2002, April). *Solving the problems of biased speech and language assessment with bilingual children.* Paper presented at the Annual Convention of the New York State Speech-Language-Hearing Association, Rochester.

Peña, E. D., & Iglesias, A. (1989, November). *System for dynamic scoring.* Paper presented to the American Speech-Language-Hearing Association, St. Louis, MO.

Peña, E. D., Iglesias, A., & Lidz, C. S. (2001). Reducing test bias through dynamic assessment of children's word learning ability. *American Journal of Speech-Language Pathology, 10,* 138–154.

Perera, K. (1986a). Grammatical differentiation between speech and writing in children aged 8 to 12. In A. Wilkinson (Ed.), *The writing of writing* (pp. 90–108). New York: Open University Press.

Perera, K. (1986b). Language acquisition and writing. In P. Fletcher & M. Garman (Eds.), *Language acquisition* (2nd ed., pp. 494–533). Cambridge, UK: Cambridge University Press.

Perfetti, C. (1997). The psycholinguistics of spelling and reading. In C. Perfetti, L. Rieben, & M. Fayol (Eds.), *Learning to spell: Research, theory, and practice across languages* (pp. 21–38). Mahwah, NJ: Lawrence Erlbaum.

Perozzi, J. (1985). A pilot study of bilingual language facilitation: Theoretical and intervention implications. *Journal of Speech and Hearing Disorders, 50,* 403–406.

Perozzi, J. A., & Chavez Sanchez, M. L. (1992). The effect of instruction in L1 on receptive acquisition of L2 for bilingual children with language delay. *Language, Speech, and Hearing Services in Schools, 23,* 348–352.

Peterson, P., & Swing, S. (1985). Students' cognitions as mediators of the effectiveness of small-group learning. *Journal of Educational Psychology, 77,* 299–312.

Piche-Cragoe, L., Reichle, J., & Sigafoos, J. (1986). *Requesting validity intervention.* Unpublished manuscript, University of Minnesota, Minneapolis.

Pidek, C. (1987). *The assignment book.* Schaumburg, IL: Communication Concepts.

Plante, E., & Vance, R. (1994). Selection of preschool language tests: A data-based approach. *Language, Speech, and Hearing Services in Schools, 25,* 15–24.

Platt, J., & Coggins, T. (1990). Comprehension of social-action games in prelinguistic children. *Journal of Speech and Hearing Disorders, 55,* 315–326.

Polmanteer, K., & Turbiville, V. (2000). Family-responsive individualized family service plans for speech-language pathologists. *Language, Speech, and Hearing Services in Schools, 31,* 4–14.

Powell, T. (1991). Planning for phonological generalization: An approach to treatment target selection. *American Journal of Speech-Language Pathology, 1*(3), 21–27.

Preece, A. (1987). The range of narrative forms conversationally produced by young children. *Journal of Child Language, 14,* 353–373.

Preferred practice patterns for the professions of speech-language pathology and audiology. (1993, March). *Asha, 35* (Suppl. II).

Prelock, P. A. (2000). Prologue: Multiple perspectives for determining the roles of speech-language pathologists in inclusionary classrooms. *Language, Speech, and Hearing Services in Schools, 31,* 213–218.

Prelock, P. A., Messick, C., Schwartz, R., & Terrell, B. (1981). Mother-child discourse during the one-word stage. *Proceedings from the Second Wisconsin Symposium on Research in Child Language Disorders.* Madison: University of Wisconsin, Department of Communicative Disorders.

Prelock, P. A., Miller, B. L., & Reed, N. L. (1995). Collaborative partnerships in a language in the classroom program. *Language, Speech, and Hearing Services in Schools, 26,* 286–292.

Prendeville, J., & Ross-Allen, J. (2002). The transition process in the early years: Enhancing speech-language pathologists' perspective. *Language, Speech, and Hearing Services in Schools, 33,* 130–136.

Prizant, B. M. (1984). Assessment and intervention of communication problems in children with autism. *Communication Disorders, 9,* 127–142.

Prizant, B. M., & Schuler, A. (1987). Facilitating communication: Language approaches. In D. Cohen & A. Donnellan (Eds.), *Handbook of autism and pervasive developmental disorders.* New York: John Wiley.

Prizant, B. M., & Wetherby, A. M. (1985). Intentional communicative behavior of children with autism: Theoretical and practical issues. *Australian Journal of Human Communication Disorders, 13,* 23–59.

Prizant, B. M., & Wetherby, A. M. (1988a). Providing services to children with autism (ages 0 to 2 years) and their families. *Topics in Language Disorders, 9*(1), 1–23.

Prizant, B. M., & Wetherby, A. M. (1988b, October). *Toward early detection of communication problems in infants and toddlers.* Paper presented at the conference of the International Association of Infant Mental Health, Providence, RI.

Proctor-Williams, K., Fey, M. E., & Frome Loeb, D. (2001). Parental recasts and production of copulas and articles by children with specific language impairment and typical language. *American Journal of Speech-Language Pathology, 10,* 155–168.

Pruess, J., Vadasy, P., & Fewell, R. (1987). Language development in children with Down syndrome: An overview of recent research. *Education and Training of the Mentally Retarded, 22,* 44–55.

Prutting, C. A. (1979). Process /pra/,ses/ n: The action of moving forward progressively from one point to another on the way to completion. *Journal of Speech and Language Disorders, 44,* 3–30.

Prutting, C. A. (1982). Pragmatic and social competence. *Journal of Speech and Hearing Disorders, 42,* 123–134.

Prutting, C. A. (1983). Scientific inquiry and communicative disorders: An emerging paradigm across six decades. In T. Gallagher & C. Prutting (Eds.), *Pragmatic assessment and intervention issues in language* (pp. 247–267). San Diego: College-Hill.

Prutting, C. A., & Kirchner, D. M. (1983). Applied pragmatics. In T. M. Gallagher & C. A. Prutting (Eds.), *Pragmatic assessment and intervention issues in language* (pp. 29–64). Austin, TX: Pro-Ed.

Prutting, C. A., & Kirchner, D. M. (1987). A clinical appraisal of the pragmatic aspects of language. *Journal of Speech and Hearing Disorders, 52,* 105–119.

Purcell, S., & Liles, B. (1992). Cohesion repairs in the narratives of normal-language and language impaired school-aged children. *Journal of Speech and Hearing Research, 35,* 354–362.

Pye, C. (1987). Pye Analysis of Language (PAL) [Computer program]. Lawrence: University of Kansas.

Raghavendra, P., & Fristoe, M. (1995). "No shoes; they walked away?": Effects of enhancements on learning and using Blissymbolics by normal three-year-old children. *Journal of Speech and Hearing Research, 38,* 174–188.

Randall-David, E. (1989). *Strategies for working with culturally diverse communities and clients.* Washington, DC: Association for the Care of Children's Health.

Raphael, T. S., & Englert, C. S. (1990). Reading and writing: Partners in constructing meaning. *The Reading Teacher, 43,* 388–400.

Ray, S. (1989). Context and psychoeducational assessment of hearing impaired children. *Topics in Language Disorders, 9*(4), 33–44.

Records, N. L., & Tomblin, J. B. (1994). Clinical decision making: Describing the decision rules of practicing speech-language pathologists. *Journal of Speech and Hearing Research, 37,* 144–156.

Redmond, S. M. (2002). The use of rating scales with children who have language impairments. *American Journal of Speech-Language Pathology, 11,* 124–138.

Redmond, S. M., & Rice, M. L. (2001). Detection of irregular verb violations by children with and without SLI. *Journal of Speech, Language, and Hearing Research, 44,* 655–669.

Redmond, S. M., & Rice, M. L. (2002). Stability of behavioral ratings of children with SLI. *Journal of Speech, Language, and Hearing Research, 45,* 190–201.

Reed, V. A. (1986). An overview of children's language disorders. In V. A. Reed (Ed.), *An introduction to children with language disorders* (pp. 65–79). New York: Macmillan.

Rees, N., & Wollner, S. (1981, April). *A taxonomy of pragmatic abilities: The use of language in conversation.* Paper presented at the Annual Convention of the New York State Speech-Language-Hearing Association, Liberty, NY.

Reich, P. (1986). *Language development.* Englewood Cliffs, NJ: Prentice-Hall.

Reichle, J. (1990, April). *Intervention with presymbolic clients: Setting up an initial communication system.* Paper presented at the Annual Convention of the New York State Speech-Language-Hearing Association, Kiamesha Lake.

Reichle, J., Busch, C., & Doyle, S. (1986). The topical relationship among adjacent utterances in productively delayed children's language addressed to their mothers. *Journal of Communication Disorders, 19,* 63–74.

Reichle, J., & Karlan, G. (1985). The selection of an augmentative system in communication intervention: A critique of decision rules. *Journal of the Association for Persons with Severe Handicaps, 10,* 146–156.

Reichle, J., Piche-Cragoe, L., Sigafoos, J., & Doss, S. (1988). Optimizing functional communication for persons with severe handicaps. In S. Calculator & J. Bedrosian (Eds.), *Communication assessment and intervention for adults with mental retardation* (pp. 239–264). San Diego: College-Hill.

Reid, D. K., Hresko, W. P., & Hammill, D. D. (2001). Test of Early Reading Ability. Austin, TX: Pro-Ed.

Rein, R., & Kernan, C. (1989). The functional use of verbal perseveratives by adults who are mentally retarded. *Education and Training in Mental Retardation, 24,* 381–389.

Remington, B., & Clarke, S. (1993a). Simultaneous communication and speech comprehension. Part 1: Comparison of two methods of teaching expressive signing and speech comprehension skills. *Augmentative and Alternative Communication, 9,* 36–48.

Remington, B., & Clarke, S. (1993b). Simultaneous communication and speech comprehension. Part II: Comparison of two methods of overcoming selective attention during expressive sign training. *Augmentative and Alternative Communication, 9,* 49–60.

Rescorla, L. (1989). The Language Development Survey: A screening tool for delayed language in toddlers. *Journal of Speech and Hearing Disorders, 54,* 587–599.

Rescorla, L. (1990, June). *Outcomes of expressive language delay.* Paper presented at the Symposium for Research in Child Language Disorders, Madison, WI.

Rescorla, L. (1991). Identifying expressive language delay at age two. *Topics in Language Disorders, 11*(4), 14–20.

Rescorla, L., & Goossens, M. (1992). Symbolic play development in toddlers with expressive specific language impairment (SLI-E). *Journal of Speech and Hearing Research, 35,* 1290–1302.

Rescorla, L., & Ratner, N. B. (1996). Phonetic profiles of toddlers with specific expressive language impairment (SLI-E). *Journal of Speech and Hearing Research, 39,* 153–165.

Restrepo, M. (1998). Identifiers of predominantly Spanish-speaking children with language impairment. *Journal of Speech, Language, and Hearing Research, 41,* 1398–1411.

Restrepo, M. A., & Silverman, S. W. (2001). Validity of the Spanish Preschool Language Scale-3 for use with bilingual children. *American Journal of Speech-Language Pathology, 10,* 382–393.

Reutzel, D. R. (1985). Story maps improve comprehension. *The Reading Teacher, 38,* 400–404.

Rhyner, P. M., Kelly, D. J., Brantley, A. L., & Krueger, D. M. (1999). Screening low-income African American children using the BLT-2S and the SPELT-P. *American Journal of Speech-Language Pathology, 8,* 44–52.

Riccio, C. A., & Hynd, G. W. (1996). Neuroanatomical and neurophysiological aspects of dyslexia. *Topics in Language Disorders, 16*(2), 1–13.

Rice, M. L. (1986). Mismatched premises of the communicative competence model and language intervention. In R.

Schiefelbusch (Ed.), *Language competence: Assessment and intervention* (pp. 261–281). San Diego: College-Hill.

Rice, M. L., Buhr, J. C., & Nemeth, M. (1990). Fastmapping word-learning abilities of language-delayed preschoolers. *Journal of Speech and Hearing Disorders, 55,* 33–42.

Rice, M. L., Buhr, J., & Oetting, J. B. (1992). Speech-language-impaired children's quick incidental learning of words: The effect of a pause. *Journal of Speech and Language Research, 35,* 1040–1048.

Rice, M. L., Cleave, P. L., & Oetting, J. B. (2000). The use of syntactic cues in lexical acquisition by children with SLI. *Journal of Speech, Language, and Hearing Research, 43,* 582–594.

Rice, M. L., & Oetting, J. B. (1993). Morphological deficits of children with SLI: Evaluation of number marking and agreement. *Journal of Speech and Hearing Research, 36,* 1249–1257.

Rice, M. L., Oetting, J. B., Marquis, J., Bode, J., & Pae, S. (1994). Frequency of input effects on word comprehension of children with specific language impairment. *Journal of Speech and Hearing Research, 37,* 106–122.

Rice, M. L., Snell, M. A., & Hadley, P. A. (1990). The Social Interactive Coding System (SICS): An on-line, clinically relevant descriptive tool. *Language, Speech, and Hearing Services in Schools, 21,* 2–14.

Rice, M. L., Snell, M. H., & Hadley, P. A. (1991). Social interactions of speech and language-impaired children. *Journal of Speech and Hearing Research, 34,* 1299–1307.

Rice, M. L., & Wexler, K. (1996). Toward tense as a clinical marker of specific language impairment in English-speaking children. *Journal of Speech and Hearing Research, 39,* 1239–1257.

Rice, M. L., Wexler, K., & Hershberger, S. (1998). Tense over time: The longitudinal course of tense acquisition in children with specific language impairment. *Journal of Speech, Language, and Hearing Research, 41,* 1412–1431.

Richgels, D., McGee, D., Lomax, R., & Sheard, C. (1987). Awareness of four text structures: Effects on recall of expository text. *Reading Research Quarterly, 22,* 177–196.

Riddle, L. S. (1992). The attention capacity of children with specific language impairment. *Dissertation Abstracts International, 53*(6-B).

Rieke, J., & Lewis, J. (1984). Preschool intervention strategies: The communication base. *Topics in Language Disorders, 5*(1), 41–57.

Rinehart, S. D., Stahl, S. A., & Erickson, L. G. (1986). Some effects of summarization training on reading and studying. *Reading Research Quarterly, 12,* 422–438.

Ripich, D., & Griffith, P. (1988). Narrative abilities of children with learning disabilities and nondisabled children: Story structure, cohesion, and propositions. *Journal of Learning Disabilities, 21,* 165–173.

Ripich, D., & Panagos, J. (1985). Assessing children's knowledge of sociolinguistic rules for speech therapy lessons. *Journal of Speech and Hearing Disorders, 50,* 335–345.

Ripich, D., & Spinelli, F. (1985). *School discourse strategies.* San Diego: College-Hill.

Rispoli, M., & Hadley, P. (2001). The leading-edge: The significance of sentence disruption in the development of grammar. *Journal of Speech, Language, and Hearing Research, 44,* 1131–1143.

Rittle-Johnson, B., & Siegler, R. S. (1999). Learning to spell: Variability, choice, and change in children's strategy use. *Child Development, 70,* 332–348.

Rivers, K. O., & Hedrick, D. L. (1992). Language and behavioral concerns for drug-exposed infants and toddlers. *Infant-Toddler Intervention: The Transdisciplinary Journal, 2*(1), 63–71.

Roberts, J. E., Medley, L. P., Swartzfager, J. L., & Neebe, E. C. (1997). Assessing the communication of African American one-year-olds using the Communication and Symbolic Behavior Scales. *American Journal of Speech-Language Pathology, 6*(2), 59–65.

Roberts, J. E., Prizant, B., & McWilliam, R. A. (1995). Out-of-class versus in-class service delivery in language intervention: Effects on communication interactions with young children. *American Journal of Speech-Language Pathology, 4*(2), 87–94.

Robertson, C., & Salter, W. (1997). *Phonological Awareness Test (PAT).* East Moline, IL: Linguisystems.

Robertson, S. B., & Weismer, S. E. (1997). The influence of peer models on the play scripts of children with specific language impairment. *Journal of Speech, Language, and Hearing Research, 40,* 49–61.

Robertson, S. B., & Ellis Weismer, S. (1999). Effects of treatment on linguistic and social skills of toddlers with delayed language development. *Journal of Speech, Language, and Hearing Research, 42,* 1234–1248.

Robinson, L. A., & Owens, R. E. (1995). Functional augmentative communication and positive behavior change: A case study. *Augmentative and Alternative Communication, 11*(4), 207–211.

Rodino, A. M., Gimbert, C., Perez, C., Craddock-Willis, K., & McCabe, A. (1992, October). *"Getting your point across": Contractive sequencing in low-income African American and Latino children's personal narratives.* Paper presented at the 16th Annual Boston University Conference on Language Development, Boston.

Rogers-Warren, A., & Warren, S. (1985). Mands for verbalization: Facilitating the display of newly trained language in children. *Behavior Modification, 4,* 361–382.

Roller, E., Rodriguez, T., Warner, J., & Lindahl, P. (1992). Integration of self-contained children with severe speech-language needs into the regular education classroom. *Language, Speech, and Hearing Services in Schools, 23,* 365–366.

Rom, A., & Leonard, L. B. (1990). Interpreting deficits in grammatical morphology in specific language impaired children: Preliminary evidence from Hebrew. *Clinical Linguistics and Phonetics, 4,* 95–105.

Romer, L., & Schoenberg, B. (1991). Increasing requests made by people with developmental disabilities and deaf-blindness through the use of behavior interruption strategies. *Education and Training in Mental Retardation, 26,* 70–78.

Romski, M., & Sevcik, R. (1989). An analysis of visual-graphic symbol meanings for two non-speaking adults with severe mental retardation. *Augmentative and Alternative Communication, 5,* 109–144.

Romski, M., Sevcik, R., & Pate, J. (1988). Establishment of symbolic communication in persons with severe retardation. *Journal of Speech and Hearing Disorders, 53,* 94–107.

Rondal, J., Ghiotto, M., Bredart, S., & Bachelet, J. (1987). Age-relation, reliability, and grammatical validity of measures of utterance length. *Journal of Child Language, 14,* 433–446.

Rondal, J., Ghiotto, M., Bredart, S., & Bachelet, J. (1988). Mean length of utterance of children with Down syndrome. *American Journal of Mental Deficiency, 93,* 64–66.

Roseberry, C., & Connell, R. (1991). The use of an invented language rule in the differentiation of normal and language-impaired Spanish-speaking children. *Journal of Speech and Hearing Research, 34,* 596–603.

Roseberry-McKibbin, C. A. (1994). Assessment and intervention for children with limited English proficiency and language disorders. *American Journal of Speech-Language Pathology, 3*(3), 77–78.

Rosegrant, T. J., & Cooper, W. (1987). Talking Text Writer [Computer program]. New York: Scholastic.

Rosen, C. & Gerring, J. (1986). *Head trauma: Educational reintegration.* San Diego: College-Hill.

Rosenkoetter, S. E. (1995). *It's a big step.* Topeka, KS: Bridging Early Services Task Force, Coordinating Council on Early Childhood Developmental Services.

Rosin, M., Swift, E., Bless, D., & Vetter, D. (1988). Communication profiles of adolescents with Down syndrome. *Journal of Childhood Communication Disorders, 12,* 49–64.

Rosin, P., & Gill, G. (1997). *Changing perspectives: Assessing your preadolescent children's communication skills—Implications for practicing clinicians.* Workshop presented at the University of Wisconsin, Madison.

Rosinski-McClendon, M., & Newhoff, M. (1987). Conversational responsiveness and assertiveness in language-impaired children. *Language, Speech, and Hearing Services in Schools, 18,* 53–62.

Ross, B. L. (1989). *The impact of individual differences in scripts memory for script-related stories.* Unpublished master's thesis, University of Utah, Salt Lake City.

Ross, B. L., & Berg, C. A. (1989). *The use of personal scripts in remembering new events across adulthood.* Paper presented at the meeting of the Society for Research in Child Development, Kansas City, MO.

Ross, B. L., & Berg, C. A. (1990). Individual differences in script reports: Implications for language assessment. *Topics in Language Disorders, 10*(3), 30–44.

Roth, F. (1986). Oral narrative abilities of learning-disabled students. *Topics in Language Disorders, 7*(1), 1–30.

Roth, F., & Spekman, N. (1984a). Assessing the pragmatic abilities of children: Part 1. Organizational framework and assessment parameters. *Journal of Speech and Hearing Disorders, 49,* 2–11.

Roth, F., & Spekman, N. (1984b). Assessing the pragmatic abilities of children: Part 2. Guidelines, considerations, and specific evaluation procedures. *Journal of Speech and Hearing Disorders, 49,* 12–17.

Roth, F., & Spekman, N. (1985, June). *Story grammar analysis of narratives produced by learning disabled and normally achieving students.* Paper presented at the Symposium on Research in Child Language Disorders, Madison, WI.

Roth, F., & Spekman, N. (1986). Narrative discourse: Spontaneously generated stories of learning-disabled and normally achieving students. *Journal of Speech and Hearing Disorders, 51,* 8–23.

Roth, F., & Spekman, N. (1989a). Higher order language processing and reading disabilities. In A. Kamhi & H. Catts (Eds.), *Reading disabilities: A developmental language perspective.* San Diego: College-Hill.

Roth, F., & Spekman, N. (1989b). The oral syntactic proficiency of learning disabled students: A spontaneous story sampling analysis. *Journal of Speech and Hearing Research, 32,* 67–77.

Roth, F. P. (2000). Narrative writing: Development and teaching with children with writing difficulties. *Topics in Language Disorders, 20*(4), 15–28.

Roth, F. P., & Clark, D. M. (1987). Symbolic play and social participation abilities of language-impaired and normally developing children. *Journal of Speech and Hearing Disorders, 52,* 17–29.

Roth, F. P., Spekman, N.J., & Fye, E. C. (1991, November). *Written syntactic patterns of stories produced by learning disabled students.* Paper presented at the Annual Convention of the American Speech-Language-Hearing Association, Atlanta, GA.

Rotholz, D. A., Berkowitz, S. F., & Burberry, J. (1989). Functionality of two modes of communication in the community by students with developmental disabilities: A comparison of signing and communication books. *Journal of the Association for Persons with Severe Handicaps, 14,* 227–233.

Routman, R. (1991). *Invitations: Changing as teachers and learners, K–12.* Portsmouth, NH: Heinemann.

Rowland, C., & Schweigert, P. (1989a). Tangible symbols: Symbolic communication for individuals with multisensory impairments. *Augmentative and Alternative Communication, 5,* 226–234.

Rowland, C., & Schweigert, R. (1989b). *Tangible symbol systems for individuals with multisensory impairments* [Videotape and manual]. Tucson, AZ: Communication Skill Builders.

Rubin, H. (1988). Morphological knowledge and early writing ability. *Language and Speech, 31,* 337–355.

Rubin, H., Patterson, P. A., & Kantor, M. (1991). Morphological development and writing ability in children and adults. *Language, Speech, and Hearing Services in Schools, 22,* 228–235.

Rumsey, J. M., Rapoport, M. D., & Sceery, W. R. (1985). Autistic children as adults: Psychiatric, social, and behavioral outcomes. *Journal of the American Academy of Child Psychiatry, 24,* 465–473.

Russell, N. (1993). Educational considerations in traumatic brain injury: The role of the speech-language pathologist. *Language, Speech, and Hearing Services in Schools, 24,* 67–75.

Russell, S. C., & Kaderavek, J. N. (1993). Alternative models for collaboration. *Language, Speech, and Hearing Services in Schools, 24,* 76–78.

Rutter, M. (1985). Infantile autism and other pervasive disorders. In M. Rutter & L. Hersov (Eds.), *Child and adolescent psychiatry: Modern approaches* (pp. 545–566). London: Blackwell.

Salvia, J., & Ysseldyke, J. (1988). *Assessment in special and remedial education* (4th ed.). Boston: Houghton Mifflin.

Salzinger, S., Feldman, R. S., Hammer, M., & Rosario, M. (1991). Risk for physical child abuse and the personal consequences for its victims. *Criminal Justice and Behavior, 18,* 64–81.

Sameroff, A., & Feise, B. (1990). Transactional regulation and early intervention. In S. Meisels & P. Shonkoff (Eds.), *Early intervention: Handbook of early childhood intervention.* New York: Cambridge University Press.

Samuel, A. (2001). Knowing a word affects the fundamental perception of the sounds within it. *Psychological Science, 12,* 348–351.

Sanders, J. (1986). *Microcomputer applications for speech-language services in the schools.* San Diego: College-Hill.

Sarno, M. T., Buonaguro, A., & Levita, E. (1986). Characteristics of verbal impairment in closed head injured patients. *Archives of Physical Medicine and Rehabilitation, 67,* 400–405.

Sattler, J. M. (1988). *Assessment of children* (3rd ed.). San Diego: Author.

Saunders, K., & Spradlin, J. (1989). Conditional discrimination in mentally retarded adults: The effect of training the component simple discriminations. *Journal of the Experimental Analysis of Behavior 52,* 1–12.

Savage, R. (1991). Identification, classification, and placement issues for students with traumatic brain injury. *Journal of Head Trauma Rehabilitation, 6,* 1–9.

Savage, R., & Wolcott, G. (1988). *An educator's manual: What educators need to know about students with traumatic brain injury.* Southborough, MA: National Head Injury Foundation.

Saville-Troike, M. (1986). Anthropological considerations in the study of communication. In O. L. Taylor (Ed.), *Nature of communication disorders in culturally and lingually diverse populations* (pp. 47–72). San Diego: College-Hill.

Sawyer, D. (1987). Test of Awareness of Language Segments. Rockville, MD: Aspen.

Sawyer, J. (1973). Social aspects of bilingualism in San Antonio, Texas. In R. Bailey & J. Robinson (Eds.), *Varieties of present-day English* (pp. 226–235). New York: Macmillan.

Scarborough, H., Wyckoff, J., & Davidson, R. (1986). A reconsideration of the relationship between age and mean utterance length. *Journal of Speech and Hearing Research, 29,* 394–399.

Scheffner Hammer, C. (1998). Toward a "thick description" of families: Using ethnography to overcome the obstacles to providing family-centered early intervention services. *American Journal of Speech-Language Pathology, 7*(1), 5–22.

Scheffner Hammer, C., Pennock-Roman, M., Rzasa, S., & Tomblin, J. B. (2002). An analysis of the Test of Language Development—Primary for item bias. *American Journal of Speech-Language Pathology, 11,* 274–284.

Scherer, N., & Olswang, L. (1989). Using structured discourse as a language intervention technique with autistic children. *Journal of Speech and Hearing Disorders, 54,* 383–394.

Schery, T., & O'Connor, L. (1992). The effectiveness of school-based computer language intervention with severely handicapped children. *Language, Speech, and Hearing Services in Schools, 23,* 43–47.

Schetz, K. (1989). Computer-aided language/concept enrichment in kindergarten: Consultation program model. *Language, Speech, and Hearing Services in Schools, 20,* 2–10.

Schiff-Myers, N. (1992). Considering arrested language development and language loss in the assessment of second language learners. *Language, Speech, and Hearing Services in Schools, 23,* 28–33.

Schiff-Myers, N., Coury, J., & Perez, D. (1989, May). *A "bilingual" evaluation of a bilingual child: How necessary is it?* Paper presented at the Annual Convention of the New Jersey Speech-Language-Hearing Association, Parsippany.

Schmidt, H. D., & Rodgers-Rhyme, A. (1988). *Strategies: Effective practices for teaching all children.* Madison: Wisconsin State Department of Public Instruction, Bureau of Exceptional Children.

Schneider, P. (1996). Effects of pictures versus oral presentation of stories on story retellings by children with language impairment. *American Journal of Speech-Language Pathology, 5*(1), 86–96.

Schober-Peterson, D., & Johnson, C. (1989). Conversational topics of 4-year-olds. *Journal of Speech and Hearing Research, 32,* 857–870.

Schopler, E., & Mesibov, G. (1987). *Neurobiological issues in autism.* New York: Plenum.

Schreibman, L. (1988). *Developmental clinical psychology and psychiatry: Vol. 15. Autism.* Newbury Park, CA: Sage.

Schuler, A. L., & Prizant, B. M. (1987). Facilitating language: Prelanguage approaches. In D. J. Cohen & A. M. Donnellan (Eds.), *Handbook of autism and pervasive developmental disorders* (pp. 301–315). New York: John Wiley.

Schultz, M. M. (1986). *The semantic organizer: A prewriting strategy for first grade students.* Unpublished doctoral dissertation, University of Connecticut, Storrs.

Schumaker, J., & Deshler, D. (1988). Implementing the Regular Education Initiative in secondary schools: A different ball game. *Journal of Learning Disabilities, 21,* 36–42.

Schwartz, R., Chapman, K., Terrell, B., Prelock, P., & Rowan, L. (1985). Facilitating word combination in language-impaired children in discourse structure. *Journal of Speech and Hearing Disorders, 50,* 31–39.

Schwejda, P. (1986). Predictive Linguistic Program: Development Copy. Version 1. 6.86 [Computer program]. Adaptive Peripherals.

Scott, C. M. (1984a). Adverbial connectivity in conversations of children 6 to 12. *Journal of Communication and Language, 11,* 423–452.

Scott, C. M. (1987). *Summarizing text: Context effects in language disordered children.* Paper presented at the First International Symposium, Specific Language Disorders in Children, University of Reading, England.

Scott, C. M. (1988a). Producing complex sentences. *Topics in Language Disorders, 8*(2), 44–62.

Scott, C. M. (1988b). A perspective on the evaluation of school children's narratives. *Speech, Language, and Hearing Services in Schools, 19,* 67–82.

Scott, C. M. (1995). A discourse approach to syntax teaching. In D. F. Tibbits (Ed.), *Language intervention: Beyond the primary grades. For clinicians by clinicians.* Austin, TX: Pro-ed.

Scott, C. M. (1999) Learning to write. In H. W. Catts & A. G. Kamhi (Eds.), *Language and reading disabilities* (pp. 224–258). Boston: Allyn and Bacon.

Scott, C. M. (2000). Principles and methods of spelling instruction: Applications for poor spellers. *Topics in Language Disorders, 20*(3), 66–82.

Scott, C. M., & Erwin, D. L. (1992). Descriptive assessment of writing: Process and products. *Best Practices in School Speech-Language Pathology, 2,* 87–98.

Scott, C. M., Nippold, M. A., Norris, J. A., & Johnson, C. J. (1992, November) *School-age children and adolescents: Establishing language norms.* Paper presented at the Annual Convention of the American Speech-Language-Hearing Association, San Antonio.

Scott, C. M., & Rush, D. (1985). Teaching adverbial connectivity: Implications from current research. *Child Language Teaching and Therapy, 1,* 264–280.

Scott, C. M., & Stokes, S. L. (1995). Measures of syntax in school-age children and adolescents. *Language, Speech, and Hearing Services in Schools, 26,* 309–319.

Segal, E., Duchan, J., & Scott, P. (1991). The role of inter-clausal connectives in narrative structuring: Evidence from adults' interpretations of simple stories. *Discourse Processes, 14,* 27–54.

Segebert DeThorne, L., & Watkins, R. V. (2001). Listeners' perceptions of language use in children. *Language, Speech, and Hearing Services in Schools, 32,* 142–148.

Seidenberg, P. L. (1988). Cognitive and academic instructional intervention for learning disabled adolescents. *Topics in Language Disorders, 8*(3), 56–71.

Seidenberg, P. L. (1989). Relating text-processing research to reading and writing instruction for learning disabled students. *Learning Disabilities Focus, 5,* 4–12.

Seidenberg, P. L., & Bernstein, D. K. (1986). The comprehension of similes and metaphors by learning-disabled and nonlearning-disabled children. *Language, Speech, and Hearing Services in Schools, 17,* 219–229.

Selman, R. L., Beardslee, W., Schultz, L. H., Krupa, M., & Podorefsky, D. (1986). Assessing adolescent interpersonal negotiation strategies: Toward the integration of structural and functional models. *Developmental Psychology, 22,* 450–459.

Sena, R., & Smith, L. (1990). New evidence on the development of the *big. Child Development, 61,* 1034–1052.

Seung, H., & Chapman, R. (2000). Digit span in individuals with Down syndrome and in typically developing children: Temporal aspects. *Journal of Speech, Language, and Hearing Research, 43,* 609–620.

Sevcik, R. A., & Romski, M. A. (1986). Representational matching skills of persons with severe retardation. *Augmentative and Alternative Communication, 2,* 160–164.

Sevcik, R. A., Romski, M. A., Watkins, R. V., & Deffebach, K. P. (1995). Adult partner-augmented communication input to youth with mental retardation using the System for Augmenting Language (SAL).

Sevcik, R. A., Romski, M. A., & Wilkinson, K. M. (1991). Roles of graphic symbols in the language acquisition process for persons with severe cognitive disabilities. *Augmentative and Alternative Communication, 7,* 161–170.

Sewell, T. E. (1987). Dynamic assessment as a nondiscriminatory procedure. In C. Schneider Lidz (Ed.), *Dynamic assessment: An interactional approach to evaluating learning potential* (pp. 426–443). New York: Guilford.

Seymour, H. N. (1992). The invisible children: A reply to Lahey's perspective. *Journal of Speech and Hearing Research, 35,* 640–641.

Seymour, H. N., Ashton, N., & Wheeler, L. (1986). The effect of race on language elicitation. *Language, Speech, and Hearing Services in Schools, 17,* 146–151.

Seymour, H. N., Bland-Stewart, L., & Green, L. J. (1998). Difference versus deficit in child African American English. *Language, Speech, and Hearing Services in Schools, 29*(2), 96–108.

Shadden, B. B. (1992, March). *Discourse analysis procedures used with adults.* Paper presented at the Conference on Pragmatics: From Theory to Therapy, State University of New York, Buffalo.

Shelton, B., Gast, D., Wolery, M., & Winterling, V. (1991). The role of small group instruction in facilitating observational and incidental learning. *Language, Speech, and Hearing Services in School, 22,* 123–133.

Shewan, C. (1988). 1988 omnibus survey: Adaptation and progress in times of change. *Asha, 30*(8), 27–30.

Shewan, C., & Malm, K. (1989). The status of multilingual/multicultural service issues among ASHA memhers. *Asha, 31*(9), 78.

Shipley, K., & Banis, C. (1989). *Teaching morphology developmentally* (rev. ed.). Tucson, AZ: Communication Skill Builders.

Shipley, K., Maddox, M., & Driver, J. (1991). Children's development of irregular past tense verb forms. *Language, Speech, and Hearing Services in Schools, 22,* 115–122.

Shriberg, L. D., & Kwiatkowski, J. (1985). Continuous speech sampling for phonologic analysis of speech-delayed children. *Journal of Speech and Hearing Disorders, 50,* 323–334.

Shriberg, L. D., Kwiatkowski, J., Best, S., Hengst, J., & Terselic-Weber, B. (1986). Characteristics of children with speech delays of unknown origin. *Journal of Speech and Hearing Disorders, 51,* 140–161.

Shriberg, L. D., Kwiatkowski, J., & Snyder, T. (1989). Tabletop versus microcomputer-assisted speech management: Stabilization phase. *Journal of Speech and Hearing Disorders, 54,* 233–248.

Shriberg, L. D., & Widder, C. (1990). Speech and prosody characteristics of adults with mental retardation. *Journal of Speech and Hearing Research, 33,* 627–653.

Siegel-Causey, E., & Downing, J. (1987). Nonsymbolic communication development: Theoretical concepts and educational strategies. In L. Goetz, D. Guess, & K. Stremel-Campbell (Eds.), *Innovative program design for individuals with sensory impairments* (pp. 15–48). Baltimore: Paul H. Brookes.

Silliman, E. R. (1993, June). *Integrating language and literacy programming. Building collaborative partnerships.* Paper presented at the Conference of the Rochester City School District, Rochester, NY.

Silliman, E. R., Bahr, R., Beasman, J., & Wilkinson, L. C. (2000). Scaffolds for learning to read in an inclusion classroom. *Language, Speech, and Hearing Services in Schools, 31,* 265–279.

Silliman, E. R., Diehl, S. F., Aurillo, M. K., Wilkinson, L. C., & Hammargren, K. M. (1995). Getting the point: A narrative journey into the Athabaskan culture. *Topics in Language Disorders, 15*(4), 30–53.

Silliman, E. R., Wilkinson, L. C., & Hoffman, L. P. (1993). Documenting authentic progress in language and literacy learning: Collaborative assessment in classrooms. *Topics in Language Disorders, 14*(1), 58–71.

Silverman, F. (1989). *Communication for the speechless* (2nd ed.). Englewood Cliffs, NJ: Prentice-Hall.

Simeonsson, R. J., Olley, J. G., & Rosenthal, S. L. (1987). Early intervention for children with autism. In M. Guralnick & F. Bennett (Eds.), *The effectiveness of early intervention for at-risk and handicapped children* (pp. 275–296). New York: Academic Press.

Simner, M. (1983). The warning signs of school failure: An updated profile of the at-risk kindergarten child. *Topics in Early Childhood Special Education, 3*(4), 17–28.

Simon, C. S. (1984). *Evaluating communicative competence: A functional-pragmatic procedure.* Tucson, AZ: Communication Skill Builders.

Simon, C. S. (1985). *Communication skills and classroom success: Therapy methodologies for language-learning disabled students.* San Diego: College-Hill.

Simon, C. S. (1987). *Classroom Communication Screening Procedure for Early Adolescents: A handbook for assessment and intervention.* Tempe, AZ: Communi-Cognitive Publications.

Sininger, Y., Klatzky, R., & Kirchner, D. (1989). Memory scanning speed in language-disordered children. *Journal of Speech and Hearing Research, 32,* 289–297.

Skarakis-Doyle, E., & Mullin, K. (1990). Comprehension monitoring in language disordered children: A preliminary investigation of cognitive and linguistic factors. *Journal of Speech and Hearing Disorders, 55,* 700–705.

Skarakis-Doyle, E., & Prutting, C. (1988). Characteristics of symbolic play in language disordered children. *Human Communication Canada, 12*(1), 7–17.

Slackman, E., Hudson, J., & Fivush, R. (1986). Actions, actors, links, and goals: The structure of children's event representations. In K. Nelson (Ed.), *Event knowledge: Structure and function in development.* Hillsdale, NJ: Lawrence Erlbaum.

Sleight, C., & Prinz, P. (1985). Use of abstracts, orientations, and codes in narratives by language-disordered and nondisordered children. *Journal of Speech and Hearing Disorders, 50,* 361–371.

Smith, M. (1985). Managing the aggressive and self-injurious behavior of adults disabled by autism. *Journal of the Association for Persons with Severe Handicaps, 4,* 228–232.

Smitherman, G. (1985). What go round come round: Keep in perspective. In C. Brookes (Ed.), *Tapping potential: English and language arts for the black learner* (pp. 41–62). Urbana, IL: Black Caucus of the National Council of Teachers of English.

Snow, C. E. (1989). Imitativeness: A trait or a skill? In G. E. Speidel & K. E. Nelson (Eds.), *The many faces of imitation in language learning* (pp. 73–90). New York: Springer Verlag.

Snow, C. E. (1990). The development of definitional skill. *Journal of Child Language, 17,* 697–710.

Snow, C. E., & Goldfield, B. A. (1983). Turn the page please: Situation-specific language acquisition. *Journal of Child Language, 10,* 551–569.

Snow, C. E., Midkiff-Borunda, S., Small, A., & Proctor, A. (1984). Therapy as social interaction: Analyzing the contexts for language remediation. *Topics in Language Disorders, 4*(4), 72–85.

Snow, C. E., Perlman, R., & Nathan, D. (1987). Why routines are different: Toward a multiple-factors model of the relation between input and language acquisition. In K. E. Nelson & A. van Kleeck (Eds.), *Children's language* (Vol. 6). Hillsdale, NJ: Lawrence Erlbaum.

Snow, C. E., Scarborough, H. S., & Burns, M. S. (1999). What speech-language pathologists need to know about early reading. *Topics in Language Disorders, 20*(1), 48–58.

Snowling, M. (1994). Towards a model of spelling acquisition: The development of some component skills. In *Handbook of spelling: Theory, process, and intervention* (pp. 111–128). Chichester, UK: John Wiley.

Snowling, M., & Frith, U. (1986). Comprehension in "hyperlexic" readers. *Journal of Experimental Child Psychology, 42,* 392–415.

Snyder, L. E., Dabasinskas, C., & O'Connor, E. (2002). An information processing perspective on language impairment in children: Looking at both sides of the coin. *Topics in Language Disorders, 22*(3), 1–14.

Snyder, L. S., & Downey, D. M. (1997). Developmental differences in the relationship between oral language deficits and reading. *Topics in Language Disorders, 17*(3), 27–40.

Snyder, L. S., & Godley, D. (1992). Assessment of word-finding disorders in children and adolescents. *Topics in Language Disorders, 13*(1), 15–32.

Snyder-McLean, L., & McLean, J. (1987). Effectiveness of early intervention for children with language and communication disorders. In M. Guaralnick & J. Bennett (Eds.), *The effectiveness of early intervention for at-risk and handicapped children* (pp. 213–274). New York: Academic Press.

Sohlberg, M. M., Mateer, C. A., & Stuss, D. T. (1993). Contemporary approaches to the management of executive control dysfunction. *Journal of Head Trauma Rehabilitation, 8,* 45–58.

Sonnenmeier, R. M. (1992, March). *Script-based language intervention: Learning to participate in life events.* Paper presented at the Conference on Pragmatics: From Theory to Therapy, State University of New York, Buffalo.

Sparks, S. N. (1989). Speech and language in maltreated children: Response to McCauley & Swisher (1987). *Journal of Speech and Hearing Disorders, 54,* 124–126.

Spector, C. (1990). Linguistic humor comprehension of normal and language-impaired adolescents. *Journal of Speech and Hearing Disorders, 55,* 533–541.

Spekman, N. (1981). Dyadic verbal communication abilities of learning disabled and normally achieving fourth and fifth grade boys. *Learning Disability Quarterly, 4,* 139–151.

Spinelli, F., & Terrell, B. (1984). Remediation in context. *Topics in Language Disorders, 5*(1), 29–40.

Spragle, D., & Micucci, S. (1990). Signs of the week: A functional approach to manual sign training. *Augmentative and Alternative Communication, 6,* 29–37.

Sprott, R. A., & Kemper, S. (1987). The development of children's code-switching: A study of six bilingual children across two situations. In E. F. Pemberton, M. A. Sell, & G. B. Simpson (Eds.), *Working Papers in Language Development, 2,* 116–134.

Staab, C. (1983). Language functions elicited by meaningful activities: A new dimension in language programs. *Language, Speech, and Hearing Services in Schools, 14,* 164–170.

Stahl, S., Osborn, J., & Lehr, F. (1990). *Beginning to read: Thinking and learning about print by Marilyn Jager Adams: A summary.* Urbana, IL: Center for the Study of Reading.

Stainback S., & Stainback, W. (Eds.). (1992). *Curriculum considerations in inclusive classrooms: Facilitating learning for all students.* Baltimore: Paul H. Brookes.

Stainback W., & Stainback, S. (Eds.). (1990). *Support network for inclusive schooling: Interdependent integrated education.* Baltimore: Paul H. Brookes.

Stanovich, K. (1986). "Matthes effects" in reading: Some consequences of individual differences in acquisition of literacy. *Reading Research Quarterly, 4,* 360–407.

Stanovich, K., Cunningham, A., & Cramer, B. (1984). Assessing phonological awareness in kindergarten children: Issues of task comparability. *Journal of Experimental Child Psychology, 38,* 175–190.

Stark, J. (1985, April). *Learning disabilities and reading: Myths and realities.* Paper presented at the Annual Convention of the New York State Speech-Language-Hearing Association, Kiamesha Lake.

Stein, N. (1982). What's in a story: Interpreting the interpretations of story grammars. *Discourse Processes, 5,* 319–335.

Stein, N., & Glenn, C. (1979). An analysis of story comprehension in elementary school children. In R. Freedle (Ed.), *New directions in discourse processing* (Vol. 2, pp. 53–120). Norwood, NJ: Ablex.

Steiner, S., & Larson, V. L. (1991). Integrating microcomputers into language intervention with children. *Topics in Language Disorders, 11*(2), 18–30.

Stephens, I., Dallman, W., & Montgomery, A. (1988, November). *Developmental sentence scoring through age nine.* Paper presented at the Annual Convention of the American Speech-Language-Hearing Association, Boston.

Stephens, M., & Montgomery, A. (1985). A critique of recent relevant standardized tests. *Topics in Language Disorders, 5*(3), 21–45.

Sternberg, R. J. (1987). Most vocabulary is learned from context. In M. G. McKeown & M. E. Curtis (Eds.), *The nature of vocabulary acquisition* (pp. 89–105). Hillsdale, NJ: Lawrence Erlbaum.

Stickler, K. R. (1987). *Guide to analysis of language transcripts.* Eau Claire, WI: Thinking Publications.

Stockman, I. (1996). *Is language sampling a workable alternative to identifying language impaired minority children?* Paper presented at the 17th Annual Symposium on Research in Children with Language Disabilities, Madison, WI.

Stockman, I., & Vaughn-Cooke, F. (1986). Implications of semantic category research for the language assessment of nonstandard speakers. *Topics in Language Disorders, 6*(4), 15–25.

Stockman, I. J. (1996). The promise and pitfalls of language sample analysis as an assessment tool for linguistic minority children. *Language, Speech, and Hearing Services in Schools, 26,* 355–366.

Stothard, S. E., Snowling, M. J., Dishop, D. V., Chipchase, B. B., & Kaplan, C. A. (1998). Language-impaired preschoolers: A follow-up into adolescence. *Journal of Speech, Language, and Hearing Research, 41,* 407–418.

Stowe, L. (1988). Thematic structures and sentence comprehension. In G. Carlson & M. Tanenhaus (Eds.), *Linguis-*

tic structure in language processing (pp. 319–358). Dordrecht, The Netherlands: Reidel.

Stremel-Campbell, K., & Campbell, C. (1985). Training techniques that may facilitate generalization. In S. Warren & A. Rogers-Warren (Eds.), *Teaching functional language: Generalization and maintenance of language skills* (pp. 309–339). Baltimore: University Park Press.

Study: English language hard for dyslexics. (2001, March 16). (Rochester, NY) *Democrat and Chronicle*, 4A.

Sturm, J. M., & Nelson, N. W. (1997). Formal classroom lessons: New perspectives on a familiar discourse event. *Language, Speech, and Hearing Services in Schools, 28*, 255–273.

Sturner, R. A., Layton, T. L., Evans, A. W., Heller, J. H., Funk, S. G., & Machon, M. W. (1994). Preschool speech and language screening: A review of currently available tests. *American Journal of Speech-Language Pathology, 3*, 25–36.

Stuss, D. T., & Benson, D. F. (1986). *The frontal lobes*. New York: Raven Press.

Summers, J. A., Brotherson, M. J., & Turnbull, A. P. (1988). The impact of handicapped children on families. In E. W. Lynch & R. B. Lewis (Eds.), *Exceptional children and adults* (pp. 504–544). Glenview, IL: Scott, Foresman.

Summers, P. A., Larson, G. W., Miguel, S. A., & Terrell, S. L. (1996). Test-retest comparisons using the CELF-RST and BLT-2S with kindergarteners. *Language, Speech, and Hearing Services in Schools, 27*, 324–329.

Sussman, J. (1993). Perception of formant transition cues to place of articulation in children with LI. *Journal of Speech, Language, and Hearing Research, 36*, 1286–1299.

Sutton-Smith, B. (1986). The development of fictional narrative performances. *Topics in Language Disorders, 7*(1), 1–10.

Swank, L. K. (1994). Phonological coding abilities: Identification of impairments related to phonologically based reading problems. *Topics in Language Disorders, 14*(2), 56–71.

Swiffin, A. L., Arnott, J. L., Pickering, J. A., & Newell, A. F. (1987). Adaptive and predictive techniques in a communication prothesis. *Augmentative and Alternative Communication, 3*, 181–191.

Swisher, L., & Demetras, M. J. (1985). The expressive language characteristics of autistic children compared with mentally retarded or specific language-impaired children. In E. Schopler & G. B. Mesibov (Eds.), *Communication problems in autism* (pp. 147–162). New York: Plenum.

Swisher, L., Plante, E., & Lowell, S. (1994). Nonlinguistic deficits of children with language disorders complicate the interpretation of their nonverbal IQ scores. *Language, Speech, and Hearing Services in Schools, 25*, 235–240.

Swisher, L., Restrepo, M. A., Plante, E., & Lowell, S. (1995). Effect of implicit and explicit "rule" presentation on bound-morpheme generalization in specific language impairment. *Journal of Speech and Hearing Research, 28*, 168–173.

Swisher, L., & Snow, D. (1994). Learning and generalization components of morphological acquisition by children with specific language impairment: Is there a functional relation? *Journal of Speech and Hearing Research, 37*, 1406–1413.

Tager-Flusberg, H. (1985). The conceptual basis for referential word meaning in children with autism. *Child Development, 56*, 1167–1178.

Tager-Flusberg, H. (1989). Putting words together: Morphology and syntax in the preschool years. In J. Gleason (Ed.), *Language development* (pp. 139–171). Columbus, OH: Macmillan.

Tannock, R. (1988a). Control and reciprocity in mothers' interactions with Down syndrome and normal children. In K. Marfo (Ed.), *Parent-child interaction and developmental disorders: Theory, research, and intervention* (pp. 163–180). New York: Praeger.

Tannock, R. (1988b). Mothers' directiveness in their interactions with their children with and without Down syndrome. *American Journal on Mental Deficiency, 93*, 154–165.

Tarone, E. (1988). *Variation in interlanguage*. London: Edward Arnold.

Tattershall, S. (1987). Mission impossible: Learning how a classroom works before it's too late. *Journal of Childhood Communication Disorders, 2*(1), 181–184.

Taylor, O. L. (1986a). Language differences. In G. Shames & E. Wiig (Eds.), *Human communication* (2nd ed., pp. 385–413). New York: Merrill/Macmillan.

Taylor, O. L. (1986b). Teaching Standard English as a second dialect. In O. L. Taylor (Ed.), *Treatment of communication disorders in culturally and lingually diverse populations* (pp. 153–178). San Diego: College-Hill.

Taylor, O. L. (1989). Old wine in new bottles: Some things change yet remain the same. *Asha, 31*(9), 72–73.

Taylor, O. L. (1990). Cross-cultural communication: An essential of effective communication. (ERIC Document Reproduction Service No. ED 325 593)

Taylor, O. L., Payne, K., & Anderson, N. (1987). Distinguishing between communication disorders and communication differences. *Seminars in Speech and Language, 8*, 415–427.

Terrell, B. Y., & Hale, J. E. (1992). Serving a multicultural population: Different learning styles. *American Journal of Speech-Language Pathology, 1*(2), 5–9.

Terrell, S. L., Arensberg, K., & Rosa, M. (1992). Parent-child comparative analysis: A criterion-referenced method for the nondiscriminatory assessment of a child who spoke a relatively uncommon dialect of English. *Language, Speech, and Hearing Services in Schools, 23,* 34–42.

Thal, D. J. (1989). *Language and gestures in late talkers.* Paper presented at the Biennial Meeting of the Society for Research in Child Development, Kansas City, MO.

Thal, D., Jackson-Maldonado, D., & Acosta, D. (2000). Validity of a parent-report measure of vocabulary and grammar for Spanish-speaking toddlers. *Journal of Speech, Language, and Hearing Research, 43,* 1087–1100.

Theadore, G., Maher, S. R., & Prizant, B. M. (1990). Early assessment and intervention with emotional and behavioral disorders and communication disorders. *Topics in Language Disorders, 10*(4), 42–56.

Thomas, C., Englert, C. S., & Morsink, C. (1984). Modifying the classroom program in language. In C. V. Morsink (Ed.), *Teaching special needs students in regular classrooms* (pp. 239–276). Boston: Little, Brown & Co.

Thomas, J. (1989). A standardized method for collecting and analyzing language samples of pre-school and primary children in the public schools. *Language, Speech, and Hearing Services in Schools, 20,* 85–92.

Tolchinsky-Landsmann, L., & Levin, I. (1985). Writing in preschoolers: An age related analysis. *Applied Psycholiguistics, 6,* 319–339.

Tomasello, M. (1987). Learning to use prepositions: A case study. *Journal of Child Language, 14,* 79–98.

Tomasello, M., & Farrar, M. J. (1986). Joint attention and early language. *Child Development, 57,* 1454–1463.

Tomblin, J. B. (1991). Examining the cause of specific language impairment. *Language, Speech, and Hearing Services in Schools, 22,* 69–74.

Tomblin, J. B., & Buckwalter, P. R. (1998). Heritability of poor language achievement among twins. *Journal of Speech, Language, and Hearing Research, 41,* 188–199.

Tomblin, J. B., Records, N. L., Buckwalter, P., Zhang, X., Smith, E., & O'Brien, M. (1997). Prevalence of specific language impairment in kindergarten children. *Journal of Speech, Language, and Hearing Research, 40,* 1245–1260.

Torgesen, J. K. (1980). Conceptual and educational implications of the use of efficient task strategies by learning disabled children. *Journal of Learning Disabilities, 13,* 19–26.

Torgeson, J. (1985). Memory processes in reading disordered children. *Journal of Learning Disabilities, 18,* 350–357.

Trabasso, T., & Van Den Broek, P. (1985). Causal thinking and the representation of narrative events. *Journal of Memory and Language, 24,* 612–630.

Treiman, R. (1993). *Beginning to spell.* New York: Oxford University Press.

Treiman, R. (1994). Use of consonant letter names in beginning spelling. *Developmental Psychology, 30,* 567–580.

Treiman, R. (1997). Spelling in normal children and dyslexics. In B. Blachman (Ed.), *Foundations of reading acquisition and dyslexia: Implications for early intervention* (pp. 191–218). Mahwah, NJ: Lawrence Erlbaum.

Treiman, R., & Bourassa, D. C. (2000). The development of spelling skill. *Topics in Language Disorders, 20*(3), 1–18.

Treiman, R., & Cassar, M. (1997) Spelling acquisition in English. In C. A. Perfetti, L. Rieben, & M. Fayol (Eds.), *Learning to spell: Research, theory, and practice across languages* (pp. 61–80). Mahwah, NJ: Lawrence Erlbaum.

Troia, G. A., Graham, S., & Harris, K. R. (1999) Teaching students with learning disabilities to mindfully plan when writing. *Exceptional Children, 65,* 235–252.

Tucker, J. (1985). Curriculum-based assessment: An introduction. *Exceptional Children, 52,* 199–204.

Turner, L., & Bray, N. (1985). Spontaneous rehearsal by mildly mentally retarded children and adolescents. *American Journal of Mental Deficiency, 78,* 640–648.

Tyack, D., & Gottsleben, R. (1977). *Language sampling, analysis, and training: A handbook for teachers and clinicians.* Palo Alto: Consulting Psychologists Press.

Tyack, D., & Gottsleben, R. (1986). Acquisition of complex sentences. *Language, Speech, and Hearing Services in Schools, 17,* 160–174.

Tyler, A., & Nagy, W. (1987). *The acquisition of English derivational morphology* (Technical Report No. 407). Urbana, IL: Center for the Study of Reading.

Udvari, A., & Thousand, J. (1995). Promising practices that foster inclusive education. In R. Villa & J. Thousand (Eds.), *Creating an inclusive school* (p. 95). Alexandria, VA: Association fo Supervision and Curriculum Development.

Uhry, J., & Shepherd, J. (1993). Segmentation/spelling instruction as part of a first-grade reading program: Effects on several measures of reading. *Reading Research Quarterly, 28,* 218–233.

U.S. Bureau of the Census. (1990). *The Hispanic population in the United States: March 1990.* Washington, DC: Author.

Vace, N. N. (1987). Word processor versus handwriting: A comparative study of writing samples produced by mildly mentally handicapped students. *Exceptional Children, 54,* 156–165.

Vallecorsa, A. L. & Garris, E. (1990). Story composition skills in middle-grade students with learning disability. *Exceptional Children, 57,* 48–54.

Vanderheiden, G. C., & Kelso, D. P. (1987). Comparative analysis of fixed-vocabulary communication acceleration techniques. *Augmentative and Alternative Communication, 3,* 196–206.

Vanderheiden, G. C., & Lloyd, L. L. (1986). Communication systems and their components. In S. Blackstone (Ed.), *Augmentative communication* (pp. 49–162). Rockville, MD: American Speech-Language-Hearing Association.

van der Lely, H. K., & Harris, M. (1990). Comprehension of reversible sentences in specifically language-impaired children. *Journal of Speech and Hearing Disorders, 55,* 101–117.

van der Lely, H. K., & Howard, D. (1993). Children with specific language impairment: Linguistic impairment or short-term memory deficit? *Journal of Speech and Hearing Research, 36,* 1193–1207.

van Kleeck, A. (1984). Metalinguistic skills: Cutting across spoken and written language and problem-solving skills. In G. Wallach & K. Butler (Eds.), *Language learning disabilities in school age children* (pp. 128–153). Baltimore: Williams & Wilkins.

van Kleeck, A. (1994). Potential cultural bias in training parents as conversational partners with their children who have delays in language development. *American Journal of Speech-Language Pathology, 3*(1), 67–78.

van Kleeck, A. (1995). Emphasizing form and meaning separately in prereading and early reading instruction. *Topics in Language Disorders, 16*(1), 27–49.

van Kleeck, A., Gillam, R. B., & McFadden, T. U. (1998). A study of classroom-based phonological awareness training for preschoolers with speech and/or language disorders. *American Journal of Speech-Language Pathology, 7*(3), 65–76.

Varnhagen, C. K., McCallum, M., & Burstow, M. (1997). Is children's spelling naturally stage-like? *Reading and Writing: An Interdisciplinary Journal, 9,* 451–481.

Venn, M. L., Wolery, M., Fleming, L. A., DeCesare, L. D., Morris, A., & Cuffs, M. S. (1993). Effects of teaching preschool peers to use the mand-model procedure during snack activities. *American Journal of Speech-Language Pathology, 2*(1), 38–46.

Vetter, D. (1982). Language disorders and schooling. *Topics in Language Disorders, 2*(4), 13–19.

Vicker, B. (1985). *Recognizing and enhancing the communication skills of your group home clients.* Bloomington: Indiana Developmental Training Center.

Violette, J., & Swisher, L. (1992). Echolalic responses by a child with autism to four experimental conditions of sociolinguistic input. *Journal of Speech and Hearing Research, 35,* 139–147.

Von Berger, E., Wulfeck, B., Bates, E., & Fink, N. (1996). Developmental changes in real-time sentence processing. *First Language, 16,* 192–222.

Wagner, J. R., & Rice, M. L. (1988, November). *The acquisition of verb-particle constructions: How do children figure them out?* Paper presented at the Annual Convention of the American Speech-Language-Hearing Association, Boston.

Wagner, R., Torgesen, J. K., & Rashotte, C. (1999). Comprehensive Test of Phonological Processing (CTOPP). Austin, TX: Pro-Ed.

Wagner, R. E., & Torgeson, J. (1987). The nature of phonological processing and its causal role in the acquisition of reading skills. *Psychological Bulletin, 101,* 192–212.

Wales, R. (1986). Deixis. In P. Fletcher & M. Garman (Eds.), *Language acquisition* (pp. 401–428). Cambridge, UK: Cambridge University Press.

Wallach, G. (1980). So you want to know what to do with language disabled children above the age of six. *Topics in Language Disorders, 1*(1), 99–113.

Wallach, G. P., & Butler, K. (1995). Language learning disabilities: Moving in from the edge. *Topics in Language Diorders, 16*(1), 1–26.

Wallach, G., & Liebergott, J. W. (1984). Who shall be called "learning disabled"?: Some new directions. In G. Wallach & K. Butler (Eds.), *Language learning disabilities in school age children* (pp. 1–14). Baltimore: Williams & Wilkins.

Wallach, G., & Miller, L. F. (1988). *Language intervention and academic success.* San Diego: College-Hill.

Wanska, S., Bedrosian, J., & Pohlman, J. (1986). Effects of play materials on the topic performance of preschool children. *Language, Speech, and Hearing Services in Schools, 17,* 152–159.

Warren, S. F. (1985). Clinical strategies for the measurement of language generalization. In S. Warren & A. Rogers-Warren (Eds.), *Teaching functional language* (pp. 197–224). Baltimore: University Park Press.

Warren, S. F. (1988). A behavioral approach to language generalization. *Language, Speech, and Hearing Services in Schools, 19,* 292–303.

Warren, S. F., Gazdag, G. E., Bambara, L. M., & Jones, H. A. (1994). Changes in the generativity and use of semantic relationships concurrent with milieu language intervention. *Journal of Speech and Hearing Research, 37,* 924–934.

Warren, S. F., & Kaiser, A. (1986a). Generalization of treatment effects by young language-delayed children: A longitudinal analysis. *Journal of Speech and Language Disorders, 51,* 239–251.

Warren, S. F., & Kaiser, A. (1986b). Incidental language teaching: A critical review. *Journal of Speech and Hearing Disorders, 47,* 42–52.

Warren, S. F., & Rogers-Warren, A. (1985). Teaching functional language: An introduction. In S. Warren & A. Rogers-Warren (Eds.), *Teaching functional language* (pp. 3–24). Baltimore: University Park Press.

Warren, S. F., Yoder, P. J., Gazdag, G. E., Kim, K., & Jones, H. A. (1993). Facilitating prelingual communication skills in young children with developmental delay. *Journal of Speech and Hearing Research, 36,* 83–97.

Washington, J. A., & Craig, H. K. (1994). Dialectal forms during discourse of poor, urban African American preschoolers. *Journal of Speech and Hearing Research, 37,* 816–823.

Washington, J. A., Craig, H. K., & Kushmaul, A. J. (1998). Variable use of African American English across two language sampling contexts. *Journal of Speech, Language, and Hearing Research, 41,* 1115–1124.

Watkins, R. V., Kelly, D. J., Harbors, H. M., & Hollis, W. (1995). Measuring children's lexical diversity: Differentiating typical and impaired language learners. *Journal of Speech and Hearing Research, 38,* 1349–1355.

Watkins, R. V., & Pemberton, E. F. (1987). Clinical applications of recasting: Review and theory. *Child Language Teaching and Therapy, 3,* 311–328.

Watkins, R. V., & Rice, M. L. (1989, November). *Verb particle acquisition in language-impaired and normally developing children.* Paper presented at the Convention of the American Speech-Language-Hearing Association, St. Louis.

Watkins, R. V., & Rice, M. L. (1991). Verb particle and preposition acquisition in language-impaired preschoolers. *Journal of Speech and Hearing Research, 34,* 1130–1141.

Watson, D., Omark, D., Gronell, S., & Heller, B. (1986). *Nondiscriminatory assessment: A practitioner's handbook.* Sacramento: California State Department of Education.

Wayman, K. I., Lynch, E. W., & Hanson, M. J. (1990). Home-based early childhood services: Cultural sensitivity in a family systems approach. *Topics in Early Childhood Special Education, 10*(4), 56–75.

Webster, P. E., Plante, A. S., & Couvillion, L. M. (1997). Phonological impairment and prereading: Update on a longitudinal study. *Journal of Learning Disabilities, 30,* 365–375.

Wehmeyer, P., & Kelcher, K. (1995). The ARC's Self-Determination Scale: Adolescent Version. Arlington, TX: The ARC of the United States.

Weiner, F. (1988). Parrot Easy Language Sample Analysis (PELSA) [Computer program]. State College, PA: Parrot Software.

Weiner, F., & Lewnau, L. (1979 November). *Nondiscriminatory speech and language testing of minority children: Linguistic interferences.* Paper presented at the Annual Convention of the American Speech-Language Association, Atlanta.

Weismer, S., & Hesketh, L. J. (1993). The influence of prosodic and gestural cues on novel word acquisition by children with specific language impairment. *Journal of Speech and Language Research, 36,* 1013–1025.

Weismer, S. E., & Hesketh, L. J. (1996). Lexical learning by children with specific language impairment: Effects of linguistic input presented at varying speaking rates. *Journal of Speech and Learning Research, 39,* 177–190.

Weismer, S., & Murray-Branch, J. (1989). Modeling versus modeling plus evoked production training: A comparison of two language intervention methods. *Journal of Speech and Hearing Disorders, 54,* 269–281.

Weiss, A., & Nakamura, M. (1992). Children with normal language skills in preschool classrooms for children with language impairments: Differences in modeling style. *Language, Speech, and Hearing Services in Schools, 23,* 64–70.

Weiss, B., Weisz, J., & Bromfield, R. (1986). Performance of retarded and nonretarded persons on information-processing tasks: Further tests of the similar structure hypothesis. *Psychological Bulletin, 100,* 157–175.

Weistuch, L., & Brown, B. B. (1987). Motherese as therapy: A programme and its dissemination. *Child Language Teaching and Therapy, 3,* 57–71.

Weistuch, L., & Lewis, M. (1986). *Effect of maternal language intervention strategies on the language of delayed two to five year olds.* Paper presented at the Conference of the Eastern Psychological Association, New York.

Wellman, H. (1985). The origins of metacognition. In D. Forest-Pressley, G. MacKinnon, & T. Waller (Eds.), *Metacognition, cognition, and human performance* (pp. 1–31). New York: Academic Press.

Wells, G. (1985). *Language development in the pre-school years.* New York: Cambridge University Press.

Wentzel, M. (2000, November 29). UR first to identify autistic gene. (Rochester, NY) *Democrat and Chronicle,* 1A, 10A.

Westby, C. E. (1984). Development of narrative language abilities. In G. Wallach & K. Butler (Eds.), *Language learning disabilities in school-age children* (pp. 103–127). Baltimore: Williams & Wilkins.

Westby, C. E. (1985). Learning to talk—Talking to learn: Oral-literate language differences. In C. Simon (Ed.), *Communication skills and classroom success: Therapy methodologies for language-learning disabled students.* San Diego: College-Hill.

Westby, C. E. (1988). Children's play: Reflections of social competence. *Seminars in Speech and Language, 9*(1), 1–14.

Westby, C. E. (1990). The role of the speech-language pathologist in whole language. *Language, Speech, and Hearing Services in Schools, 21,* 228–237.

Westby, C. E. (1992). Narrative assessment. *Best Practices in School Speech-Language Pathology, 2,* 53–64.

Westby, C. E. (1995). Culture and literacy: Frameworks for understanding. *Topics in Language Disorders, 16*(1), 50–66.

Westby, C. E. (1997). There's more to passing than knowing the answers. *Language, Speech, and Hearing Services in Schools, 28,* 244–287.

Westby, C. E., & Roman, R. (1995). Finding the balance: Learning to live in two worlds. *Topics in Language Disorders, 15*(4), 68–88.

Westby, C. E., Van Dongen, R., & Maggart, Z. (1989). Assessing narrative competence. *Seminars in Speech and Language, 10,* 63–76.

Weston, D. R., Ivins, B., Zuckerman, B., Jones, C., & Lopez, R. (1989). Drug exposed babies: Research and clinical issues. *Zero to Three, 9*(5), 1–7.

Wetherby, A. K., Cain, D. H., Yonclas, D. G., & Walker, V. G. (1988). Analysis of intentional communication of normal children from the prelinguistic to the multiword stage. *Journal of Speech and Hearing Research, 31,* 240–252.

Wetherby, A. K., & Prizant, B. M. (1989). The expression of communicative intent: Assessment issues. *Seminars in Speech and Language, 10,* 77–94.

Wetherby, A. K., & Prizant, B. M. (1990). *Communication and Symbolic Behavior Scales—Experimental edition.* San Antonio, TX: Special Press.

Wetherby, A. K., & Prizant, B. M. (1991). Profiling young children's communicative competence. In S. Warren & J. Reichle (Eds.), *Causes and effects in language assessment and intervention* (pp. 217–253). Baltimore: Paul H. Brookes.

Wetherby, A. K., & Prizant, B. M. (1993). Communication and Symbolic Behavior Scales. Chicago: Riverside.

Wetherby, A. M., Prizant, B. M., & Hutchinson, T. A. (1998). Communicative, social/affective, and symbolic profiles of young children with autism and pervasive developmental disorders. *American Journal of Speech-Language Pathology, 7*(2), 79–91.

Wetherby, A. K., & Prutting, C. A. (1984). Profiles in communicative and cognitive-social abilities in autistic children. *Journal of Speech and Hearing Disorders, 27,* 364–377.

Wetherby, A. K., & Rodriguez, G. (1992). Measurement of communicative intentions in normally developing children during structured and unstructured contexts. *Journal of Speech and Hearing Research, 35,* 130–138.

White, T. G., Power, M. A., & White, S. (1989). Morphological analysis: Implications for teaching and understanding vocabulary growth. *Reading Research Quarterly, 24,* 283–304.

Whitehurst, G. L., Fischel, J. E., Lonigan, C. J., Valdez-Menchaca, M. C., Arnold, D. S., & Smith, M. (1991). Treatment of early expressive language delay: If, when, and how. *Topics in Language Disorders, 11*(4), 55–68.

Wiederholt, J. L., & Bryant, B. R. (2001). Gray Oral Reading Test. Austin, TX: Pro-Ed.

Wiegel-Crump, C. A., & Dennis, M. (1986). Development of word-finding. *Brain and Language, 27,* 1–23.

Wiig, E. H. (1990). Language disabilities in school-age children and youth. In G. H. Shames & E. H. Wiig (Eds.), *Human communication disorders: An introduction* (3rd ed., pp. 193–220). New York: Merrill/Macmillan.

Wiig, E. H. (1995). Teaching prosocial communication. In D. F. Tibbits (Ed.), *Language intervention: Beyond the primary grades. For clinicians by clinicians.* Austin, TX: Pro-Ed.

Wiig, E. H., Jones, S. S., & Wiig, E. D. (1996). Computer-based assessment of word knowledge in teens with learning disability. *Language, Speech, and Hearing Services in Schools, 27,* 21–28.

Wiig, E. H., & Semel, E. M. (1984). *Language assessment and intervention for the learning disabled* (2nd ed.). New York: Merrill/Macmillan.

Wiig, E. H., & Wilson, C. C. (1994). Is a question a question? Passage understanding by preadolescents with learning disabilities. *Language, Speech, and Hearing Services in Schools, 25,* 241–250.

Wiig, E. H., Zureich, P. Z., & Chan, H. H. (2000). A clinical rationale for assessing rapid automatized naming with language disorders. *Journal of Learning Disabilities, 33,* 359–374.

Wilcox, K., & McGuinn-Aasby, S. (1988). The performance of monolingual and bilingual Mexican children on the TACL. *Language, Speech, and Hearing Services in Schools, 19,* 34–40.

Wilcox, M. J., Kouri, T., & Caswell, S. (1990). Partner sensitivity to communication behavior of young children with development disorders. *Journal of Speech and Hearing Disorders, 55,* 679–693.

Wilcox, M. J., Kouri, T., & Caswell, S. (1991). Early language intervention: A comparison of classroom and individual treatment. *American Journal of Speech-Language Pathology, 1*(3), 49–62.

Wilkinson, G. S. (1995). *Wide Range of Achievement Test-3.* Wilmington, DE: Jastak Associates.

Wilkinson, I., & Milosky, I. (1987). School-age children's metapragmatic knowledge of requests and responses in the classroom. *Topics in Language Disorders, 7*(2), 61–70.

Wilkinson, K. M., & Romski, M. A. (1995). Responsiveness of male adolescents with mental retardation to input from nondisabled peers: The summoning power of comments, questions, and directive prompts. *Journal of Speech and Hearing Research, 38,* 1045–1053.

Wilkinson, K. M., Romski, M. A., & Sevcik, R. A. (1994). Emergence of visual-graphic symbol combinations by youth with moderate or severe mental retardation. *Journal of Speech and Hearing Research, 37,* 883–895.

Williams, F., Cairns, H., & Cairns, C. (1971). *An analysis of the variations from standard English pronunciation in the phonetic performance of two groups of nonstandard-English speaking children.* Austin: University of Texas, Center for Communication Research.

Williams, J. P. (1986, August). *Reading comprehension: Categorization, macrostructures, and finding the main idea.* Paper presented to the American Psychological Association, Washington, DC.

Williams, J. P. (1988). Identifying main ideas: A basic aspect of reading comprehension. *Topics in Language Disorders, 8*(3), 1–13.

Williams, R., & Wolfram, W. (1977). *Social dialects: Differences vs. disorders.* Washington, DC: American Speech-Language-Hearing Association.

Williams, T. (1989). A social skills group for autistic children. *Journal of Autism and Developmental Disorders, 19,* 143–156.

Wilson, B. A. (1996). *Wilson Reading System Dictation Book, Steps 1-6.* Milbury, MA: Wilson Language Training Corporation.

Windsor, J., & Hwang, M. (1999a). Children's auditory lexical decisions: A limited processing capacity account of language impairment. *Journal of Speech, Language, and Hearing Research, 42,* 990–1002.

Windsor, J., & Hwang, M. (1999b). Testing the generalized slowing hypothesis in specific language impairment. *Journal of Speech, Language, and Hearing Research, 42,* 1205–1218.

Windsor, J., Scott, C. M., & Street, C. K. (2000). Verb and noun morphology in the spoken and written language of children with language learning disabilities. *Journal of Speech, Language, and Hearing Research, 43,* 1322–1336.

Wing, C. (1990). A preliminary investigation of generalization to untrained words following two treatments of children's word-finding problems. *Language, Speech, and Hearing Services in Schools, 21,* 151–156.

Winner, E. (1988). *The point of words.* Cambridge, MA: Harvard University Press.

Winograd, P. N., & Niquette, G. (1988). Assessing learned helplessness in poor readers. *Topics in Language Disorders, 8*(3), 38–55.

Wixson, K., Bosky, A., Yochum, M., & Alvermann, D. (1984). An interview for assessing students' perceptions of classroom reading tasks. *The Reading Teacher, 37,* 346–352.

Wolf, M., Bally, H., & Morris, R. (1986). Automaticity, retrieval processes, and reading: A longitudinal study in average and impaired readers. *Child Development, 57,* 988–1000.

Wolf, M., & Segal, D. (1992). Word finding and reading in the developmental dyslexias. *Topics in Language Disorders, 13*(1), 51–65.

Wolfram, W. (1985). The phonologic system: Problems of second language acquisition. In J. M. Costelli (Ed.), *Speech disorders in adults* (pp. 59–76). Austin, TX: Pro-Ed.

Woltosz, W. (1988). *Words+, Inc.* Pittsburgh, PA: Adaptive Communication Systems.

Wong, B. Y. (1986). A cognitive approach to teaching spelling. *Exceptional Children, 53,* 169–173.

Wong, B. Y. (2000). Writing strategies instruction for expository essays for adolescents with and without learning disabilities. *Topics in Language Disorders, 20*(4), 244.

Wong, B. Y., Butler, D. L., Ficzere, S. A., & Kuperis, S. (1996). Teaching low achievers and students with learning disabilities to plan, write, and revise compare and contrast essays. *Journal of Learning Disabilities, 12*(1), 2–15.

Wong, B. Y., Butler, D. L., Ficzere, S. A., & Kuperis, S. (1996). Teaching low achievers and students with learning disabilities to plan, write, and revise opinion essays. *Journal of Learning Disabilities, 29*(2), 197–212.

Woodcock, R. W. (1998). Woodcock Reading Mastery Test—Revised. Circle Pines, MN: American Guidance Services.

Work, R. S., Cline, J. A., Ehren, B. J., Keiser, D. L., & Wujek, C. (1993). Adolescent language programs. *Language, Speech, and Hearing Services in Schools, 24,* 43–53.

Wren, C. (1985). Collecting language samples from children with syntax problems. *Language, Speech, and Hearing Services in Schools, 16,* 83–102.

Wysocki, K., & Jenkins, J. R. (1987). Deriving word meanings through morphological generalization. *Reading Research Quarterly, 22,* 66–81.

Ylvisaker, M. (1986). Language and communication disorders following pediatric head injury. *Journal of Head Trauma Rehabilitation, 1,* 48–56.

Ylvisaker, M., & DeBonis, D. (2000). Executive function impairment in adolescence: TBI and ADHD. *Topics in Language Disorders, 20*(2), 29–57.

Ylvisaker, M., & Feeney, T. (1995). Traumatic brain injury in adolescence: Assessment and reintegration. *Seminars in Speech and Language, 16,* 32–44.

Ylvisaker, M., & Feeney, T. (1996). Executive functions after traumatic brain injury: Supported cognition and self-advocacy. *Seminars in Speech and Language, 17,* 217–232.

Ylvisaker, M., & Szekeres, S. (1989). Metacognitive and executive impairments in head-injured children and adults. *Topics in Language Disorders, 9,* 34–49.

Ylvisaker, M., Szekeres, S. F., & Feeney, T. (1998). Cognitive rehabilitation: Executive functions. In M. Ylvisaker (Ed.), *Traumatic brain injury rehabilitation: Children and adolescents* (pp. 221–269). Boston: Butterworth-Heinemann.

Yoder, D. (1985, June). *Communication and the severely-profoundly retarded.* Paper presented at the Conference on Communication and the Developmentally Disabled: The State of the Art in 1985, Buffalo, NY.

Yoder, P. J., & Davies, B. (1990). Do parents' questions and topic continuations elicit replies from developmentally delayed children? A sequential analysis. *Journal of Speech and Hearing Research, 33,* 563–573.

Yoder, P. J., Davies, B., Bishop, K., & Munson, L. (1994). Effect of adult continuing *wh-* questions on conversational participation in children with developmental disabilities. *Journal of Speech and Hearing Research, 37,* 193–204.

Yoder, P. J., & Feagans, L. (1988). Mothers' attributions of communication to prelinguistic behavior of infants with developmental delays and mental retardation. *American Journal of Mental Retardation, 93,* 36–43.

Yoder, P. J., Kaiser, A. P., & Alpert, C. L. (1991). An exploratory study of the interaction between language teaching methods and child characteristics. *Journal of Speech and Hearing Research, 34,* 155–167.

Yoder, P. J., Kaiser, A. P., Alpert, C., & Fischer, R. (1993). Following the child's lead when teaching nouns to preschoolers with mental retardation. *Journal of Speech and Hearing Research, 36,* 158–167.

Yoder, P. J., Spruytenburg, H., Edwards, A., & Davies, B. (1995). Effect of verbal routine contexts and expansions on gains in the mean length of utterance in children with developmental delays. *Language, Speech, and Hearing Services in Schools, 26,* 21–32.

Yoder, P. J., Warren, S. F., Kim, K., & Gazdag, G. E. (1994). Facilitating prelinguistic communication skills in young children with developmental delay: III. Systematic replication and extension. *Journal of Speech and Hearing Research, 37,* 841–851.

Yoder, P. J., Warren, S. F., & McCathren, R. B. (1998). Determining spoken language prognosis in children with developmental disabilities. *American Journal of Speech-Language Pathology, 7*(4), 77–87.

Yopp, H. K. (1998). The validity and reliability of phonemic awareness tests. *Reading Research Quarterly, 23,* 159–177.

Yorkston, K., Honsinger, M., Dowden, P., & Marriner, N. (1989). Vocabulary selection: A case report. *Augmentative and Alternative Communication, 5,* 101–108.

Yorkston, K., Smith, K., & Beukelman, D. (1990). Extended communication samples of augmented communicators: I. A comparison of individualized versus standard single-word vocabularies. *Journal of Speech and Hearing Disorders, 55,* 217–224.

Yoshinaga-Itano, C., & Snyder, L. (1985). Form and meaning in the written language of hearing impaired children. *Volta Review, 87*(5), 75–90.

Young, J. (1988). *Developing social conversational skills: An intervention study of preverbal handicapped children with their parents.* Unpublished master's thesis, Ohio State University, Columbus.

Zhang, Y., Brooks, D. W., Fields, T., & Redelfs, M. (1995). Quality of writing by elementary students with learning disabilities. *Journal of Research on Computing in Education, 27,* 483–499.

Zimmerman, I. L., Steiner, V. G., & Pond, R. E. (1992). Preschool Language Scale (3rd ed.). San Antonio, TX: Psychological Corporation.

Zitnay, G. A. (1995). Foreword. In D. G. Stein, S. Brailowsky, & B. Will (Eds.), *Brain repair* (pp. v–vi). New York: Oxford University Press.

Author Index

Subject Index